CYTOGENETICS

CYTOGENETICS

By

Dr. S. Sundara Rajan
Prof. and Head
Department of Botany
St. Joseph's College, Bangalore

ANMOL PUBLICATIONS PVT. LTD.
NEW DELHI - 110 002 (INDIA)

ANMOL PUBLICATIONS PVT. LTD.
4374/4B, Ansari Road, Daryaganj
New Delhi - 110 002
Ph.: 23261597, 23278000
Visit us at: www.anmolpublications.com

Cytogenetics

First Published, 2000
Reprint 2004

PRINTED IN INDIA

Published by J.L. Kumar for Anmol Publications Pvt. Ltd., New Delhi - 110 002 and Printed at Mehra Offset Press, Delhi.

CONTENTS

Preface

Inheritance of characters from parents to offspring is the key that life has managed to provide itself in order to maintain the essential continuity eversince its origin. The vehicles for hereditary characters and the patterns of inheritance are the essential aspects of a cytogenetic study. Cytological study provides the analysis of the structural basis of inheritance, while Genetics deals with the mechanisms of inheritance. A basic understanding of Cytogenetics is essential for all students of life sciences (Botany and Zoology), Agriculture, pharmacy and even medicine.

The book 'Cytogenetics' is essentially a text book meant for the use of B.Sc., B.Sc (Hons) and M.Sc., students studying Botany, Zoology, Microbiology, Biotechnology etc. There are 25 Chapters dealing with all aspects of Cytogenetics. Examples are chosen both from plants and animals to focus on the genetic concepts. There is a separate chapter on Microbial Genetics to deal with the genetic mechanisms of microbes. A separate chapter deals with the breeding mechanisms in plants and animals. Genetic diseases in human beings and the methods of improvement of human race (Eugenics) are discussed in chapters 23 and 25 respectively.

The language used in the book is straight and simple clearly focussing on the essential aspects. Constructive criticisms and useful suggestions are welcome.

I am thankful Mr. J.L. Kumar, M.D and Mr. H.S. Negi Director, (Sales), Anmol Publications Pvt. Ltd., New Delhi for publishing this book.

P.G. Dept. of Botany
St. Joseph's College
BANGALORE - 560 025.

Dr. S. SUNDARA RAJAN
Professor and Head

1

INTRODUCTION

One of the most important sub divisions of biological sciences is cytogenetics dealing with the study of cell and its hereditary potentialities. Cytogenetics is in a sense a hybrid science from the historical point of view. Etymologically analysed, it comprises cytology and genetics which were thought to be discrete branches of Biology. The fusion of cytology and Genetics as an integral study was achieved only recently and now it is reinforced by discoveries arising out of electron microscopy, tissue culture, microbilogy and biochemistry.

CYTOLOGY

Historically the beginnings of cytology dates back to the earlier part of the 17th century with the invention of microscope and the discovery of cell. For quite some time the microscope was thought to be a curiosity (because of the structure and philosophy of science at that time) rather than a useful instrument for the scientific study of living beings. Nevertheless the observations of Robert Hooke (1635 - 1703) Grew (1641 - 1712) and Malpigi (1628 - 1694) did lead tom an understanding of the fundamental fact that all organisms-plants as well as animals hae a common structural basis and that they are composed of cells. These that all living beings are cellular. Although, it was a Frenchman H.J. Dutrochet who for the first time in 1824 gave the idea of cell theory, the credit for formulating the cell theory generally goes to a German botanist M.I.Schleiden and a German Zoologist T. Schwann. These two scientists clearly outlined the basic concepts of the cell theory in 1839.

The theory of Schleiden and Schwann was simple, direct and elementary and it clearly focussed the study of biology on the cell as the basic unit of all organisms. Thus the study of cell or cytology progressed rapidly and supported the 19th century biologists, it lead to the opening of an immense and varied field of biological research.

In the current sense, cytology or cell biology as it is now called deals with the study of cells from morphological biochemical, physiological, embryological, genetical and even pathological point of view. In recent years modern cell biology has gone beyond the light microscopic structure of the cell. By the application of new methods and tools like electron microscopy, ultra centrifugation etc, quite a number of sub cellular structures have been discovered and studied in detail - probing further, biologists have analysed the architectural pattern of the molecules that comprise the living matter.

This has lead to a new branch of biology - the molecular biology - a science dealing with the ultra structural organisation of the living matter. Molecular biology attempts to explain the phenomena of metabolism, variation, mutation etc., in terms of changes of macromolecules such as proteins, nucleic acids etc.

The following list gives the names of some important scientists and their discoveries with reference to the study of cell.

Name	Year	Contribution
Robert Hooke	1665	Discovered the plant cell
Mirabel	1808	Plants consist of membranous cellular tissues
R.J.H. Dutrochet	1824	All organisms are cellular
F.V. Raspail	1825	Founder of cytochemistry
Turpin	1826	Reported cell division
R. Brown	1831	Described the nucleus in plant cells
Von Mohl	1835	Described the cell division
M.J. Schleiden	1838	Proposed cell theory
T. Schwann	1839	Proposed cell theory
J.E. Purkinje	1840	Named cell contents as protoplasm
K. Nageli	1846	New plant cells arise from pre-existing cells
W. Hofmeister	1849	Studied fertilisation in plants and nuclear divisions in stamens
R. Virchow	1855	All cells arise from pre-existing cells
Shultze	1861	Called protoplasm as the physical basis of life
Gregor Mendel	1865	Founded the science of Genetics
Haeckeel	1866	Named plastids in plant cells
George	1867	Discovered the organnel which was later called golgi complex
F. Mischer	1871	Discovered Nucleic acids
H. Fol	1873	Discovered spindle and astral fibres
O. Hertwig	1876	Discovered that fertilisation involves the fusion of sperm and ovum
E.G. Balbiani	1881	Discovered the giant salivary gland chromosomes in the larva of *Chronomus*
W. FLemming	1882	Introduced the term mitosis
Strassburger	1882	Described mitosis in plant cells
Schimper	1883	Introduced the term chloroplast

Van Benden	1887	Discovered centrioles
Waldeyer	1888	Introduced the term chromosomes
Boveri T.	1892	Described oogenesis and spermatogenesis in *Ascaris* (round worm)
Benda	1898	Named the mitochondrion
G. Golgi	1898	Described the Golgi complex
C.E. Meclung	1902	Identified sex chromosomes in hemiptera
Sutton W.S.	1902	Proposed the chromosome theory of heredity
E. Buchner	1903	Awarded Nobel prize for the discovery of Enzyme
F. Meves	1904	Demonstrated the occurrence of mitochondria in plant cells
J.B. Farmer	1905	Coined the term meiosis along with J.E. Moore
R.G. Harrison	1907	Developed tissue cultural technique
A. Kossel	1910	Obtained Nobel prize for the chemistry of the nucleus
R.M. Willstatler	1915	Got Nobel prize for research work on chlorophyll
R. Feulgen and H. Rossenbeck	1924	Developed feulgen technique for staining DNA
T. Svedberg	1926	Discovered ultra centrifuge and got Nobel prize
O.H. Warburg	1931	Discovered respiratory enzymes and got Nobel prize
M. Knoll and E. Ruska	1932	Invention of first electron microscope
T.H. Morgan	1933	Chromosome function in heredity. Got Novel prize
O.T. Avery C.H. Mcleod and H. Mc.Carthy	1944	Importance of DNA in the inheritance of bacterial cells
F. Zernike	1953	Invention of phase contrast microscope. Got Nobel prize
H.A. Krebs	1953	Discovery of citric acid cycle in aerobic respiration. Got Nobel prize
F.A. Lipmann	1953	Discovery of Co-enzyme A and its role in intermediary metabolism. Got Nobel prize
J.D. Watson and F.H.C. Crick	1953	Proposed the double helix model for DNA molecule and got Nobel prize

G.W. Beadle and E.L. Tatum	1958	One gene one enzyme hypothesis
S. Ochoa	1959	Synthesis of polyribonucleotide *in vitro*. Received Nobel prize
A. Korneberg	1959 -	Synthesis of polydeoxy ribonucleotides *in vitro*. Received Nobel prize
M. Calvin	1961	Discovered the dark reduction cycle in photosynthesis and Got the Nobel prize.
M.W. Nirenberg and H.G. Khorana	1968	Received Nobel prize for work on genetic code

Cytology and related sciences : The study of cell has helped biologists to understand various life processes like growth, metabolism, differentiation etc., at the cellular levels. Due to its wide application in various fields, cytology has given birth to various applied branches of biology. Some of these are -

Cytogenetics : This deals with the cytological and molecular basis of heredity, variation, mutation, morphogenesis etc.

Cytotaxonomy : In this branch, cytological details are used in solving taxonomic problems. Individuals of same species or related species have many similarities in chromosome morphology. Cytology also gives proof for the origin of certain taxonomic units or groups.

Cell physiology : This branch deals with functional aspects of cell. Study of nutrition, metabolism, growth, reproduction, division etc., come under the perview of cell physiology.

Cytochemistry : Chemical analysis of the cell is the subject matter of this branch. Analysis of carbohydrates, proteins, fats, nucleic acids, etc., in the cell are dealt within this branch.

Molecular biology : This is the most modern branch of biology. It deals with the molecular configuration and architecture of the living matter and helps to analyse and understand the molecular basis for various life processes. It also attempts to provide a molecular basis for the various inborn errors in metabolism. Molecular biology has provided many significant answers to various problems of biology.

Cytopathology : Study of cells and the analysis of cell structure at the microscopic and the submicroscopic level has helped us to study various diseases. As most of the diseases are ultimately caused by alteration in enzyme functioning, a study of their activity at the cellular level is vital to the understanding of the disease.

Cytoecology : While ecology deals with the study of organisms in relation to their environment, cytoecology deals with cytological characters of individuals in different environmental conditions. Ecological habitat and geographical distribution have their effect on the cytological features of organisms.

GENETICS

Like begets like and organisms do not arise *de novo* are two important and interdependent concepts in biology. While the former explains the similarity between offspring and parent, the latter explains that life comes from preexisting life.

In earlier times it was thought that certain organisms arise from non living source. Even Aristotle believed in this. It was Louis Pasteur who provided conclusive proof to discard spontaneous generation of living organisms. This theory that organisms arise from pre existing ones, gave the idea of parents and offspring and perhaps also paved the way for the study of inheritance of characters from one generation to the other.

While the offspring resemble their parents to a great extent, they also have some characters of their own.

The fact that the offspring resemble their parents is due to inheritance, while the differences encountered are due to variations. The science of genetics mainly deals with variation and inheritance of characters and their causes in living beings.

It is believed that ancient Indians and Egyptians had some idea of the inheritance of characters and reproduction, long before the dawn of the Christian era. There are reports to indicate that they were carrying out breeding in plants and animals. Breeding procedures for date palms were practised by Egyptians. Genetics in its present form however is a product of modern biology. It had its origin in the latter part of the 19th century.

Though the scientists of eighteenth and early nineteenth century tried to study the inheritance of characters in living beings from one generation to another generation, the actual understanding of the process was made possible only after the discovery of details of sexual reproduction.

The first person to experiment with hybridization was a German botanist Kolreuter, who studied the inheritance of characters in a cross of two tobacco plants. He observed that the offspring resembled both the partners.

The most important name in Genetics perhaps is that of Gregor Mendel, the Austrian monk. He is regarded as the father of Genetics. It is he, who for the first time studied the inheritance in detail and applied mathematics to biology.

The name of Devries, Tschermark and Correns are to be remembered as the rediscoverers of the Mendelian laws of inheritance.

The names of Charles Darwin, Lamarck and Weismann are also important for the contribution made towards the inheritance of characters. Darwin however had an erroneous interpretation regarding the inheritance of characters.

The discovery of chromosomes, cell division and genes are some of the milestones in the history of Genetics.

Present day Genetics is a very important branch of biological and medical science and finds application in various fields. The following are some of the branches of science which are related to Genetics.

Cytogenetics : Genetic studies at the cellular level is dealt with here.

Biochemical genetics : Biochemical analysis of hereditary units and inheritance patterns are studied in this branch.

Physiological Genetics : The functional aspects of inheritance (for ex. transmittence of certain functional defects) are studied.

Population Genetics : Application of genetic laws at the population level, growth of populations and quantitative study of genetic traits and their survival in populations are dealt with in this branch of genetics.

Eugenics : For a long time inheritance of characters was studied in all organisms except human beings. Genetic laws were propounded even for human beings based on inheritance pattern in other organisms. But as the study of Genetics progressed it was extended even to the study of human beings. Eugenics may be said to be the study of human genetics and the application of laws of genetics for the improvement of human race.

Significance of the study of Cytogenetics : Before we proceed with the study of cytogenetics, it is relevant to ask and answer a few questions. Of what importance is the study of cytogenetics? Is it merely to quench the academic thirst or can it be pressed into human service?

The answer to the above questions are very simple indeed. Perhaps no other branch of biology is as useful to human beings as a detailed study of cytogenetics. Speaking from academic point of view the study of cytogenetics helps us to understand the very basis of some of the vital life processes like cell division, growth, metabolism etc. It also provides us answers to the problems of inheritance of parental characters, origin and sustenance of heritable variations, bases of mutagenic change in the genetic material etc. Cytogenetics also provides a clue to the origin and diversification of different taxonomic groups of organisms.

From the point of view of applied aspect the uses of cytogenetics are manifold. The services of cytogenetics are sought after in Agriculture, Medicine etc.

One of the major menaces to the world agriculture is plant diseases. They take a heavy toll of our agricultural produces. Among the many methods employed to combat the plant diseases, the breeding of disease resistant varieties is perhaps the most important and the most effective. A through knowledge of the reproductive behaviour, chromosome structure and heritable traits of plants is of paramount importance in breeding.

Cytogenetics is also of great use in the field of medicine. A new branch of medical science has sprung up solely with the aid of cytogenetics. Biomedical science as it is called, aims to find out the causes and remedies for human diseases employing the tools of cytogenetics.

Cytogenetics also provides a clue to the understanding of many of the heritable human diseases like hemophilia, colour blindness etc. It is with the aid of cytogenetics again the Rh factor in the blood has come to light. Only those couples who have Rh positive factor in the blood are advised to marry. A marriage between a Rh negative female and a Rh positive male may prove fatal to the children. It brings about in infants an inborn disease called - *Erythroblastosis foetalis.* In western countries, the would be couple are generally subject to blood test before marriage and are advised about the feasibility or otherwise of the wedlock. Such a practise however is yet to come into existence in our country.

Many of the genetic diseases and the inborn errors of metabolism have their cytogenetic basis. Several of the syndrome diseases in man like Down's syndrome or Mongolism, Klienfetler's syndrome etc., all share a cytological basis in that they are the result of chromosomal abnormalities. Down's syndrome may be recognised by the physical abnormalities of the face, eyelids, tongue and other parts of the body. This is due to the presence of one extra chromosome in one of the autosomal assembly. In Klienfelter's syndrome, the testes are abnormally small and this is due to an additional 'X' chromosome in an otherwise 'XY' individual.

Many inborn errors of metabolism (metabolic diseases) like Alkaptonuria (black urine), Phenyl ketonuria, sickle celled anemia etc., can be understood only in terms of their cytogenetic basis.

Genetic counselling or advice based on the genetic characters and the probable inheritance is gaining currency rapidly. By studying a family pedigree, a counsellor will be able to advice on the type of future inheritance.

Genetic councelling of prospective parents with a defective history, has helped them to decide whether to have children or not. The counsellor will advice them on the percentage probability of the defect being carried to their offspring.

To sum up, it can be easily said that cytogenetics is gaining vast importance in recent years in the field of human medicine. With the incidence of infections or environmentally borne diseases being forcefully eradicated, the importance of genetic or systemic diseases need hardly be emphasised. Knowledge of the cause and inheritance of these disease is not only compatible with the hope of control, but one of the main foundations on which the control is based upon.

Some milestones in the History of Genetics

Name	Year	Contribution
Empedocles - Aristotle	200 BC	Semen theory Semen is highly purified blood
Harvey	1651	Living beings originate from egg.
Hartsoekes and	1694	Supported preformation theory
Datempotius	1692	"Observed" miniature human being in a sperm's head
Charles Darwin	1809-1882	Pangenesis theory
August Weismann	1889	Germplasm theory
Gregor Mendel	1822-1884	Laws of Heredity; regarded as father of Genetics
Hertwig	1875	Discovered fertilization
Flemming	1879	Described longitudinal splitting of chromosomes
Genden E.W.	1883	Gametes of round worm have half the number of chromosomes as the body cells
Waldeyer Tschermark	1888	Coined the term chromosome
Devries and Correns	1900	Rediscovering of Mendelian laws
Landsteiner	1900	Blood groups
Devries	1901	Mutation in *Oenothera*
McClung	1902	Sex chromosomes
Bateson. W	1906	Coined the term genetics
Bateson and Punnet	1906	Linkage in peas
Johanssen	1909	Coined the word gene
T.H. Morghan	1910	Sex linkage in *Drosophila*
Bridges	1923	Chromosomal aberrations
Beadle and Tatum	1941	Biochemical genetics in *Neurospora*

Some milestones in the History of Genetics

Name	Year	Contribution
Stern	1931	Cytological proof of crossing over
Avery, Mcclead and McCarty	1944	DNA - genetic material
Muller	1946	Radiation genetics·
Chargaff	1950	Base pairs are equal in proportion in DNA
Watson and Crick Ochoa and	1953	Molecular model of DNA
Kornberg	1959	DNA synthesis
Jacob and Monad	1961	Operon concept
Nirenberg, Holley and Khorana	1968	Genetic code
Palade	1974	Ultra structure of cells.

2

THE CELL

One of the marvels of nature is the creation of tiny yet potent biological compartments called cells. There is virtually no living being in the biological world save for Viruses which is not cellular. Either one, two or many millions of cells go to make the body of the living beings. A cell may be defined as the 'structural and functional unit of a living being. It is the minimal biological unit capable of maintaining and propagating itself. The study of cell comes under the perview of cytology, physiology and anatomy; while anatomy deals mainly with the structural aspects, the other two lay emphasis both on structure and function.

History

The word cell has been derived from the Latin word *cellula* meaning a small compartment. The term in the present sense was first used by Robert Hooke (1665) in his book *Micrographic.*

There has been some mention about cell in ancient Indian literature also. Parasara (1st century BC) in his book *Vrkshayurveda* refers to invisible compartments in the leaf and names them *Rasakosha.* He further opines that each cell has a sap *(Rasa),* not visible to the naked eye *(Anavah)* and has two boundaries *(Kalavestitena),* some of the cells have a colouring matter *(Ranjakayukta).*

The credit however of discovering the cell goes to Robert Hooke (1965), since it s difficult to establish the discovery to the ancient Indians in the absence of complete text of Parasara and the general apathy among Indians to their scientific heritage. Robert Hooke who constructed the first compound microscope observed the sections of cork and opined that they contain honey comb like compartments. German Biologists M.J. Schleiden and T.S. Schwann(1838) established the '*cell theory'* that all organisms are made up of cells.

Dutrochet in 1824 separated the cells from *Mimosa* plant. He boiled the leaves in nitric acid to isolate the cells. Turpin and Meyers (1830) observed that every tissue is an assemblage of cells.

One of the significant discoveries of the cell came from Robert Brown (1830). He discovered the presence of a spherical body in the centre of every cell, which he named *'nucleus'*

In the year 1835-37, Purkinje and Mohi independently discovered that protoplasm is an important constituent of every cell and it plays an important role in every cell activity including division. Golgi (1838) discovered the golgi apparatus. Balbiani (1881) discovered chromosomes in the salivary glands of *Chironomus*. At about the same time, Flemming (1882) studied cell division in detail and gave the name *Mitosis*.

Endoplasmic reticulum was discovered by Porter in 1945, while Benda gave the name mitochondria to organelles originally discovered by Hemming. Lysosomes were discovered in 1955 by de Duve.

Shape of Cell

The shape of the cell may be variable as in the case of *Amoeba* or fixed. When the shape is fixed or permanent, all conceivable shapes are found-they may be spherical, rectangular, flattened, polygonal, oval, triangular, cone like, columnar etc. As in *Acetabularia,* the body of the plant made of a single cell is differentiated into a rhizoid like base, a long and slender stalk and an umbrella like cap. Certain cells, like the Ascospores of *Claviceps* are acicular (needle like).

Size

There is a great range of variation among cells in size also. Some of them are not visible to the naked eye, some are barely visible, while some are macroscopic This smallest cell size can be encountered in *Coccus* bacteria (0.2 to 0.5m), while the largest size of cell is seen in Ostrich egg (nearly 15 cms). The table given below summarises the variations in cell size.

Table 1 (Adopted from U. Sinha and S. Sinha, 1976)

Cell type	Size
Fibre cell of *Linum*	550mm (length)
Egg of ostrich	170 x 35mm
Egg of Hen	60 x 45mm
Human egg	0.1mm = 100μm
Amoeba	100μ
Sea urchin egg	70μ
RBC	7μ
Typhoid bacillus	2.4 x 0.5μ

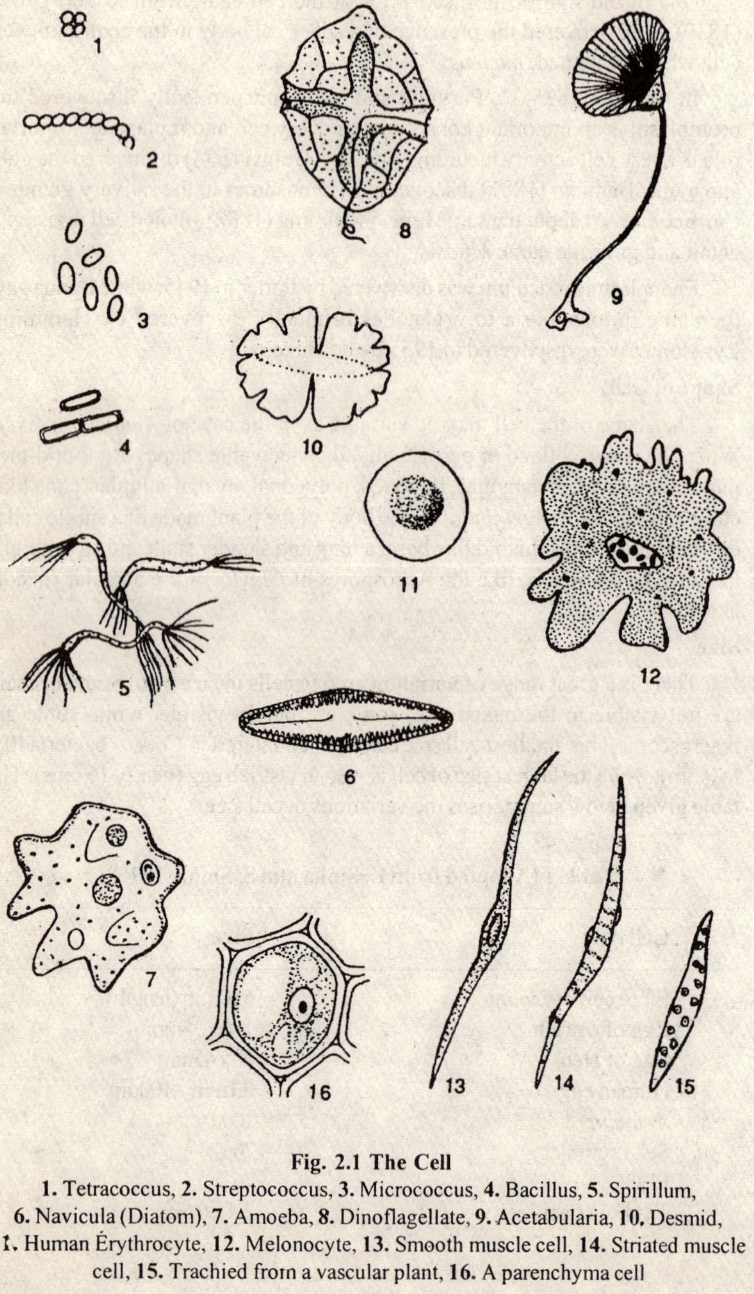

Fig. 2.1 The Cell

1. Tetracoccus, **2.** Streptococcus, **3.** Micrococcus, **4.** Bacillus, **5.** Spirillum, **6.** Navicula (Diatom), **7.** Amoeba, **8.** Dinoflagellate, **9.** Acetabularia, **10.** Desmid, **11.** Human Érythrocyte, **12.** Melonocyte, **13.** Smooth muscle cell, **14.** Striated muscle cell, **15.** Trachied from a vascular plant, **16.** A parenchyma cell

E. Coli	1.5 x 0.7μ
Diplococcus pneumonieae	200 x 100nm
*Influenze virus	100nm
*TMV	300 x 15nm
*T_3 bacteriophage	45nm,

(Even though Viruses cannot be regarded as cells, they have been mentioned as they are independent entities).

The factors governing the cell's size are -a) ratio between the volume of nucleus and volume of cytoplasm, b) ratio of cell surface to cell volume and c) the rate of metabolism.

Gross Morphology of the cell

A generalised plant cell has an outermost envelope called the cell wall. This is absent in animal cells. Internal to this is the plasma membrane. This encloses the nucleus and other cytoplasmic inclusions suspended in cytoplasm. The chief cytoplasmic inclusions are -Ribosomes, Lysosomes, Mitochondria, Plastids, Golgi complex, Endoplasmic reticulum, Vacuole and non living inclusions like crystals, raphides etc.

Prokaryotic and Eukaryotic cells

In primitive organisms like certain bacteria, blue green algae etc., the nucleus is not properly organised hence such cells are called *Prokaryotic,* while in evolved organisms, the nucleus is organised. Such cells are called *Eukaryotic.* The following are some of the fundamental differences between eukaryotic and prokaryotic cells.

1. Nucleus : Nuclear membrane is absent in prokaryotic cells, while eukaryotic cells have a definite bounding membrane. The nuclear material does not form definite chromosomes in prokaryotic cells. The DNA is circular and lies in a tangled mass. In Eukaryotes, the chromenema forms definite number of chromosomes and is associated with proteins.

2. Cytoplasmic organelles : Mitochondria, endoplasmic reticulum, Golgi complex, lysosomes and centrioles are absent in prokaryotes. The enzymatic functions associated with mitochondria are carried out by the infolding of the cell membrane at several points. Eukaryotes have all the organells mentioned above.

3. Cell wall : Chemically the cell wall of prokaryotes is composed of amino sugars and muramic acid. These are absent in the cell wall of eukaryotes (plants).

4. Flagella : The flagella of eukaryotes have eleven fibres with (2 + 9 arrangement) 2 central and 9 peripheral fibres, while prokaryotic flagella do not exhibit this arrangement.

5. Plastids : These are absent in prokaryotes. In photosynthetic prokaryotes the chlorphyll is associated with the lamellae, but the lamellae are not enclosed by any membrane. Ir. contrast to this, in all eukaryotes, the chlorophyll pigment is found in definite organelles called chloroplasts.

In addition to the above differences, the streaming movement of cytoplasm may also be added, which is present in eukaryotes, but absent in prokaryotes.

Table 2. Comparison between Prokaryotic and Eukaryotic Cells
(Adopted from De Robertis Et al 1980)

	Character	Prokaryotic	Eukaryotic Cells
1.	Nuclear membrane	Absent	Present
2.	DNA	Naked and circular	Combined with proteins
3.	Chromosomes	Single	Multiple
4.	Nucleolous	Absent	Present
5.	Cell division	amitosis (fisson)	Mitosis or meiosis
6.	Ribosomes	70s (50s + 30s)	80s (60s + 40s)
7.	Endomembrane system	Absent	Present
8.	Mitochondria	Definite organelle absent enzymes of respiration and photosynthesis stored in the folds of plasma membrane	
9.	Choloroplast	Absent	Present
10	Cell wall	Non cellulosic (present in plants only)	Cellulosic
11.	Exocytosis and endocytosis	Absent	Present
12.	Flagella	No definite arrangement of fibrills	9 + 2 fibrillar arrangement

PROKARYOTIC CELL

The prokaryotic cells are generally smaller and vary in size in different members. In mycoplasma it is about 0.12)μm while in *Oscillatoira,* a filamentous blue green the size is 40 x 5\μ. A great majority of them, however are about μ in size. Among the bacteria the smallest are to be found among cocci (0.1 μ) while the largest are the spirilla (60 x 6~m). The various components of the prokaryotic cell are described below.

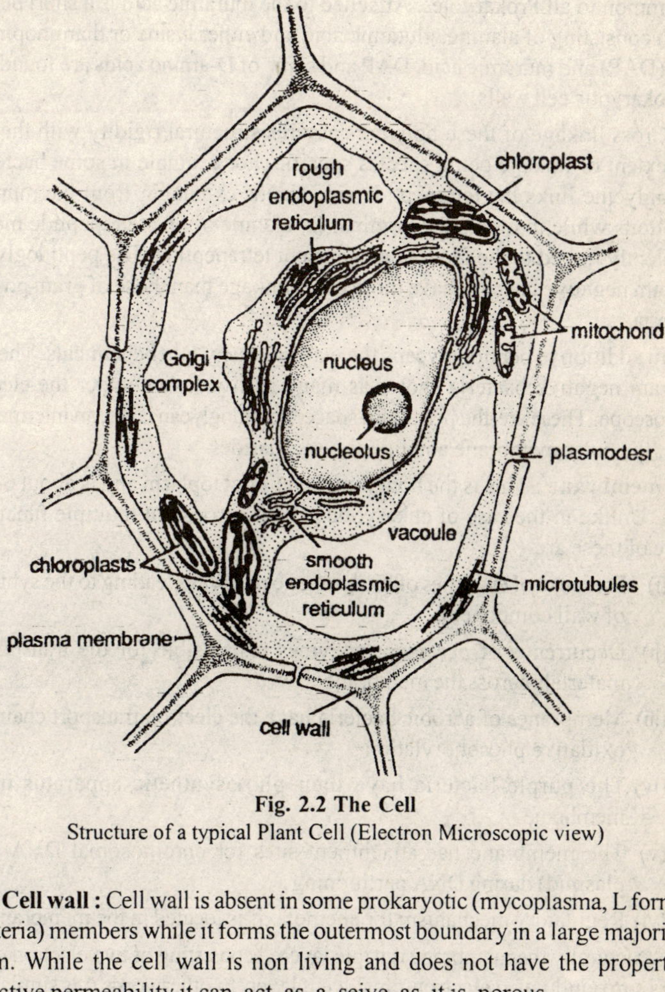

Fig. 2.2 The Cell
Structure of a typical Plant Cell (Electron Microscopic view)

Cell wall : Cell wall is absent in some prokaryotic (mycoplasma, L forms of bacteria) members while it forms the outermost boundary in a large majority of them. While the cell wall is non living and does not have the property of selective permeability it can act as a seive as it is porous.

In some prokaryotes the space between the cell membrane and cell wall is filled with some enzymes and metabolites consituting the periplasm.

Chemically the cell wall is made up of strong fibres of hetropolymers called *mucopeptides ofpeptidogycans.* They are also refered to as *glycopeptide, muropeptide, murein etc.*

The peptidoglycans consist of alternating units made up of N acetyl glucosamine and N acetyl muramic acid with 1-4 linkages. This type of a linkage is common to all Prokaryotes. Attached to the muramic acid is a short peptide chain consisting of alanine, glutamic acid and either lysine or diaminopimelic acid (DAP) and muramic acid. DAP and some of D-amino acids are found only in prokaryotic cell walls.

Cross linkage of these polymers assures structural rigidity with the type and extent of linkage being species specific. For example in some bacteria a pentaglycine links the tetrapeptide side chains extending from the muramic acid units while in others the terminal D- alanine of one tetrapeptide may be covalently linked to the DAP of an adjacent tetrapeptide. The peptidoglycans of gram negative bacteria have more cross linkage than those of gram positive bacteria.

In addition to peptiodglycans the wall has many other chemicals. The wall of gram negative bacteria shows as many as five layers under the electron microscope. These are-the periplasm space, Peptidoglycan layer, an intermediate zone, the outer membrane and lipopolysaccharides.

Cell membrane : This is the bounding layer of cytoplasm and is about 6-8nm thick. Unlike in the case of eukaryotic cells it carries out multiple functions. Some of these are -

(i) Presence of enzymes of biosynthetic pathways leading to the synthesis of wall components

(ii) Occurrence of *permease* enzymes responsible for the transport of materials across the membrane

(iii) Membranes of aerobic bacteria have the electron transport chain and oxidative phosohorylation

(iv) The purple bacteria have their photosynthetic apparatus in the membrane

(v) The membrane has attachment sites for chromosomal DNA (also plasmid) during DNA partitioning

(vi) Regulatory mechanism for chemotaxis is located in the membrane.

Structurally the membrane is triple layered consisting of two electron dense layers surrounding an electrontranslucent layer. In otherwords it is similar to a unit membrane. The architecture and chemical coposition is similar to the fluid mosaic model proposed by Singer and Nicolson (1972) (For details see later in the chapter).

Cytoplasm : Cytoplasm does not appear to have an organized structure when observed under electron microscope. It may be regarded as a concentrated solution containing a host of metabolites, enzymes, amino acids, inorganic ions, sugars, vitamins etc. Cytoplasm plays an important role in intermediary metabolism. There is no cytoskelcton.

Flagella (see bacteria)

Capsule (see bacteria)

Pili (see bacteria)

Surface layers : These are present in all gram negative and gram positive bacteria. Three main types of S layers have been reported in prokaryotic cells (bacteria) The S layers are composed of single homogenous peptides with occasional carbohydrates as minor components. These layers are believed to act as macromolecular sieves preventing the entry of toxic molecules and also to protect the peptidoglycans of the wall from the action of lytic enzymes.

Nucleoid : This represents the genetic material of prokaryotic cells. It is similar in all prokaryotes. (for details see - bacteria) The molecular structure of DNA is same as in eukaryotic cells.

Inclusion bodies : These are storage granules and other particles distributed in the cytoplasm. There are two kinds of inclusion bodies-membrane enclosed and membraneless (Shiviey 1974).

Membrane enclosed bodies : These are enclosed by a non unit type of membrane 2-4nm thick and made up of proteins. The inclusion bodies encountered in the prokaryotic cells are chlorosomes, carboxysomes, magnetosomes, gas vacuoles, polyhydroxybutyrate (PHB) granules, sulphur granules and glycogen granules.

PHB granules occur in cyanobacteria, sulphur granules are found in Thiorhodaccae and glycogen granules in *Clostridium* spp.

Chlorosomes have been demonstrated in photosynthetic bacteria belonging to chlorlobiaceae. (Cruden and Stanier, 1970). These are different from chromatophores in being non-membranous.

Carboxysomes are seen in cyanobacteria (Murphy et al 1974).

Magnetosomes are particles which help the bacterium in orienting itself in relation to the magnetic behaviour of the surroundings. Reported to occur in *Aquaspirillum magnetotacticum* (Balkwill et al 1980), the magnetosomes allow the bacteria to punise the most efficient aerotactic behaviour.

Non membranous Inclusion bodies : Phycobilisomes, cyanophycin granules (found in cyanobacteria), polyglucoside granules and several crystalline substances belong to this group.

In addition to the above there are R - bodies (retractile stuctures) demonstrated in bacteria by Lalucat and Mayer (1978). These are supposed to be similar to kappa particles of *Paramecium*.

Ribosomes (see bacteria)

Mesosomes (see bacteria)

Chromatophores : These are present in the photosynthetic bacteria belonging to the families Rhodospirillaceae, Chromatiaceae and Cyanophyceae. Chromatophores vary in form and have vesicles, tubes, bundles, stacks or thylakoids etc.

EUKARYOTIC CELL

Cell Wall

The cell wall is the characteristic feature of the plant cells. It is made up of non living matter and is believed to be secreted by the plasma membrane. The structure and composition of the cell wall not only varies in different plants, but in different types of cells of the same plant. Often, there might be variety in the cell wall composition at different stages of growth of the cell. The cell wall is very rigid and maintains the shape of the cell acting as a boundary. A unique feature of the cell wall is its permeability which is due to the presence of small pores.

Gross structure

Three layers are distinguishable in the cell wall. these are the *primary cell wall, middle lamella* and the *secondary cell wall.* The primary cell walls of adjacent cells are separated by middle lamella. Secondary wall is deposited after a certain period of development.

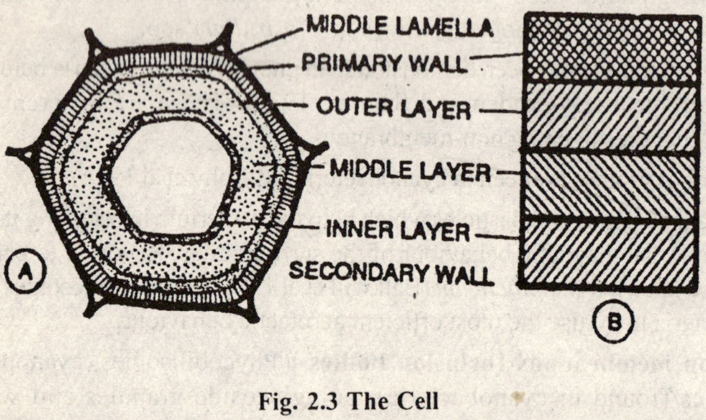

Fig. 2.3 The Cell
Arrangement of wall layers. **A.** Cross section, **B.** Arrangement of fibrils

The primary wall is secreted by the plasma membrane. In some instances like the leaves, fleshy stems, roots etc., the cells have only the primary wall and the middle lamella. The primary wall is formed during the early stages of growth and is about 1 to 3nm in thickness. Chemically the primary wall is composed of cellulose, hemicellulose and pectic compounds. The young primary wall is plastic and is prone to changes. Often it may be lignified.

The Middle lamella is the intercellular substance binding together the primary and the secondary walls. The middle lamella is formed during cell division and is amorphous and colloidal in nature. Chemically the middle lamella is composed of pectin, cellulose, calcium and magnesium pectate.

The secondary wall is deposited on the primary wall after cell maturation. It is very rigid and does not alter its shpae. The thickness varies from 5 - 10nm. The secondary wall usually has three layers viz., *outer layer, middle layer* and *inner layer*.

Chemically the Secondary wall is composed of cellulose, non cellulosic polysaccharides and hemicelluloses.

Ocassionally a *tertiary cell wall* may also be found as in the tracheids of some gymnosperms. This is a very thin layer and is composed of *xylan,* instead of cellulose. The secondary wall acquires different types of thickenings.

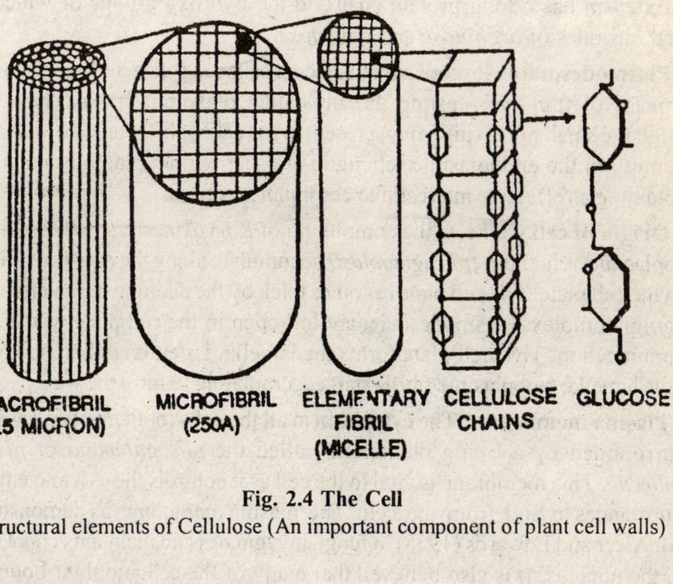

Fig. 2.4 The Cell
Structural elements of Cellulose (An important component of plant cell walls)

Ultra structure of the cell wall

The cell wall is mainly composed of cellulose. Cellulose is a polymer of glucose molecules. Approximately each molecule of cellulose consists of about 3000 glucose residues joined together by 1-4 oxygen bridges. These cellulose chains are oriented along the axis of the cell. About 100 of these cellulose chains bundle together to form *micellels* or *elementary fibrils*. Each micelle is about 100Å in diameter. Many hundreds of these micelles of these stack together to form *microfibrils*. Each microfibril is 200Å to 300Å in diameter. The micorfibril is visible only under eletron microscope. About 2000 of these microfibrils join together to constitute the *macrofibril* which is about 0.5μ in width. The macrofibrils are visible under the light microscope.

In secondary walls, the microfibrils are more orderly and compact than in the primary walls. The space between fibrils is filled by an interfibrillar substance usually the matrix. The matrix is filled by non cellulosic polysaccharides - such as pectin, hemicellulose, xylans etc.

The primary cell wall of dicotyledons contains many complex polysaccharides such as *xyloglucans, arabinogalactans* and *rhamnogalacturonans.* These are linked to the cellulose fibril and to one another by covalent linkages.

In certain walls, a glycoprotein called extensin is present. It is similar to collagen in being rich in 4 - hydroxyproline.

Extensin has a long protein chain, to the hydroxy groups of which are linked, residues of *arabinose* and *galactose.*

Plasmodesmata : Protoplasts of adjacent cells are connected to one another by means of thin cytoplasmic threads called plasmodesmata. These pass through the small pores (pit fields) present in the cell wall. Tubules which are in continuity in the endoplasmic reticulum are seen within plamodesmata thus maintaining an effective intercellular communication.

Origin of cell wall : At the completion of *Karyokinesis,* small vesicles of endoplasmic reliculum *(phragmoplast)* accumulate along the equatorial line to form the cell plate. The cell plate becomes thick by the addition of material from the golgi complex. Plasmodesmata are left open in the cell plate to maintain communication. This cell plate forms the lamella. Later, on either side of the middle lamella, cytoplasmic fibrils start accumulating to form the wall.

Plasma membrane : The cytoplasm in all the cells (both plant and animal) is surrounded by a living membrane called the *plasmalemma* or *plasma membrane.* This membrane is vital to the cell as it controls the exit and entry of all substances to and from the cell. The plasma membrane, as demonstrated by McAlear and Edwards (1958) in fungi, invaginates and maintains connection with the nucleus. It is also believed that many of the cell and their bounding membrane is same as the plasma membrane These organelles are nucleus, mitochondria, chloroplasts etc.

The presence of the cell membrane is proved by the following evidences.

1. On injury to a cell, when protoplasm flows out, it remains as a discreet unit.
2. Observations under electron microscope have revealed the presence of a boundary membrane over the surface of cytoplasm.

Size of the membrane : It is about 75Å thick and is composed of three concentric layers. The middle layer is about 35Å in thickness, while the outer layers on either side or 20Å thick.

Chemical composition : Membranes from different sources show variations in chemical composition. Essentially however all membranes are lipoproteinanceous. The components are held together in a thin sheet by non convalent bonds. The ratio of protein to lipids varies depending on the type (Golgi membrane, plasma membrane etc) of membrane, type of organism (eukaryote, prokaryote, etc.) and the type of cell (epidermis, phoelm etc.). In adition to these two, certain membranes also have carbohydrates.

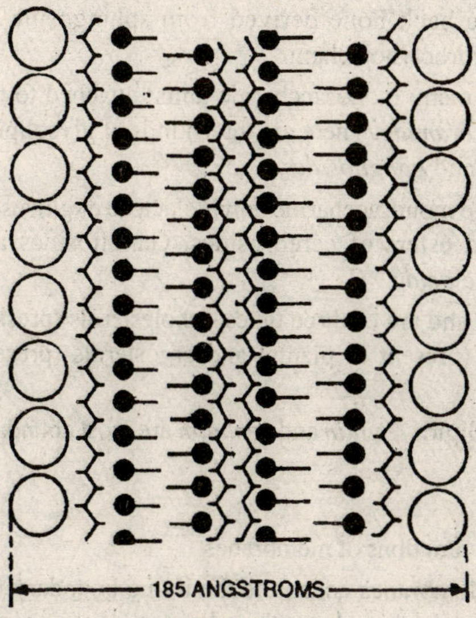

Fig. 2.5 The Cell
Diagrammatic representation of a cell membrane having two unit membranes

Membranes have three dfferent categories of proteins. These are - structural *proteins, functional proteins* (enzymes) and *carrier proteins.* Structural proteins maintain the structural frame work of the membranes. The average molecular weight of structural proteins found in membranes in 3×10^4. Enzymes catalyzing various physiological activities are found in the membrane of mitochondria, endoplasmic reticulum etc. *Carrier proteins* are known to form a complex with the substances and help them to pass through the membrane.

The protein composition of different membranes vary (as has been pointed out already). For instance plasma membranes have 50% while mitochondrial membranes have 75% proteins.

The proteins present in plasma membrane are categorized into two viz. *integral proteins* and *peripheral proteins.* While integral proteins form the back bone of the membrane, peripheral proteins have a weak association maintained by weak electrostatic interaction. The integral proteins are hydrophobic in nature as they have to penetrate the hydrophobic lipids to form the basic structure of the membrane. These proteins do not easily disassociate from the membrane and it requires harsh chemical procedures to accomplish it.

The integral proteins have a hydrophilic portion also which protrudes out of lhe lipoid bilayer. Peripheral proteins are associated either with the hydrophilic head of lipids or hydrophilic part of the integral proteins.

The Lipids of membranes are of several types, but all of them share a common character in being *amphipatic* i.e. having both *hydrophilic* and *hydrophobic* portions within a molecule. There are three categories of membrane lipids-they are phosopholipids, glycolipids and sterols. While most membrane lipids are phospholipids, cholesterol does not have phosphates.

Phospholipids are of two categories viz. *phosphoglycerides* and *sphingophospholipids*. Phosplioglycerides have a glycerol back bone, while sphingophospholpids have the back bone derived from sphingosine an aminoalchobol having a long hydrocarbon chain.

Glycolipids contain one or many monosaccharide units attached to the lipids based on *sphingenine* or *ceramide*. There are three kinds of glycolipids viz., *Cerebrosides, sulphatides* and *gangliosides*.

Cerebrosides contain a single monosaccharide unit (galactose or glucose). Sulphatides are sulphuric acid esters of cerebrosides. Gangliosides are glycosphingolipids having *sialic acid*.

Sterols are steroid alcohols and are of three types - cholesterols (present in animal tissues), phytosterols (present in plants) and ergosterols (present in eukaryotic microorganisms).

Among the glycerophospholipids *lecithin* and *cephalin* are most abundant in higher plants and animals.

Membrane functions

The following are the major functions of membranes.

1. **Compartmentalization:** Membranes constitute the living boundary for cytoplasm and cell contents. As unbroken sheets they divide the living mater into self sustaining units to effectively coordinate and regulate the activities.

2. **Regulation of movement:** In a biologically active cell many susbstances enter and many others go out of the cell. However, if the entry and exit is unregulated, it is deleterious to the cell. Hence plasma membrane regulates and decides which substances are to be allowed and which should not. This unique property of the cell membrane called selective permeability or differential permeability is responsible for most of the physiological activities of the cell.

3. **Communication:** All the membranes have certain special substances (on their surface) called receptor molecules which mediate and control the message from one to another. The receptor molecules vary in different membranes. These molecules combine with substances (ligands) of different types and generate signals (in the form of cyclic AMP) directed to the interior of the cell. The best studied ligands are the hormones and neurotransmitters.

4. **Interaction between cells:** It is the responsibility of the plasma membrane as the living boundary between cells to effectively coordinate actions between cells since an organism consists of differnt types of cells and many a time the actions have to be coordinated to achieve harmony.

5. **Energy transformations :** Membranes are intimately associated with the inter conversion of energy. For instance, in green plants the light energy has to be converted into chemical energy. Similarly the chemical energy stored in carbohydrates has to be converted into energy currency i.e. ATP molecules. The machinery for energy capture and conversion is hidden in the membranes of mictochondria and chloroplasts.

6. **Locus for biochemical functions :** Membranes provide the structural framework for the location of various enzymes. The scaffolding of the membrane interconnecting the various organelles helps in the coordination of activities. Such an effective coordination of activities is best illustrated in the mitochondrial membrane where the various components of the electron transport chain work together as they are located in an orderly fashion.

7. **Other activities :** Membranes also function in various other capacities such as providing mechanical strength, involving in cell movement secretion etc., and also acting as electrical insulators.

Structure of the membrane : The molecular structure of the membrane has been interpreted in various ways by different cell biologists in order account for their known function. Various models have been proposed for the molecular structure of the membrane. These fall into two basic categories, viz., bilayer models and micellar or subunit models. The bilayer models are believed to have protein and lipid to be arranged in the form of layers, while the subunit models assume the presence of a number of independent subunits. We shall discuss a few of these models. The chart below summarises the list of various models.

MEMBRANE MODELS

- Bilayer models
  - Lipid membrane Model
  - Sandwich Models
    - (a) Danielli Davson model
    - (b) Unit membrane model
    - (c) Greater membrane odel
    - (d) Kavanau's model
- Micellar models
  - Models in which protein penetrate into the lipid layer
    - (a) Benson's model
    - (b) Lenard and Singer' model
    - (c) Mosaic membrane model
    - (d) The fluid mosaic model

BILAYER MODELS

Lipid membrane model : Overtoil (1895) discovered that fat soluble subsatances easily pass through the membrane indicating their affinity to the lipids. Hober (1910) and Fricke (1925) found out that the low electrical conductivity of the Iving cell is due to the presence of lipids. The experiments of Mudd and Mudd (1931) in placing an oil droplet which adheres to the cell surface provided the presence of lipids in the cell membrane. It was Gorter and Grendel (1925) who suggested a structural model based on lipids. They studied the erythrocyte (RBC) membrane and concluded that it is composed of two layers of liqid molecules whose polar groups are situated on the outside of the membrane.

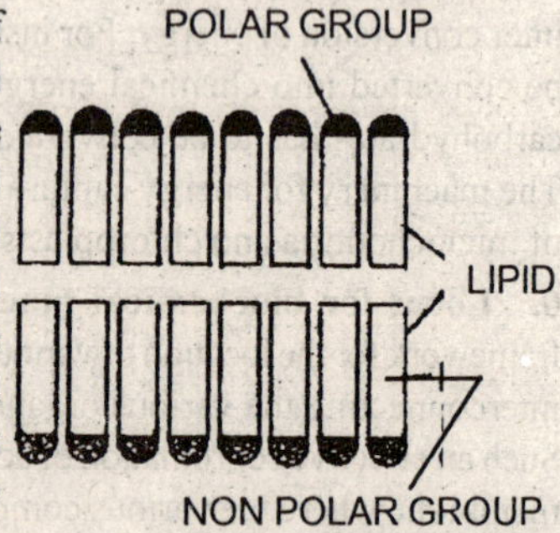

Fig. 2.6 The Cell
The lipid membrane model of Forter and Grendel

Sandwich models : In these models the lipid layers are supposed to be sandwiched between the two protein layers on either surface. The polar groups of the lipids adhere to the proteins on either side. The following are some of the models based on sandwich principle.

(a) Danielli Davson model : The study of surface tension of cells by Daniell and Harvey (1935) and Harvey and Cole (1931) indicated that there must be more to the structure of the membrane than merely being made up of lipids. In 1935, Hugh Davson and James Denielli proposed that the plasma membrane is a lipid layer sandwiched between layers of globular proteins. In a way the Danielli model was the first structural interpretation to account for the physiological properties of the membrane.

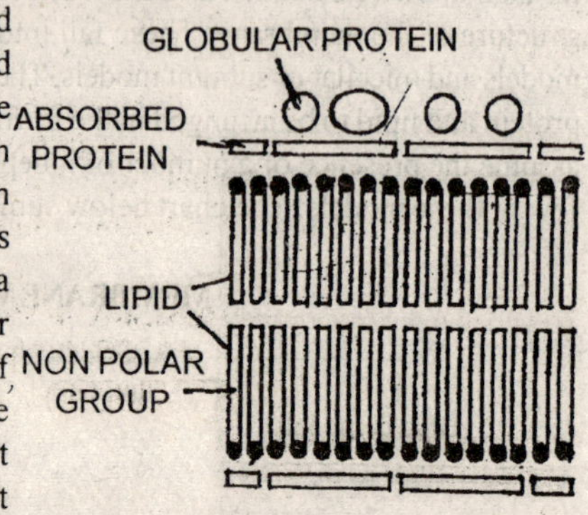

Fig. 2.7 The Cell
The Danielli-Davson model

Over the years various modifications have been proposed for the model. Danielli (1938) opined that there could be two kinds of globular proteins on the surface and diagonally arranged proteins in contact with the lipid layer. In order to account for the permeability, certain small pores were visualised in the lipid layers with an inner lining of protein molecules providing an inner hydrophilic surface.

The following are some other variations in the protein lipid arrangement.

1. Proteins are in the form of folded chain.
2. Proteins are in coiled from on both sides of the lipid layer.
3. Proteins are asymmetrically arranged i.e., one side has globular proteins and the other side a folded β chain.
4. Globular proteins are found on either side.
5. Helical proteins extend into the pores between the lipid molecules.

Nature of lipids in the membrane

The lipids are mainly phospholipids with their polar groups pointing outwards - *lecithin* alternates with a steroid molecule (*cholesterol*). Each lecithin molecule consists of two glycerol chains with the part containing *phosphate* and *choline,* the polar head is bent like a walking stick.

(b) The unit membrane model : The specimens of membrane fixed in osmium tetroxide for the purpose of electron microscopic observation reveal the occurrence of *two lines,* presumably indicating their double membrane nature. This observation originally made in 1950's by Humberto Fernandez Moran and David Robertson led to the unit membrane model. Robertson used a new fixative potassium permanganate. He discovered that each of the dense line possessed a sub structure having a trilaminar appearence. Each membrane is composed of two thin eletron dense lines of 20Å, with the intervening space of about 35Å. The inner and outer layers are non identical. The outer is a mucoid protein, while the inner surface is a non mucoid protein. The unit membrane model is similar to Danielli Davson model except that protein layers are asymmetrical. Membrane of cell organelles, plasma membrane and endoplasmic reticulum are thought to be similar in havingo the unit membrane structure. But current studies have shown that arrangement of lipids and proteins vary in different membranes. Further, the Robertson model is based on the study of myelin which is a non typical membrane.

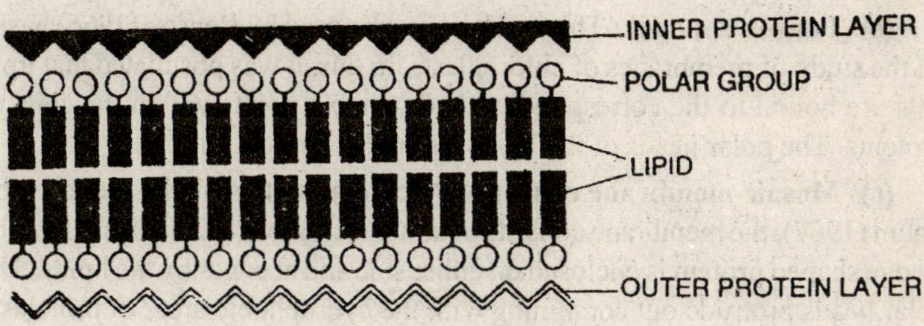

Fig. 2.8 The Cell
The unit membrane model of Robertson

(c) The Greater membrane model : This is similar to the trilaminar sandwich model except that the outer and inner surface proteins are different. The inner surface has an unconjugated structural protein adhering to polar heads of lipids. The outer surface also has structural proteins, on which is superimposed a *glycoprotein*. To this glycoprotein are attached side chains of oligosaccharides.

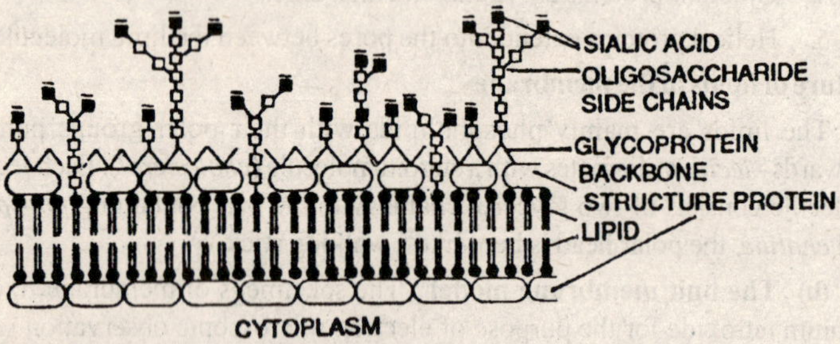

Fig. 2.9 The Cell
The greater membrane model

(d) Kavanau's lipid pillar model : According to Kavanau J.L. (1965), the lipid layer exists in two forms. Kavanau's model is essentially similar to Danielli Davson model. The two types of lipid structures are *pillars* and *flattened discs*. Pores are present between pillars to faciliate the passage of ions. Membranes with pillar lipids are thicker than those with discs. Internally the pillars have non polar tails, while the surface is made up of polar phospholipids. Proteins are present on either side of lipids.

Models based on protein penetration of lipids

(a) Lenard and Singer's model : This is based on the protein arrangement in the membrane. About 25 to 30% of proteins are helical while the rest are irregular coils.

(b) Benson's model : This model was proposed by Benson (1966) based on the study of membranes of chloroplasts. In this, it was postulated that lipid tails are bound to the corresponding hydrophobic points within the coils of proteins. The polar heads of the lipids lie on the surface.

(c) Mosaic membrane concept : According to this model proposed by Baum (1967), the membrane consists of units, each about 80Å in diameter. The wedge shaped protein is enclosed on either side and at edges by the lipids. The polar heads protrude out combining with the hydrophobic areas of proteins.

(d) The Fluid mosaic model : The molecular model of the plasma membrane proposed by Singer and Nicolson (1972) emphasises on the dynamism of membrane organisation and visualises it to be a semifluid like structure with a mosaic arrangement of lipids and proteins. The fluid mosaic model, though essentially based on bilayer models, rejects the idea of continuous bilayer.

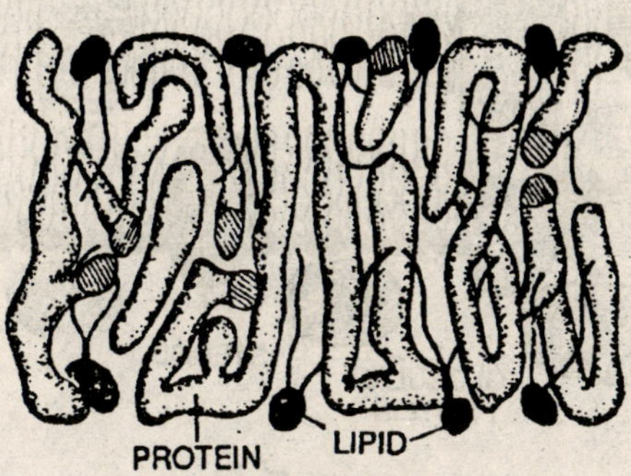

Fig. 2.10 The Cell
Membrane model of Benson

Instead of forming continuous external layer adhering to the hydrophilic heads of the phospholipids, as in the Danielli model; the proteins constitute discontinuous particles often penetrating deeply into the lipid layer. In a way the protein units could be compared to floating incebergs in a sea of phospholipids. The countinuity of the bilayer is not maintained because of complete or incomplete interruption by proteins. While the Danielli model assumes a hydrophilic bonding between lipids and proteins, the Singer Nicolson model regards it to be hydrophobic.

The membrane proteins in the fluid mosaic model are of two types distinguishable by their intensity of lipid association. These are the *integral* or *intrinsic proteins* and the *extrinsic* or *pheripheral proteins.* ITie integral proteins penetrate deep into the lipid layer and are the hydrophobic as they have to coexist in the hydrophobic environment of fatty acids. The integral proteins are *amphipatic.* While their tips are hydrophilic; the central portion is hydrophobic. These proteins are difficult to extract from the membranes.

The peripheral proteins which are weakly associated whith the membrane can be easily extracted. They are hydrophilic and never penetrate the interiors of the lipid bilayer. They form weak bonds either with the polar heads of lipids or with the hydrophilic surfaces of integral proteins. One of the best evidences for a broken surface layer of proteins comes with the using of phospholipases. These phosphate degarding enzymes very easily percolate into the membrane, which would have been impossible, if there were to be an unbroken surface envelope of proteins.

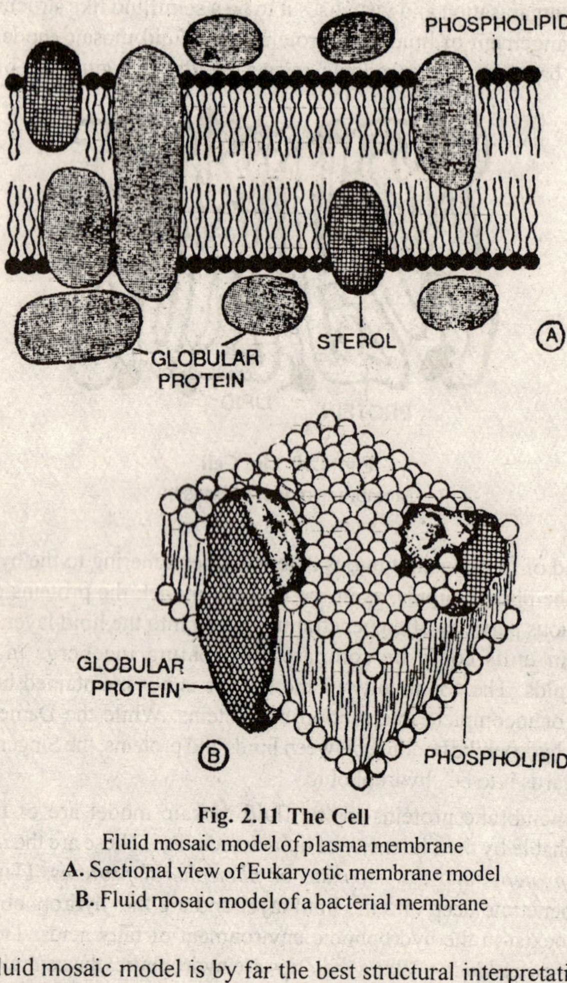

Fig. 2.11 The Cell
Fluid mosaic model of plasma membrane
A. Sectional view of Eukaryotic membrane model
B. Fluid mosaic model of a bacterial membrane

The fluid mosaic model is by far the best structural interpretation of the membrane which satisfactorily explains all its (membrane's) known functions.

MICELLAR MODELS

According to Fernandez Moran (1963) the membrane is corpuscular in nature consisting many repeating units. These units called *globular units* or elementary particles range in diamiter form 40 - 70Å and form closely packed repeating units. The membrane structure may be globular or unit membrane in different organelles or under different metabolic conditions. According to some cell biologists, the corpusular nature is an artifact.

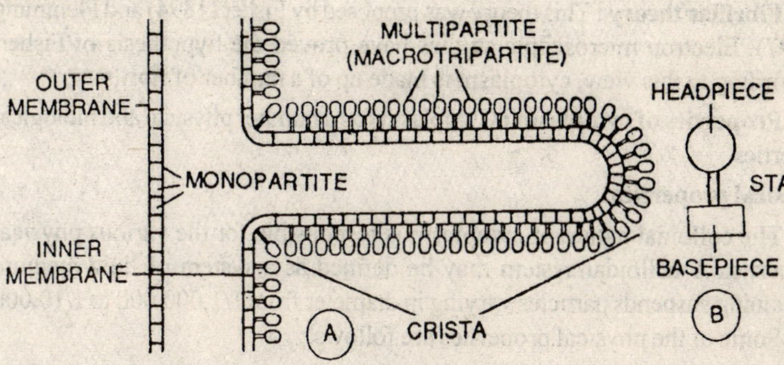

Fig. 2.12 The Cell
Green's model of repeating units
A. Crysta of a mitochondrion, **B.** Repeating unit

Green (1970) suggests that membranes made up of repeating units are of two types viz., *monopartite* and *multipartite* The monopartite membranes have repeating units flush with the membrane surface, while the multipartite have repeating units projecting from the membrane sufrace. Each repeating unit has a base, a stalk and a head. In monopartite, the repeating units correspond only to the base of the repeating unit of a multipartite membrane. The inner membrane of mitochondria corresponds to the multipartite membrane.

Of the two types of membrane stuctures, it is difficult to say which model is correct There seems to be evidence for both the bilayer and micellar models. While electron micrographs have shown the trilaminar structure for the unit membrane, the inner membranes of chloroplast and mitochondria have revealed the repeating globular sub units. It is quite likely that different membranes show different structure or the combination of both actually constitutes the membrane structure.

Cytoplasm

The colloidal substance in the cell, internal to the plasma membrane (without the inclusions) is called cytoplasm. The cytoplasm is usually granular and has many substances either dissolved or suspended in it The suspended particles may be in the solid or semi solid condition. There are several theories regarding the structure of the cytoplasm. Some of these are-

Reticular theory : Cytoplasm is made up of network of fibrils or particles.

Alveolar theory : According to Butschill (1892), cytoplasm consists of a number of droplets or alveoli. It gives an appearence of oil droplets floating on water.

Granular theory : According to Altmann (1893), Cytoplasm is composed of a number of minute granules suspended in a matrix.

Fibrillar theory : This theory was proposed by Fisher (1894) and Flemming (1897). Electron microscopic studies have proved the hypothesis of Fisher. According to this view, cytoplasm is made up of a number of fibrils.

Properties of cytoplasm : Cytoplasm has a number physical and biological proerties.

Physical properties

The colloidal nature of cytoplasm is responsible for the various physical properties A colloidal system may be defined as a system of liqid medium containing suspends particles varying in diameter from 1/1,000,000 to 1/10,000 nm. Some of the physical properties are follows.

Phase reversal : Cytoplasm may be differentiated into a *sol state* and *gel state.* Sol state is the liquid state and the gel state is the semi solid state. These two phases are interchangeable. This capacity is known as phase reversal.

Elasticity : Depending on the circumstances, the cytoplasm can extend or contract subject to a certain limit. This is known as elasticity.

Cohesiveness : The suspended particles in cytoplasm have mutual attraction, thus exhibiting cohesiveness.

Contractility : It is the capacity of peripheral cytoplasm to absorb or remove water from cell to the exterior. This is manifested very well by guard cells.

Viscosity : The suspended particles of cytoplasm are responsible for its viscous nature.

Brownian movement : The suspended particles of cytoplasm are in a state of to and fro movement called Brownian movement

In addition to this, cytoplasm also exhibits movements (seen in the plasmodium of slime molds) and 'cyclosis or streaming movements (seen in the leaf cells of *Elodea).*

Biological properties

Growth, respiration, excretion, nutrition, reproduction, metabolism, irritability etc., are some of the important biological activities of cytoplasm.

Chemical composition of cytoplasm : 90% of cytoplasm is water. The remaining 10% is constituted by organic and inorganic compounds.

About 40 or more inorganic constituents are found in cytoplasm. These are found in the form of ions (either cations or anions). Some of the common inorganic constituents are - Oxygen (62%), Hydrogen (10%), Carbon (18%) and Nitrogen (3%). The less common inorganic contituents are Calcium (0.25%), Phosphorus (1.2%), Sodium (0.1%), Magnesium (0.7%), Iodine (015%) and Chlorine (0.15%).

Among the various organic substances proteins, carbohydrates, lipids, hormones, vitamins and nucleic acids are most important.

Cytoplasmic Inclusions : Cytoplasm has a number of living and non living inclusions. The living inclusions are - Nucleus, mitochondria,. plastids, endoplasmic reticulum, golgi complex, lysosome, centrioles, microbodies, etc.

Nucleus

This is the most important organelle of the cell which regulates all its activities. It was discovered by Robert Brown in 1831.

Position : Usually it is present at the centre of the cell, but in some instances as in mature parenchyma cells, the nucleus is peripheral. In *Acetabularia,* the nucleus occupies various positions, though mainly present at the basal region.

Shape, size and number : The shape is variable depending on the cell type. Though the nucleus is generally spherical, ellipsoidal or flattened ones also may be seen in certain cells. The surface is generally smooth but as in leucocytes it may have small infoldings.

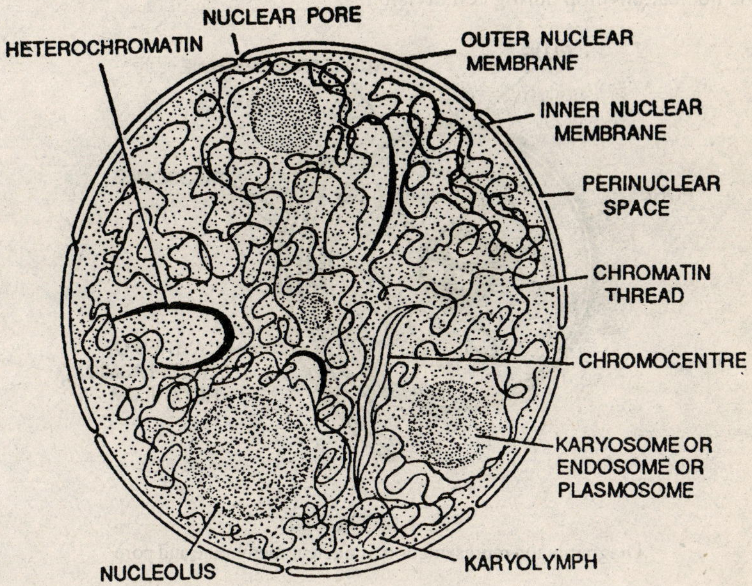

Fig. 2.13 The Cell
Structure of the nucleus

The size of the nucleus is also variable depending on the cell; the size of the nucleus being directly proprolional to that of cytoplasm. The following formula or Heywig may be used to determine the size of the nucleus in a particular cell.

$NP = Vn/Vc - Vn$

When NP = nucleoprotein index, Vn is the volume of the nucleus and Vc is the volume of the cell.

Most of the cells are uninucleate, while some *(Paramecium)* may be binucleate or multinucleate *(Cladophora)*. In certain fungi like *Mucor,* where there are no septa dividing the plant body into cells, numerous nuclei occur indicating a coenocytic condition.

Ultrastructure of the nucleus : Ultrastructurally the nucleus has the following parts - 1. Nuclear membrane, 2. Karyolymph or Nuclear sap, 3. Chromonemata, 4. Nucleolus and 5. Endosomes.

Nuclear membrane : In all eukaryotic organisms, a limiting membrane envelops the nucleus. This membrane helps in effective communication between nucleus and cytoplasm. The elements of endoplasmic reticulum contribute to the nuclear envelop during cell division.

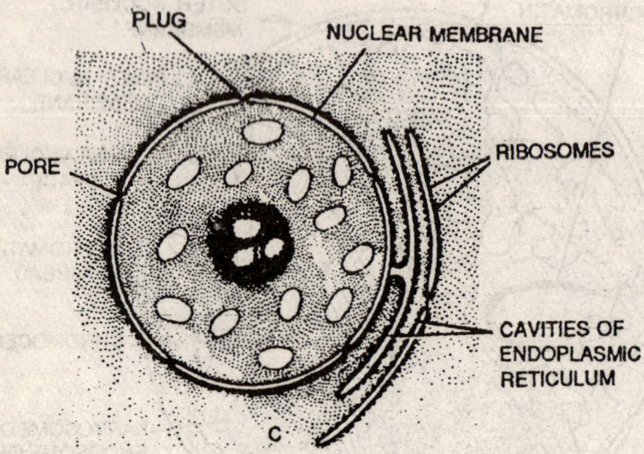

Fig. 2.14 The Cell
Diagrammatic representation of nuclear membrane and pore

Electron microscopic studies have revealed the nuclear membrane to be a double membrane with a number of pores. According to Watson (1959) these pores called *nuclear pores* are octogonal in shape. The outer nuclear membrane is called endokaryotheca. Each membrane is about 75 - 90Å thick and they enclose a space between them about 100 - 150Å (De Robertis et al 1970). This space is called the *perinuclear space* or *cisterna.* The outer membrane is rough due to the presence of RNA particles. Internally the nuclear membrane is followed by a supporting membrane called *fibrous lamina* (300Å thick).

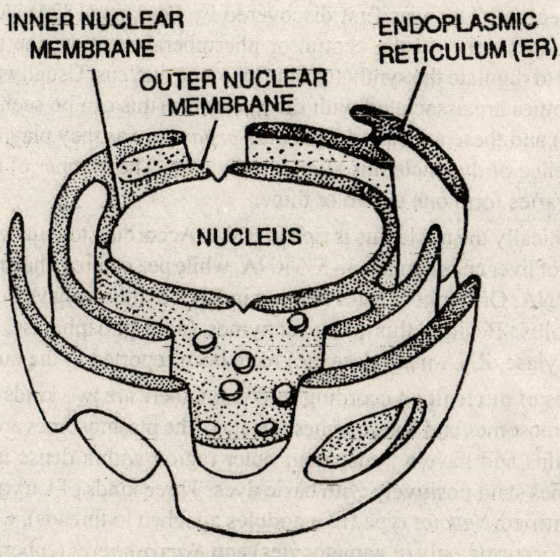

Fig. 2.15 The Cell
Three dimensional view of nuclear membrane complex

The nuclear pores are 600Å wide and are enclosed by rings called *annuli.* These together constitute the pore complex. In some instances, the pore complex is covered by a membrane to regulate the premeability.

Nuclear sap (Karyolymph) : The interphase nucleus consists of a homogenous matrix of fluid substances enclosing a network. Primarily the Karyolymnh is proteinaceous, but also has nucleic acids, enzymes and minerals. It is quite probable that in plants the nuclear sap contributes to the spindles.

Chromonemata : Enclosed in the Karyolymph and visible in the interphase nucleus are found a number of fibrillar structures constituting a network called *chromonemata* or *chromatin fibrils.* These stain positively with basic fuchsin stain. Some coarse granules are deposited on the chromatin network. These are a called *chromocentres* and constitute the points of condensation of chromosomes. During cell division the chromatin network breaks up into specific number of chromosomes. Two regions can be identified in the chromatin material. These are *heterochromatic* region and *euchromatic* region.

The heterochromatic region stains darkly and shows numerous bead like structures called *chromomeres.* The heterochromatic region has less DNA. This region is believed to be genetically and metabolically inert. The light staining region of the chromatin is called the euchromatic region. This region contains more of DNA and is supposed lo be genetically active.

Nucleolus : This was first discovered by Fontana (1874). A spheroidal body, situated either in the central or pheripheral position, the nucleolus is supposed to regulate the synthetic activity of the nucleus. Usually two or more chromosomes are associated with the nucleolus (this can be seen during late prophase) and these are called *nucleolar organisers* as they play a role in the reappearence of the nucleolus after cell division. The number of nucleoli per nucleus varies form one to two or three.

Chemically the nucleolus is rich in RNA. According to Palade (1963), the nucleous of liver cells contain 3 - 5% RNA, while pea embroys have 10 - 20% of nuclear RNA. Orthophosphates helping in RNA synthesis have been reported in nucleolus. Besides this many enzymes (acid phosphatase, nucleoside phosphorylase, RNA methylase etc) have been reported in the nucleolus.

Types of nucleoli : According to Wilson, there are two kinds of nucleous viz., Plasmosomes and Karyosomes (Ocata). The plasmosomes are positive to acidic stains and have a transparent outer region with a dense interior. The karyosomes stain positively with basic dyes. Three kinds of karyosomes have been identified-*Netknot* type (like nodules attached to threads), *Chromosome nucleoli* (occuring only in gametocytes) and *Karyospheres* (spheriodal bodies with basic chromatin).

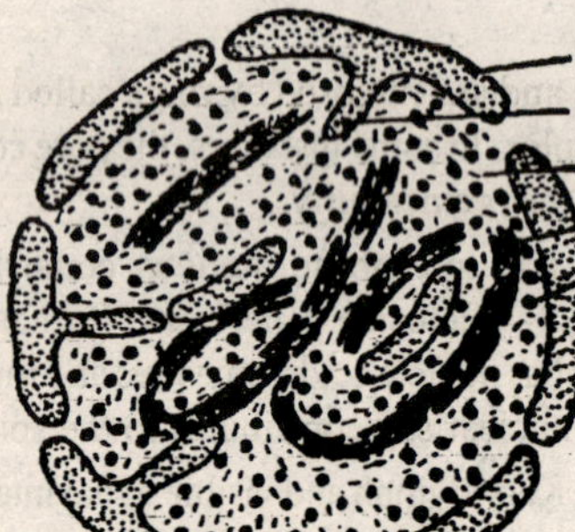

Fig. 2.16 The Cell
Schematic representation of Ultra structure of nucleus

In some instances, plasmosomes and karyosomes combine to form amphinucleoli; these are common in molluscan eggs.

Fine structure of the nucleolus : Detailed analysis of the nucleolus has revealed the presence of three regions. These are granular region, fibrillar region and amorphous region. The granular region occuring at the peripheral region of the nucleolus is composed of granules of 150-250Å thick. This region has ribonucleic acid and proteins. The fibrillar region also known as nucleolonema is composed of fibrils 50-80Å in length. The amorphous region has low electron density and is the one to disappear first at the time of cell division.

There is no limiting membrane to the nucleolus and the organisation is maintained by the calcium ions.

Functions of nucleolus

1. It is the active site of RNA synthesis
2. It is the source of ribosoinal RNA
3. It produces precursors of ribosomes
4. According to Maggio (1990), protein synthesis takes place in the nucleolus. But this may not be totally true.

Endosomes : These are granular structures present in the karyolymph and are smaller in size than the nucleolus.

Chemical composition of Nucleus : The main constituents of nucleus are nucleoprolcins, besides enzymes and inorganic salts. The following gives the total distribution of nucleoproteins in the mammalian liver cells-DNA 9%, RNA 1%, Histones 11%, Residual proteins 14%, and other acidic proteins 65%.

Nucleic Acids : These are the most important constituents of the nucleus playing a vilal role in the inheritance of characters from one generation to-the other. There are two types of nucleic acids-Deoxyribose nucleic acid (DNA) and Ribose nucleic acid (RNA). While both constitute the genetic material in different organisms, it is predominantly the DNA which is the genetic material in most of the organisms. The following are some of the important milestones in the discovery of Nucleic acids.

1. Meischer (1869) isolated nucleic acids and called them nuclein.
2. Hertwig (1884) suggested a heriditary role to the nuclein.
3. Kossel (1884) recognised purines and pyrimidines in the nucleic acids.
4. Feulgen (1912) devised basic fuchsin dye positive only to DNA.
5. Astbury and Bell (1938) showed that the bases in DNA molecule are arranged one above the other.
6. Avery, Macleod and Macarty (1944) presented evidence for DNA to be the genetic material.
7. Chargaff (1950) showed that DNA contains equal amount of puriness and pyrimidines.
8. Wilkins et al (1950) identified the molecular distances between the bases.
9. Furberg (1952) opined that DNA is a coil of single chain.
10. Pauling and Corey (1952) suggested that DNA is a helix of three chains.
11. Waston and Crick (1953) demonstrated the double helix model for DNA molecule.

12. Meselson and Stahl (1958) demonstrated the semi conservative replication of DNA molecule.
13. Jacob and Monad (1961) postulated the presence of RNA in protein

Deoxy Ribose nucleic Acid (DNA) DNA is the main genetic material in almost all organisms except for certain Viruses.

Mitochondria : (Gr. *mito* = thread, *chondiron* = granule)

Popularly called 'power house' of cells, these granular or filamentous organelles are present in all eukaryotes. They are characterised by their special structure, and unique physiological function concerning intracellular energy transformation.

Historically, mitochondria were first observed by Altmann (1894) who called them *bioblasts.* The present name was coined by Benda (1897) who developed the crystal violet staining. Bensely and Hoerr (1934) first isolated the liver cell mitochondria. The discovery that mitochondria are seats of cellular respiration was made by Hogeboom *et al* in 1948.

It is difficult to observe mitochondria in living cells due to their low refractive index, but they can be studied under phase contrast microscope after staining with a dilute solution of janus green. Mitochondria may be isolated from cells by centrifugation between 20,000 g -40.000 g.

Shape : Generally mitochondria are granular or filamentous, even through the shape is variable. During certain conditions a long mitochondrion may swell at one end lo become club shaped or look like a tennis racket (De Robertis et al 1970). Mitochondria may also become vesicular.

Size : Size also is variable. The width is about 0.5μm and the length may reach a maximum of 7μm. The si/e depends on the osmotic pressure.

Distribution : In general, mitochondria are distributed evenly in the cytoplasm, but in some instances they may accumulate around the nucleus or at the periphery of the cytoplasm. During cell division, mitochondria accumulate near the spindles. The distribution of mitochondria within the cell is in relation to the energy demand. For example in skeletal muscles they are grouped like rings or braces around the I-band of the myofibril.

Orientation : Mitochondria have more or less a specific orientation. In cylindrical cells, their long axis is parallel to the long axis of lhe cell. In leucocytes, mitochondria are arranged radially in respect to the centrioles.

Number : Mitochondria are absent in prokaryotic cells. The quantity of mitochondria per cell varies, but in liver cells it is estimated that mitochondria contains 30-35% of the total protein content of the cell. A normal liver cell contains about 1000-1500 mitochondria. Some oocytes coniain an many as 300000 mitochondria.

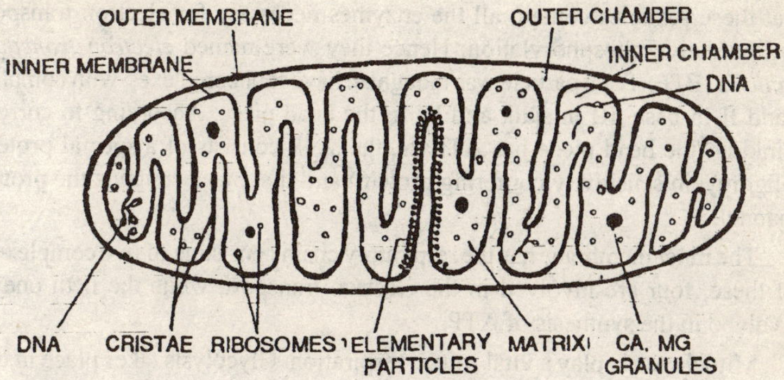

Fig. 2.17 The Cell
Diagrammatic representation of a section through a mitochondrion (ETPs are not shown on all christae)

Structure of mitochondria : The mitochondrion is enveloped by two membranes viz, *inner membrane* and *outer membrane.* The outer membrane is 6nm thick; internal to this is the inner membrane. Separating these two is a space (outer chamber) filled wilh a watery fluid. This space is 40-70Å thick. The inner membrane is folded into finger like projections called *cristae.* This membrane encloses the inner chamber or matrix, usually filled by dense protinaceous material. The matrix may be homogenous or may have a granular substance. The cristae of the inner membrane facing matrix is called the M side, while the other side is called the C side. The cristae have an inner space called the intercristae space which is in continuity with the intermembrane space.

Within the mitochondrial matrix are small ribosomes and a circular DNA. The ribosomes are of 70s type and similar to those of bacteria. These can synthesise proteins (Tyier 1973). The DNA called mDNA may be circular as in most of the animal cells or linear as in plant cells. Rabinowitch (1968) has demonstrated that the mitochondrial DNA has more G-C content than the nuclear DNA.

The mitochondrial DNA can replicate itself as it has DNA ploymerase. It is due to this, that mitochondria can replicate themselves.

The inner membrane ; The inner membrane has numerous nail like or tennis racquet like projections protruding into the matrix. Each particle is about 70-100A^0 in diameter. The particles are placed apart a distance of 100A^0 and each is attached to the inner membrane by a short stalk,of 35-50A^0 long. The number of these particles per mitochondrion ranges from 10^4-10^5. These are called elementary particles, F_1 *particles* or *subunits.* It was formerly believed that these particles contain all the enzymes necessary for electron transport and oxidative phosphorylation. Hence they were named *electron transport panicles* (ETP). Each particle was thought to have four complexes, with complex I and II in base, III in stalk and IV in the head piece. According to current thinking, the head piece has ATPase, the stalk consists of a special protein (oligomycin sensitivity confering protein) and the piece contains the proton channel.

The inner membrane has the respiratory chain consisting of five complexes. Of these, four are involved in the electron transport, while the fifth one is involved in the synthesis of ATP.

Mitochondria play a vital role in respiration. Glycolysis takes place in the *cytosol* (cytoplasm) while the enzymes of the Kerbs cycle are found in the matrix, those of oxidative phosphorylation are found in the inner membrane.

Biogensis of mitochondria : Each mitochondrion lasts for about a week or little more. There are three views regarding the origin of mitochondria-a) origin from cell membranes, b) Division of pre existing mitochondria and c) *de novo* origin.

According to Robertson (1964), mitochondria in muscle cells arise by the infloding of the plasma membrane. This infolding joins another piece and forms a vesicular structure. In the nerve fibres of cray fish, endoplasmic reticulum may form mitochondria.

According io Luck and Rich (1964), mitochondria are capable of self feproduction. DNA, protein synthesis, DNA polymerase and all the other essential, features for self repliciation are present in mitochondria.

Harvey (1951) supports a *de novo origin* for mitochondria. Centrifugal separation of sea-urchin eggs into two halves, a nucleated half (without mitochondria) and a non nucleated half (with mitochondira) showed that the nucleated half produced the mitochondria.

Are mitochondria symbolic organisms? The many similarities between a bacterial cell and mitochondria made many people (Lloyd 1974; Borst 1977, O'Brien 1977 believe that the mitochondrion was once an autonomous entity which later entered into a symbiolic association with an anaerobically respiring host cell. The host cell derived its energy only from glycolysis. Subsequently with the association, the host cell started respiring aerobically. De Robertis (1970) opines that in evolutionary terms it is possible that a symbiotic relationship could have evolved into the present semiautonomus condition of the mitochondria.

The same theory has been Proposed for chloroplasts also, as they also have all (the independent attributes of mitochondria.

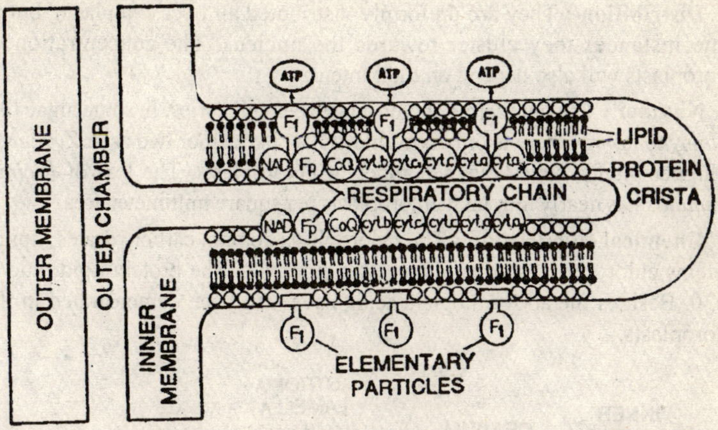

Fig. 2.18 The Cell
Arrangement of complexes (I-IV) in the ETP (old view)

PLASTIDS : These are living cytoplasmic inclusions found in most of the plants except for some bacteria and some fungi.

The plaslids are of three categories viz., chromoplasts, leucoplasts and chloroplasts.

Chromoplasts : These are pigmented plastids. The pigments are non chlorophyllous like, carolenes, xanthophylls, fucoxathin, phycoerythrin etc. In photosynthetic bacteria, the chromoplasts have bacteropchlorophyll.

Leucoplasts : They are colourless plastids. They lack pigments and are usually present in cells which do not receive direct light. Leucoplasts may be seen in the storage leaves of onion. Leucoplasts that store starch are called *amyloplasts,* those that store oil are called elaioplasts and the ones storing proteins are called *aleuroneplasts.*

Chloroplasts : These are by far, the commonest and the most plastids. As the primary sites for trapping and converting solar energy they are very vital for the existence of not only the green plants, but for the whole living world.

Shape : Chloroplasts have varied shapes. The algal chloroplasts exhibit an array of shapes. They may be cup shaped *(Chlamydomonas),* girdle shaped *(Utothrix),* reticulate *(Hydrodictyon),* stellate *(Zygnema),* ribbon shaped *(Spirogyra)* or discoid. They are generally spherical or ovoid in higher plants.

Size : There is a great variety in siz.e. Normally they are about 1μm thick and 4-6μm in length. Chloroplasts ofpolyploid cells are generally larger than in the diploid cells. Cells in the shaded area have longer chloroplasts but with less intensity in colouration.

Distribition : They arc uniformly distributed all over cytoplasm, but in some instances they cluster towards the nucleus. The concentration of chloroplasts will also depend on light intensity.

Number : The number of choloroplasts per cell varies. In some algae like *Chlamydomonas,* there is only one chloroplast per cell or two as in *Zygnema.* In higher plants, cells have a number of chloroplasts. The leaf of *Ricinus communis* has nearly lour lakh chloroplasts per square millimeter area.

Chemical composition : The chloroplasts contain carbohydrates, lipids, proteins chlorophyll, carotenoid and xanthophylls. The protein lipid ratio is 40:30. Besides the above, nucleic acids have also been demonstrated in the chloroplasts.

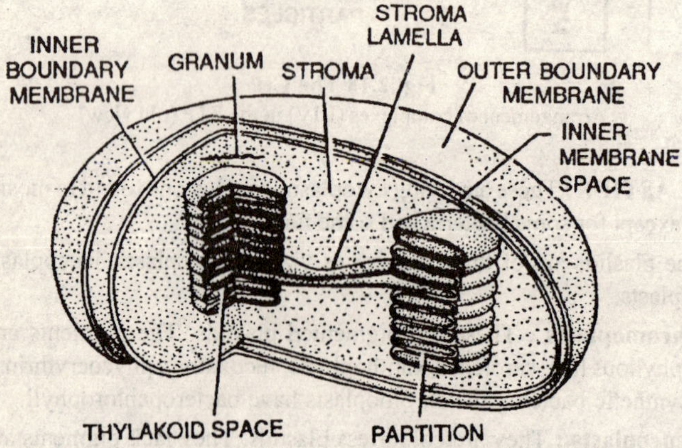

Fig. 2.19 The Cell
Model of Unltrastructure of chloroplasts

Ultra structure of the chloroplasts : The chloroplast has a covering of two membranes with an inner membrane space. These membranes are smooth and there are no perforations or particles. The membranes are differentially permeable (Mudrak).

A section of the chloroplast reveals an intricate system of membranes enclosed in a granular matrix. These membranes are called lamellae and the surrounding matrix-the *stroma.* In a sectional view, the lamellae can be seen packed and these stacks are called *thylakoids.* In the chloroplasts of higher plants, the thylakoids themselves form highly compact bundles called *grana.* Some thylakoids of granum extend into the stroma and maintain contact with other grana. These are *called-Stroma thylakoid* or *stroma lamellae* or *intergrana.*

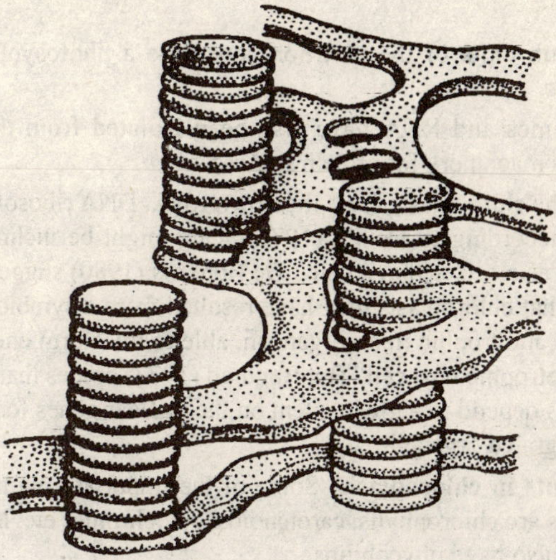

Fig. 2.20 The Cell
Three dimensional view of Grana (enlarged view)

The chloroplasts of algae lack the granum arrangement and in cyanobacteria (blue green algae), the thylakoids lie naked in cytoplasm without any envelope. In such instances, pigments are uniformly distributed on or in the lamellae.

The stroma has in addition to the lamellae - granules (globuli), lipid droplets, starch grains and vesicles.

Structure of the lamellae : All the photosynthetic pigments are concentrated in the chloroplast lamellae. The lamellae as well as the outer membranes are composed of lipoprotein sub units, each sub unit according to Weir and Benson has a protein core surrounded by a lipid sheath. The chloroplast membranes have a single layer of sub units, whereas in thylakoids it is double due to the juxtaposition of the membranes. The appressed areas are called partitions. These are hydrophobic in nature The space between the two membranes of thylakoid (fret membrane) is called *fret channel.* The space between two thylakoids is called *loculus* while the ends of disc shaped thylakoids are called *margins.* These areas (loculus, fret channel) are hydrophilic. The chlorophyll molecules are concentrated in the fret channel ie., in the space between the two membranes of thylakoids. The chlorophyll molecules may be entirely in the space or the *heads* may be in the fret channel while the *tails* are buried in the sub units, occasionally the entire chlorophyll molecule may be found in the fret membrane. Other pigments like cytochromes, carotenoids, etc., are also found in the fret membranes.

Four sub units of the partition constitute a photosynthetic unit or a *quantosome.*

Ribosomes and RNA have also been isolated from the chloroplasts indicating a machinery for protein synthesis.

Since the chloroplasts, have their own RNA, DNA ribosomes and protein synthesis, according to Deviln (1975) "One might be inclined to view the chloroplast as a cell within a cell". De Robertis (1980) suggests "It has been suggested that chloroplasts may have resulted from a symbiotic relationship between an autotrophic microorganism, able to tmasform energy from light, and a heterotrophic host cell" But Bogorad (1977) opines that the chloroplast components depend to a great extent on the nuclear genes for their assembly into an integrated organelle.

Pigments in chloroplast : Some of the important pigments present in chloroplasts are chlorophylls, carotenoids, cytochromes etc. In algal cells the thylakoids also have phycobilins.

Chlorophylls : These are the most important pigments involved in the basic photochemical reaction that sustains life. Atleast nine types of chlorophylls have been identified so far - chlorophylls *a. b. c. d* and *e.* Bacterio Chlorophylls a and b and the chlorobium chlorophylls 650 and 660μm.

Among the chlorophylls, chlorophyll *a* and *b* are best known and most widely distributed. These are absent in pigmented bacteria. Chlorophylls *c, d* and e are found only in algae in combination with chlorophyll a. Bacteriochlorophylls and chlorobium chlorophylls are found only in photosynthetic bacteria.

The chlorophyll molecule is a complex structure basically made up of a 'head' and 'tail' resembling a tennis racquet. The 'head' is a *porphyrin* structure made of four *Pyrrole rings* attached to each other at the centre by an isocyclic ring containing Mg atom at the centre. Extending from one of the pyrrole rings is the 'tail' - the alcoholic chain *(phytol).* The emperical formula for the chlorophyll molecule is CH, O,N Mg. The phytol chain is esterified on the C atom of one of the pyrrole rings and has only one double bond.

Chlorophyll *a* and *b* differ structurally in having different atomic groupings at the C atom in the pyrrole ring. In chlorophyll a C atom has a methyl group, while chlorophyll *b* has an aldehyde group; besides the two pigments have different absorption spectra. The peaks are as follows

Chlorophyll *a* 429, 410 and 660nm

Chlorophyll *b* 430,453 and 442nm

(The above spectra are for chlorophyll in *vitro)*

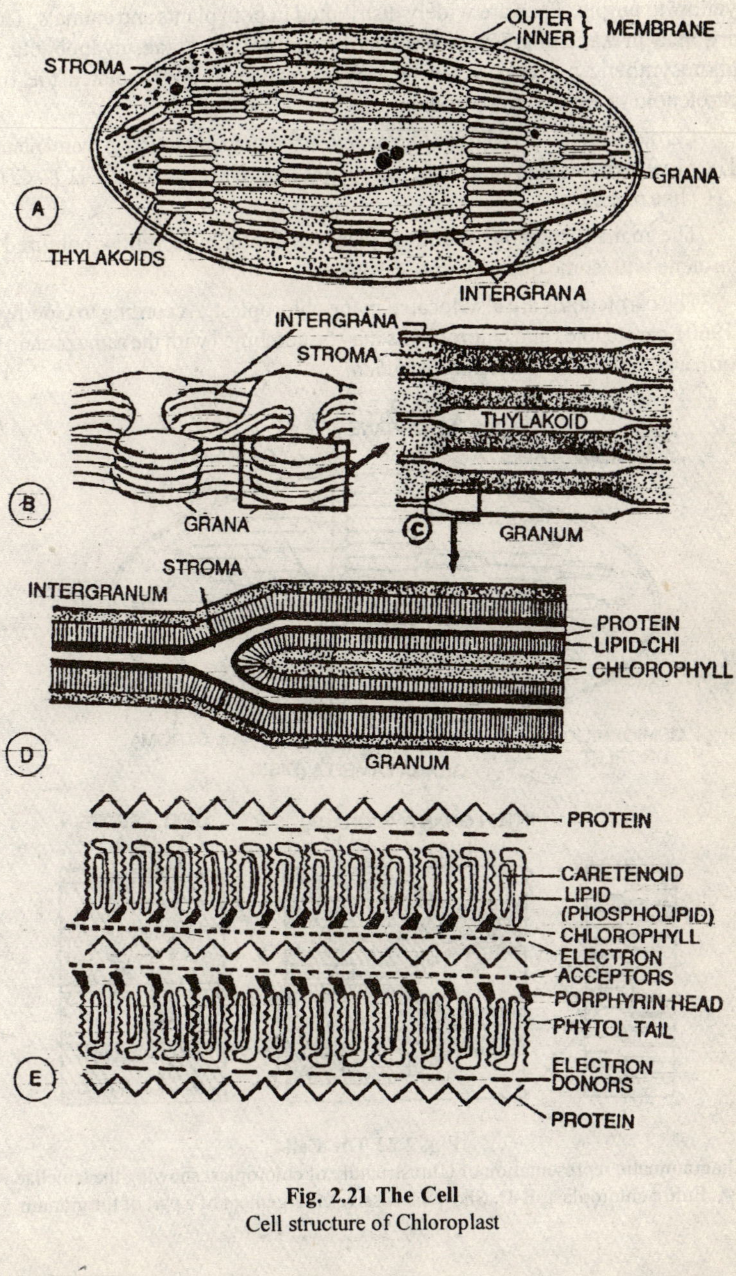

Fig. 2.21 The Cell
Cell structure of Chloroplast

Carotenoid pigments : These are lipid compounds ranging in colour from yellow to purple. They are widely distributed in both plants and animals. They are also present in microorganisms including red algae, cyanobacteria, photosynthetic bacteria, fungi, etc. Wackenroder (1931) isolated the first carotenoid - carotene from tissue.

Carotenoids are derivatives of *lycopene* a red pigment found in many plants. They (carotenoids) are known to have eight isoprene ($CH_2 = C[CH_3] - CH = CH_2$) like residues.

The main carotenoid found in plants is the orange yellow coloured β carotene with some quantity of α carotene.

The carotenoids are also located in the chloroplast. According to Goodwin (1960), carotenoids and chlorophylls may be combined with the same protein to form a complex known as *photosynthein.*

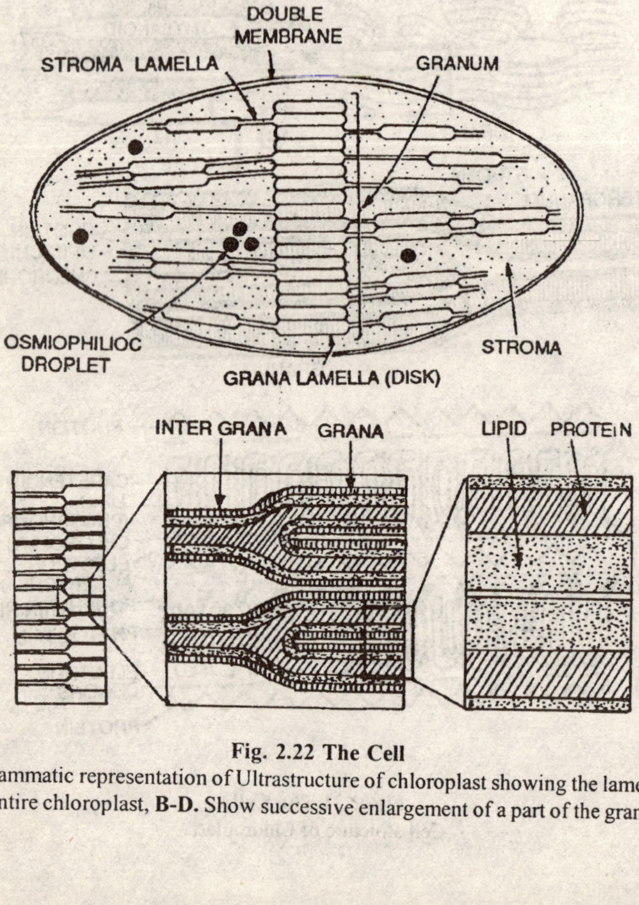

Fig. 2.22 The Cell
Diagrammatic representation of Ultrastructure of chloroplast showing the lamellae. **A.** Entire chloroplast, **B-D.** Show successive enlargement of a part of the granum

Carotenoids protect the chorophyll form photooxidation and transfer the light energy they absorb to chlorophyll *a*.

Phycobilins: These are found only in algae. There are two types of pycobilins - the *Phycoreythrin* (red) and *Phycocyanin* (blue) These pigments are strongly associated with a protein and consequently it is difficult to isolate the pigments in the pure state.

Like carotenoids phycobilins are also involved in the transfer of light energy (they absorb) to the chlorophyll.

The absorption spectra of phycobilins presents an intersting study considering the fact that they act as accessory pigments in photosynthesis. R - phycoerythrin has peaks at 495, 540 and 545nm, while R - phycocyanin has peaks at 550 and 615nm.

ENDOPLASMIC RETICULUM : The cytoplasm in the cells of most of the plants and animals is traversed by a network of anastamosing fibrillar structures called endoplasmic reticulum (ER). Originally known as ergastoplasm, the current name ER was given by Porter and Kaallman (1952). The ER is connected to the outer nuclear membrane with the ER space opening into the perinuclear space between two membranes. The ER is known to be connected with the plasma membrane.

Morphologically the ER consists of three types of structures viz., *Cistemae, Vesicles* and *Tublllues*.

The **Cisternae** *are* elongated cyllindrical unbranched structures arranged parallel to one another respresenting a lamellated structure. They are 40 - 50μm in diameter. Cisternae are generally found in cells active in synthesis.

The **Vesicles** or sacs or oval bodies, attached to the membrane and have a diameter of 25-500μm. These are abundant in pancreatic cells.

The **Tubulues** are branched irregularly and are of diverse shapes having a size of 50 - 100μm. The tubules are abundant in cells which are active in the synthesis of steroid compounds. They are also found in the epithelical cells of retina.

Ultra structure : All the three components of ER are bounded by a unit membrane 50 - 60Å thick. The membrane is trilamenar like the other unit membranes. Palade (1956) has observed some secretory granules in the cavity of endoplasmic reticulum. The membrane has two outer layers of protein enclosing two layers ofphospholipids. However the ER membrane is symmetrical unlike in other organelles (mitochondria).

Types of ER : Two types of ER have been observed in the cells (same or different). These are - smooth ER (agranular) and rough ER (granullar).

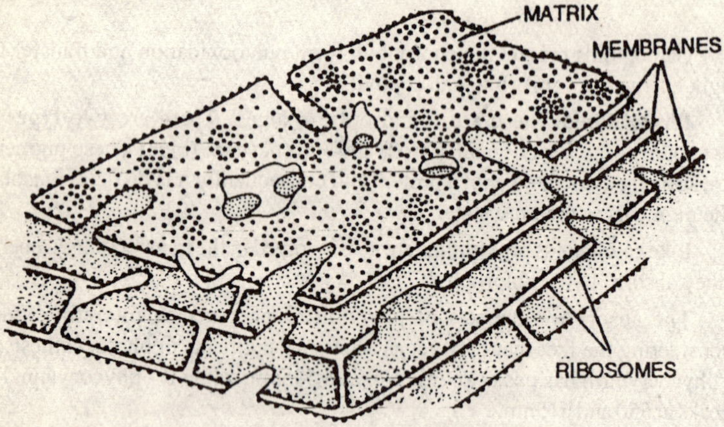

Fig. 2.23 The Cell
Three dimentional view of endoplasmic reticulum

The membrane of smooth ER are not granular due to the absence of ribosomes. Smooth ER in mainly seen in tubules. The tubules measure about 500 - 1000Å in length. Agranular ER is seen in cells involved in lipid or steroid synthesis. Cells active in protein synthesis do not have agranular ER. Agranular reticulum of muscle cells is called *sarcoplasmic reticulum* and it forms lace like sleeve around myofibrils. In the pigmented cells of retina, the agranular ER occurs in the form of tightly packed tubules and vesicles called *myeloid bodies.*

The rough ER has a granular surface due to the presence of a large number of ribosomes attached to it. Since ribosomes are actively involved in protein synthesis rough ER is conspicuous in cells that are actively involved in protein synthesis e.g. meristematic cells, plasma cells, goblet cells etc. The rough ER stains positively by basic dyes.

The cells (Spermatocytes) of certain vertebrates show an unnsual type of ER. Usually ER membrane does not have pores or openings. But in the instance mentioned above pores or annuli have been reported resembling the ones found in the nuclear membrane. There is a diaphragm across the octogonal symmetry (Manul 1968).

The ER performs many vital cellular functions. These are

(a) Enzymatic activities
(b) Transport of synthetic products
(c) Storage of metabolities
(d) Formation of nuclear envelope
(e) Intracellular impulse conduction etc.

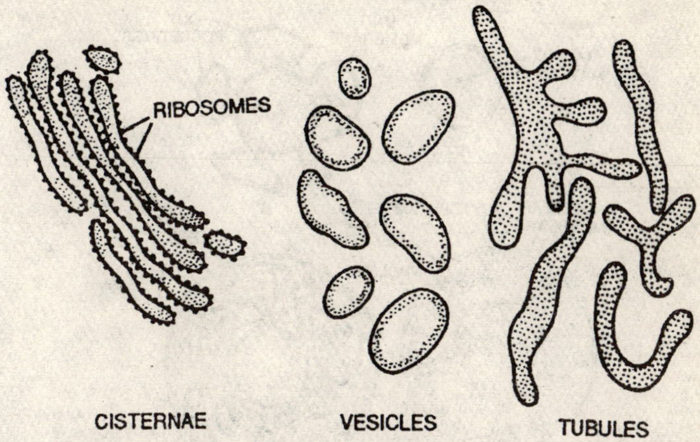

Fig. 2.24 The Cell
Various components of endoplasmic reticulum

Microsomes : These are structures that result due to the homogenization of the membranes. The cell membranes break up into fragments, round off and form microsomes. Microsomes are actually fragments of ER. They can be isolated by high speed centrifugation (100,000g) when they settle after nuclear and ribosomal fractions. Observed under electron microcope they appear as membrane bound vesicles of 500- 1500 Å in diameter. It should be understood however that microsomes are not natural structures found in the intact cell. They are the result of homogenization of cell. The microsome fraction contains fragmented membranes.

Origin of ER : The origin is uncertain, invagination of the plasma membrane might give rise to a canalicular system. But evidences for this hypothesis are yet to come (Dallmes et al,1966).

RIBOSOMES : These are dense granular nuclecoprotein structures occuring in cytoplasm, matrix of mitochondria and chloroplasts. In many instances ribosomes are attached to the ER. Observed first in plant cells in 1953 by Robinson and Brown while studying bean roots, these were later discovered in animal cells also. Ranging in diameter from 150 - 200Å they have RNA and protein in equal quantities.

Ribosomes are isolated by differential centrifugation depending on sedimentation coefficient. The sedimentation coefficient is expressed in terms of *svedberg units*. The S units are related with the size and weight of the ribosome molecules.

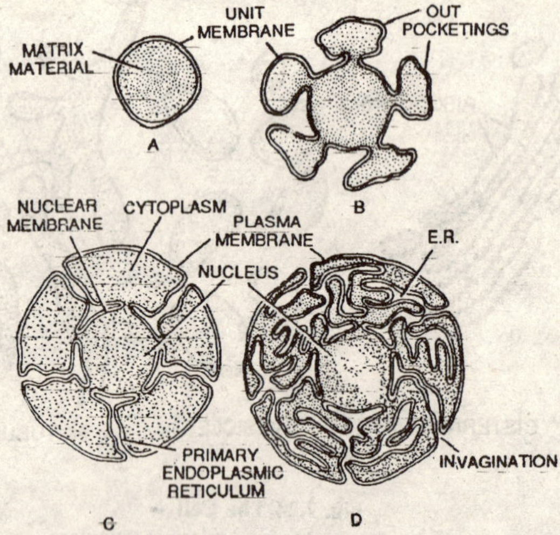

Fig. 2.25 The Cell
Stages in the origin of Endoplasmic reticulum

Types of ribosomes : Two types of ribosomes have been identified based on the sedimentation coefficient which shows how soon a cell organelle can sediment under centrifugation. If the organelle is heavier, its sedimentation coefficient is more. The two types of ribosomes are - *70s ribosomes* and *80s ribosomes*.

The 70s ribosomes are comparatively smaller and have a molecular weight of 2.7 x 10^6 daltons (Dalton is a unit of molecular weight; one dalton = weight of one H atom = 1) According to Huxley and Zubay (1960) the size of a 70s particle is 170 x 170 x 200Å. These ribosomes occur in prokaryotic cells as well as in chloroplasts of eukaryotic cells. The 70s ribosomes have two sub units - a large 50s sub unit and a small 30s sub unit.

The 80s ribosomes have a moleculer weight of 4 x 10^6 daltons, and are predominantly found in eukaryotic cells. There are two sub units in an 80s ribosome. These are - 60 and 40s.

Ribosomes may occur singly as isolated units when they are called *monosomes*. When they occur in clusters or groups, they are called *polyribosomes*. *Tbe* polyribosomes may have a sedimentation coefficient of 100s - 600s.

The number of ribosomes per cell varies, it may be 10,000 (bacterial cell) or up to 10 million (eukaryotic cell).

Ribosomes of chloroplasts and mitochondria have their own protein synthesis. They have a sedimentation coefficient of 55s with two sub units 40s and 30s.

Ultra structure of ribosomes : Ribosomes are oblate or spheroidal structures having two sub units (a large and a small). The large sub unit is dome like and the smaller subunit is placed above like a cap. The 70s ribosome has two units 50s and 30s as already mentioned. The 50s sub unit has a diameter of 140 - 160A^{0}and is pentagonal in shape. In the center of this sub unit occurs a round area of 40 - 60A^0. According to Fernando (1968), there is a pore like transparent area in the centre which prohibits the entry of proteolytic enzymes.

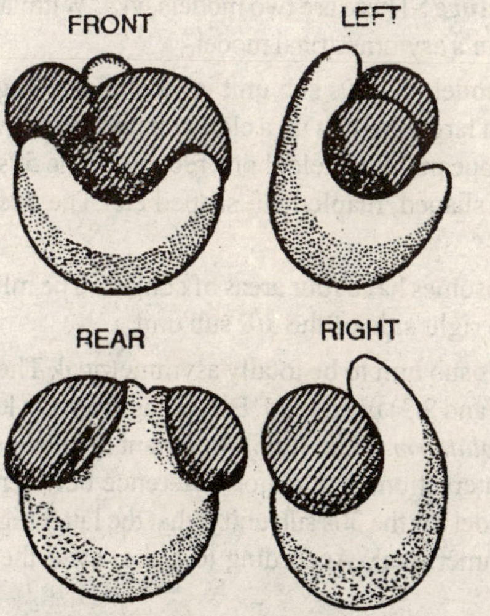

Fig. 2.26 The Cell
Ribosome - different views

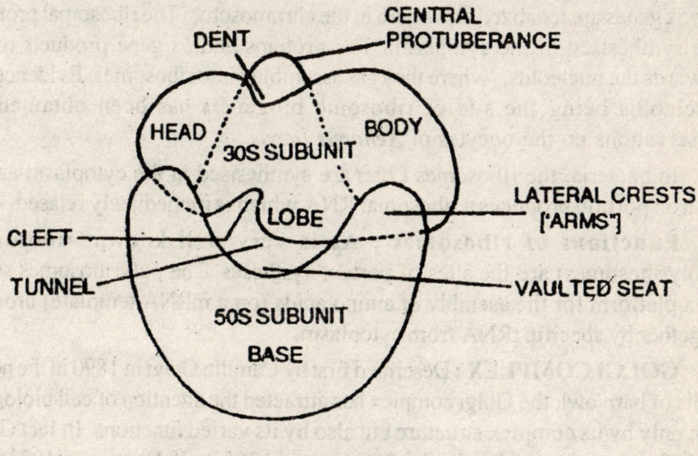

Fig. 2.27 The Cell
Witlmann's model of prokaryotic ribosome

The pores have been found in 50s sub units of 80s ribosomes also. The smaller sub units of both the types of ribosomes are often divided into two portions which remain connected to each other by a strand of 30 - 69A^0 Thickness.

Models for ribosomes structure : There are two models, viz., Wittmann's quasi symmetrical model and Lake's asymmertrical model.

According to Wittmann's model, the 30s sub unit is an elongate slightly bent stucture, having a head and a larger body with a cleft in between; with two parts protruding uniequally. It appears like a telephone receiver. The 50s sub unit is variously shaped - round shaped, maple leaf .shaped etc. The 50s sub unit has three protruberances.

The two sub units of 70s ribosomes have four areas of contact. The mRNA binding. region is located on the right side of the *30s* sub unit.

Lake's model regards the 30s sub unit to be totally asymmetrical. The sub unit is divided into two parts (1/3 and 2/3) unequally. Extending from the lower 2/3 region is a portion called the *platform*. This cleft is important in the sense of location of codon - anticodon interaction. The major difference between the Wittmanns model and Lake's model for the 30s sub unit is that the latter regards the 30s sub unit as totally asymmertrical. According to Lake, even the 50s subunit is asymmetrical.,

Biogensis of ribosomes : The synthesis of eukaryotic ribosome is a complicated process involving several areas of the cell. The genes coding for 18s, 28s and 58s RNA are in the nucleolar organizing part of the chromosomes; the 5s genes are localized eleswhere in the chromosome. The ribosomal proteins are synthesised in the cytoplasm. The proteins and 5s gene products move towards the nucleolus, where they are assembled into ribosomes. Evidence for nucleolus being the site of ribosome biogeneis has been obtained by observations on the oocytes of *Xenopus laevis*.

In bacteria, the ribosomes (70s) are synthesised in the cytoplasm as the cistron portion produces a ribosomal RNA which is immediately relased.

Functions of ribosomes : As is very well known, ribosomes (polyribosomes) are the sites of portein systheses. The polyribosomes serve as a platform for the asembly *of* amino acids (on a mRNA template) brought together by specific tRNA from cytoplasm.

GOLGI COMPLEX : Described first by Camillo Golgi in 1890 in the nerve cells of barn owl, the Golgi complex has attracted the attention of cell biologists not only by its complex structure but also by its varied functions. In fact Golgi complex was observed earlier by St George in 1865 itself. Nassonov (1923) and Bowen (1929) established the secretory function in the Golgi apparatus.

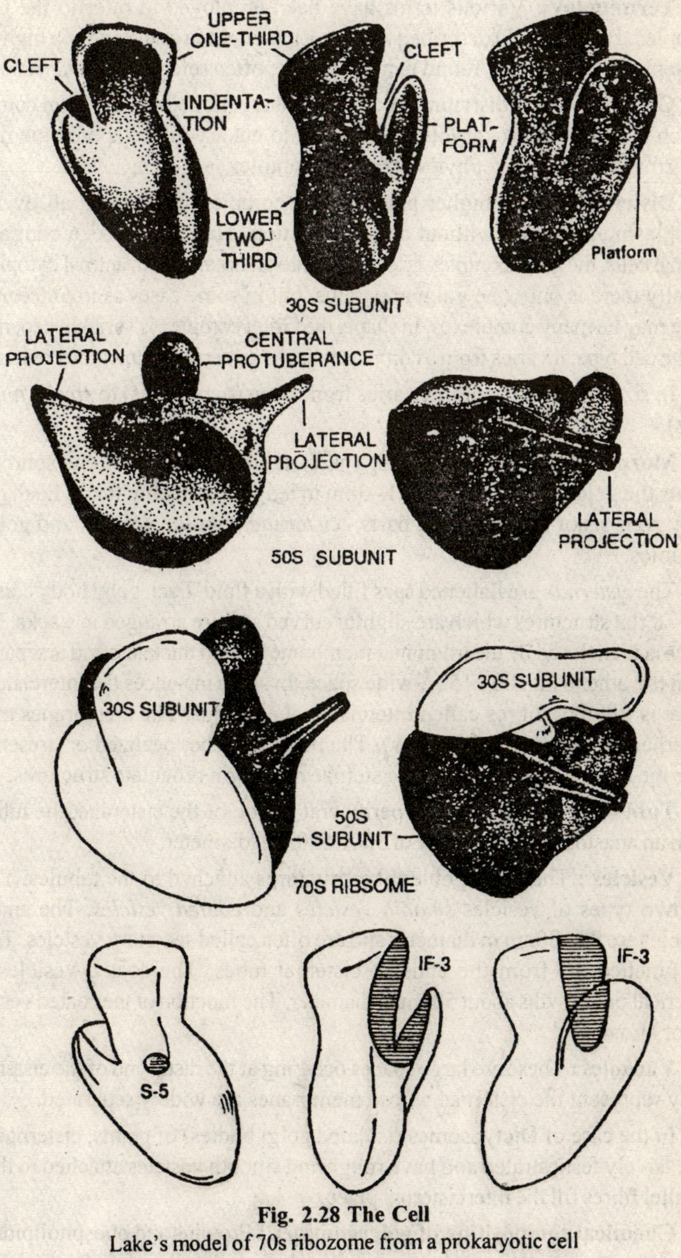

Fig. 2.28 The Cell
Lake's model of 70s ribozome from a prokaryotic cell

Terminoloy : Various terms have been employed to refer to the Golgi complex. Baker (1953) described them as Lipochondria as they have a high lipid content. Golgi complex found in plant cell are often refered to as *Dictyosomes.*

Occurrence and distribution : All the eukaryotic cells have a golgi complex which is absent in prokaryotic cells. Even in eukaryotic cells of some fungi, spenrmatozoids of bryophytes etc. golgi complex is absent.

Distribution : In higher plants, golgi complex is scattered all over the cytoplasm apparently without any localization (Hall 1974). As a contrast in animal cells, the golgi complex is localized into an organelle. In animal cytoplasm, usually there is only one golgi apparatus, but in some cases as in *Storeomyxa* there may be many complexes. In shape, the Golgi complex is variable depending on the cell type; it varies from a compact mass to dispersed filamentous reticulum.

In size, the golgi complex varies from large (nerve cells) to small (muscle cells).

Morphology : The morphology is variable depending on the source. In plants the golgi bodies are about I - 3nm in length and 0.5nm thick. Each golgi body consists of the following parts - *cisternae, tubules, vesicles* and golĝian vacuoles.

The *cisternae* are flattened sacs filled with a fluid. Each golgi body consists of 4 - 8 flat structures which are slightly curved and are arranged in stacks. Each cisterna is enclosed by the trilaminar membrane 6nm in thickness and is separated from the other by a 100 - 150Å wide space. In some instances the intercisternal space is filled by fibres called intercistemal elements. The membranes of the cisternae are *fenestrated* (porous). The pores may be localized or present all over the cistemae. Occasionally cisternae may form reticulate structures.

Tubules: Arising from the peripheral region of the cisterane, the tubules form an anastomosing network of 300 - 500Å in diameter.

Vesicles : These are goblet like structures attached to the tubules. There are two types of vesicles *smooth vesicles* and *coated vesicles.* The smooth vesicles are 20 - 80nm in diameter and are often called secretory vesicles. These are pinched off from the ends of cistetnal tubes. The coated vesicles are spherical outgrowths about 50nm in diameter. The function of the coated vesicles is not known.

Vacuoles : These are large spaces occuring at the distal end of the cisternae. They represent the cisternae whose membranes are widely separated.

In the case of Dictyosomes (isolated golgi bodies) of plants, cisternae are extensively fesnestrated and have rough and smooth vesicles attached to them. Parallel fibres fill the intercisternal place.

Chemical composition of golgi complex : Proteins and phospholipids are in equal concentration. Golgi material in the nerve cells consists of cephalin and lecithin. Giroud has reported Vitamin C in the golgi complex.

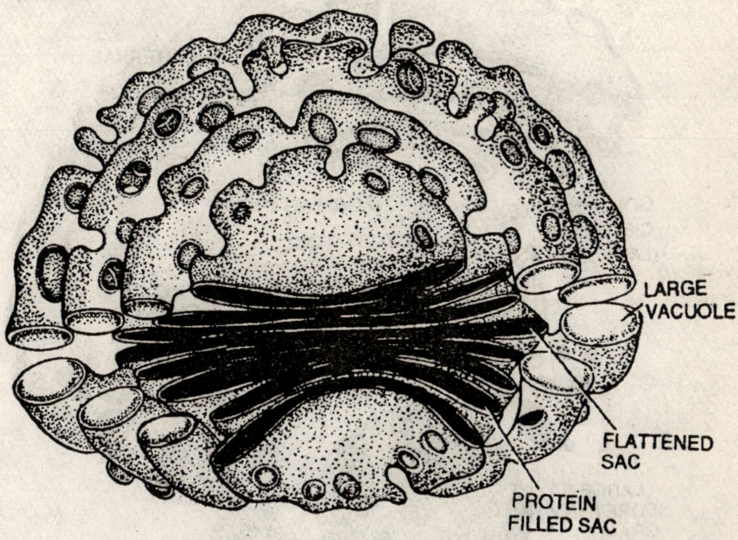

Fig. 2.29 The Cell
Golgi Complex

Functions of the golgi complex : The following are some of the functions attributed to the golgi complex -

1. Absorption of compounds
2. Sites of enzyme production
3. Sites of hormonal production
4. Sites of protein storage
5. Forms acrosome during sperm maturation
6. Forms intracellular crystals
7. Formation of plant cell wall - the golgi bodies synthesise pectin, hemiceullulose and cellulose microfibrils. They also help in the formation of cell plate during mitosis.

Origin of golgi complex : Evidences indicate that the golgi bodies are produced from the membranes of the smooth ER. Earlier it was thought that they arise *de novo* or from the phragmoplasts of the cell wall. Both these theories are found to be incorrect.

Lysosomes : (*Gr.Lyso* = digestive, *soma* = body). First discovered in 1949 as dense round bodies, the lysosomes were called *pericanalicular bodies.* It was de Duve, (1955) who gave the present name.

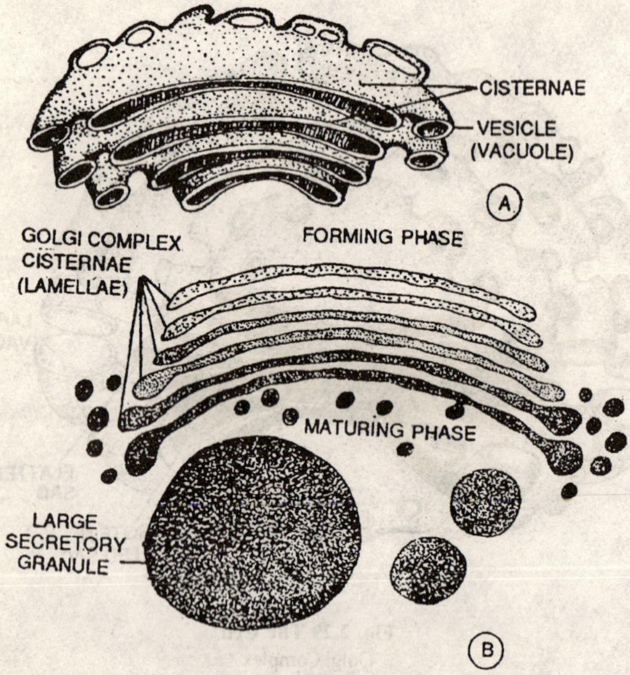

Fig. 2.30 The Cell
Golgi Complex (another view) **A.** Steroscopic view, **B.** Section view

Occurence : Lysosomes are found in most of the animal cells and few plant cells. The hepatic cells, pancreatic cells, kidney cells etc. posses large number of lysosomes. According to Matile (1969) the lysosomes in plant cell are membrane bound. Generally lysosomes are absent in the prokaryotic cells. Slime molds also have lysosomes.

Lysosomes are pleomorphic as seen in the meristematic cells of the root. The diameter may be 0.4 to 0.8μ; but in some mammalian kidney cells lysosomes as long as 5μ have been found.

Ultra structure : Lysosomes are saccate structures filled with digestive enzymes. Each lysosome has two parts, viz., *limiting membrane* and *inner dense mass.*

The **limiting membrane** is not double membraned like in other organelles. It is single and composed of lipoproteins. The membrane however is bilayered like any unit membrane.

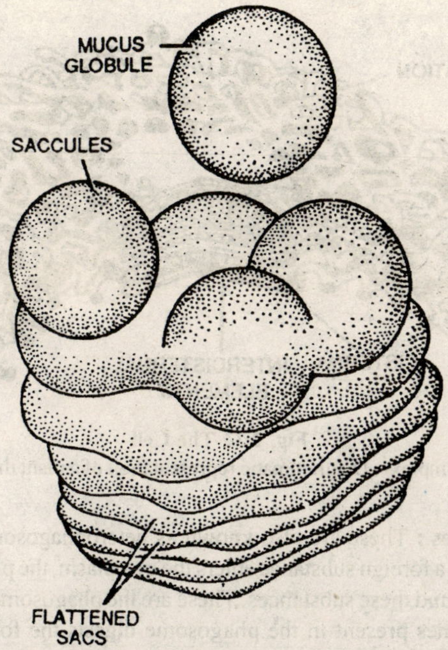

Fig. 2.31 The Cell
Golgi Complex with mucucus globules

The **inner dense mass** is the core of lysosomes; it is mostly enzymatic. The membrane is impermeable to substrates the enzymes of which are present in the lysosomes. Occassionally certain substances called *labilizers* destabilize the membrane causing the enzymes to come out. Alternatively, there are substance called *stabilizers* which stabilize the membrane. The limited permeability of the membrane prevents excessive digestion of cellular components by the lytic enzymes of lysosomes. The enzymes present in the lysosomes are - Nucleases, Phosphatases, Lipases, Glycosidases, and Sulphatases.

Polymorphism : Lysosomes are ploymorphic assuming various shapes depending on the cell type and situation. Basically there are two types of lysosomes viz. *Primary lysosomes and secondary lysosomes.* The secondary lysosomes are of three categories - *Phagosomes, residual bodies* and *autophagic vaculoes.*

Primary lysosomes : There are sac like structures produced directly from ER from the Glogi bodies.

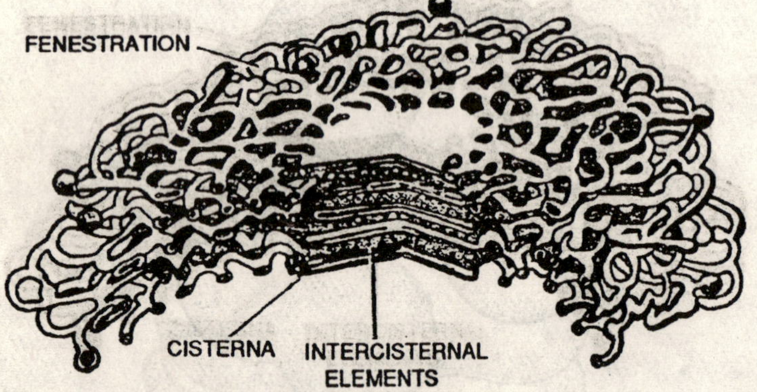

Fig. 2.32 The Cell
Golgi Complex – Diagrammatic representation of a plant dictyosome

Phagosomes : These are also known as heterophagosomes or digestive vaculoes. When a foreign substance enters the cytoplasm, the plasma membrane forms a sac around these substances. These are the phagosomes or pinosomes. The lytic enzymes present in the phagosome digests the foreign substance. The phenomenon is called *Phagocytosis* or *pinocytosis.*

Residual bodies : After the digested material has passed out of the lysosomes, the undigested material remains within the lysososmes. Such lysosomes with residual substrate are called residual bodies. Residual bodies may remain within the cell or very often they are pushed out of the cell by exocytosis.

Autophagic vaculoe : Occasionally, a lysosome may digest a part of the cell (ER, mitochondria, etc.). This is a mechanism to digest a part of the cell without destroying the entire cell. Liver cells show autophagic vacuoles or autophagosomes under starvation.

Origin of lysosomes

(a) *Extra cellular origin* : Vacuoles absorbed due to'pinocytosis or phagocytosis may become secondary lysosomes after fusing with primary lysosomes.

(b) *Origin from golgi bodies* : There are enough evidences to show that lysosomes are produced from golgi bodies at the height of their secretory activity.

(c) *Origin from ER* : According to Novikoff (1965), the rough ER gives rise to the lysosomes.

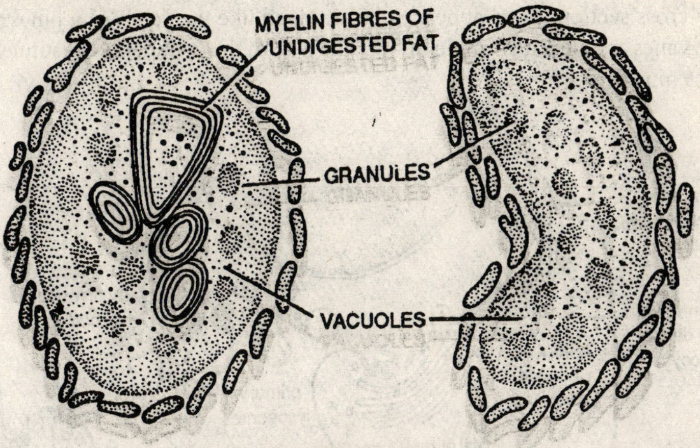

Fig. 2.33 The Cell
Lysosome – Structure

Major functions of lysosomes : The main function of the lysosomes is digestion of intracellular substances. According to Hirsch and Coh (1964), lysosomes help in destroying the dead cells from the tiusse. Recently it has been found out that in some animals (frog), lysosomes play an important role in metamorphosis. Lysosomes also perhaps help in the formation and destruction of bone cells.

CENTROSOMES : The centromes are found in the centre of the cell near the nucleus. These are present in all animal cells and lower plants like Dinoflagellates, *Euglena* and *Chlamydomonas,* etc. Van Benden (1887) disocvered centrosomes.

The centrosomes play an important role in organising the mitotic apparatus in flagellated animals, while in flagellated plants they function as basal granules of flagella.

Size : In mature centrosomes the diameter is 1600Å - 2500Å while the length is about 160A^0. Giant centrioles have been found in spermatocytes or oocytes of certain organisms.

The centrosome has two parts, viz., *centrioles* and *centrosphere*

Centrioles : These range in number from one to two and are made up of RNA. Electron microsocopic observation has revealed the centrioles to be paired cylindrical structures 3000 - 5000Å long and 1200 - 1500Å in diameter. These are open at one or both ends and placed at right angles to each other. Each cylinder is composed *of* nine fibres spaced equally and running parallel to the cylinder axis. Each fibre is in turn made up of three *microtubules (triplet).*

In a cross section, these appear to be arranged like the vanes of a pin wheel. The vanes are tiled at an angle of 40⁰. The wall of the cylinder is constituted by these nine triplet fibres.

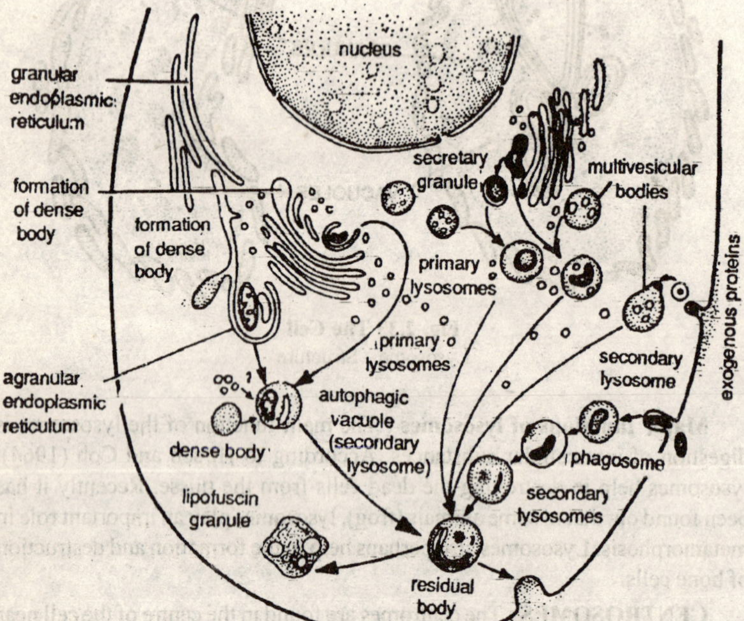

Fig. 2.34 The Cell
Polymorphism in Lysosomes

The microtubule triplet in a fibre can be designated as A,B and C of which A is innermost. Each microtubule wall is 50A⁰ in diameter and the lumen in 120 - 130A⁰ (the total diametre varies from 180 - 200A⁰). The length of each microtubule is about 560A⁰. At the innerside of each triplet fibre a dense line runs and it is called *triplet base* connecting A and C tubules. In addition to this, a dense RNA region called *foot* is present.

Centrosphere : The dense granlar region of cytoplasm surrounding the centrioles is called the centrosphere.

Structure : Structurally the microtubules are lipoproteinaceous (Fulton 1971).

Origin: They have a multiple origin.

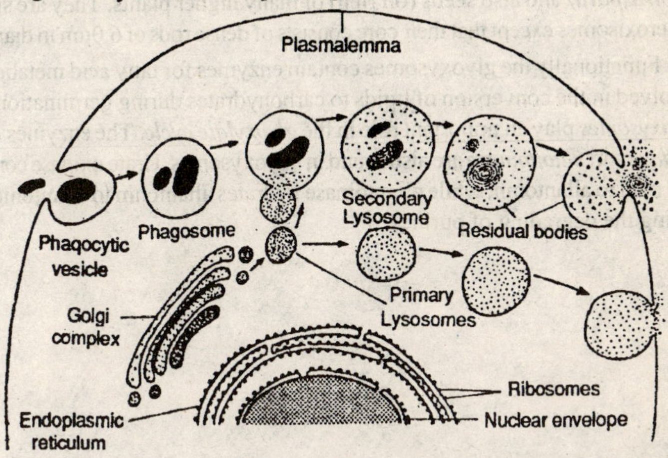

Fig. 2.35 The Cell
Origin and phases of Lysosomes

Functions : Centrosomes appear to play an important part in cell division. people believe that centrioles play an important part in the formation of spindle. They however constitute the mitotic pole in higher animals. In primitive animals which are ciliated, centrioles seem to help in the generation of cilia.

Microbodies : The cells of plants, fungi, certain protozoa and liver cells of vertebrates contain certain small granular structures associated with ER, mitochondria and chloroplasts. These spherical bodies ranging in size from 0.2μ to 1.5μ have a central crystalline core and are called *microbodies*.

Recent studies have revealed the presence of two types of microbodies viz., **Peroxisomes** and **Glyoxysomes**.

Peroxisomes are found in animal cells and also in the leaves of higher plants. These particles participate in the oxidation of substrates resulting in the formation of hydrogen peroxide. In plants, peroxisomes are involved in photorespiration.

Structurally peroxisomes are variable in shape and size but are generally circular. They have an envelope of a single membrane made up of proteins and lipids enclosing a granular matrix. In certain instances, the matrix is crystalline or amorphous. The peroxisomes catalyze the H_2O_2 production. In plants, the peroxisomes contain enzymes of glycolate pathway.

Glyoxosomes are found in the cells of yeast and certain other fungi *(Neurospora)* and also seeds (oil rich) of many higher plants. They are similar to peroxisomes except that their core consists of dense rods of 6.0μm in diameter.

Functionally the glyoxysomes contain enzymes for fatty acid metabolism, involved in the conversion of lipids to carbohydrates during germination. The *glyoxysomes* play an important role in lhe *glyoxylate cycle.* The enzymes *Urate oxidase* and *allantoinase* are also found in glyoxysomes. Urate oxidase converts uric acid to allantonin, while allantoinase hydrates allantonin to allantonic acid during the degrading of purines.

3

MICROSCOPY

The study of cell biology involves the use of a number instruments. The rapid strides made by cell biology would not have been possible but for the pivotal role played by these instruments in unraveling the mysterious world of microcosm. For instance, if there were to be no microscope the whole of the microbial world would be non available to us and we would not be in a position to explain the various diseases that confront us; for we would not know what microbes are. In this chapter we will try to understand the various instruments and their working mechanism. Microbiological instruments may be basically categorized into two - those that are used for visual observation and those that are used for analytical purposes. Visual observation of microbes is made possible by the use of microscopes while a wide array of instruments such as spectrophotometers, centrifuges, nephelometers, autoclaves inoculation chambers etc., are used for various analytical purposes.

In this chapter we shall study the various optical instruments (microscopes) used in cell biological study.

Microscopy

The most important tool of a biologist is the microscope. The invention of light microscope in the sixteenth century is perhaps the single most important contribution ever made to the advancement of biology.

The present day microscope used in biological laboratories has been developed over the course of several centuries. Ancient Romans, Greeks and Indians had known lenses of glass and quartz. In the 14th century itself spectacles and single lenses were used as magnifiers. Zacharias Jensen, a Dutch astronomer added one more lens and constructed a true telescope. Campini, an Italian scientist found out that lens can be ground to the desired curvature. Since the curvature of the lens increases its magnifying power, microscope thereafter became a very powerful tool in the hands of biologists.

Antony Van Leeuwenhoek (1632 - 1723), some times wrongly credited with the invention of the microscope, used his single lens microscope to observe several minute objects like insects, mold, pond water, saliva etc. It was Robert Hooke (1665) an Englishman who developed an instrument that could truly be referred to as the forerunner of the modern day microscope.

The microscope opened up to biologists (hitherto unknown to them) an exciting microcosm - the universe of microorganisms. Bacteria, cells, detailed structure of tissues, all became visible under the microscope. New fields of biology like cytology, embryology owe their existence to the single most powerful tool of biology - the microscope.

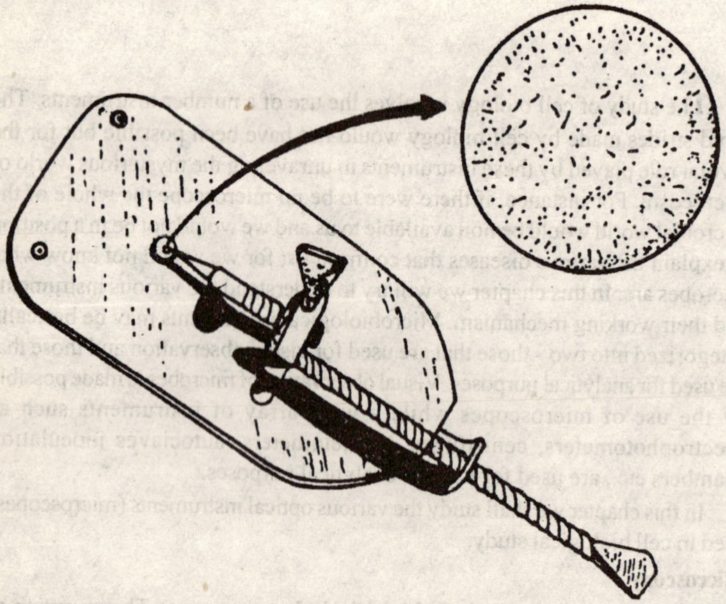

Fig. 3.1 Microscopy
Van Leeuwenhoek's Microscope. A simple lens of high magnification, this was the forerunner of the modern microscope

The working of a microscope

The main function of the microscope is to produce a large and clear image of the object. Clarity is very often referred to as the resolving power of the microscope.

In order to understand the functioning of the microscope, it will be necessary to understand as to how our own eye resolves and produces an image of the object.

The lens of the eye focuses the light reflected by an object and projects an image on the retina. The retina is a granular matrix consisting of light sensitive cells called rods and cones. These cells convert the light impulses falling on them into nerve impulses producing a sensation of vision in the brain. The *rods* and *cones* are placed five microns apart, hence the eye cannot resolve details of an object, less than five microns in size. When an object is brought closer to the eye it grows larger, but when it is brought too close, the lens of the eye cannot focus the image and the object appears blurred.

The shortest viewing distance of human eye is about 25 cms. At this distance, the limit of resolution is about 0.2 mm. Objects lying together closer than 0.2 mm will not be seen separately by the human eye.

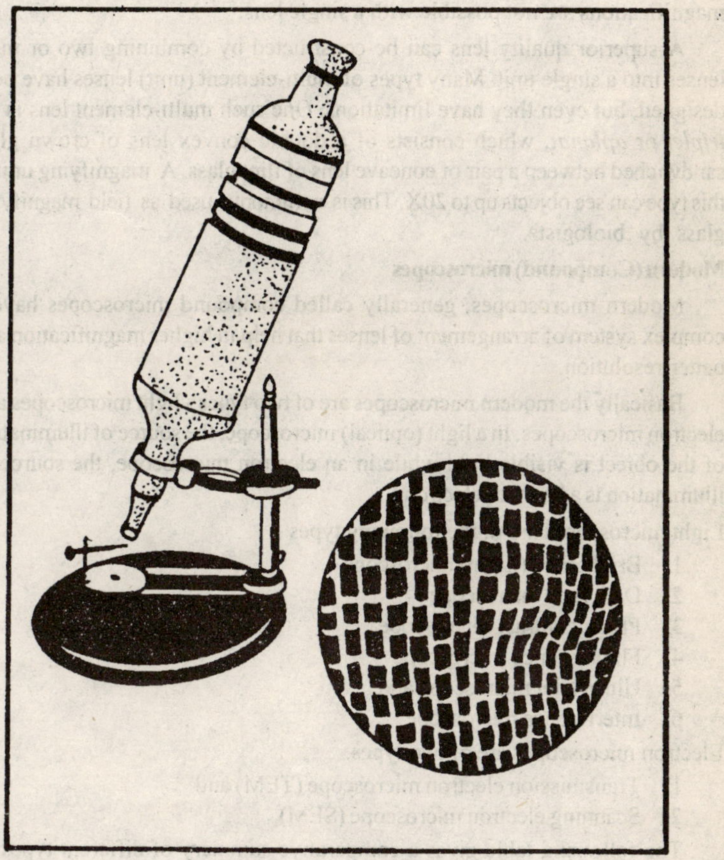

Fig. 3.2 Microscopy
Hooke's Microscope and cork cells

Simple Microscope

The simple microscope is nothing but a single convex lens or a combination of more than one lenses functioning like a single lens. This type of lens when placed between an object and the eye allows the object to come closer, thus forming an enlarged image on the retina. Since the image is larger, the eye is able to resolve finer details that could not be distinguished without the lens.

The magnification obtained with a simple lens can be calculated as follows.

$M = 250/f \quad + \quad 1$

Where f is the focal length of the lens in mm, and 250 is the distance of normal vision also in mm.

A single convex lens can be used for magnification upto 3X. Higher magnifications are not possible with a single lens.

A superior quality lens can be constructed by combining two or more lenses into a single unit. Many types of multi-element (unit) lenses have been designed, but even they have limitations. One such multi-element lens is the *triplet* or *aplanat*, which consists of a double convex lens of crown glass sandwiched between a pair of concave lens of flint glass. A magnifying unit of this type can see objects up to 20X. This is commonly used as field magnifying glass by biologists.

Modern (Compound) microscopes

Modern microscopes, generally called compound microscopes have a complex system of arrangement of lenses that help in higher magnification and better resolution.

Basically the modern microscopes are of two types - light microscopes and electron microscopes. In a light (optical) microscope, the source of illumination of the object is visible light while in an electron microscope, the source of illumination is a beam of electrons.

Light microscopes are of the following types -

1. Bright field (Light) microscope
2. Dark field microscope
3. Phase contrast microscope
4. Fluorescence microscope
5. Ultraviolet microscope and
6. Interference microscope

Electron microscopes are of two types.

1. Transmission electron microscope (TEM) and
2. Scanning electron microscope (SEM)

The following table gives a comparative summary of different types of microscopes.

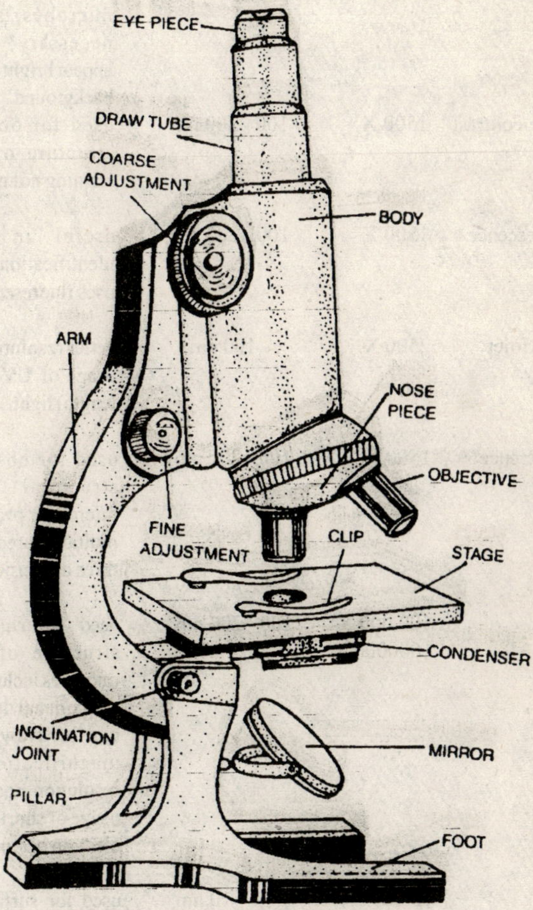

Fig. 3.3 Microscopy
A Compound Microscope

Table Comparison of different types of microscopes

No.	Type of Microscope	Maximum	Resolution Magnification	Remarks (uses)
1.	Bright field	1500 X	100 - 200 nm	used for visual observation of microbes; staining is necessary to view the specimens

2.	Dark field	1500 X	100 - 200 nm	used for seeing live microbes; staining not necessary; specimens appear bright against a dark background.
3.	Phase contrast	1500 X	100 - 200 nm	used for observing the structure of microbes; staining not necessary.
4.	Fluorescence	1500 X	100 - 200 nm	useful in diagnostic identification of microbes; uses fluorescent staining.
5.	Ultraviolet	2500 X	100 nm	better resolution due to the usage of UV (short wave length) light.
6.	Interference	1500 X	100 - 200 nm	used for observation of structural details of microbes; produces sharp multicoloured image with three dimensional view.
7.	TEM	500,000 X-1000000 X	100 - 200 nm	used for study of ultra structure of cells and microbes including viruses. Anatomical details of cells can be viewed; highest magnification and resolution possible due to usage of short wave length electron beam.
8.	SEM	10,000 - 1000000 X	1 - 10 nm	used for surface viewing of microbes, pollen grains and other objects; surface architecture at the ultra structural level can be seen, three dimensional image is produced.

Bright Field (Light) Microscope

The bright field microscope or light microscope or compound microscope is the most common and the most indispensable instrument in the biology laboratory.

Basically the microscope has two types of parts. The mechanical parts provide the structural framework of the microscope and support the optical parts. The optical parts are involved in the magnification of the object. The following is a detailed description of the various parts of a light microscope.

Base, Pillar and Inclination Joint

The base and the attached pillar serve to support the entire microscope. The base is generally *'V'* (horse shoe) shaped or some times 'U' shaped. Usually the pillar and the base are made heavy in order to minimize vibration. The inclination joint joins the arm of the microscope to the pillar. The joint permits the tilting of the microscope to any degree as desired by the observer.

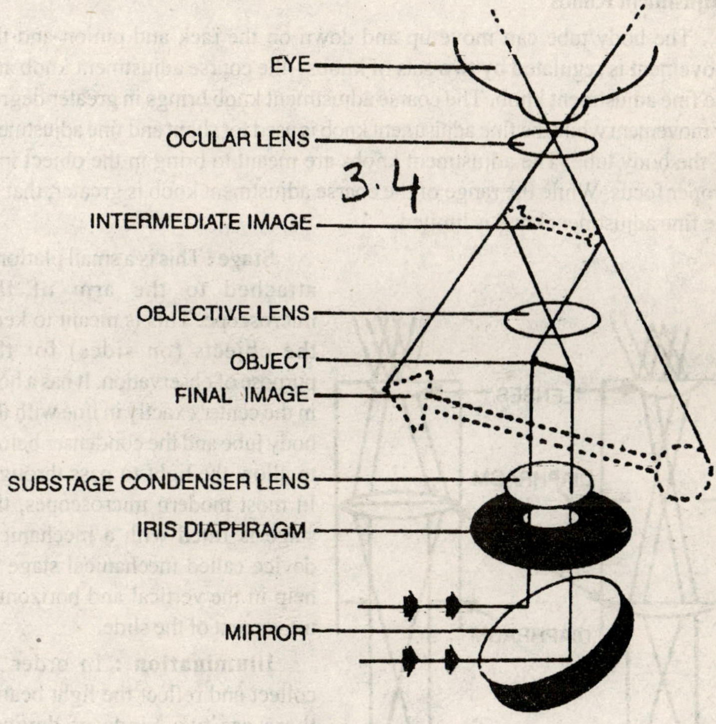

Fig. 3.4 Microscopy
Optical system of the compound microscope

Arm and body tube

The arm is a slightly bent solid piece of iron which is attached at one end to the pillar by the inclination joint. The other end of the arm has the body tube to which the principal optical systems are attached. The body tube is a cylindrical structure and at the point of attachment to the arm there is a graduated rack and pinion which helps in the movement of the body tube up and down.

Draw tube, revolving nose piece

Fitting properly inside the upper end of the body tube is the draw tube, which may be drawn up. "The ocular lens fits into the draw tube. The purpose of the draw tube is to adjust tube length so that the objective lens and the ocular are at a specified distance.

The revolving nose piece is a circular rotating disc attached to the body tube. Objective lenses are attached to this.

Adjustment Knobs

The body tube can move up and down on the rack and pinion and the movement is regulated by two sets of knobs - the course adjustment knob and the fine adjustment knob. The coarse adjustment knob brings in greater degree of movement while the fine adjustment knob is used for slight and fine adjustment of the body tube. The adjustment knobs are meant to bring in the object into proper focus. While the range of the coarse adjustment knob is greater, that of the fine adjustment knob is limited.

Stage : This is a small platform attached to the arm of the microscope. This is meant to keep the objects (on sides) for the purpose of observation. It has a hole in the center exactly in line with the body tube and the condenser below to allow the light to pass through. In most modern microscopes, the stage is fitted with a mechanical device called mechanical stage to help in the vertical and horizontal movement of the slide.

Illumination : In order to collect and reflect the light beams there are two kinds of devices attached to the base of the microscope. These are - mirror or an artificial illumination (built in illumination).

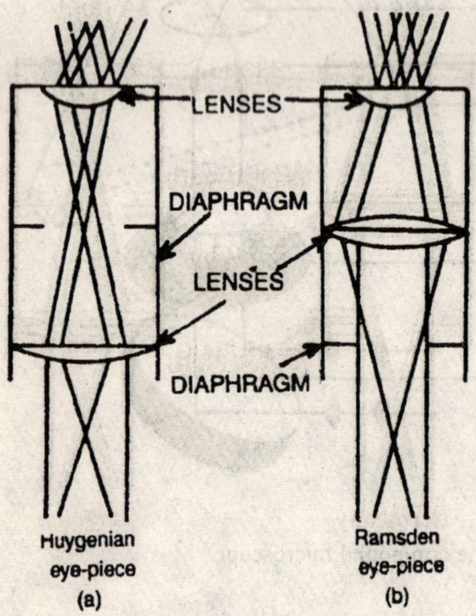

Fig. 3.5 Microscopy
Types of eye-pieces

The mirror collects the light either from a natural source (sun light) or an artificial source (electric light) and reflects the rays into the microscope. The mirror has both sides reflective - one side is plain, the other side is concave. Usually concave side is used when natural light is focussed and plain side is used while focussing artificial light.

In some of the compound microscopes there is provision of built in illumination (instead of a mirror) which has a devise to use 8 or 12 volt bulb and provide direct illumination to the stage.

Sub stage Condenser; Iris diaphragm

The light either reflected by the mirror or by a built in source will be diffuse and does not have sufficient density. In order to condense the light and focus it on to the object, there is a sub stage condenser. This consists of a condensing lens. The condensing lens may be fixed or in some microscopes it can also move up and down for suitable adjustment on a rack and pinion. The condenser helps to focus all the light on the object. Beneath the condenser there is an *iris diaphragm* which regulates the quantity of light entering into the condenser. The iris diaphragm may be closed and opened with the help of a lever to regulate the entry of light.

Optical parts

There are two sets of optics or lenses in a compound microscope. These are eye pieces (ocular) and objectives.

Eye pieces (Ocular) : The ocular or eye piece is a short tube with two lenses which fits into the upper part of the draw tube. The main function of the eye piece is to magnify the image of the object formed by the objective. Eye pieces are marked 5X, 10X, 15X etc.

The eye piece commonly used is the 10X Huygenian eye piece with monocular tube. These eye pieces are also referred to as negative oculars. The positive ocular or Ramsden eye pieces are constructed with convex surfaces of both lenses facing inwards.

Objective lenses : These are attached to the revolving nose piece and are very important as they affect the quality of the image seen by the observer. Based on their type of construction objectives are classified into *achromatic, apochromatic and fluorite.* The first one is simple in construction and less expensive, while the other two are complicated more expensive and used in costly microscopes. These two are also corrected for most of the common aberrations that occur in the lenses.

The objectives are of the following four types based on their magnification - 10X(Low), 40X(Medium), 60X(High) and 100X(Oil immersion). Several microscope manufacturers use different colored rings to distinguish individual objectives. They can also be distinguished based on their length; low power being the shortest and oil immersion, the longest.

The oil immersion lens in used for very high magnification. The lens is so named because a drop of a highly refractive liquid (refractive index same as glass) is added on the slide while viewing through an oil immersion objective.

The main functions of the objective lenses are - 1. Concentration of light rays coming from the object, 2. Forming the image of the specimen and 3. Magnifying the image.

Magnification : A microscope is primarily used to enlarge or magnify the object that is being viewed which can not otherwise be seen by the naked eye. Magnification may be defined as the degree of enlargement of an object provided by the microscope. Magnification by a microscope is the product of the individual magnifying ability of the oculars and the objectives. For example if the ocular is 10X, and objective is 40X, the specimen is magnified 400 times. If an oil immersion objective (100X) is used along with 10X ocular, the specimen is magnified 1000 times. The following factors play an important role in magnification.

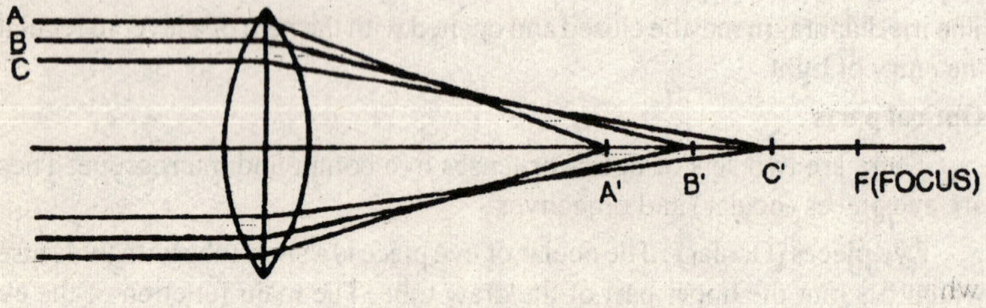

Fig. 3.6 Microscopy
Spherical aberration

(i) Optical tube length
(ii) Focal length of the objective lens
(iii) Magnifying ability of the ocular

Total magnification can be calculated as follows:

Total magnification = Optical tube length / Focal length of the objective X magnification of ocular

Resolving power

Theoretically if the magnifying power of the ocular and objectives are increased it should be possible to get higher and higher magnifications. By using high powered lenses a magnification up to 3000 can be obtained but the image will be blurred and details are not clear. This is due to the fact that in a microscope not only the lenses, but the wave length of the illumination is also important and this decides the resolving power of the microscope.

Resolving power of a microscope is defined as its *ability to distinguish between two particles situated very close.* In a magnified image the object should not only be larger but the details should also be clear. This is possible when a microscope has the ability to see two points situated very close as two distinct entities. In other words, resolving power may be said to be the minimum distance at which two structural entities of an object can be visualized as discrete individual structures even in the magnified image.

(The above explanation may be illustrated clearly with a comparison with the human eye. Human eye functions on the same principal as that of light microscope i.e. we see objects because of the light reflected by them. The human eye has a resolving power about 0.25 mm in the sense, two dots situated 0:25 mm (or more) apart can be seen as two dots; any thing closer will look like a single dot).

The resolving power of a microscope depends on two factors - the wavelength of the light used for illumination and the numerical aperture (NA) of the objective.

In optical light (bright field) microscopes, the wave length of the light used falls in the visible range (400 - 750nm). Within this range if light of shorter wave length is used the resolution will be higher. For example blue light has a shorter wavelength than red light. Greater resolution can be achieved by using a blue light as a source of illumination than a red light.

The second factor that decides the resolving power (RP) is the numerical aperture of the objective. NA is defined as the property of a lens that decides the quantity of light that can enter into it. It depends on two factors.

(i) Refractive index of the medium that fills the space between the specimen and the front of the objective lens and

(ii) The angle of the most oblique rays that can enter the objective lens (The more divergent or oblique rays that an objective can admit, greater is the resolving power).

NA can be mathematically calculated by the following formula

NA = n sin f Where

n = refractive index of the medium

f = angular aperture. This is defined as the angle between the most divergent rays passing through the lens and optical axis of the lens. Rays cannot enter the objective if their angle of divergence from the normal rays (straight rays) is greater than half the angular aperture.

Using NA, the resolution power of the microscope can be calculated as follows.

RP = Wave length of light / 2 x NA

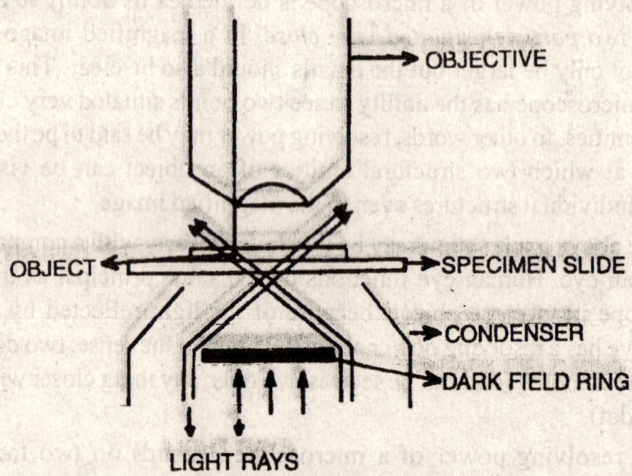

Fig. 3.7 Microscopy
Dark field microscope

For instance if a yellow light of wave length 580nm with NA of 1.0 is used RP will be as follows:

RP = 580/2x1 = 290nm

If a blue light is used the RP will be still higher (i.e. it can resolve objects smaller than 290nm).

Limit of resolution : This may be defined as the shortest distance between two objects when they can still be distinguished as two separate entities. Highest resolution in a light microscope is possible with the shortest wave length light (visible) and with the objective having highest NA. This can be expressed as follows:

$d = \lambda / 2\text{NA}$

Where d = resolution and λ = wave length. For instance if we use green light (520nm wave length) and an objective with 1.3 NA the resolution may be calculated as follows:

$\text{d} = {}^{520}/_{2 \times 13} = 200\text{nm}$

From the above it can be calculated that the smallest particle that can be seen by light microscope is the one not smaller than 0.2 μm in dimension.

Working Principle (higher magnification) **of Oil Immersion Lens**

When an objective lens (less than 100X) other than oil immersion is used it is referred to as a dry objective; in the space between the specimen and the front of objective there is only air. Air has a refractive index of 1.0. Rays whose angular divergence from the center of the optical axis is greater than half the angular aperture can not enter the objective lens and are lost. If a drop of oil (Cedar wood oil) is placed in between the specimen and the objectives lens, many rays whose angle of divergence is more, also can enter the objective lens as the refractive index of oil about 1.5. Thus NA of the objective is increased which results in better resolution and higher magnification.

Types of Condensers : Three types of condensers are in use in microscopes. These are

***Abbe's Condenser* :** This is the simplest one fitted to a microscope. There are two lenses in this, but both are not corrected for any chromatic or spherical aberration. This type of condenser is good only for low power viewing. At higher magnifications, the images of the specimens get blurred due to improper focussing.

***Aplanatic Condenser* :** In this, there is a third lens added to the original two, to correct the spherical aberration only and not chromatic. Aplanatic condenser gives a good image when used with monochromatic light

***Achromatic Condenser* :** This focuses most of the incident light on the object and allows very little light to escape and produce glare. The NA of the condenser generally equals that of the objective. In this condenser both spherical and chromatic aberrations are corrected.

Aberrations in the objectives

The surfaces of objective lenses are spherical and such surfaces can not form perfect images. This is due to variations in refraction and focus by the peripheral parts of the objectives. These cause defects or aberrations in the images. Aberrations in objectives are of two types - *Spherical aberrations and Chromatic aberrations.*

Spherical aberrations result due to passing of lenses-which cannot be brought to the same focus as those which pass through near the optical axis. As a result the image gets distorted.

Chromatic aberration occurs due to the splitting of light into its individual component colours as it would happen when it passes through a prism. These monochromatic beams of various wavelengths are not recombined to the same focus due to varying refraction of lens. The result is a hazy image.

Correction of aberrations : Aberrations may be corrected by using better quality lenses or by the combination of lenses with varying dispersive qualities. A lens system corrected for chromatic aberration of two colours is called *achromatic* and the one corrected for three different colours is called *apochromatic.* Crown glass with low dispersive power is used for convex lenses while flint glass with high dispersive power is used for concave lenses. A combination of the two will result in an achromatic lens system.

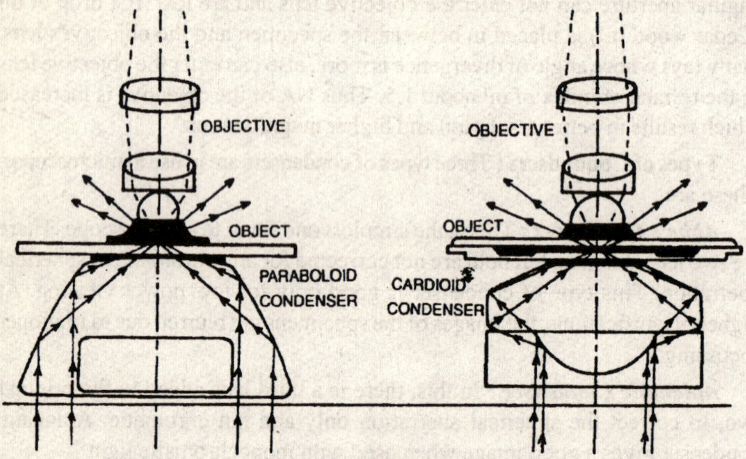

Fig. 3.8 Microscopy
Two types of dark field condensors

Spherical aberrations are corrected by the proper use of iris diaphragm to keep out peripheral rays. Additionally the lens may be ground to a shape which will permit the peripheral and axial rays to have a common focus.

DARK FIELD MICROSCOPE

There are several alternative type of microscopes other than bright field microscope that increase the contrast between the background and the specimen without staining, thus allowing for visualization of living specimens. One such microscope is dark field microscope.

Principle : In a dark room dust particles in the air are practically invisible. But if a beam of light crosses the room the dust immediately becomes visible as bright particles in light. This is due to the fact that the dust particles refract the rays of light and direct some of them towards the observer. By this method of indirect illumination against a dark background, particles are visible.

In a dark field microscope also, the specimen under observation is brightly illuminated against a dark background. In other words, the images of specimens appear as luminary bodies against a dark background. This is in contrast with bright field microscope where the specimens will be darker against a light background.

The dark field condenser : The dark field microscope is essentially a light microscope, but with a different condenser. The normally used Abbe condenser is replaced by dark field condenser. In a dark field condenser, the centre of the top lens is opaque, so that none of the central rays of light can pass through, and the specimen on the stage is illuminated only with the peripheral oblique rays. The light rays are focussed in such a way that they do not reach the specimen directly (as in the ordinary microscope) but instead the light rays traverse across the specimen horizontally almost at right angle to the objective lens. As a result of this the field appears dark but the specimen stands out as a bright refractive structure in the same way as a dust particle in a beam stands out due to its shining.

In normal operations of dark field microscopy a modified version of Abbe condenser with low power objectives would suffice. But for higher magnifications, special dark field condensers with cardoid and paraboloid lenses are employed. In some instances ordinary light may not be enough. Sources of intense light such as *carbon arc* lamps may become necessary. Utmost care should be taken to use perfectly clean and scratch free glass slides and cover slips. Many a time unwanted particles or dust are capable of reflecting light and may illuminate the background which should always remain dark.

Uses of dark field microscope : The dark field microscope is used for examination of live, unstained preparations of microbes or other specimens suspended in fluid. It is highly useful for the study of very small bacteria which are generally invisible under ordinary microscope. Motility of microbes also can be observed since they (microbes) are in live condition and are not killed.

PHASE CONTRAST MICROSCOPE

In bright field microscopes, transparent protoplasmic contents cannot be differentiated unless they are stained. This is due to the fact that when light rays pass through both medium and the specimen, there is very little difference or contrast in their refractive indices. As a result, the alteration in the rays that pass through the specimen or the medium will be almost same when viewed under light microscope. In order to increase the contrast between the specimen and the background or to bring about differences in the refraction of the rays that pass through the specimen and those that pass through the medium, dyes (stains) are used that selectively stain different cell organelles. Staining however leads to cellular death and when we observe a stained specimen we will not be seeing a live specimen.

Phase contrast microscope is a special microscope that enables the viewer to see transparent protoplasmic components without staining and without killing. Originally developed by Frederick Zernike (1933) hence called *Zernike microscope,* Phase contrast microscope is the ideal instrument for observation of living protozoans and other transparent microbes, without staining. Frederick Zerinke was awarded-Nobel Prize in physics in the year 1953 for the discovery of phase contrast principle.

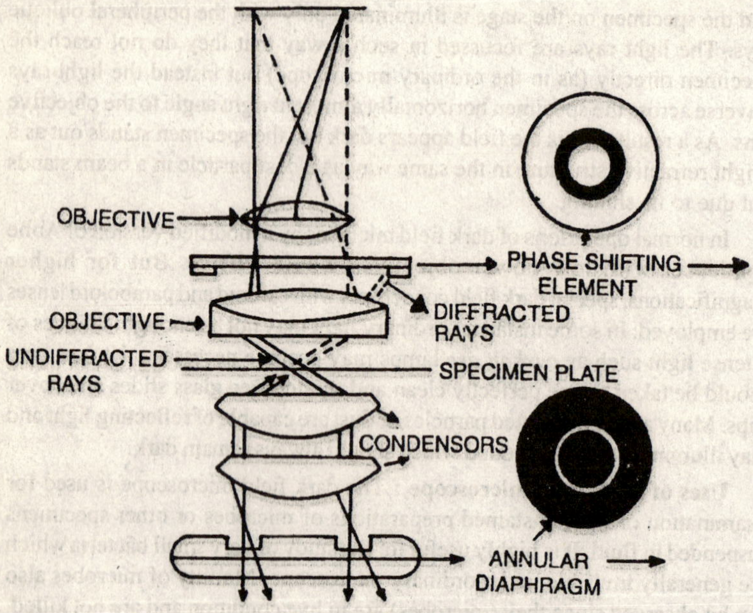

Fig. 3.9 Microscopy –
Phase contrast microscope

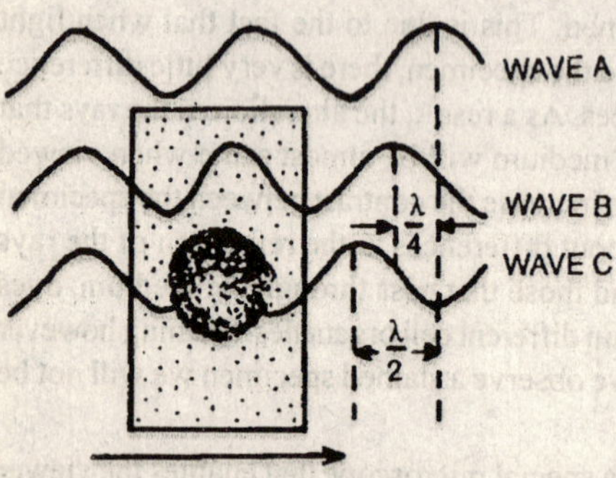

Principle : In order to understand the principle behind the working of a phase contras microscope we must first understand how image contrasts are produced and the variable behaviour of the light rays as they pass through an object

Fig. 3.10 Microscopy
The retardation of phases of light waves

Objects in a microscopic field can be categorized into two - *Amplitude objects* and *Phase objects*. Amplitude objects show up as dark objects under the microscopic view because of the reduction in the intensity (amplitude) of the rays that pass through. Phase objects which are transparent on the other hand allow the light rays to pass through without any reduction in their intensity. But when the light rays are passing through a transparent object, some rays will have retardation by about one quarter wave length. This retardation is called *phase shift.* But the phase shift will not cause any change in amplitude; thus the objects appear transparent. The 1/4 wave length phase shift is utilized in the phase contrast microscope to create image contrast.In order to understand this, First we should understand what happens to the rays when they pass through a transparent object.

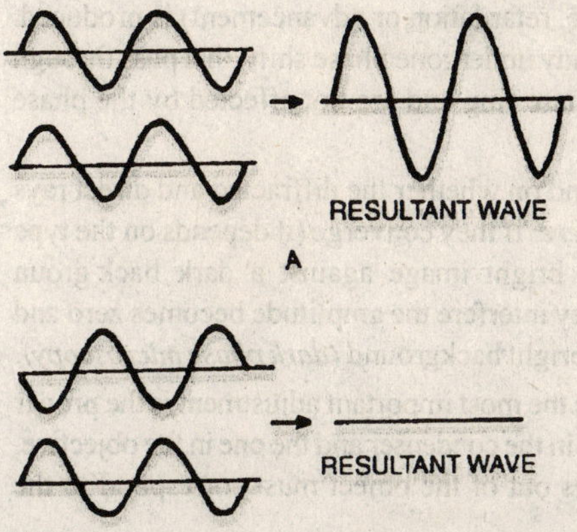

Fig. 3.11 Microscopy
Additive and destructive interference of light waves

Behaviour of rays : Light rays passing through a transparent object emerge out in two different ways - *direct* and *diffracted.* The rays that pass through the object in a straight line are called direct rays and are unaltered in amplitude and phase. The rays that are bent and slowed down as, they pass through due to differences in density of the medium, are called diffracted rays. It is this relationship between the rays that is made use of in the phase contrast microscope.

If the direct rays and diffracted rays of an object can be brought into the same phase (the crest of both light waves coincide) with each other, the resultant increase in amplitude is due to the sum of both the converaged rays and is called *coincidence.* As a result of the increased amplitude, the object looks very bright in the field. On the other hand if the direct and diffracted rays are out of phase (i.e. the crest of one wave coincides with the *trough* and *not the crest* of another wave) it is said to be *reverse phase* and their amplitudes cancel each other and the object looks dark. This is called *interface.* Both these phenomena (coincidence and interference) are used in a phase contrast microscope.

The phase contrast set up

The basic construction of a phase contrast microscope is like a bright field microscope only except for two special attachments. These are-(i) a special type condenser and (ii) a phase plate.

The condenser has a special diaphragm consisting of an *annular stop*. This annular stop can be compared to a solid rod kept loosely at the centre of a cylinder. The annular stop allows only a hollow cone of light rays to pass through the condenser and light the object on the slide.

The phase plate is a special optical disc located in the rear focal plane of the objective. It has a special phase ring coated with a material that can either advance or retard the direct rays depending on its construction.

The rays of light (direct rays) that emerge from the object as solid lines converge on the phase ring within the objective. Here, depending on the coated material the desired phase shift (i.e. retardation or advancement) is produced. The diffracted rays (that have already undergone phase shift) that pass through the object on the slide miss the phase ring and are not affected by the phase plate.

The resultant image will depend on whether the diffracted and direct rays are allowed to *converge* and *interfere*. If they converge (it depends on the type of phase ring) it will result in a bright image against a dark back groun (*bright phase microscopy*) or if they interfere the amplitude becomes zero and it results in a dark image against a bright background *(dark phase microscopy)*.

In a phase contrast microscope the most important adjustment is the proper alignment of the two rings - the one in the condenser and the one in the objective. The ring of direct light that comes out of the object must correspond to the phase ring in the objective.

How an unstained preparation can be seen under a phase contrast microscope? In any specimen or cell there will be difference in thickness between the structures of components. When the light rays pass through these there will be variable refraction of the rays and these phase changes are converted into visible differences of light intensity (due to the phase ring). Even some structures which are difficult to stain and observe under light microscope become conspicuous in a phase contrast microscope because small phase changes result in interference of light waves resulting in high contrast images.

FLOURESCENCE MICROSCOPE

Flourescence microscope involves staining of the specimens with special flourescent dyes and is an indispensible instrument in diagnostic microbiological laboratories.

A flourescence microscope differs from an ordinary light microscope in the following respects.

(i) Light source is a mercury vapour lamp

(ii) A dark field condenser is used instead of the normal Abbe condenser

(iii) Three sets of filters are employed to alter the light rays that pass through the instrument and reach the eye.

The Principle of flourescence

Light exists as a form of energy and is transmitted in the form of waves. When a wave of light encounters any obstruction like when it reaches molecules of a substances the electrons of the molecule at the outer orbit get excited and oscillate in resonance with the light waves. When a substance absorbs light it essentially absorbs energy. This energy that is absorbed can not just disappear. It should be transmitted out in some form or it should be converted to some other form of energy as it happens in photosynthesis. When light is transmitted by the energized (excited) molecules it is said to be *Photoluminiscence.* In photoluminiscence, the light absorbed is not transmitted immediately. There is always a time lapse between absorption and emission. If the time lapse is greater than 10 (1/10,000) seconds it is said to be *Photoluminiscence.* If on the other hand the time lapse is less than 10 seconds it is known as *fluorescence.*

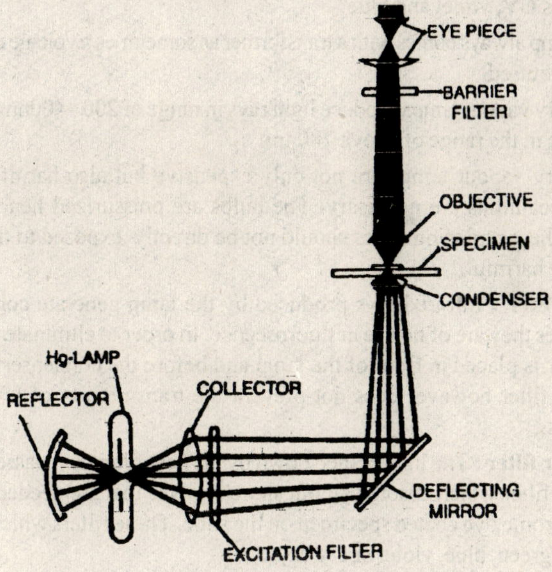

Fig. 3.12 Microscopy

Fluorescence microscope diagrammatic representation of the path of rays and action of excitation and barrier filters

When a fluorescent dye is applied to a molecule it absorbs a wave length of light (excitation wave length) and emits a light ray of a different wave length (emission wave length). In other words, the wave length of light changes as it emerges out of a fluorescent compound. Usually the emission light will have a longer wavelength. For instance, When the flourescent dye *fluorescein isothiocyanate* is illuminated with blue light, it emits green light. This is due to the fact that light rays of shorter wavelength have more energy than those of longer wavelength and emission light always has less energy.

Microbiological specimens to be observed under a flourscence microscope are coated with fluroscent componds (flourochromes) such as Auramine O, Acridine orange, Fluoroscein, etc.

Parts of a Fluroscence microscope

The principles of magnification and resolution of a fluoroscence microscope are no different from a bright field microscope. The essential components are light source, heat filter, exciter filter.condenser and barrier filter.

Light source : This is provided by a bright mercury vapour arc lamp. As against the normal incandescent bulb, this lamp provides shorter wave length light rays such as UV, violet and blue.

The lamp always comes with a transformer as sometimes a voltage of 18,0000 volts are required.

Mercury vapour lamps produce light rays in range of 200 - 400nm (UV) and visible ravs in the range of above 780nm.

Mercury vapour lamps are not only expensive but also harmful. Hence several precautions are necessary. The bulbs are pressurized hence there is danger of their explosion. Eyes should not be directly exposed to the bulb as the rays are harmful.

Heat filter : Infrared rays produced by the lamp generate considerable heat, besides they are of no use in fluoroscence. In order to eliminate these rays a heat filter is placed in front of the lamp and before the condenser to absorb heat. Heat filter however does not prevent the transmission of UV and the visible rays.

Exciter filter : The light cooled down by the heat filter next passes through the exciter filter which absorbs all but shorter waves that are needed to excite the flurochrome dye coated specimen on the slide. These filters which are dark allow only green, blue, violet or UV rays.

Condenser : For best results always a dark field condenser is used, because in a dark background even mild fluoroscence can be easily detected-Anolher advantage of this condenser is that it deflects majority of the UV rays thus protecting the observer's eyes. In order to achieve this the NA of the objective is always kept at 0.05 less than that of the condenser.

Barrier filter : This is situated in the body tube of the microscope between the objectives and the eye piece to remove all remnants of the exciting light so that only the fluoroscence is seen. When excitation is by UV, the exciter filters are dark and barrier filters will be almost colourless. On the other hand, if blue excitation is used, the barrier filters are either yellow or deep orange in colour.

Hints for using the microscope : The following points are to be kept in mind while using a fluorescent microscope for best results.

1. *Warm up :* Fluorescent micrscopes require a warm up period. The illumination is low when turned on but reaches the maximum in about two minutes. Optimum illumination is obtained in about 30 minutes. It is better to switch on the light 45 minutes before using.
2. *Check of mercury lamp :* The life expectancy of a mercury arc lamp is about 400 hours. Hence it is necessary that a log should be maintained regarding the number of hours that the instrument is used. A check should be made after approximately 200 hours of usage.
3. *Selection of filter:* Proper combination of exciter and barrier filters are necessary to acilieve best results. The most frequently used filters are

   Bluish Schott BG12 - Exciter filter
   Yellowish Schott OG I - Barrier filter

Examination : For preliminary exmination like locating a particular part or cell of the specimen, it is better to use ordinary illumination and use the mercury arc illumination only for precise observation. If the specimen has to be observed under oil immersion, special low fluorsecing immersion oil is to be used. Ordinary immersion oil used for bright field microscopy should not be used.

Safety measures : Fluorescent microscope can be harmful and injurious if not used properly. The following precautions are necessary to avoid any harm to the user.

1. The pressurized mercury arc bulb may explode under certain circumstances. But the equipment is designed to prevent this. However lamp should not be inspected when it is hot. The lamp is safe when relatively cold. Usually 15 - 20 minutes is sufficient to cool the lamps.
2. Do not expose your eyes directly to the mercury lamp. the equipment is designed in such a way as to prevent the scattering of the rays. Please note that the unfiltered rays from the lamp contain UV as well as infrared rays both of which are harmful to the eyes.
3. Make sure that both the filters (of the suitable type) are in their place before looking into the microscope. Removal of any one or both is harmful to the to the eyes.

ULTRAVIOLET MICROSCOPE

In Ultraviolet microscope, the optics are specially meant to transmit or reflect UV light (200 - 350nm). As the source of illumination (UV) is having a shorter wave length, UV microscopes have a better resolving power than light microsopes. It is not possible to look into a UV microscope directly as the rays are injurious. Hence the images of the object are either photographed or projected on using UV sensitive TV cameras.

INTERFERENCE MICROSCOPE (Stereomicroscope)

The interference is essentially based on the same principle as that of phase contrast microscope. In both the microscopes the principle of increased or decreased amplitude due to the interference between *out of phase* light waves and *in phase* light waves is used to produce contrast in the image. While a single beam of light passing through the object is made use of in phase contrast microscope, there are two beams of light that combine after passing through the specimen. This produces an interference pattern. Interference microscopes are more versatile in comparison with phase contrast microscopes as they have objectives of higher NA and also use colour to increase the contrast.

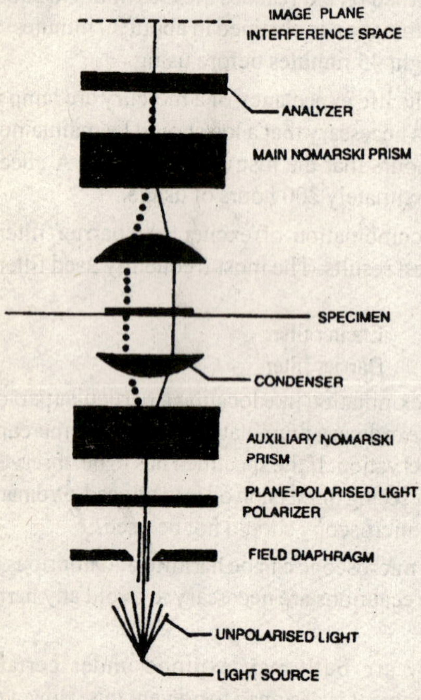

Fig. 3.13 Microscopy
The Nomarksi Interference microscope

One of the most frequently used interference microscope is a *Nomarski Differential Interference Contrast(NDIC) Microscope* which can produce a high contrast, almost three dimensional image of transparent objects. The special features of a NDIC microscope are a polarizing filler, and interference contrast condenser and a prism analyzer plate.

In *the-*. NDIC microscope. a beam of polarized light is split into two beams at right angles to each other; are made to travel through the specimen and are combined and forced through an analyzer. The resultant interference pattern will produce a pseudo three dimensional image. This is due to the fact that the two beams of light passing through the specimen produce a sterescopic effect. The degree or level of three dimensional configuration that is visualized is a function of the varations of refractive indices at the surface of the specimen. In other words, higher the difference of refractive index at the surface, more will be the contrast in the image of the specimen. Edges of specimen such as cell walls with a high refractive index variation are very well defined under a NDIC microscope. Images seen through the NDIC microscope are normally brilliantly coloured (non - stained) because of the phase changes of light waves that pass through the various components of an object such as a microbial cell. Qualitative observations of specimens are best made through an interference microscope, because the images have a high contrast and high topographic relief due to the three dimensional effect.

ELECTRON MICROSCOPY

The microscopes which are based on visible light as a source of illumination have their own limitations. In spite of the numerous modifications there is a limit to the resolving power of these microscopes. The maximum resolution that the light microscopes can achieve is the wave length of the light waves. A particle smaller than the wavelength of visible light can not be resolved under the light microscope.

The development of electron microscope in the late 1940's however has changed the situation dramatically. Using a source of electrons for illumination which have a much shorter wave length than that of light rays, the electron microscope has opened up before biologists a hitherto unknowen exquisite subcellular architecture of the world of microcosm.

The electron microscope is a remarkable research tool of the 20th century. Its power of magnification runs into 100000X or a resolving power of 10^{-9} centimeters. Experiments that eventually lead to the development of electron microscope began as early as 1920. The First prototype model was developed for physical applications.

Principle of working

As the name indicates, in an electron microscope, a beam of electrons is used as a source of illumination, instead of a beam of light as in light microscopes. In order to understand the working mechanism of an electron microscope, we must first understand some elementary facts about electrons and their behaviour.

Electrons are negatively charged subatomic particles having a mass of 9.1×10^{-28} grams. An integral part of all atoms, electrons orbit round the atomic nucleus at velocities for exceeding 50,000 kms per second. When the atoms of a metal are excited by heat energy to an extent where the electron velocity exceeds the attraction of the nucleus, they (electrons) fly off from the clutches of the nucleus and are lost. When a melal, like tungsten is heated by applying a high voltage current, electrons come out in a continuous stream and this can be directed to form a high velocity electron beam.

Louis de Bragile (1924) working on electrons opined that electrons being particulate must behave like light waves and should have both a fixed wave length and frequency. He used the following formula to caculate the wave length λ (lambda) of the matter

$$\lambda = h / mv$$

where *h is* planck's constant, *m is mass* and *v* is velocity. Calculations based on this equation have shown that electrons accelerated to a potential of 60,000 volts have a wave length of 0.05 Å (Angstorm) or 105 times smaller than that of visible light. Hence an electron beam should be able to resolve (theroretically) particles 105 times smaller than that of the wave length of light.

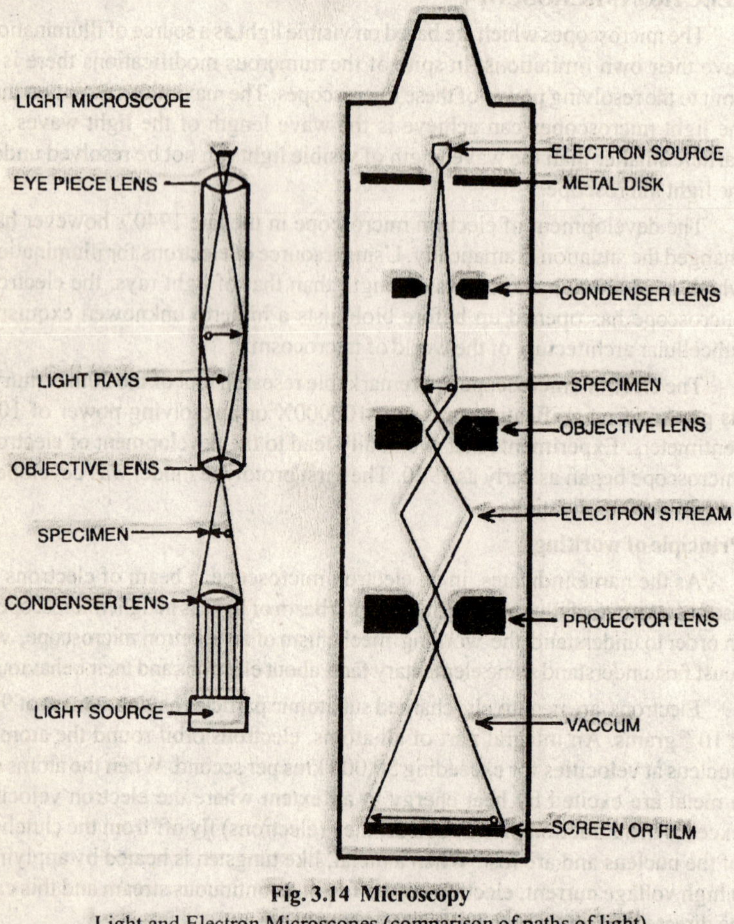

Fig. 3.14 Microscopy
Light and Electron Microscopes (comparison of paths of light)

The discovery that electrons have wave motion and they can be focussed on to an object in the form of a beam (like light ray) in a magnetic field provided the impetus for the development of electron microscope. By the late 1930's a system of magnetic coils capable of focussing an electron beam had been designed. It was also shown that by regulating the current flowing through the magnetic coils, the magnification can be regulated. Theoretically, an enhancement of resolution power equivalent to the wave length of a beam of electrons should be possible in an electron microscope.

But there are practical limitations in the design of magnetic coils (equivalent to lenses in a light microscope) used for focussing the beam of electrons. The main problem is the one of the distortion produced when the angle of illumination is more than a few tenths of a degree. As a result, to catch the beam of electrons, the numerical aperture of objectives has to be much lesser than that of light microscopes. The actual resolving power of electron micrtoscopes is only about 0.05nm; far less than the theoretical potential of 0.002nm. But even then, 0.05nm is much much smaller when compared with 100nm that is the limit in a light microscope.

Basic construction of an electron microscope

The modern electron microscopes have a common basic construction pattern with standard components such as

(i) Electron generator (gun)
(ii) Electromagnetic coils (lenses) - 3 sets
(iii) Screen (for viewing) and
(iv) Vacuum pump

The electron generator is the source of illumination. Also called electron gun, it is a tungsten filament, which when heated by electric current emits a stream of electrons. The electrons accelerated by the high voltage energy are forced through a *collimating* aperture which renders the rays in parallel lines and fashions them into a beam. From there the beam passes through the condenser. The condenser 'lens' is a magnetic coil which corrects the aberrations (bending) in the beam and directs them towards the object. The strength of the magnetic lens depends on the amount of current that is allowed to flow through it. Greater the flow of current, greater will be the strength of the magnetic field and greater will be the bending effect on the rays of electron. In other words, by varying the magnetic field strength,the beam can be properly focussed on to the object.

The specimen to be observed must be exceedingly thin (at least 200 times thinner than the ones used for routine optical observation) and must be supported on an equally exceedingly thin but strong film or metallic grid. As the electron microscope always functions only in a vaccum, the specimen must be absolutely dry. Specimen supporting grid is usually a collodion film or Fonnvar or polymerized plastic plus a screen grid of copper having 200 meshes to an inch. The specimen is kept below the condenser and the electron beam passes through it and is scattered depending on the varying refractive index of the specimen. From there, the electron beam (coming out of the specimen) passes through the second set of magnetic coils (objective lens) which focus the electrons and form an intermediate image. A third set of magnetic lenses (equivalent to the oculars) - the projection lenses, produce the final image.The final image however cannot be directly viewed as the rays of electrons are harmful to the eye. They are either projected on to a fluorescent screen for viewing or allowed to expose a photographic plate kept for that purpose.

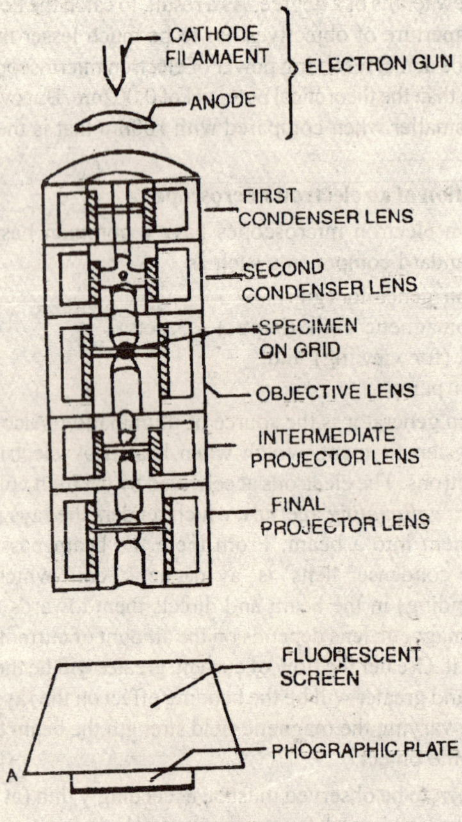

Fig. 3.15 Microscopy

The transmission electron microscope

The entire electron mcroscope must be in a vacuum or otherwise the electrons get scattered due to collisions with air molecules and fail to get focussed. Hence the equipment unit is housed in a single unit which is continuously evacuated with a high speed vacuum pump.

Types of electron microscopes

There are two basic types of electron microscopes. There are - the *Transmission electron microscope* (TEM) and *Scanning electron microscope* (SEM).

Transmission Electron Microscope (TEM)

In a TEM, the beam of electrons passes through the specimen forming an image of the detailed structure of the specimen. This is similar to the light microscope in construction except for

(i) source of illumination is a beam of electrons (not visible light)

(ii) There are a series (usually three sets) of electromagnets for focussing the beam of electrons. These are called magnetic lenses (not made out of glass)

The general construction pattern of TEM is same as that explained above. TEM is for sstudying the structural details of the various components present in a cell or microbe.

The specimens form a contrasting image with all the structural details. Depending on their refractive index, the components of a specimen bring about varying degrees of scattering of the electron rays. Generally however biological specimens do not produce a great degree of scattering of electrons,hence the contrast is low. Staining is resorted to improve the contrast-But instead of dyes used for staining in light microscopy, electron dense heavy metal salts are used for staining in electron microscopy.

Some problems are encountered while viewing a specimen through TEM. Many a time artifacts appear which can be easily mistaken to be a component of a cell. (An *artifact* is the appearance of something in an image due to causes within the optical system or due to the preparation of a specimen and does not represent any component of the specimen under view). Proper preparation of the specimen, correct adjustment of the electron beams, accurate vaccumization will help in reducing the chances of artifact appearance.

Preparation of specimen for TEM

The biological specimens to be examined have to be specially prepared in order to obtain proper structural details with high magnification, but at the same time avoiding the appearance of artifacts. The following steps are necessary before the specimens are ready for observation under TEM.

Dehydration and Fixation : Under light microscopy specimens are kept in water or oilier liquids for observation. But in an electron microscope, the specimens have to be absolutely dry. Any water present, the specimen would boil (as it is in a vacuum) resulting in disintegrating the structural organization of the specimen. Additionally the specimen also has to be fixed in its proper orientation. Fixation and dehydration have to be carried out in several stages in order to prevent distortion.

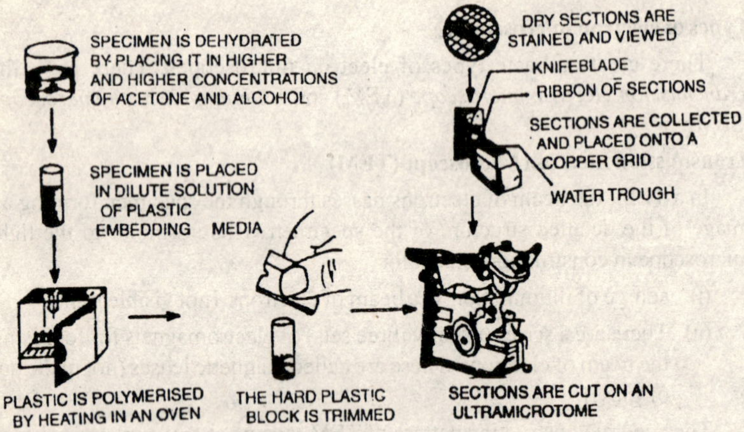

Fig. 3.16 Microscopy
Preparation of specimen for viewing through TEM

Ultra Sectioning : From the point of view of magnification obtained in an electron microscope, microbes are too thick for viewing. Hence normally they are cut into thin sections using an ultra microtome. The ultra microtome has a device which advances the fixed specimen on a diamond or glass knife surface at a known thickness so that sections of uniform thickness are cut. The microbes are usually embedded in a plastic resin to facilitate sectioning.

Staining : In order to enhance the contrast, the specimens are stained with heavy metal containing compounds such as phosphotungstic acid. The staining can be negative or positive. In *negative staining,* the sectioned specimen in dipped in heavy metal solution which sfains the background and not the specimen. The specimens are then visualized in relief against a dark background.

Freeze etching : This is a special technique employed mainly to reveal the details of structure in microbes. In freeze etching, various biochemically defined layers are made visible, including the organelle details. In this technique (instead of using fixatives to preserve the cell structure) the specimens are rapidly struck with a knife blade. At this temperature (freezing) biological specimens are hard to cut, but they crack along the lines of their natural weakness i.e. they are fractured. The fractured specimen is then *etched* i.e. the water (ice) is allowed to evaporate from the surface. This evaporation raises the surface layers of the specimen. A replica, then is made of the freeze etched specimen, by exposing it to vapours of heavy metal (platinum) at 45^0 angle to produce a shadow effect. The specimen then is rotated at 90, and exposed to vapourized carbon. This produces a replica of the surface of the specimen. After removing the remmants of biological material, the carbon replica is viewed under electron microscope. Surface details (internal as well external) of organelles can be clearly visualized by the freeze etching technique.

Scanning Electron Microscope (SEM)

SEM is primarily used for visualizing the surface architecture of the specimen (pollen grains, hairs, membranes, etc.) rather than the internal details. In a SEM, an electron beam is scanned across the surface and a three dimensional image is produced.

The construction plan and working principle of a SEM is different from that of TEM. In SEM, an accelerated beam of electrons is produced from the electron gun and is focussed on the specimen by the condenser lens. The magnetic lenses of a SEM are so constructed as to produce an extremely thin beam of electrons.

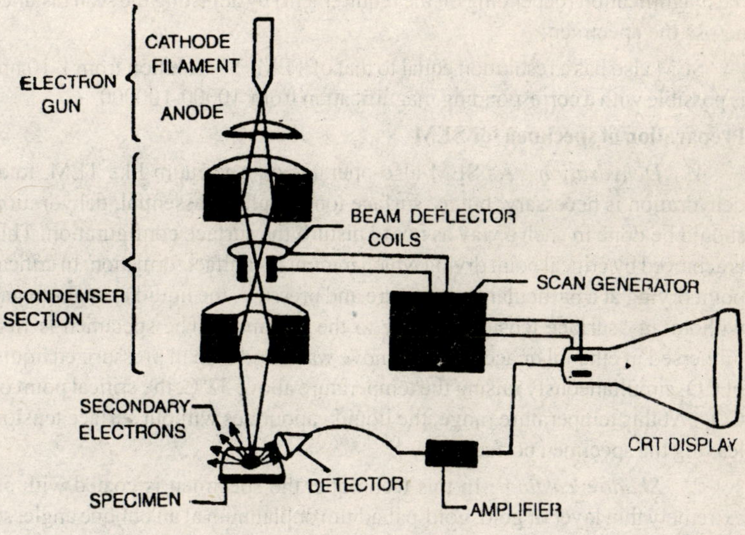

Fig. 3.17 Microscopy
The Scanning electron microscope

The primary electron beam as it strikes the specimen, forces, out electrons from the surface (of the specimen). These are the secondary electrons and are transmitted to a collector. During this process some of the primary electrons also are reflected and transmitted to the collector, but their (primary electrons) number is far less than the secondary electrons. As a result the image signal is developed more by the secondary electrons than by the primary electrons. The electrons are then transmitted from the collector to a detector which has a substance that emits light when struck by electrons. The light so emitted is converted to an electrical current which is used to control the brightness of an image on a CRT (Cathode Ray Tube) screen.

The secondary electrons deflected out of the specimen will be a replica of the refractive index of the surface and thus produce an image on the CRT screen revealing all the topographical details. Image contrast mainly depends on surface topography which determines the number of secondary electrons reaching the detector. The image on the CRT screen will be three dimensional.

Magnification of the image of the specimen in SEM is not achieved through the lenses as in a light microscope or TEM. It is dependent upon the ratio of the length of the scan across the specimen surface to the length of the scan of CRT. For instance if the electron beam scans 100 nm across of specimen and the image on CRT is 100 nm, the magnification is 100000 times. Thus one can decide the magnification (depending on the requirement) by adjusting the scan distance across the specimen.

SEM also has a resolution equal to that of TEM. A resolution from 1-10 nm is possible with a corresponding magnification from 10000-100000.

Preparation of specimen for SEM

1. *Dehydration* : As SEM also operates on a vacuum like TEM, total dehydration is necessary, but as surface topography is essential, dehydration should be done in such a way as not to disturb the surface configuration. This is achieved by critical point drying which minimizes artifact formation. In critical point drying at a particular temperature and pressure, the liquid changes to gas without any surface tension damage to the specimen. The specimen is first immersed in ethanol or acetone to remove water and then in pressurized liquid of CO_2 simultaneously raising the temperature above 32°C, the critical point of CO_2 . At this temperature range, the liquid vapourizes without surface tension leaving the specimen perfectly dry.

2. *Shadow casting* : In this technique, the specimen is coated with an extremely thin layer of gold, gold-palladium or platinum at an oblique angle, so that the specimen produces a shadow on the uncoated side. The shadow technique results in the production of a three dimensional topographic image of the specimen. Coating is done with a device called *a sputter coater*. In some cases double shadowing also can be done by coating the materials from two different angles.

3. *Surface replica:* In this technique, widely used for the study of architectural pattern of the wall surface of spores, pollen etc, a thin layer of a coherent material is coated on to the specimen which is then floated on to a water surface, from where it is transferred on to a strong acid or alkali.

This dissolves the specimen without damaging the replica. The replica is then dried and kept on the metal grid for viewing.

Biological applications of electron microscope

1. Viewing of ultra structure of the cell organelles is made possible.
2. Structural details of large biomolecules such as proteins can be studied.
3. Minute details of the topographic architecture is possible which is of systematic value as in the case of pollen grains.

Limitations of electron microscope

Even though electron microscope is a great advancement over the light microscopes in terms of higher magnification and better resolution, there are certain limitations and light microscopes have their own useful role to play in the microbiological laboratory. The limitations imposed by electron microscope are.-

1. Hydrated specimens are not to be used, hence live specimens cannot be observed
2. Dehydration even if carefully done will cause some distortion

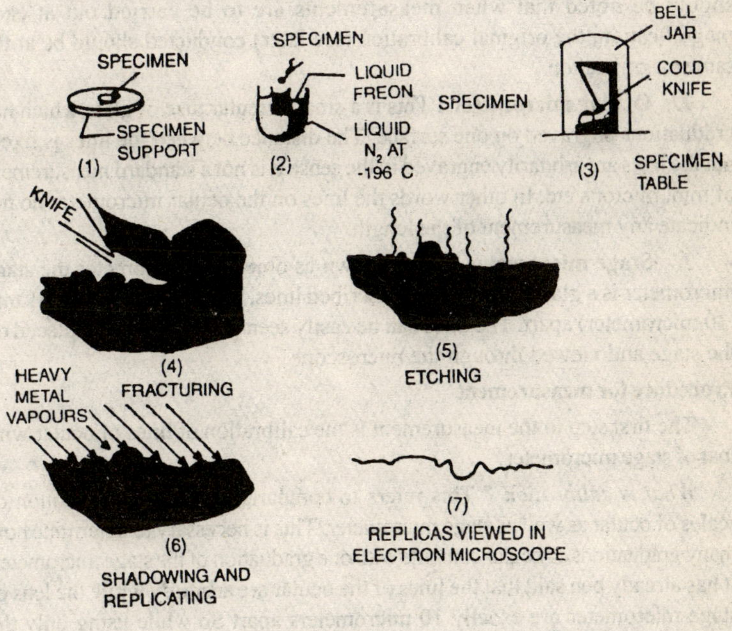

Fig. 3.18 Microscopy
Procedure for freeze etching replicas

3. Artifacts may appear
4. As electrons have a low penetration power extremely thin sections are necessary.

MICROMETRY

Micrometry or microscopic measurements refer to measurements of microbes (length, breadth) seen under the light microscope. Many a time the size of the microbes is an essential criterion besides their morphological characters. The following are necessary to carry out microscopic measurements.

1. A good microscope with 10X eye piece and 10X, 40X and 100X objectives
2. Ocular micrometer
3. Stage micrometer

1. A good microscope (with straight tube) : is necessary to carry out the measurements.

The eye piece may be 10X or 15X with objectives of 10, 40 and 100. It should be noted that when measurements are to be carried out at each magnification, the original calibration (see later) conducted should be at the same magnification.

2. Ocular micrometer : This is a small circular disc of glass which has graduations engraved on one surface. The distance between the lines is fixed, but the lines are arbitarily engraved in the sense it is not a standard measurement of mm, microns etc. In other words the lines on the ocular micrometer do not indicate any measurement of the length.

3. Stage micrometer : Also known as objective micrometer the stage micrometer is a glass slide that has inscribed lines, which are exactly 0.01 mm (10 micrometer) apart. The lines can be easily seen when the slide is placed on the stage and viewed through the microscope.

Procedure for measurement

The first step in the measurement is the calibration of lines of ocular with that of stage micrometer.

What is calibration ? This refers to comparison or super imposition of scales of ocular as well as stage micrometer. This is necessary to determine how many graduations of ocular coincide with one graduation of the stage micrometer. It has already ben said that the lines of the ocular are arbitrary while the lens of stage micrometer are exactly 10 micrometers apart So while using only the ocular micrometer for measurement it becomes necessary to know as to what is the distance between graduations.

At this stage it can be said, that instead of the cumbersome procedure of calibration why not use only the stage micrometer which has the measurements

? This is difficult because the microbes then have to be mounted directly on the stage micrometer which is always not possible. Hence calibration of ocular with the stage micrometer and removing the stage micrometer.

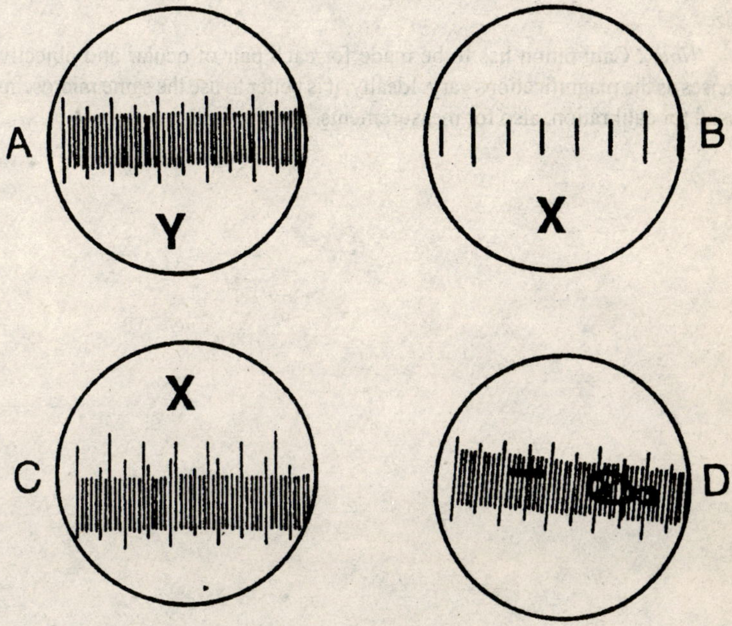

Fig. 3.19 Microscopy
Calibration of ocular micrometer

Procedure for calibration

The first step is the installation of ocular micrometer into the ocular lens. This can be done by unscrewing the top lens in the ocular, placing the micrometer inside thetube and screwing back the lens. In some of the latest microscopes, the ocular micrometer comes with a ring and it can easily inserted into the bottom of the ocular tube.

Next step is placing the stage micrometer on the stage of the microscope and focussing it properly. After focussing, the stage micrometer has to be adjusted so that its graduations align with the graduations of the ocular properly. After the graduations are aligned, count how many ocular divisions equal one division (0.01 mm) of the stage micrometer. If (as shown in the figure) seven ocular divisions equal one division of stage micrometer, the value for each division of ocular is 0.01/7 or 0.0014μm. In other words each ocular division is about 1.43 μm apart. Having known this, the stage micrometer may be replaced with the slide containing microbes for measurements. To determine the size of an organism all that one has to do is to count the number of graduations, the microbe measures and to multiply this number with 1.43 μm to give the actual size.

Note : Calibration has to be made for each pair of ocular and objective lenses as the magnifications vary. Ideally, it is better to use the same microscope used for calibration, also for measurements.

4

CHEMICAL BASIS OF HEREDITY

The cells have diverse chemical components of which most were known to scientists by the first quarter of the nineteeth century. These are classified into three major groups namely-carbohydrates, proteins and lipids. Of these three-proteins are most complex and diverse and many biologists through that they may constitute the basis of biological diversity.

Eventhough the other group of macromolecular compounds - Nuclei acids were discovered in 1869 by Sweedish biochemist Fredrich Miescher, it was only in 1952, their (nuclei acids) role in inheritance was proved.

Meischer collected pus filled hospital bandages and from them he isolated and purified nuclei. On chemical fractionation he found that a cellular chemical content had a very high component of phosphorous compound than what was known before. As the new compound was obrtained from nucleus, Miescher named it *nuclein.* Subsequently nuclein was isolated from many sources and due to its acidic properties, it was named nucleic acid. Upto 1952 however, interest in nuclei acids was limited to only its physiochemical studies. When its role in inheritance was proved nucleic acid became the focus of intensive research. Comparative studies of nuclei acids and proteins revealed that while proteins are of diverse types, there are only two types of nuclei acids. It was hard to believe that nuclei acids which apparently had no diversity could be the basis of heredity and not the proteins.

Presently however, there is not even an iota of doubt as to the fact that nucleic acids alone constitute the hereditary factor. Three major experiments helped provide an evidence for this.

Bacterial Transformation

Fred Griffith and English bacteriologist worked with *Diplococcus pneumococci* and found out that there are two strains in this - *Virulent and Avirulent.* When injected to experimental mice the virulent strains cause the death of the mice while avirulent strains do not casue any harm. Griffith showed that heat killed virulent strains injected into the mice along with avirulent strains cause the death of the mice and from the bodyof the mice live virulent strains can be obtained. Dawson and Sia (1931) showed that the heat killed virulent strains can transform avirulent strains on a nutrient broth. Alloway (1933) showed that even a lysed cell of virulent strain retains the ability of transformation thereby indicating that some component of the cell rather than the entire cell was involved in transformation.

Nature of the transforming agent

Three scientists - O.T. Avery, Colin Macleod and Maclyn McCarty (1944) went into serious search of the transforming agent from the lysed cells of bacteria. Even after digestion of polysaccharide coat, the cell retained the ability of transformation. This shows that the capsule has no role in transformation. Similarly protein degradation also had no adverse effect on transformation. With the two important components out of the way, it thus became clear that nucleic acids perhaps might play a role in transformation. It was shown that the DNA fraction of nucleic acids was responsible for transformation. It was also shown that if the cells are treated with DNAse (a DNA degrading enzyme), the transforming ability will be lost. Enzymes which digest RNA do not disturb transformation.

Bacteriophages and chemical basis of heredity

Bacteriophages are viruses that attack a bacterial cell and multiplty inside the (bacterial) cell. The phage attaches itself to the bacterial cell and ingects its components into the cell where replica of phages are produced. Hershey and Chase (1952) conducted an experiment to find out which component of the bacteriophage carries the genetic information necessary for the replication of viruses. They cultured the host bacterium *Escherichia coli* in a medium containing radio isotopes of Sulphur (S^{35}) and phosphorus (P^{32}). When T_2 phages attacked these cells subsequently, the labelled compounds get incorporated in phage DNA which always has radioactive phosphorus but not any sulphur. In the next set of experiment only the protein coat of T_2 phage was labelled with S^{35} and the DNA core of another was labelled with P^{32}. Hershey and Chase separated the radioactive phages by centrifugation and allowed them to infect a population of non radioactive bacteria. A few minutes after initial infection they separated the phages from bacteria by agitating the medium. After centrifugation, the host and the parasite were separated by centrifugation and their radioactivity measured. About 95% of P^{32} was found in bacteria while about 95% S^{35} was seen in phages. This experiment conclusively proved that during infection only DNA is injected into the medium. This is the reason why the non radioactive bacteria showed labelled P^{32} (as they obtained it from labelled phage DNA). For this work Hershey was awarded Nobel prize in 1969.

Thus the experiments of Hersehy and Chase. Avery, Mcleod and McCarty. Griffith etc., clearly proved that DNA constitutes the chemical basis of Heredity.

TMV and Chemical Basis of Heredity

The discovery that DNA is the hereditary material posed some problems to explain the inheritance in instances such as TMV (Tobacco mosaic virus) where there is no DNA (TMV is a RNA virus). But the absence of DNA has not prevented TMV from transmitting its characters from one generation to the other. TMV is made up of a RNA core and a helical protein coat. The protein RNA component of TMV can be easily separated by shaking the viral particles in a mixture of water and phenol. Frankek Conrad and Wichams (1955) separated the protein and RNA from TMV and reassembled the particles from the individual components thus indicating the purification process (of the components) does not affect their function. Subsequently Gierr and Shramm (1956) showed that on contact with the host only the RNA can bring about the disease and not the protein coat. In TMV therefore it is RNA which is the hereditary material. It can therefore be concluded that nucleic acids in general and DNA in particular is the hereditary material in most of the organisms and in the absence of DNA (as in some viruses) RNA can constitute the genetic material.

Nucleic Acids

These are the most important constituents of the nucleus playing a vital role in the inheritence of characters from one generation to the other. There are two types of nucleic acids - Deoxyribose nucleic acid (DNA) and Ribose nucleic acid (RNA). While both constitute the genetic material in different organisms, it is predominantly the DNA which is the genetic material in most of the organisms. The following are some of the important milestones in the discovery of Nucleic acids.

1. Meischer (1869) isolated nuclei acids and called them nuclein.
2. Hertwig (1884) suggested a heriditary role to the nuclein
3. Kossel (1884) recognised purines and pyrimidines in the nucleic acids.
4. Feulgen (1912) devised basic fushsin dye positive only to DNA.
5. Astbury and Bell (1938) showed that the bases in DNA molecule are arranged one above the other.
6. Avery, Macleod and Macarty (1944) presented evidence for DNA to be the genetic material.
7. Chargaff (1950) showed that DNA contains equal amount of purines and pyrimidines.
8. Wilkins *et al* (1950) identified the molecular distance between the bases.
9. Furberg (1952); DNA is a coil of single chain.
10. Pauling and Corey (1952); DNA is a helix of three chains.
11. Watson and Crick (1953) demonstrated the double helix model for DNA molecule.
12. Meselson and Stahl (1958) demonstrated the semi conservative replication in DNA.

13. Jacob and Monod (1961) postulated the presence of RNA in protein synthesis.

DEOXY RIBOSE NUCLEIC ACID (DNA)

DNA is the main genetic material in almost all organisms except for certain viruses. In prokaryotes like *Escherichia coli,* the genetic material is a single giant molecule of *DNA* is mainly concentratedin the nucleus, it has also been reported in cytoplasmic organelles like chloroplast, mitochondria etc.

Chemical Composition of DNA

DNA extract from many living organisms has revealed it to be a complex macromolecule. It is a long chain polymer cmposed of monomers (units) called nucleotides. Each nucleotide in turn is composed of three sub units. These are - (a) nitrogen base, (b) sugar and (c) phosphate.

Nitrogen bases

The nitrogen bases are of two kinds viz., pyrimidines and purines. Both pyrimidines and purines are heterocyclic compounds, with a basic six membered ring in which one or the other carbon position is replaced by nitrogen.

The pyrimidines have a basic six membered ring of benzene in which, position 1' and 3' are replaced by nitrogen. There are two kinds of pyrimidines - *Cytosine* and *Thymine.* Structurally cytosine has a single six membered ring with a hydroxyl group at the 2' position and an amino group at the 6' position *(2 hydroxy, 6 amino pyrimidine).* Thymine also has a single six membered ring with hydroxyl groups at the 2' and 6' position and a methyl group attached to the 5' position *(2, 6 hydroxy 5 methyl pyrimidine).*

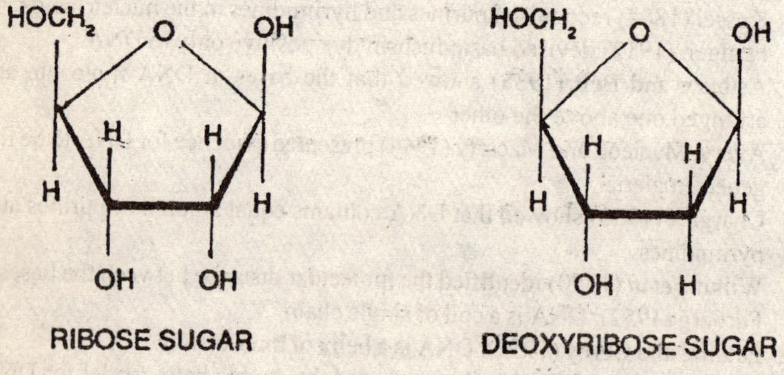

Fig. 4.1 Chemical basis of heredity
Pentose sugars of nucleic acids (left, robose; right dexyribose)

The purines have a double ringed structure. Attached to the six membered benzene ring is a 5 membered imidazole ring. The imidazole ring is joined to the hexagonal ring at 4' and 5' positions. The benzene ring has nitrogen in the 1' and 3' position (replacing Carbon).

There are two types of purines viz. *Adenine* and *suanine.* Adenine has an amino group at the 6' position (*6 aminopurine),* while guanine has an aminogroup at the 2' position and a hydroxyl group at the 6' position (2 *amino, 6 hydroxy purine).*

Sugar

The sugar molecule in DNA is basically a ribose sugar. The ribose sugar is a *Pentose Sugar.* It is a 5 membered ring. The ring consists of four carbon atoms while the 5' C atom is outside thering. Positions 1', 3' and 5' in the ring have OH groups while the 2' carbon position has only H. There is no O; hence the sugar is said to be Deoxyribose (no oxygen in the seconc carbon position).

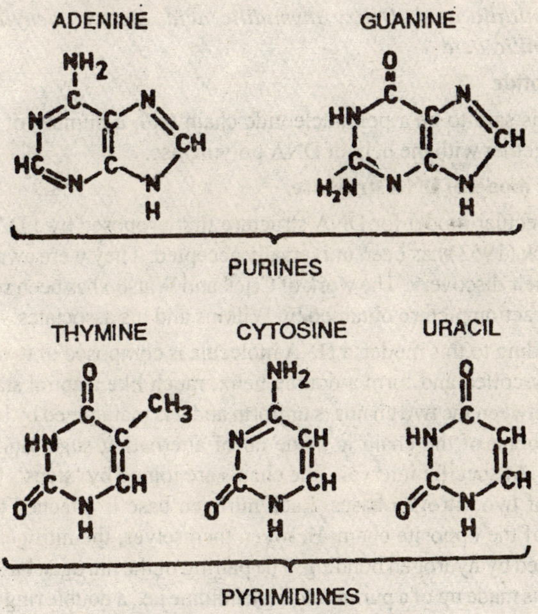

Fig. 4.2 Chemical basis of heredity
Nitrogen bases of nucleic acids

Phosphate

It has one central phosphorus with four oxygen atoms.

Nucleosides

A nitrogen base coupled with sugars forms a nucleoside. DNA has four nucleosides -

(a) Deoxycytidine
(b) Deoxythymidine
(c) Deoxyadenosine and
(d) Deoxyguanosine

The sugar molecule is attached to the nitrogen base to the 3' position in the benzene ring in the case of pyrimidines and to the 9' position of the imidazole ring in the case of purines.

Nucleotides

A nucleotide is derived from the nucleoside by the addition of phosphoric acid molecule to the latter. The phosphate group is usually linked to the two sugar molecules above and below. The linkage is with the 3'C atom of one deoxyribose sugar and with the 5' C atom of another. DNA has four nucleotides - *Deoxycytidilic acid, Deoxy thymidilic acid, Deoxy adenylic acid* and *Deoxyguanilic acid.*

Polynucleotide

DNA is said to be a polynucleotide chain with a number of nucleotides joining together with the help of DNA polymerase.

Molecular model of DNA structure

A molecular model for DNA structure first proposed by J.D.Watson and F.H.C Crick (1953) has been universally accepted. They were awarded Nobel prize for their discovery. The work of Crick and Watson has been supported by X-ray diffraction picture obtained by Wilkins and his associates.

According to this model, a DNA molecule is composed of two chains that are spirally coiled and form a double helix, much like a spiral stairway. The distance between the two chains is uniform and it is maintained by base pairing. The back bone of the chain is made up of alternating sugar and phosphate molecules. At specific intervals, the chains are joined by 'steps'. Each step is made up of two nitrogen bases. Each nitrogen base is attached to the sugar molecule of the opposite chain. Between themselves, the nitrogen bases of a set are joined by hydrogen bonding. The pairing of the nitrogen bases is always specific. It is made up of a purine and a pyrimidine i.e., a double ring and a single ring. Two purines would occupy too much space and can not be accomodated between two chains; similarly two pyrimidines would form a short step and leave a gap between two chains. Hence the pairing is always between a purine and pyrimidine. Because of this pairing,in a DNA molecule, the total purine content is always equivalent to total pyrimidine content.

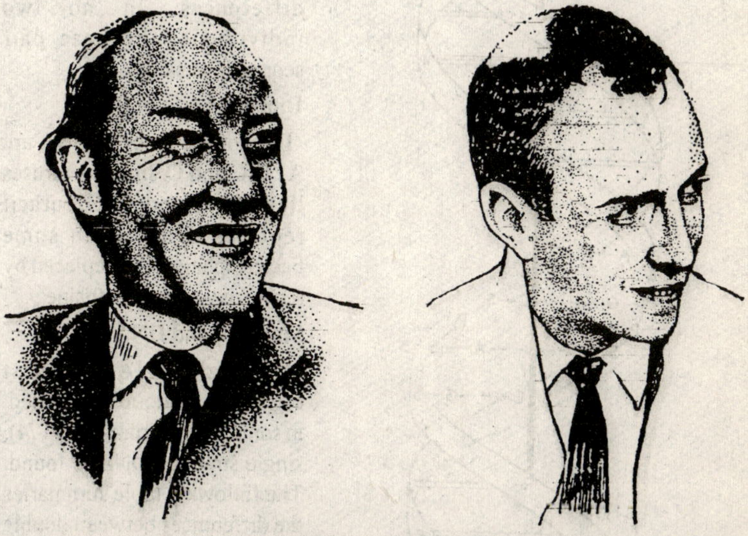

Fig. 4.3 Chemical basis of heredity
F.H.C. Crick (left) and J.D. Watson (right)

The purine, pyrimidine base pairing is further specific. It is always Adenine with Thymine and Guanine with Cytosine. Adenine and Thymine are joined by two hydrogen bonds through atoms attached to position 6' and 1'. Cytosine and Guanine are joined by three hydrogen bonds at positions 6' 1' and 2', the bonding with hydrogen is weak; but this facilitates easy separation of two strands during replication. According to Crick and Watson, the helix has a diametre of 20 A^0 and there is one complete turn to the helix at every 34 A^0 and has a stack of 10 nucleotides at every turn.

One unique character of DNA is its unity and yet infinitismal variety. The DNA structure mentioned above is uniform in all organisms, whether it is man or virus. At the same time it is also true that DNA is the genetic material that decides the characters of individual organisms. Then how does DNA decide the individuality? The answer lies in the base pair sequence. The combination of A/T, G/C is uniform, but their sequence is not; for instance in one individual it may be AT, G/C, GC, AT, GC AT etc. There is no limit to the variety in which base pair sequences are arranged.

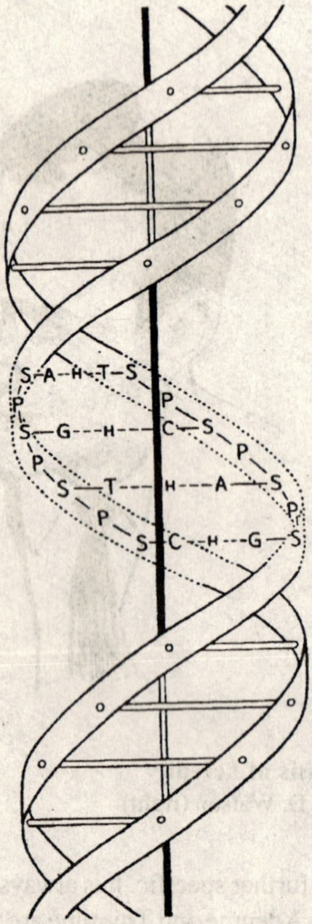

Fig. 4.4 Chemical basis of heredity
The double helix model of DNA

This is the secret of individual differences. In no two individuals, the base pair sequence is same.

Unusual bases in DNA

The normal bases in DNA are A, T, G and C. In some viruses like PBS1 and PBS2 uracil replaces thymine. In some bacteriophages C is replaced by 5 hydroxy methyl cytosine.

Single strand DNA

Although DNA in most organisms is double stranded, in some phage viruses (ϕ x 174), single stranded DNA is found. The following table summaries the differences between double stranded DNA and single stranded DNA.

	Character	Double Strand DNA	Single Strand DNA
1.	U.V. Absorption	Constant from 10-80°C and then rises rapidly	Steady increase from 20° to 90°C
2.	Action of formaldehyde	Resistant	Not Resistant
3.	Ratio of	equal, A=T and 1.33:0.98:0.75	A:T:G:C is
4.	Shape	Linear	Circular
5.	Respiration	Two strands separate and replication begins	Becomes double (replicative form) temporarily.

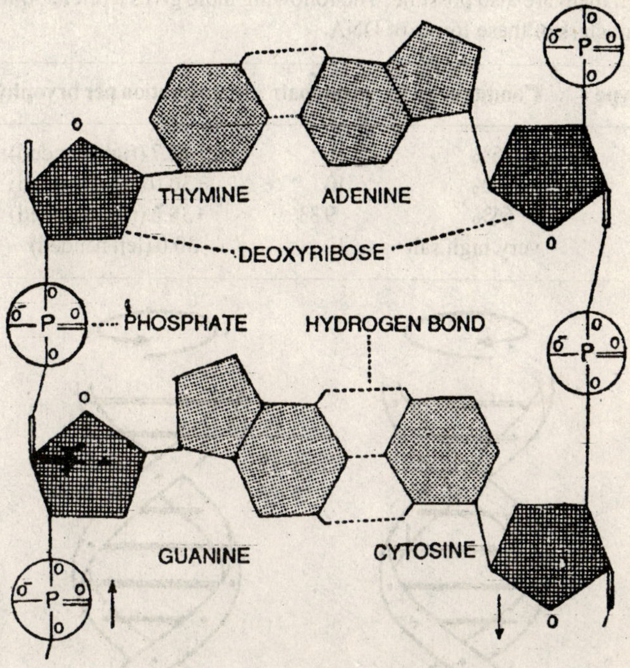

Fig. 4.5 Chemical basis of heredity
Arrangement of nucleotides in a segment of the DNA model

Alternative forms of DNA double helices

The structure of DNA molecule described above as visualized by crick and Watson assumes that the helical coiling of the molecule is right handed and this form of DNA has been called the B-form. Subsequent researches however have indicated that other types of coiling are also possible for the DNA helex. These alternative forms of DNA differ from one another inthe following respects.

1. Number of residues per turn (*n*) and
2. Spacing of residues along the helix (*h*)

The existence of DNA as double helix has also been confirmed by experiments used for measuring the number of base pairs per turn of the helix and this works out to be 10.4 instead of 10 in the B-DNA. This leads to the modification of angle of rotation from 36 to 34.6. Thus it is possible that there could be structural variants of DNA with varying values for *n* and *h*. Three structural variants of DNA A,B and C are known since a long time and transitions between them are also possible. The following table gives a brief summary of the characters of these forms of DNA.

Helix type	Condition	Basepair	Rotation per bryophytes
A	75%	11	+32.7 (right handed)
B	92%	10	+36.0 (right handed)
C	66%	9.33	+38.6 (right handed)
Z	very high salt	12	-30.0 (left handed)

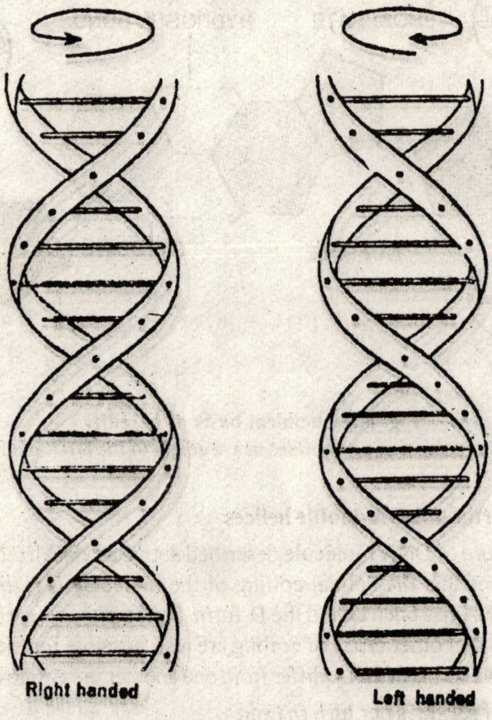

Fig. 4.6 Chemical basis of heredity
Two helices, one showing right handed coil as found in B-DNA and the other showing left handed sense as found in Z-DNA

The forms of DNA are assumed to be found in all molecules depending on the surrounding conditions. In addition to the above D and E forms of DNA are also found very rarely with only 8 and 7.5 base pair per turn. These are found only in some molecules of DNA lacking in Guanine. In contrast A,B and C forms are found in all molecules irrespective of DNA sequence.

Z-DNA

This type of DNA was first synthesized artifically but subsequently has been reported from living cells also. As this molecule follows a zig-zag course it is called Z-DNA. The resemblances and differences between B-DNA and Z-DNA are as follows -

Resemblances between B-form and Z-form

1. Both are double helical
2. The two strands are antiparallel in both forms
3. Both forms exhibit A=T and G=C pairing

Differences between Z-DNA and B-DNA

1. Z-DNA is left handed while B-DNA is right handed
2. The phosphate back bone is regular in B-DNA while it is zig in Z-DNA.
3. In Z-DNA sugar residues have alternating orientations as a result of which repeating units are dinucleotide whereas in B-DNA they are monocleotides.
4. Z-DNA has 12 bp for every twist of 360⁰ while B-DNA has only 10bp.
5. As more base pairs are accommodated in one helix in Z-DNA the angle of twist is 60⁰ as against 36⁰ in B-DNA.
6. One complete helix is 45A⁰ in Z-DNA while it is 34A⁰ in B-DNA
7. The diameter of the helix is 18A⁰ in Z-DNA while it is 20A⁰ n B-DNA

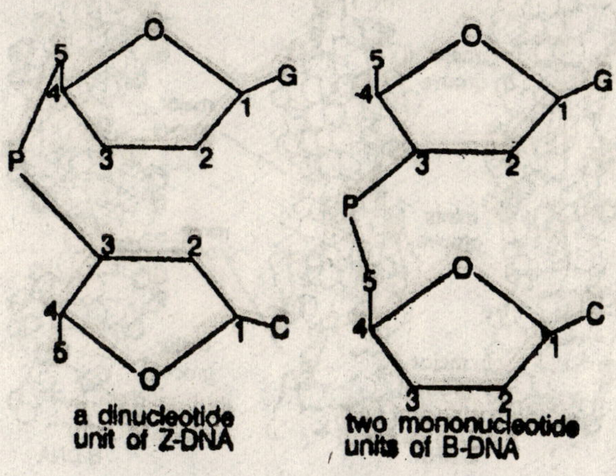

Fig. 4.7 Chemical basis of heredity

Orientation of adjacent sugar residues in Z-DNA and B-DNA showing opposite orientations in Z-DNA and same orientation in B-DNA. This results in dinucleotide units in Z-DNA as against mononucleotide units in B-DNA

The role of Z-DNA is not certain, even though it is thought to play a role in regulation of gene activity, recombination or rearrangement of DNA.

RL Model

A new model for the molecular structure of DNA has been proposed by Sasisekharan and associates (1976-89) working at the Indian Institute of Science Bangalore. According to them the right handed (R) helix of B-DNA cannot easily explain the unwinding of the coil due to topological differences. Hence they suggested a combination of right handed (R) and left handed (L) helices which they called the RL model. In this model, a B-DNA molecule will have alternating left handed and right handed segments of approximately 5 base pairs in a repeat of 10 base pairs. This model provides conformational flexibility. Many molecular biologists opine that there is strong experimental evidence for the RL model although one is not sure of the continuous length of right and left handed segments in a molecule of DNA.

Super Coiling of DNA

The double helix structure of DNA represents in linear molecule but in living conditions the molecule is a closed structure without free ends. In bacteria the DNA is circular while in eukaryotes also large loops appear to represent part of a circle. As a result of this the DNA becomes supercoiled. One supercoil

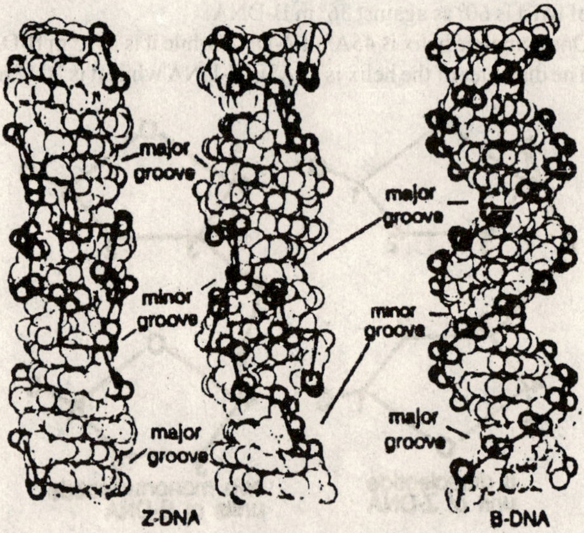

Fig. 4.8 Chemical basis of heredity

Side views of A-DNA. Two views of Z-DNA are 300 apart. Irregularity of backbone in Z-DNA is shown by heavy lines showing the path of phosphate residues, which is quite regular and smooth in B-DNA

is introduced everytime when the duplex is twisted about its axis. The super coil may be negative (winding opposite to the helix coiling) or positive (winding in the same direction as the helix coiling)

RIBONUCLEIC ACID (RNA)

The RNA is also a polymer of nucleotides. These are called ribonucleotides. Each ribonucleotide has three parts viz., a pentose sugar, a nitrogen base and a phosphate group.

The pentose sugar is a ribose sugar much like that of DNA, but with oxygen (present) attached to the 2' carbon position of the ring.

The nitrogen bases are - Adenine and guanine (purines) and cytosine and uracil (pyrimidines).

Molecular structure of RNA

Here also the back bone is made up of alternating sugar and phosphate. The single chain folds to enable the base pairs to meet here and there to form the steps. The pairing is between A-U and C-G. Occasionally the RNA may be double stranded but does not form a helix like DNA.

Single stranded RNA is the genetic material in plant viruses, poliomyletis viruses etc. Double stranded (non helical) RNA occurs as the genetic material in reoviruses.

Types of RNA

The following are the types of RNA found

(a) Genetic RNA
(b) Ribosomal RNA
(c) Messenger RNA
(d) Soluble or Transfer RNA.

Genetic RNA

In certain viruses, RNA is the only genetic material. DNA being absent. This RNA is self replicating; it is called RNA dependent RNA synthesis. The viral RNA directly functions as a messenger and produces RNA polymerase enzyme as well as proteins.

Ribosomal RNA (rRNA)

This is found in the ribosomes. It constitutes about 80% of total RNA of the cell. The base pairs of rRNA are complementary to that part of the nuclear DNA from where they are produced rRNA consists of a single strand folding upon itself at some regions. The folded regions have paired bases, while the other regions have unpaired bases. Due to this in rRNA there is no purine pyrimidine equality.

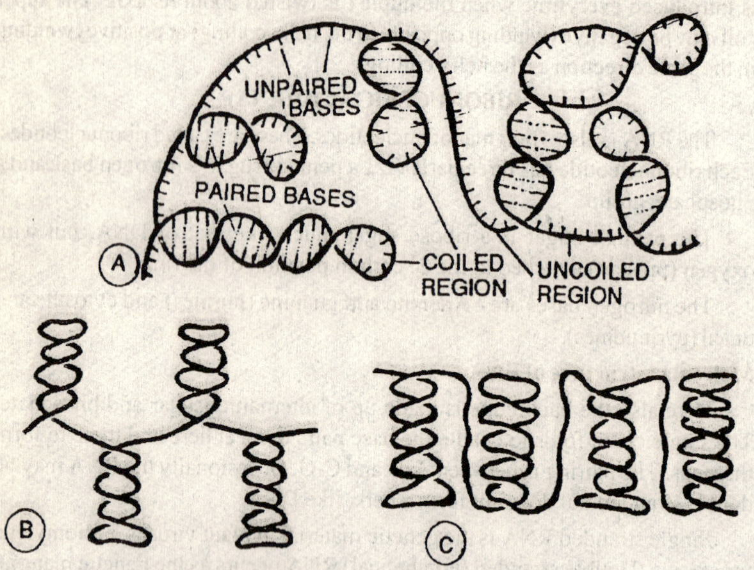

Fig. 4.9 Chemical basis of heredity
Secondary structure of ribosomal RNA (diagrammatic)
A. Extended strand, **B.** Negative interaction showing repulsion,
C. Positive interaction showing association

There are three types of rRNA bases on sedimentation and molecular weight. These are (a) rRNA with molecules weight over a million, e.g. 21s-29s rRNA, (b) rRNA with molecular weight less than a million, e.g. 12s-18s rRNA, (c) rRNA with very low molecular weight (40,000) e.g. 5srRNA.

Messenger RNA (mRNA)

mRNA carries the message from DNA to ribosomes during protein synthesis. It is about 3-5% of total RNA content of the cell.

mRNA has a molecular wieght of about 5,00,000 with a edimentation cefficient of 8s. This however is highly variable mRNA is always single stranded and there is no base pairing, even though random coiling may be observed. The mRNA molecule is produced from the coding strand and its base sequence is complementary to the coding strand. The following are some of the general features of mRNA.

1. *Cap :* This is a blocked methylated structure found at the 5' end of RNA.
2. *Non coding region :* This follows the cap and consists of 10-100 nucleotides. There are no codes for proteins in this region.

3. *Initiating codon :* This region begins the coding
4. *Coding region :* Codes for proteins and has about 1500 nucleotides.
5. *Termination codon :* The coding region is followed by a terminating codon, which stops translation.

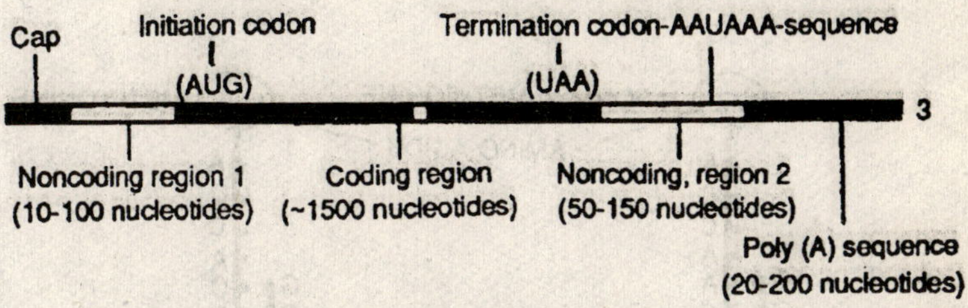

Fig. 4.10 Chemical basis of heredity
General features of eukaryotic mRNA

Transfer RNA (rRNA or sRNA)

The transfer RNA also called soluble RNA, is next in quantity to rRNA. It has a low molecular weight of about 25,000-30,000 and the sedimentation co-efficient is 3.8s. It is made up of about 70-90 nucleotides.

tRNA is synthesised in the nucleus on a DNA template. Only a minute fraction of DNA (0.025%) codes for tRNA. The tRNA molecule consists of a single strand looped around itself with the 3' end always terminating in a C-C-A sequence. Some bases are paired.

The function of tRNA is to carry aminoacids to mRNA during protein synthesis. Each aminoacid couples with a specific tRNA. Since the protein molecule consists of about 20 types of amino acids, there must at least be 20 types of tRNAs. But there could be many more, sinced there are two tRNAs for every amino acid in several cases.

Secondary structure of RNA

This refers to the arrangement of the chain of the molecule to enable it to function in a proper way. Many models have been proposed for the secondary structure of tRNA. Of these, clover leaf model proposed by Holley (1966) is most widely accepted.

According to the clover leaf model, the single chain of tRNA is folded on itself to form five arms. As a result of this folding, the 3' end and 5' end lie adjacent to each other. Each arm consists of a basal stalk, and a loop. The double stranded stalks show the typical base pairing. There could be an exceptional mismatch. The loops do not have base pairing. One of ther arms which does not have a loop is called the acceptor as this is the binding site for amino acids. The second arm is called the DNA arm. This has a synthetase site which recognises the amino acid activating enzyme. The fourth is a variable arm; it has a stem, but the loop may or may not be present. The Tψ arm has a ribosome recognition site.

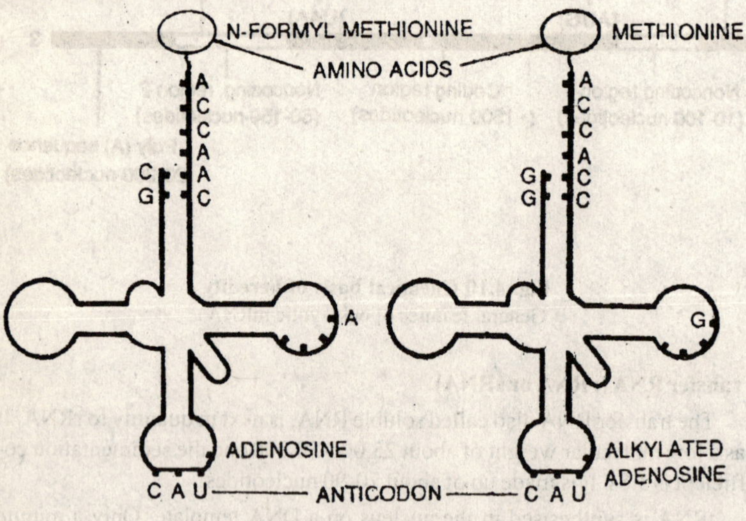

Fig. 4.11 Chemical basis of heredity
Secondary structure of tRNA (Clover leaf model)

There is also a tertiary structure to the rRNA. This is brought about by H bonding between bases, and between bases and sugar phosphate backbone.

5

REPLICATION OF DNA

The DNA molecule regulates all the activities in the cell which includes both metabolism as well as reproduction. Because of its unique structure it is able to control the synthesis of other macromolecules of the cell. At the same time when the cell reproduces, the DNA also should duplicate itself to be able to get distributed equally to the daughter cells. These two unique properties of the DNA molecule can be called *Heterocatalytic* and *Auto catalytic* functions. In the heterocatalytic function DNA regulates the synthesis of other molecules like proteins. In the autocatalytic function which is perhaps very unique to DNA it is able to make copies of itself in a precise and accurate manner. It is this ability of DNA that is responsible for the maintenance of life and inheritance of characters from one generation to another generation.

In this chapter the various aspects of DNA replication is discussed together with a brief account of the enzymes responsible for replication.

Types of Replication

Three different types of replication have been proposed at the molecular level for DNA; these are - Semiconservative, Conservative and Dispersive.

1. Semiconservative

In this model of replication the DNA helix unwinds but there is no rupture of a separated polynucleotide strands. Thus the primary helices of DNA are not completely changed. According to this mechanism the unwinding of the original strand would be followed by the synthesis of complementary strands for each of the two separated original polynucleotide strands. This mechanism was proposed by Crick and Watson the discoverers of the molecular structure of DNA. In this method of replication, after replication of the original molecule, two molecules of DNA are formed. Each one will have one parental strand and one newly synthesised strand. Thus in the semiconservative process, after replication the molecules of the next generation can be regarded as hybrids. The mechanism is called semiconservative because of the two strands of the parental molecule only one strand remains in the molecule whereas the other goes to another molecule.

2. Conservative

In this mechanism the original molecule is complr tely conserved and thus form a part of the second generation molecule. Both the strands of the parental helix will synthesis an entirely new molecule the new molecule synthesized would have both of its strands produced newly. After one generation of application 50% of the molecules will be parental and 50% newly produced molecules. This is called conservative because the original combination of both the parental strands will remain together and will not be separated.

3. Dispersive

In this method of replication the parental DNA helix breaks up at several points forming many fragments. Each fragment of the helix would replicate and recombine at random to produce two daughter molecules of DNA. This is called dispersive because the original combination of the strands is completely disturbed as they get fragmented into bits.

Evidence for the Semiconservative Mode of Replication

Of the three types of replication mentioned above there are overwhelming evidences to support the semiconservative mode of replication. Taylor *et al* (1957) demonstrated by autoradiography that the two chromatids during prohpase have one strand old and one strand new material. This clearly indicates that the replication is semiconservative. The following three experiments have clearly given experimental evidence for the semiconservative mode of replication.

1. Meselson and Sthal's Experiment

Meselson and Stahl (1958) conducted experiments on *E.coli* and demonstrated that the semiconservative mode of replication is correct. In their experiments they used the following two basic principles.

(i) They cultured *E.coli* on a culture medium containing N^{15} (N^{15} is an isotope while normal nitrogen is N^{14}). The bacteria replicated in this medium for a number of generations and as a result both the strands of the DNA molecule now contain N^{15}. In other words, the DNA of the bacterial populaton was now labelled with heavy nitrogen (N^{15}). The labelled bacteria were then transfered to a culture medium containing N^{14} and are allowed to replicate. After the first generation of replication, the molecules of DNA each one possesed one strand with N^{15} and the other strand with N^{14} (this should be the composition of the molecules if the mode of replication is semiconservative). In these molecules the N^{15} strand represents a parental strand and the lighter N^{14} strand presents a newly synthesised strand. Thus each molecule can be regarded as a hybrid DNA (having both N^{15} and N^{14}).

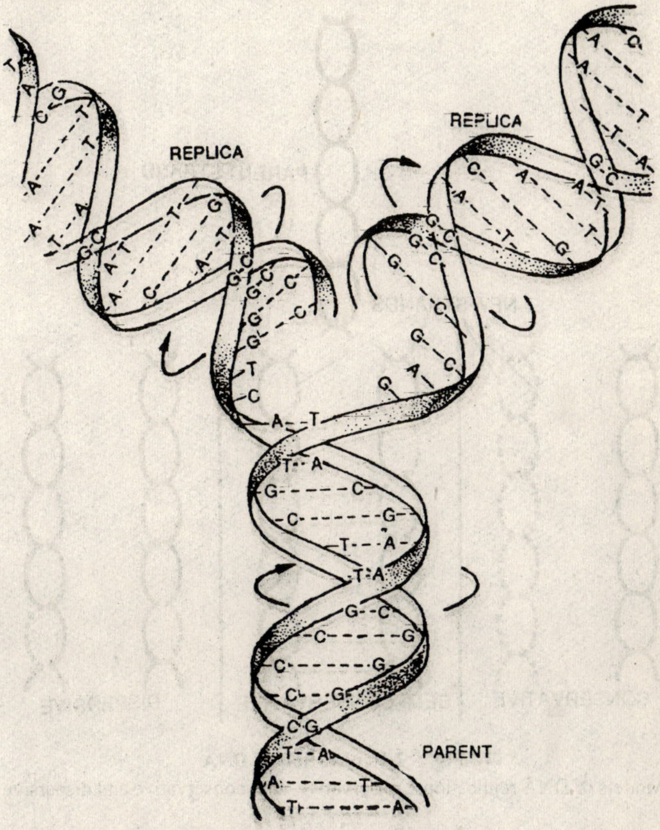

Fig. 5.1 Replication of DNA
Model of replication of DNA

(ii) Meselson and Stahl used the principal of density gradient centrifugation and prepared gradients of Caesium chloride. This density gradient is based on the fact that when heavy salt solutions are subjected to ultra centrifugation a continuous density gradient is set up (heavy would be at the bottom and lighter ones will be at the top with a range in between in the centrifuge tube). When a substance having a density within the range of this gradient is dissolved in salt solution, the substance will find place at its own level of density. Thus with this technique even very slight differences in density can be detected.

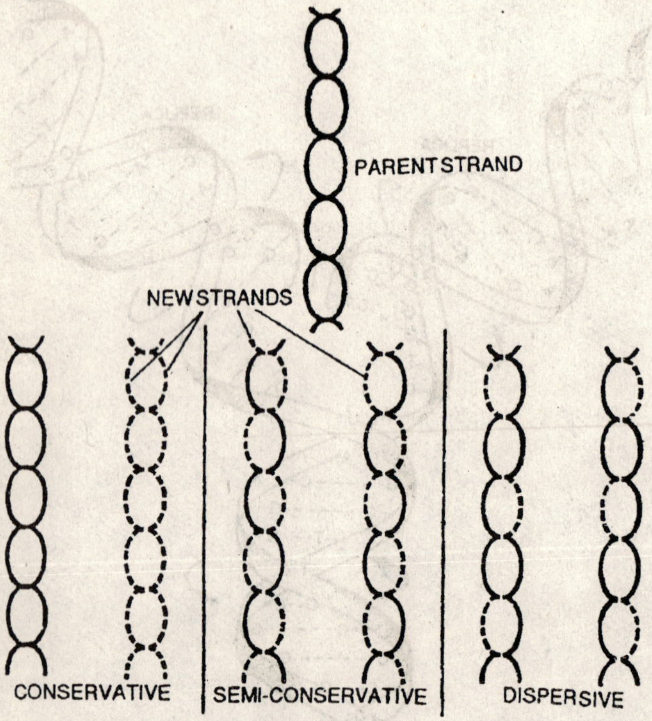

Fig. 5.2 Replication of DNA
Models of DNA replication-Conservative, semiconservative and dispersive

Based on the principles mentioned above Messelson and Stahl subjected the bacterial cultures for density gradient centrifugation. At the first instance N^{15} labelled bacteria were allowed to replicate on a medium containing N^{14}. After the first division the centifugation showed the hybrid DNA had an intermediate density and formed a band inbetween N^{14} and N^{15} indicating clearly that each molecule contains one N^{14} and N^{15}. in the second generation two bands were found one having normal N^{14} and the other having a hybrid (N^{14} and N^{15}). This is expected because the labelled nitrogen - N^{15} is getting reduced as the medium has only N^{14} and the original labelled N^{15} gradually gets decreased in the molecules. In the third generation 3/4ths of the DNA had N^{14} and 1/4th of the DNA was hybrid. If the replication continues for some more generations N^{15} would disappear.

In the above experiment if we assume that the replication is conservative there should be two bands in the centrifuge one with N^{15} and the other with N^{14}

(newly formed molecule). On the other hand if the mechanism is dispersive the molecule should spread all over the medium and should form one continuous band as both N^{14} and N^{15} in different combinations would be there in all the molecules. If the mechanism is semiconservative the first generation would show only one layer having a mixture of N^{14} and N^{15} and in the second generation there would two layers one N^{14} and the other N^{15} and N^{14}. Gradually N^{14} would show greater band width and N^{15} would decrease. (Note. In the dispersive mode also only one band is formed in the first generation and it continues to be so for the second generation also. Where as in semiconservative mode two bands are formed in the second generation).

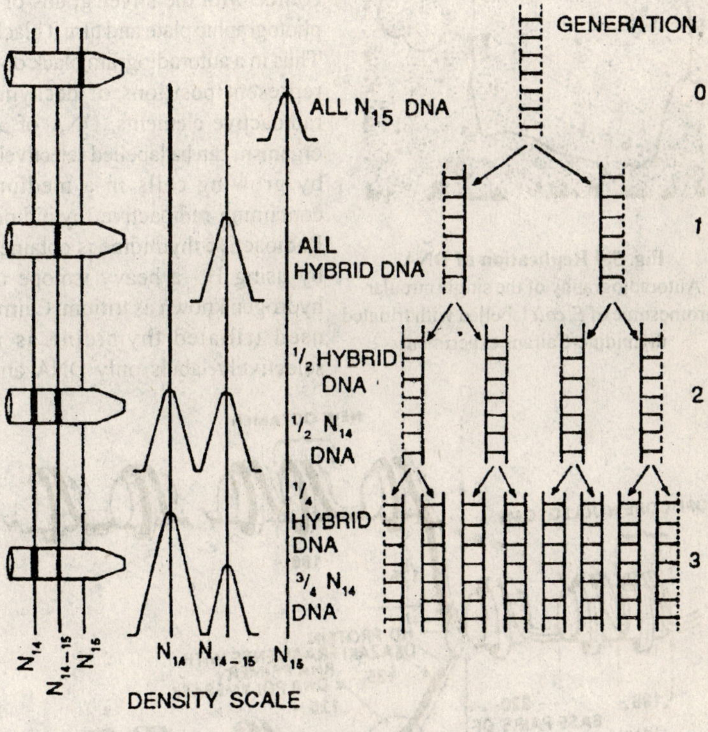

Fig. 5.3 Replication of DNA
Meselson and Stahl experiment in support of the semiconservative model of DNA replication

The above explanation clearly demonstrates that the semiconservative mode of replication proposed by Watson and Crick is the actual method of replication.

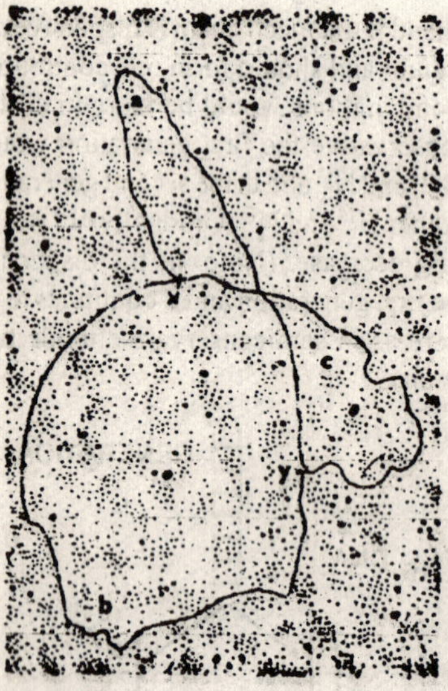

Fig. 5.4 Replication of DNA
Autoradiography of the single circular chromosome of *E.coli* labelled with tritiated thymidine-Cairans experiment

2. Cairn's autoradiographic experiment

The semiconservative mode of DNA replication has been proved in the chromosomes of *E.coli* by autoradiographic experiments conducted by Cairns.

Autoradiography is based on the fact that decaying radioactive elements emit electrons which collide with the silver grains of a photographic plate and turn it black. Thus in a autoradiogram black dots represent positions of decaying radioactive elements. DNA of an organism can be labelled selectively by growing cells in a medium containing radioactive thymidine. Radioactive thymidine is obtained by using H_3- a heavy isotope of hydrogen known as tritium. Cairns used tritiated thymidine as it selectively labels only DNA and

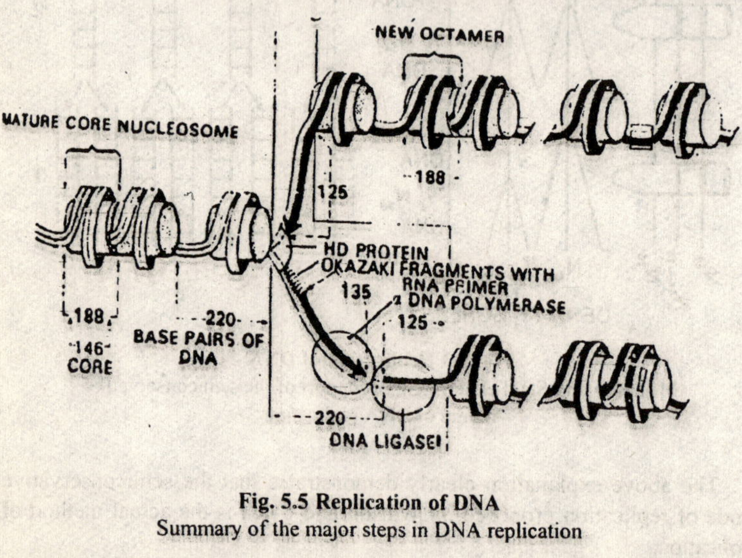

Fig. 5.5 Replication of DNA
Summary of the major steps in DNA replication

not RNA, because thymidine base is found only in DNA and not in RNA. By growing *E.coli* in the culture medium containing tritiated thymidine, radioactivity was incorporated in the daughter DNA molecules. The material (DNA) was extracted and mounted on a photographic emulsion for autoradiography. The labelled DNA exposes the film producing a diffused profile of DNA molecule. The duplicating molecule showed a replication fork. After the replication the radioactivity was found incorporated in only one strands of DNA and in the second generation both the strands become labelled and this will be clearly seen on the photographic emulsion because of the presence of black dots.

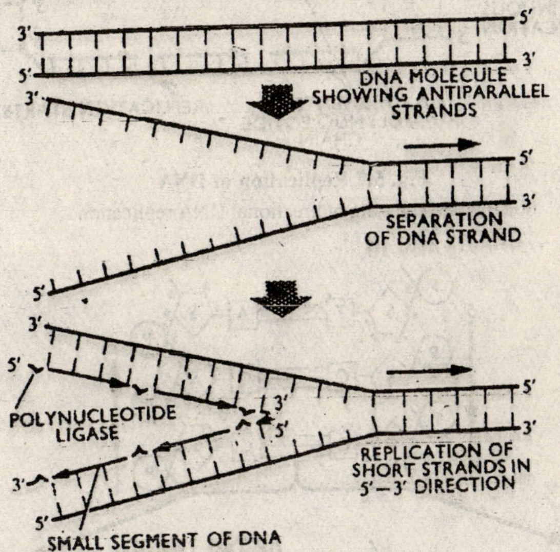

Fig. 5.6 Replication of DNA
Diagrammatic representation of discontinuous synthesis of DNA

This experiment also clearly shows the mode of replication is semiconservative because after the first replication, each molecule will have only one labelled and the other non tritiated strand. In the second generation both the strands are tritiated in some molecules and in the other hybrid - one tritiated other non tritiated strands occur.

Mechanism of replication

The mechanism of DNA replication in is as follows -

1. *Stage of replication during cell division* - It has been observed that replication takes place during interphase between two mitotic cycles. During interphase the amount of DNA doubles due to synthesis. However, DNA synthesis does not take place during the entire interphase. It is confined to the S phase.

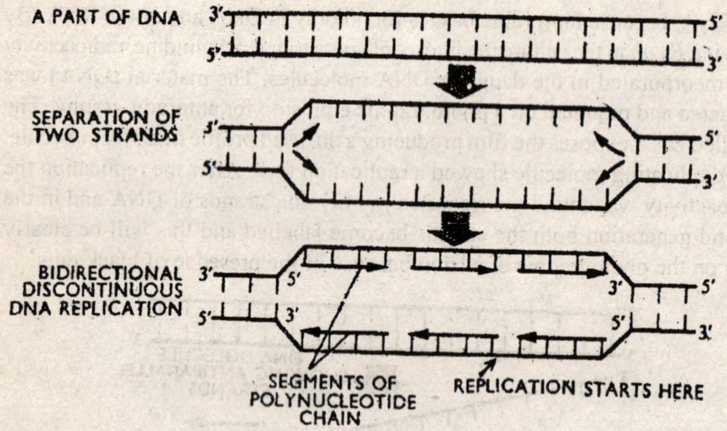

Fig. 5.7 Replication of DNA

Diagram showing bidirectional DNA replication

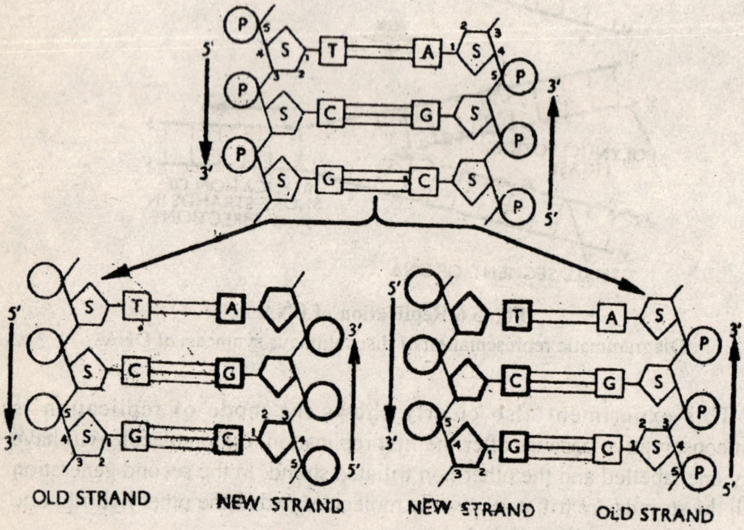

Fig. 5.8 Replication of DNA

Replication of DNA molecule. The two strands of DNA separate and each of them synthesizes its counterpart, thereby forming two similar molecules of DNA

2. *DNA Synthesising Genes* - In *E.coli* the overall process of replication requires the products of the genes *dnaA, dnaB, dnaC-D, dnaE,* and *dnaG.* The gene products of A, C and D ae required for the initiation of fresh

replication and the products of E and G are required for the fork movement for replication. The product of G appears to be necessary for initiating the synthesis of DNA fragments. The *E.coli* also possesses a gene for the origin of DNA synthesis which is about 74 minutes from the beginning. There is also a gene for the termination of the replication. There are additional genes to control the synthesis of the three DNA polymerase enzymes. PolA and polB regulate the synthesis of polymerase I and polymerase II enzymes while G and E regulates polymerase III enzyme.

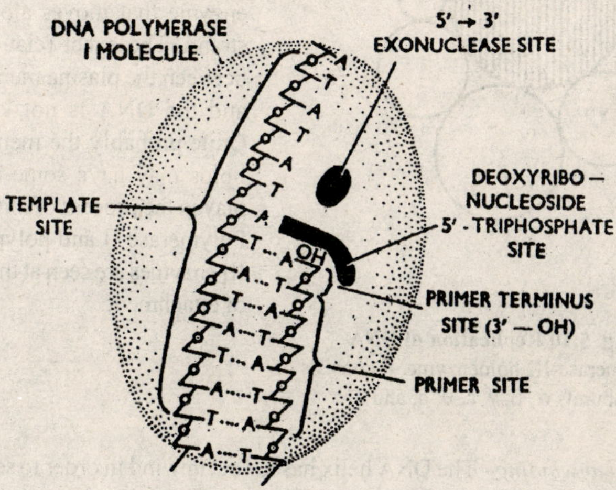

Fig. 5.9 Replication of DNA
A molecule of DNA polymerase-1 showing specific binding sites

3. *Initiation of replication with a nick* - Unlike in the case of eukaryotes when the molecules are linear in prokaryotes the DNA molecules are circular. As such there has to be break in the circle to begin replication. The DNA consists of many replicating units or replicons. According to one hypothesis replication is initiated only after a break or nick in one of the two parental strands. The cut is presumed to take place in the helix at a specific initiation point. This cut or incision is made by a specific endonuclease enzyme.
4. *Origin of replication* - Replication does not begin randomly it always begins with a specific site called *ori* site and is regulated by a gene and its product. It has been discovered that in *E.coli* the origin of replication point as about 74 minutes on the map.
5. *Role of plasma membrane* - There are evidences to indicate that *E.coli* consists of an enzyme complex at the point of attachment of DNA to the

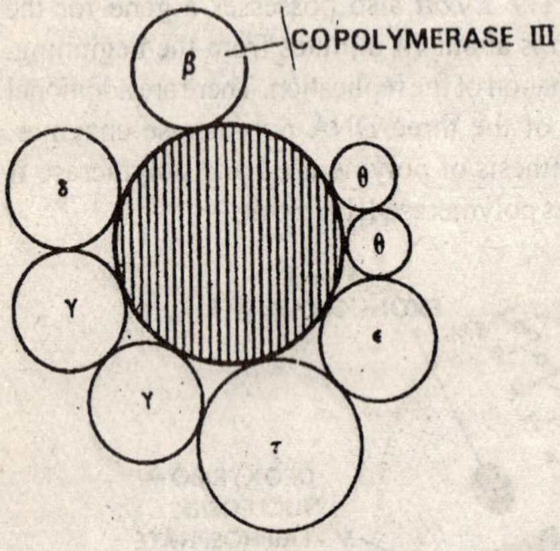

Fig. 5.10 Replication of DNA
DNA polymerase-III holoenzyme, it consists of subunits α, β, γ, ε, θ, δ, and ε

membrane. This point of attachment is known as the replicating point. The DNA thread moves through the replicating point and duplicates itself in the process. In this process the replication is exactly opposite of what is seen in eukaryotes where it is the enzyme that moves along the strand. The exact relationship between the plasma membrane and the DNA is not known. Quite probably the membrane lipids may have some role to play in the process of initiation. Polymerase II and polymerase III enzymes are seen at the point of attachment.

6. *Strand unwinding* - The DNA helix has to first unwind in order to separate the two strands for beginning the replication. A study of the unwinding process in T_2 bacteriophages shows that each DNA molecule has to undergo 20,000 rotations in unwinding during replication. As the molecule itself consists of 2 lakh nucleotide pairs, in these phages replication must go on simultaneously along with unwinding.

   The unwinding of the helix is controlled by enzyme proteins commonly referred to as DNA unwinding proteins. These proteins selectively bind to the single strands of DNA and promote unwinding of the coil. The region of the double helix where the proteins bind forms a Y shaped structure called the replication fork. It has been found out that nearly 200 molecules of the proteins are found at each fork.

   Chemical analysis of the DNA unwinding protein shows that each molecule is a tetramer having 4 sub units. Experimental evidence in *E.coli* has shown that the addition of DNA unwinding proteins to the medium increases the phase of the unwinding of the DNA molecule.

7. *Role of Swiveling Protein* - As the replication fork moves downwards along the parental strands, unwinding begins. For every ten nucleotides

there will be one rotation of unwinding. As the original configuration of the molecules is in the form of a wound helix in circular DNA molecules present in prokaryotes untwisting or unwinding imposes a strain. To some extent this strain can be releived by additional twisting called super twisting in the unreplicated part of the DNA. However this super twisting has a limit and ultimately even the supertwisting should be unwound for the replication fork to continue. The releiving of the strain imposed by unwinding in brought about by proteins called superhelix relaxing proteins. These proteins introduce small cuts in the non replicating region of DNA thereby making one strand to rotate upon the other; thus releiving the strain. The breaks can then be healed by ligation.

8. *DNA Template* - To synthesis a fresh strand of DNA apart from the enzymes the most important requirement are the nucleotides and a DNA template. The 4 nucleotides are adenine, guanine, cytosine and thymine. The previously existing DNA can serve as a template on which can be assumbled fresh nucleotides.

   The template DNA can be either single stranded or double stranded. Single stranded DNA is found naturally in some bacteriophages. Template DNA acts as a mould on which new strand of DNA is synthesised by complementary base pairing.

9. *RNA Primer* - DNA synthesis cannot be initiated on a DNA primer. DNA polymerase enzymes can initiate DNA synthesis only if there is a RNA primer. In other words synthesis of a fresh strand can begin only if there is a small piece of a strand already. This small piece which is RNA is called RNA primer. The RNA primer is a short polynucleotide chain synthesised by the DNA template close to the point of replication. In all probability this is catalysed by a modified RNA polymerase enzyme. It has been noticed that in *E.coli* RNA polymerase is necessary to begin the replication.

10. *Elongation of chain* - Synthesis of new DNA strand takes place by the addition of fresh nucleotides to the 3'-OH group of the last nucleotide in the RNA primer. This synthesis takes place in 5'→3' direction and the enzyme that catalyses this is DNA polymerase III.

    The newly synthesised DNA chain has an RNA primer attached to its 5' end. After the synthesis of the chain, the RNA primer is hydrolysed by the exonuclease activity of DNA polymerase I. The resulting gap left by the RNA primer is filled by DNA nucleotides by the catalytic activity of DNA polymerase I. The freshly formed nucleotide chain is joined to the existing chain by the lygase enzyme.

    Several opinions have been put forward to account for the presence of an RNA primer to initiate the synthesis of DNA chain. According to one opinion if any errors occur during the initial synthesis it can be eliminated when the RNA primer is removed.

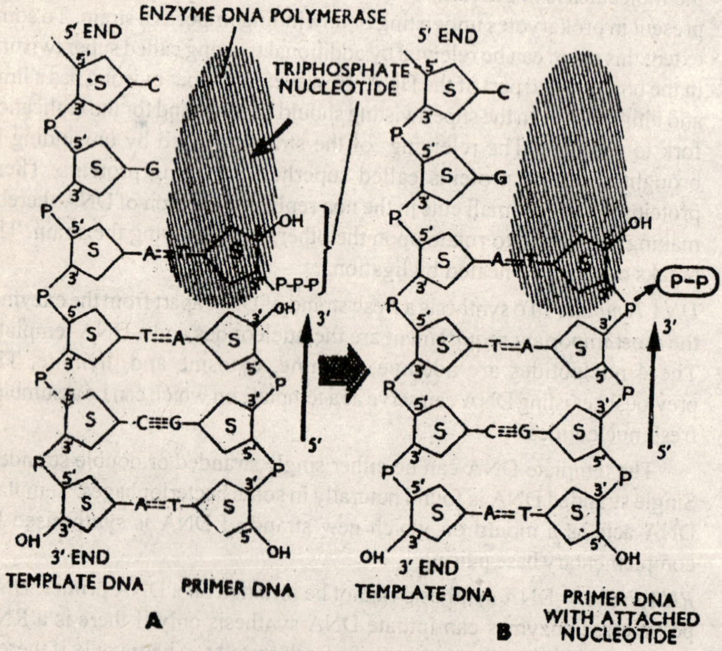

Fig. 5.11 Replication of DNA
Diagram showing action of DNA polymerase in DNA replication

11. *Direction of Replication* - It has been seen that in prokaryotes the replication may proceed in one or both directions from the point of origin. Thus replication may be unidirectional or bidirectional. Bidirectional replication has been seen in *E.coli, Bacillus subtilis, Salmolella, typhimirum, E.coli* phages etc. Unidirectional replication has been reported bacteriophages P2 and 186 and also in the mit DNA of mouse LD cells. Bidirectional replication has an advantage in that the origin is completely duplicated before the complication of replication.
12. *Formation of Replicating Forks* - At the point where the two strands get separated to initiate replication a replicative fork is found. The shape of the replicating fork is in the form of the English alphabet Y. When bidirectional replication takes place, the separated strands between the two forks appear like the bubble or a convex lens under the electronic microscope. The speed of movement of the two forks need not be the same.

In organisms like *E.coli* where the chromosome is circular there will be only two replicating forks, where as in eukaryotes there could be several thousand replicating forks. These large number of forks is due to the fact that replication begins simultaneously at many points along the length of DNA. Occasionally however even in bacteria when replication is going on at one point another replication may start at another point. This will facilitate in completing the replication in shorter period.

13. *Discontinuous Replication* (Okazaki fragments) - The duplication of the strand of DNA takes place by the movement of replication forks. Replication of the two parental strands will take place at the same time as the fork moves along. However all the DNA polymerase enzymes can enhance the length of the strands only in the 5'→3' direction. The strands of DNA on the other hand polarise in opposite directions. This naturally possess a question as to how can DNA polymerase bring about simultaneous replication. While the enzyme moves forward on one DNA strand, simultaneously it cannot move backward on the other.

Okazaki et al (1968) have provided an answer to the above problem. According to them only one strand 3'→5' is continuously replicated while the other 5'→3' replicates in a discontinuous manner and synthesize only short fragments of DNA. These short fragments have been called Okazaki fragments. The direction of synthesis of Okazaki fragments in opposite to the movement of the replicating fork. Eventually Okazaki fragments are joined together by the enzyme polynucleotide ligase. In prokaryotes the Okazaki fragments are as long as 1,000- 7,000 nucleotides.

According to another suggestion (Okazaki et al) both the strands may replicate discontinuously and the fragments formed may join up later.

Evidence obtained form *in vitro* culture of *E.coli* have shown that both the strands are synthesisd discontinuously.

Enzymes involved in DNA Replication

1. DNA Polymerases - Kornberg (1957) isolated an enzyme from *E.coli* which had the ability to polymerise the nucleotides dATP, dTTP, dCTP and dGTP to form a polynucleotide in the presence of a primer and DNA template. This enzyme was capable of synthesizing new DNA strands by proceeding in 5'→3' direction. Subsequent works of DeLucia and Carims (1969), Knippers (1970) and Gefter et al (1969) showed that in prokaryotic cells there are at least three DNA polymerases - *poly I, pol II,* and *poly III.* Kornberg's DNA polymerase is equivalent to *Pol I.*

Polymerase I - This enzyme does not seem to be necessary as bacterial mutatants lacking this are able to synthesize DNA. *Poly I* seems to be taking part in DNA repair. Structurally poll is a single polypeptide chain with a molecular weight of 1,09,000. Electron microscopic studies of the enzyme have shown that the enzyme has a number of functional sites -

(i) A template site for binding template DNA
(ii) Primer site for binding primer RNA segment
(iii) A primer terminus site for 3' - hydroxyl terminus of primer
(iv) A triphosphate site - locus for incoming deoxy ribonucleotide 5' group
(v) Exonuclease site for 5'→3' exonuclease activity.

Polymerase II - This is a single polypeptide chain with a molecular weight of 90,000, *E.coli* cell has about 40 molecules of *pol III*. It helps in 5'→3' polymerization.

Polymerase III - Discovered by Kornberg and Gefter (1972) it is the most active among all the three enzymes. The enzyme is chiefly responsible for DNA chain elongation. It has a molecular weight of 5,5000. The enzyme also acts as 5'→3' and 3'→5' exonuclease..

DNA ligase. Also known as polynucleotide ligase, this enzyme joins the two fragments by catalysing the synthesis of a phosphodiester bond between a 3'-OH group at the end of one chain and 5'→3' - OH group at the other end of the other chain. The enzyme is necessary to join Okazaki fragments which are produced after discontinuous replication.

The enzyme has been isolated from *E.coli*. It is made up of a single polypeptide chain and has a molecular weight of 70,000. Each cell of *E.coli* is known to posses 2000-4000 molecules of this enzyme. DNA ligase has the following functions.

1. Joins Okazaki fragments during DNA replication
2. Helps in sealing single strand nicks in DNA duplex
3. Joins free ends of DNA (linear molecule) to form a circular chromosome.
4. Joins the segments of DNA during recombination during meiosis.

MODELS FOR DNA REPLICATION (IN PROKARYOTES)

Jaboc and Brenner's Model

Studies with phase contrast microscope have shown that in the dividing cell, the sister chromosomes get oriented equidistantly inside the cell. In eukaryotic cell, this separation is achieved by the mitotic spindle. In prokaryotes like bacteris such a mechanism is lacking. Jacob and Brenner have proposed a model to explain the replication and separation of daughter chromosomes. According to this model, the chromosome gets attached to the mesosome at the point of origin of replication. After the completion of replication, a new membrane attachment site is formed adjacent to the old one. The strand which has acted as a template remains a circle, while the newly formed one is broken. One of the free ends of the newly formed chromosome attaches to the new binding site. During replication, the replicating fork and the enzyme system remains stationary while the DNA molecule moves along and gets replicated. Simultaneously a new membrane is synthesized between the two and the two genomes get separated. The newly synthesized DNA becomes circular eventually.

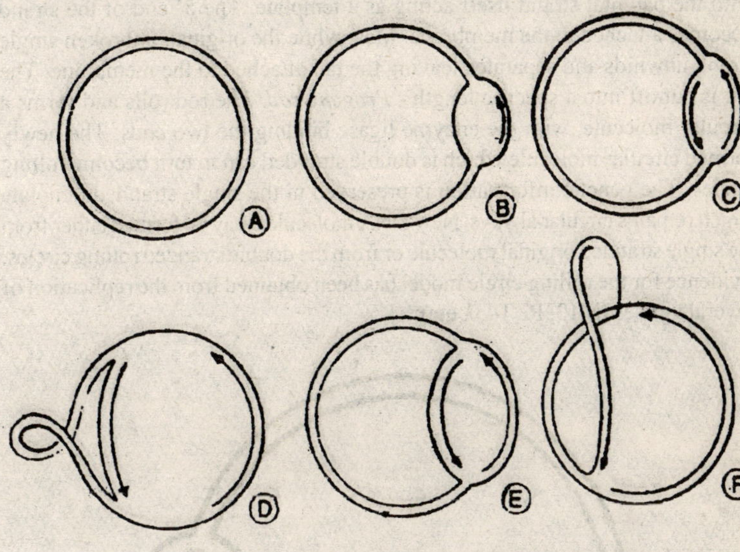

Fig. 5.12 Replication of DNA
Cairn's model for circular DNA replication

Carin's Model

At a specific point (origin) the DNA breaks and replication begins and proceeds in two opposite directions. As the replication proceeds, the DNA strand unwinds. This unilateral unwinding (the other cannot unwind freely) creates a pressure and it is transfered to the unreplicated part resulting in supertwisting. This results in the stoppage of replication. To begin replication once again a 'nick' is made in one of the strands by a swivelling protein. This facilitates rotation of the strands and the break is closed subsequently.

Yoshikawa Model

This is a modification of the Cairn's model. According to Yoshikawa, the newly formed DNA strands covalently join to the ends of original chromosome.

Rolling Circle Model

This is the model accepted for the replication of single stranded DNA in Viruses (ϕ x174). The single stranded circular DNA becomes double stranded by the synthesis of another strand starting at the origin. One strand of this duplex ring is now cut at a point by an endonuclease. As a result of this, a linear strand with 3' and 5' end is created. The 3' end serves as a primer for the synthesis of a new DNA strand. The unbroken strand is used for this purpose; with the parental strand itself acting as a template. The 5' end of the strand becomes attached to the membrane. Meanwhile the original, unbroken single strand unwinds and separates leaving the tail attached to the membrane. The tail is cut off into a specific length - *Progeny rod.* The rod rolls and forms a circular molecule, with the enzyme ligase binding the two ends. The newly formed circular molecule which is double stranded can in turn become rolling circles. The genetic information is preserved in the single stranded template which remains circular always. New DNA molecules may be formed either from the single stranded original molecule or from the double stranded rolling circles. Evidence for the rolling circle model has been obtained from the replication of several viruses (M13, P2 T4, λ etc).

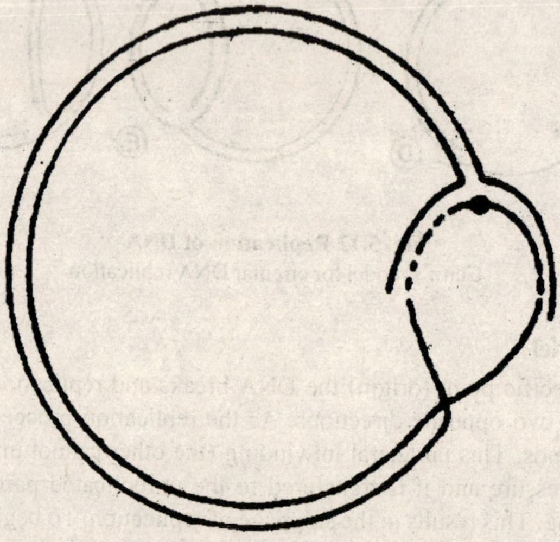

Fig. 5.13 Replication of DNA
Yoshikawa model of a circular DNA replication

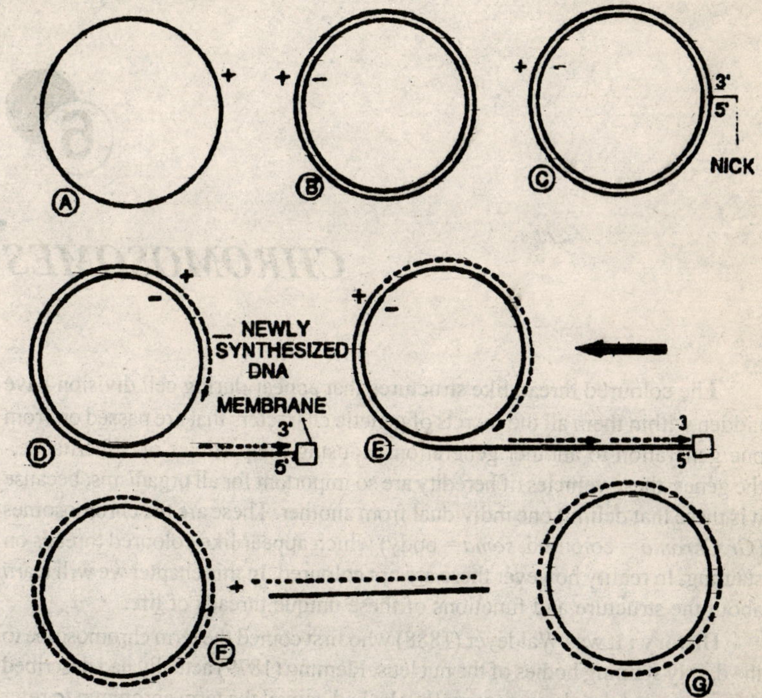

Fig. 5.14 Replication of DNA
Rolling circle model of a circular DNA replication

6

CHROMOSOMES

The coloured thread like structures that appear during cell division have hidden within them all the secrets of genetic characters that are passed on from one generation to another generation. Housing the particles of inheritance,- the genes, these vehicles of heredity are so important for all organisms; because it is these that delimit one individual from another. These are the chromosomes (*Gr.Chromo* = coloured, *soma* = body) which appear like coloured threads on staining. In reality however these are not coloured. In this chapter we will learn about the structure and functions of these unique threads of life.

History : It was Waldeyer (1888) who first coined the term chromosome to the darkly staining bodies of the nucleus. Fleming (1879) actually had described the splitting of the chromosomes, but he had coined the term chromatin to refer to them. Sutton and Boveri (1902) suggested that the chromosomes are the carriers of hereditary particles. Morgan (1933) discovered the role of chromosomes in the transmission of hereditary characters.

Chromosomes occur as a network of Fibrils called chromonema in the interphase nucleus. At the time of cell division the chromonema breaks and condensation takes place forming specific number of chromosomes.

Number of chromosomes : The number of chromosomes is constant for a given species. This number has been evolved during the course of evolution and characterises the species. Chromosome number and morphology is one of the parameters in deciding the phylogeny and interrelationship of the group as well as the individual. The number of chromosome in various species is as varied as the organisms themselves. They range from four to 500.

Ploidy of chromosomes : The total number of chromosomes present in the cell of an organism is called *ploidy.* In all sexually reproducing higher organisms the ploidy is of two types - *haploid* and *diploid.* The somatic cells contain diploid or two sets of chromosomes (2x). In these organisms during reproduction, the chromosome number would be halved in meiosis. As a result, the gametes have haploid or one set (x) of chromosomes. When two gametes fuse, the resultant zygote has two sets of chromosomes (diploid). It is this zygote which develops into the adult individual.

In lower organisms like many algae and fungi, the somatic cells have haploid chromosome numbers. In these organisms only the zygote will have diploid chromosomes. The meiotic division which halves the number of chromosomes takes place in zygote rather than during gamete formation. In some unusual cases (for details see chapter 6.) the cells have many sets (polypoid) of chromosomes, in which case it is a multiplication of the base number called x

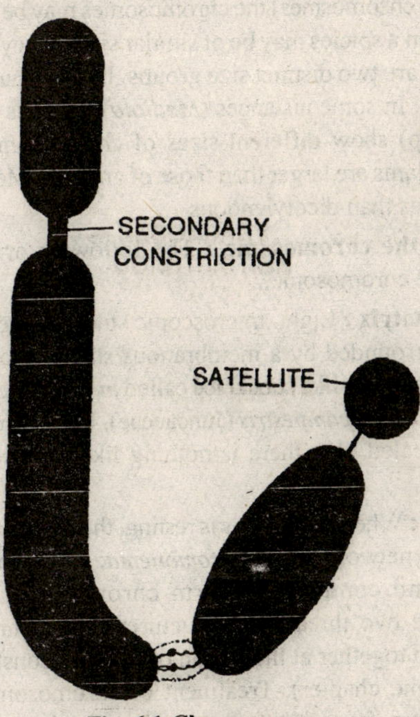

Fig. 6.1 Chromosomes
External view of a metacentric chromosome

Group	Name of the organism	Chromosome number
Protozoa	*Paramecium*	30-40
Coelenterata	*Hydra vulgaris*	32
Nematoda	*Ascaris lumbricoides*	24
Chordata	*Rana esculenta*	26
	Homo sapiens	

Fungi	*Mucor heimalis*	2
Pteridophyte	*Ophioglossum spp*	500
Gymnosperm	*Pinus ponderosa*	24
Angiosperm	*Crepis capillaris*	6
	Allium cepa	

Size of the chromosomes : There is a great variety in chromosome size and shape. In size they range from 0.1 μ to about 30 μ in length. In exceptional cases however (polytene chsomosmes) the chromosomes may be as long as 2mm. All the chromosomes in a spicies may be of similar size or they may vary. In *Yucca arakansana*, there are two distinct size groups. In some human beings there is a gradation in size. In some instances (*Mediola*) the cells at different regions (root and shoot tip) show different sizes of chromosomes. In general, the chromosomes of plants are larger than those of animals. Monocotyledons have larger chromosomes than dicotylendons.

Structure of the chromosome : The following are the parts usually associated with the chromosome.

Pellicle and matrix : Light. microscopic studies have revealed that each chromosome is surrounded by a membranous structure called *pellicle*. This membrane encloses a jelly like substance called *matrix*. The presence of matrix has been shown in *Luzùla campestris* (Juncaceae). Electron microscopic studies however have revealed, that there is nothing like a pellicle enveloping the chromosome.

Chromonema : When the nucleus is resting, the chromosomal material will be in the form of a network called *chromonema*. At the time of cell division these break up and condense to form chromosomes. The metaphase chromosomes have two thread like structures called chromatids. The two chromatids are held together at the region of primary constriction (for details see later in the same chapter). Treatment of chromosomes with a protein hydrolysing enzyme (trypsin) will reveal each chromatid to have two *subchromatids*, but there is no unanimity on this. Various chromosome models have proposed chromonema coils ranging from 2 to 32. The chromonema coils (subchromatids) were first observed by Baranetzky (1880) in the pollen mother cells of *Tradescantia*. It was Vejdovsky (1912) who First gave the name chromonema to these coils. The number of chromonema fibrils not only varies with different species, but at different growth stages in the same cell.

The chromonemal fibrils are coiled around each other in two different ways. These are *paranemic coils* and *plectonemic coils*.

The paranemic coils are loosely coiled and the threads are easily separable from one another. The plectonemic coils however are intertwined very closely so that they are not easily separable.

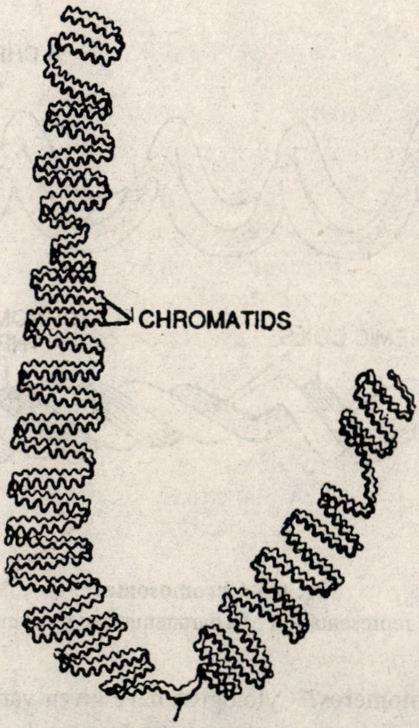

Fig. 6.2 Chromosomes
Internal structure of a metacentric chromosome

The extent of coiling in the chromonema fibrils during cell division depends on the length of the chromosomes. These coiling are of three categories-

Major Coils : Each coil consists 10-30 gyres

Minor Coils : These are at right angles to the major coils and have many more gyres than major coils

Standard or somatic coils : These are coils found in the chromonema of cells during mitosis. They are similar to major coils.

Chromomeres : The chromonema in the chromosomes particularly during mitotic prophase appears to contain alternating thick and thin regions giving a bead like appearance in a chain. The thick bead like regions are called *chromomeres* and the region in between the two chromomeres is called the *interchromomere*. The position of chromomeres in the chromonema appears to be specific to a given chromosome in an individual.

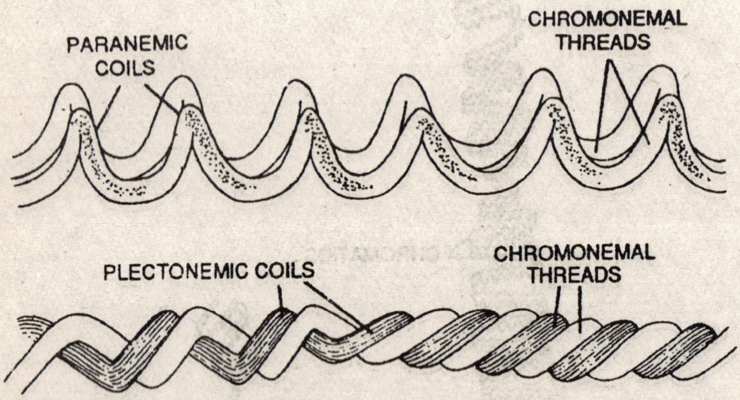

Fig. 6.3 Chromosomes
Diagrammatic representation of a paranemic and piectanomic coiling

What are chromomeres? Cytologists have given various interpretations; while some regard it as the regions of condensed nucleoplasmic material, others interpret it as regions of superimposed chromonemal coils. This view is supported by electron microscopic observations. Previously the chromomeres were mistaken for genes.

The chromomeres were first described by Balbiani in 1876 and later by Pfitzner in 1881. Belling (1928) had equated chromomeres with the genes in liliaceous plants. But McClintock (1944) has shown that genes are located in the interchromomere region of the chromonema. However in case of polytene chromosomes the chromomeric bands are associated with certain regions.

Centromere (primary constriction)

The stained chromosomes reveal a certain region or constriction which stains lightly. This is called *centromere* or *kinetochore or primary constriction*. The centromeres occupy a constant position relative to the ends of chromosomes and are responsible for the various shapes of chromosomes.

The centromere has a diametre of 0.2 μ and may occupy various positions on the chromosome. It (centromere) consists of spherules or granules (*Kinosome*)and interchromomeral fibrillae. The number of fibrillae per centromere varies. The chromonema are less coiled in the centromeric region and hence stain lightly. DNA however is present in the centromeric region (Lime-de-Faria 1955).

Most of the organisms have their chromosomes with a single centromere (*monocentric*). Certain other chromosomes have two centromeres (*dicentric*). In hemipteran insects however the chromosomes have many centromeres (polycentric). Such a centromere is said to be a *diffused centromere*. The proof for centromere being diffuse comes from the fact that when such a chromosome is fragmented by X-Rays, each bit functions like a typical chromosome, replicates itself and participates in the division cycle. Diffused centromere has also been reported in *Luzllla purpurea* of the family Juncaceae (Brown 1954). According to some cytologists chromosomes with a diffused centromere are more primitive than the ones with a localized centromere. The polycentric chromosomes found in the nematode *Ascaris megalocephala* are unique in the sense they are restricted to only those cells which constitute the germ line (Swanson 1957).

The position of the centromere in the chromosome (which is constant to a given chromosome) varies ie., it may occupy different positions. Based on this,four morphological shapes have been identified in chromosomes. These are -

1. Metacentric

The Centromere occupies a middle position with reference to the length of the chromosome. The two arms thus resulted are almost equal in length. During anaphasic movement in cell division metacentric chromosomes appear 'V shaped, eg: *Trillium, Tradescantia* etc.

2. Sub metacentric

When the centromere is located some distance away from the middle region of the chromosome, the position is said to be sub median and the chromosome sub metacentric. As a result, one arm of the chromosome will be shorter than the other. During anaphasic movement, sub metacentric chromosomes appear 'L' shaped eg: Human beings.

3. Acrocentric

In this case, the centromere is situated almost near one end of the chromosome. As a result, one arm of the chromosome will be extremely short and the other one very long. The centromere is said to occupy a subterminal position, Eg: Grass hoppers.

4. Telocentric

When the centromere is situated exactly at one end, the chromosome will be having only one long arm. Telocentric chromosomes are very rare. Truly telocentric chromosomes have been identified by Marks (1957) in certain plants, protozoa and certain mammals. Cleveland (1949) has also reported in certain protozoa inhabiting the digestive track of wood termites, the occurrence of telocentric chromosomes. The earlier report regarding chromosome IV of

Drosophila melanogaster, being telocentric has been disproved as a second arm has been seen.

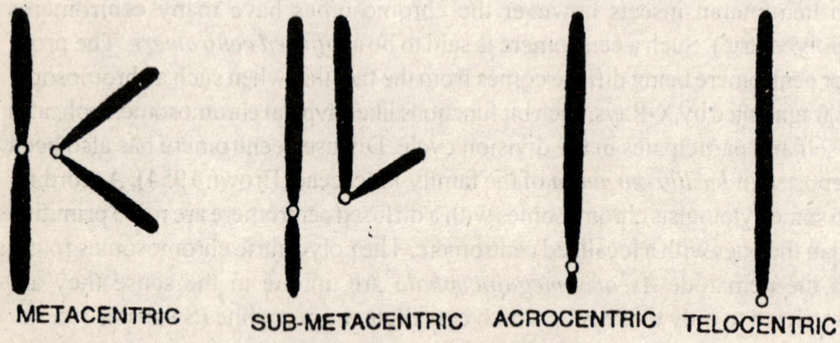

Fig. 6.4 Chromosomes
Types based on centromere position

Acentric chromosome

In certain instances, chromosomes may undergo fragmentation resulting in one fragment without a centromere. Such a chromosome fragment is said to be *Acentric*.

Arm ratio

The ratio of length between the long arm and short arm is said to be the arm ratio, which is constant for a given chromosome. The arm ratio is less in metacentric chromosomes and high in acrocentric chromosomes.

Centromeric chromomeres

The centromere should not be mistaken or equated with a chromomere as the former stains lightly and is a constriction while the latter is a swelling on the chromosome found throughout its length. Metaphase chromosomes which have two chromatids exhibit in their centromere four granular structures. These granules called *centromeric chromomeres* are about 0.5 μ in size and are arranged in a square.

Functions of centromere

1. Centromere provides mobility to the chromosome. Chromosomes lacking in centromere fail to orient themselves properly on the anaphase plate, lag behind and finally get eliminated.
2. Centromeres decide the shape of the chromosome.
3. Centromeres attach themselves to the spindle fibres during anaphasic movement.

4. The centromere divides along the longitudinal axis of the chromosome at the beginning of anaphase. Very rarely the centromere may divide at right angles to the chromosome giving rise to the pieces of centromere, each bit holding the arms parallel to each other and genetically alike (because of duplication) as they represent the replicated parts of a single chromatid.' Such chromosomes with genetically identical arms (having same genes on both arms) are called *isochromosomes* (Darlington 1939).

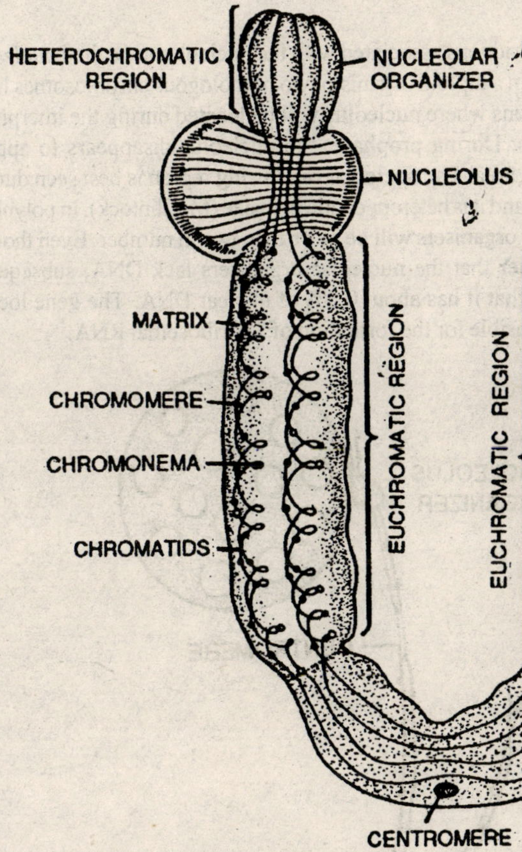

Fig. 6.5 Chromosomes
Structure of a typical chromosome showing a nucleolar organiser

Secondary constrictions

These are lightly staining areas on the chromosome other than centromere. One or more secondary constrictions may be found in the chromosomes. The part of the chromosome (arm) present beyond the secondary constriction is called a satellite. There may be one or two satellites depending on the number of secondary constrictions.

Chromosomes with satellites are called *SAT- Chromosomes* (sine acid thymonucleinico - without DNA). Generally in a genome atleast one chromosome will have a satellite.

Secondary constrictions associated with the nucleolus are called *nucleolar organisers*. Usually in a diploid organism two homologous chromosomes have additional constrictions where nucleolus will be located during the interphase stage of the nucleus. During prophase, the nucleolus disappears to appear again in the identical area. The nucleolar organising region is best seen during the pachythene stage and it is heteropycnotic in maize (McClintock). In polyploid organisms, nucleolar organisers will be more than two in number. Even though it was believed earlier that the nucleolar organisers lack DNA, subsequent studies have shown that it has about 0.3% of nuclear DNA. The gene loci at this region are responsible for the formation of 28*s* ribosomal RNA.

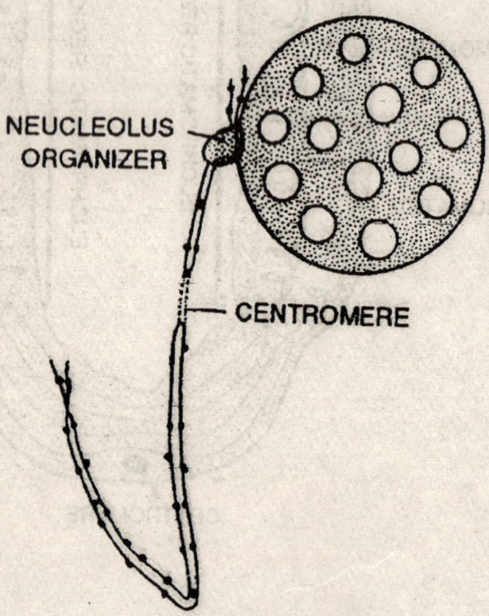

Fig. 6.6 Chromosomes
Nucleolar organiser (enlarged)

Telomeres : The terminal part of chromosomes are called telomeres which have polarity, preventing the tips of other chromosomes from fusing with it. Telomeres however attach themselves to the nuclear envelope during interphase.

CHEMICAL COMPOSITION OF CHROMOSOMES

The two main chemical components of the chromosome are nucleic acids and proteins.

Proteins : Besides nucleic acid, there are three types of proteins in the chromosomes. These are *protamines, Histones and non histone proteins.*

Protamines are basic proteins with a molecular weight less than 4,000. They are rich in amino acid, arginine and are found in the spermatozoa of salmon,herring and other fish, snails and squids. The protamines are helically bound to the DNA. Each polypeptide of protamine consists of about 28 amino acids of which 19 residues are arginine.

Histones are basic proteins associated with eukaryotic nuclear DNA in the ratio of 1:1 in quite a number of plants and animals. They are the main structural proteins of chromosomes.

Based on the amino acid sequence they are categorized into five principal classes HI(H5),H2a,H2b,H3 and H4.

Histones are charecterized by the total lack of *tryptophan,* but have an abundance of *arginine* and lysine. Other modifications of histone proteins are acetylation, methylation and phosphorylation.

Functions of Histones : They act as gene repressors; but this may be a general activity rather than being specific as most of the histones have identical composition. Histones perhaps provide a structural framework for encompassing the DNA molecule.

Synthesis of Histones : In the interphase nucleus, histones are synthesized during the 'S' phase. Some histones may also be synthesized at other stages. The eukaryotic DNA has certain genes called repetitive genes coding for histones.

Non histone proteins : These are acidic proteins with a very high molecular weight when compared with that of histones. NH proteins show great variation in structure in different species. NH proteins are known to inititate genetic activity, while histones are known to depress genetic activity.

DNA, protein association in the chromosome : There are different views regarding the association of DNA with the proteins. It is possible, according to one interpretation that the protamines occupy only the small grooves in the DNA molecule, while histones occupy both the grooves (small and large). Another view is that the histones follow the two helices of the DNA molecule coiling in the same way. According to Dupraw, the histones hold together the DNA molecule in the supercoiled position.

Euchromatin and heterochromatin : Based on the staining reaction two regions may be identified in the chromatin material. These are - *Euchromatin* and *Heteroehromatin.*

The euchromatin stains positively with the DNA specific stains (basic fuchsin) indicating a concentration of DNA. This region is genetically active and stains lightly. The euchromatic regions are supposed to represent areas of less condensation.

Heterochromatin stains more deeply than euchromatin and represents highly condensed regions on the chromosome. In the interphase nucleus, the heterochromatic regions form condensed structures called *chromocenters* or false nucleoli. The following table summarises the differences between euchromatin and heterochromatin.

		Heterochromatin	Euchromatin
1.	**Staining**	Stains deeply	stains less deeply
2.	**Coiling**	Found in the region of more coiling and condensation.	Foung in the region of less coiling and condensation.
3.	**Replication**	Late replication replication in late 'S' phase.	Early replication; replication in early 'S' phase.
4.	**Acetylation**	Does not occur	Occurs.
5.	**Effect of temperature**	Pronounced	Not affected easily.
6.	**Genetic effect**	Inert genetically but few genes are present	Genetically active. More number of genes present.
7.	**Cross over frequency**	Less	Frequent.

Types of Heterochromatin : There are two main types viz., *constitutive heterochromatin* and adaptive *heterochromatin*. The first type shows dark staining reaction (Heteropycnosis) always and in all cells, while the second type shows heteropycnosis only in certain cells or only al certain stages in the cell cycle. Constitutive heterochromatin was originally named satellite DNA (S-DNA). It is mostly inactive during protein synthesis and is repetetive from the point of view of base sequence. Adaptive heterochromatin is metabolically inert and comprises of about 2.5% of genome.

Heteropycnosis : This is the staining phenomenon seen in the chromosomes with reference to heterochromatic and euchromatic regions. The heterochromatic regions which stain deeply are said to exhibit heteropycnosis as against euchromatin which stain sightly. However it should be noted that the heterochromatin always docs not stain deeply with reference to euchromatin. While the euchromatic region is always constant in its behaviour (non heteropycnotic) towards staining (has constant coils), the heterochromatic region may stain deeply or lightly and this is known as *differential heteropycnosis*. Differential heteropycnosis is of two types-positive and negative.

The areas of heterochromatin showing positive heteropycnosis are more condensed and deeper staining than euchromatic region. In areas of positive heteropycnosis there is more of nucleic acids and proteins. Chromosomes with positive heteropycnosis in prophase appear like metaphase chromosomes.

The areas of heterochromatin showing negative heteropycnosis are possibly less condensed and stain lighter than euchromatic region. Chromosomes with negative heteropycnosis have a hazy outline and metaphase chromosomes appear like prophase chromosomes.

CHROMOSOME MODELS

The chromosome consists of DNA and proteins, but the way in which the two are arranged in the chromosome is a matter of debate. The main aspects of the chromosome structure are a) the number of strand or strands of DNA; b) whether the DNA molecule is continuous throughout the length of the chromosome or whether it is interrupted and c) what is the mode of association of protein and DNA.

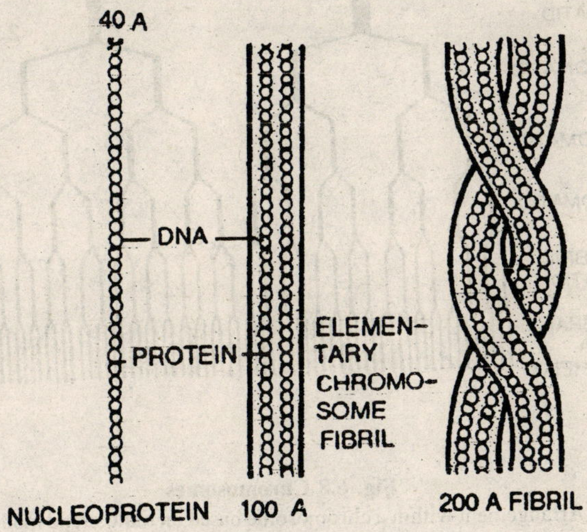

Fig. 6.7 Chromosomes
Ris' multistrand model

Various chromosome models have been proposed and these fall into two basic categories viz. *Multiple strand models* and *single strand models.*

Multiple strand models : According to this, the chromosome consists of several DNA and protein strands. The work of Nebel (1938) on radiation effect on chromosomes have shown that there are at least four sub units. Similarly some models suggest the existence of 4,8,16,32 or even 64 fibrils with each fibril having about 20-40 DNA molecules. The following are some of the multiple strand models-

Simple multistrand model : According to this model proposed by Steffensen (1961), the chromosome has 64 molecules of DNA arranged parallely and twisted around each other. If one agrees with this model, the replication of DNA would be a difficult process.

Ris multistrand model : In this model, the DNA and histone form a complex 40Å wide fibril. Two such Fibrils according to Ris (1961) combine to form an *elementary chromosome fibril*, two of these again combine to form a fibril which is 200 Å wide. These fibrils form the chromatids. Each chromatid has 16 to 32 elementary chromosome fibrils. But there is no experimental proof for this work. In fact Ris himself rejected this model later.

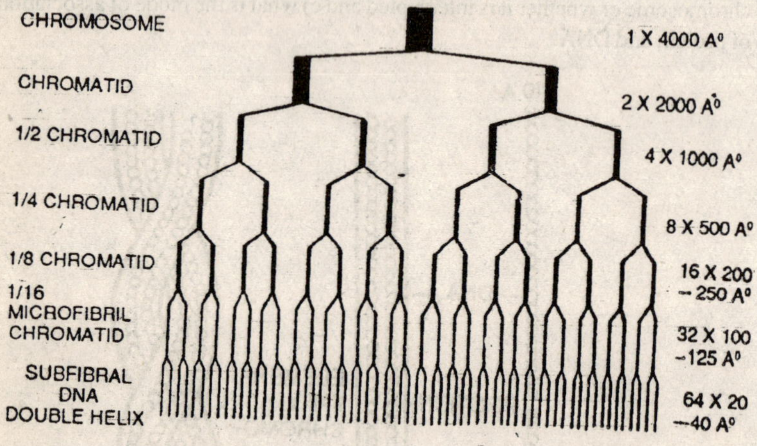

Fig. 6.8 Chromosomes
Arrangement within a chromosome based on multistrand model

Single strand models : Most of the current evidence available indicates that the chromosomes (barring the abnormal chromosome) are made up of a single strand of DNA. Experimental evidence by X-ray radiation have suggested the whole of the chromosome is composed of one single coiled molecule of DNA. The following are some of the single strand models.

The Freese-Taylor model : According to this model originally proposed by Freese (1958) and later modified by Taylor (1959), there are two chains of proteins with the DNA molecule attaching itself to these like the rungs of a ladder. The protein linkers maintain the shape of the DNA molecule. The two protein chains get closely appressed in the chromosome resulting in the coiling of DNA.

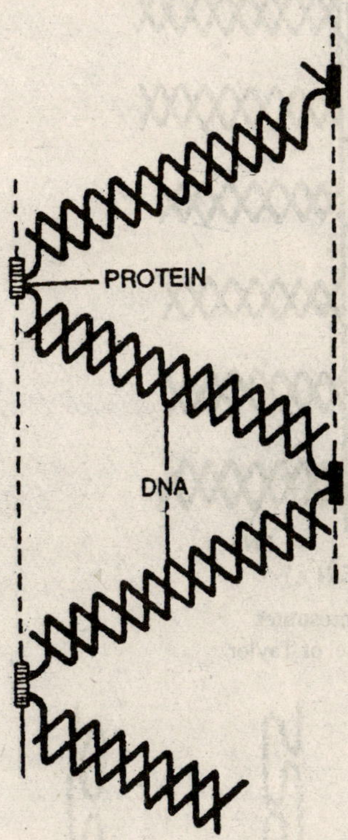

Fig. 6.9 Chromosomes
The Freese-Taylor model

The original model suggested by Taylor (1957) is called the *side chain model* or *centipede model*. According to this model, the chromosome consists of a central backbone of protein from which the loops of DNA spring up like the legs of a centipede. According to him, replication is possible when the protein backbone made up of two chains, separates longitudinally into two and in the process separates also the DNA coils, with each strand having a single strand of DNA. But this is not in conformity with the linear arrangement of the genes on the chromosome.

Nebel's coiled coil model : According to this, the chromosome is made of a single fibril which is coiled in a complex manner.

Ris' modified model : After discarding his earlier multistranded model Ris (1967) suggested, that the chromosome fibril (see his earlier model) is folded to form a 100Å wide nucleo - histone fibril. The nucleohistone fibril folds because of calcium bridges to form a 250Å wide *basic fibril*. Further folding of the basic fibril forms the chromosome.

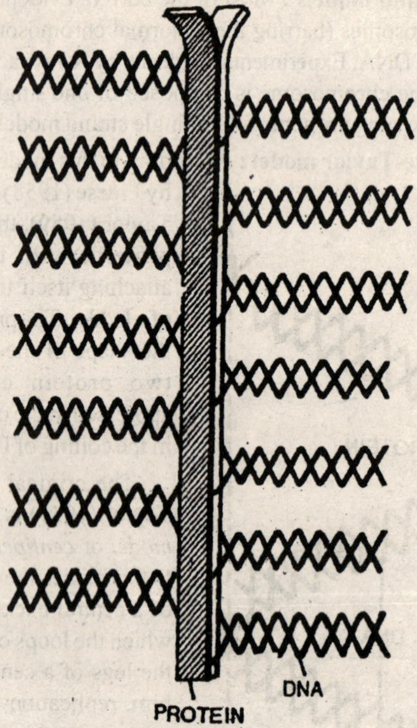

Fig. 6.10 Chromosomes
The centipede model of Taylor

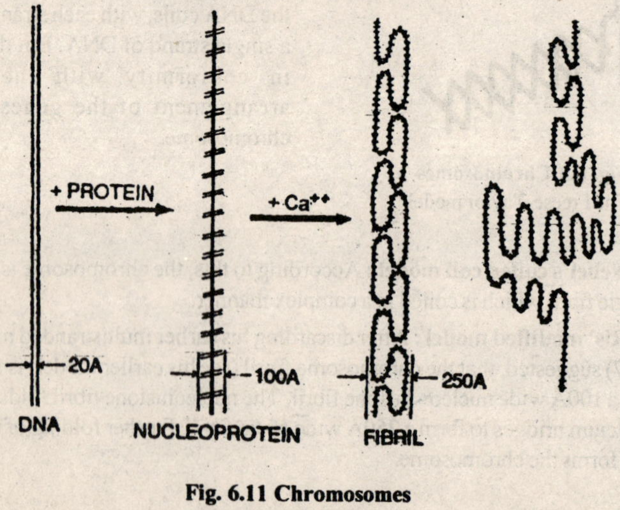

Fig. 6.11 Chromosomes
Ris' modified model

Folded fibre model of Dupraw (1966). While studying leucocyte (human) chromosomes Dupraw observed that the chromatids have folded fibres of 200-500Å width. As he did not find many free ends it was concluded that there must be a single strand of DNA which is highly folded.

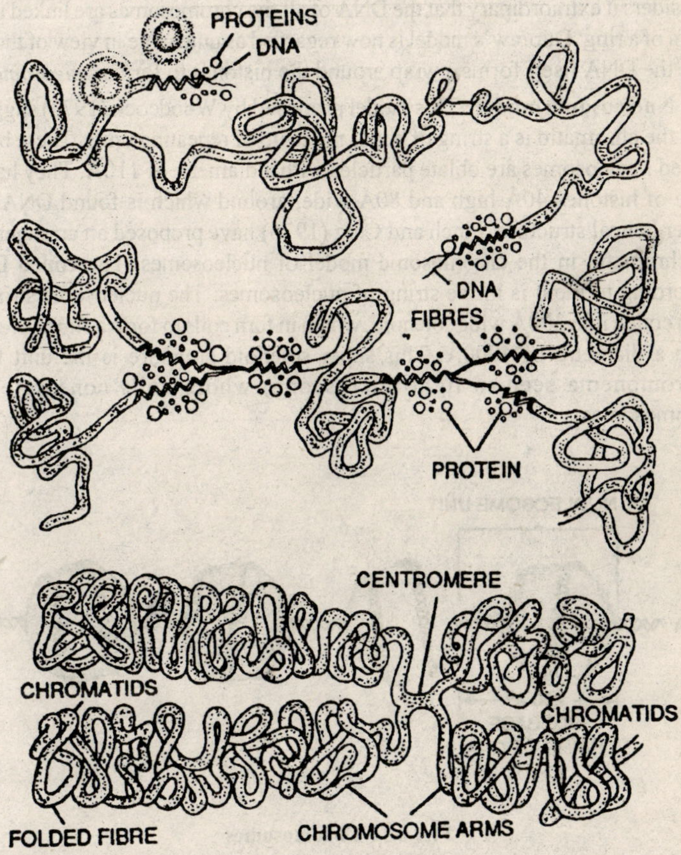

Fig. 6.12 Chromosomes
Folded fibre model of Dupraw

The essentials of Dupraw's model are basically like that of Ris' model with some variations. According to this, the 20Å DNA is packed in protein to form a fibril. The fibril gets coiled and forms a 100Å wide *type A fibre.* The DNA is packed in this fibre in the packaging ratio of 6:1 (packaging ratio is the ratio between the condensed length and the extended length). The type A fibre is coiled in the ratio of 10:1 to form type B fibre which is 200-250Å wide. The type B fibre is extensively folded to form the chromatid. This has been supported by many workers (Me Dermot 1968, Fedric 1969, Lamport 1969 etc). Though many scientists have supported Dupraw's view, White, M.J.D (1973) strikes a discordant note when he does not agree with the folded fibre model and he considers it extraordinary that the DNA of all the chromosomes are linked in the form of a ring. Dupraw's model is now regarded as untenable in view of the fact that the DNA itself forms a wrap around the histones to form *nucleosomes*.

Nucleosome model : This model proposed by Woodcock (1973) suggests that the chromatid is a string of beads made up of repeating units. These beads called nucleosomes are oblate particles with a diametre of 110Å. They have a core of histones 40Å high and 80Å wide, around which is found DNA in a super helical structure. Finch and Clug (1976) have proposed an arrangement of chromatin in the chromosome model of nucleosomes. The coiled DNA according to them is in the string of nucleosomes. The nucleosome string is then coiled into 300Å wide solenoid, which in turn coils to form a *supersolenoid* with a diametre of 4000Å. This super solenoid structure is the unit fibre (chromonema seen in light microscope) whose coils constitute the chromosomes.

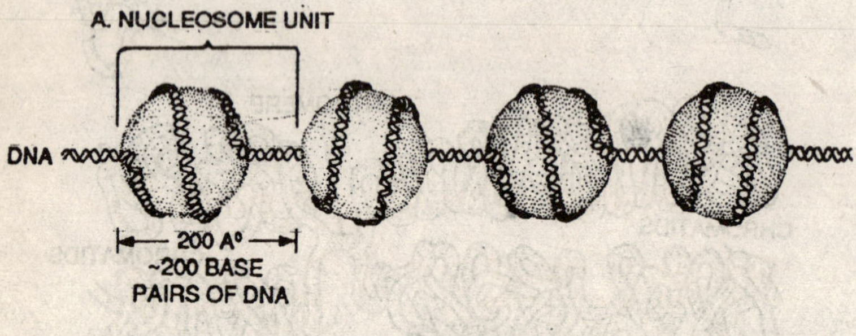

Fig. 6.13 Chromosomes
Nucleosome model

The exact nature of the chromosome arrangement of proteins and nucleic acids may be said to be still an open question.

UNUSUAL CHROMOSOMES

The above discusion on chromosomes pertains to normal ones. There are however abnormal or giant chromosomes encountered in many instances. These are – The *polytene* chromosomes in the salivary glands of fruit flies, the *lamp brush chromosomes* in the oocytes of amphibians, and the *supernumerary* or *B chromosomes*.

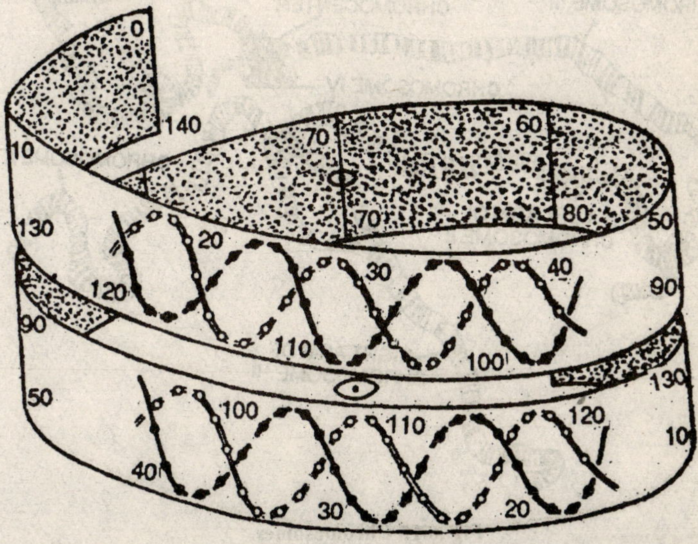

Fig. 6.14 Chromosomes
Schematic representation of DNA super helix in the nucleosome

Polytene chromosomes : These multithreaded chromosomes were first reported by Balbiani in 1881 while observing the squash of salivary cells of *Chironomous*. Subsequently they have been seen in the larvae of Dipterans (*Drosophila* etc). The name polytene was suggested by Kollar due to the appearance of many threads. Besides salivary glands the polytene chromosomes also occur in rectal epithelium and maiphigian tubules.

The nuclei in the salivary gland cells are much larger than the normal ones and are about 25 μ in diametre with the giant chromosomes larger by 50-200 times than the normal chromosomes. The polytene chromosome in the salivary cells of *Drosophila melanogaster* (Painter 1933) are about 200 μ in length. The enormous size is due to the duplication of chromonema which do not separate. According to an estimate, the polytene chromosomes have 1000 times more DNA than the normal somatic chromosomes.

Structure : Each polytene chromosome is transversely striated by alternating *bands* and *inter band regions*. In *Drosophila*, over 5000 bands have been found in the four chromosomes of the salivary gland cells. The bands take an intense stain (Feulgen) while the inter band regions stain less intensely.

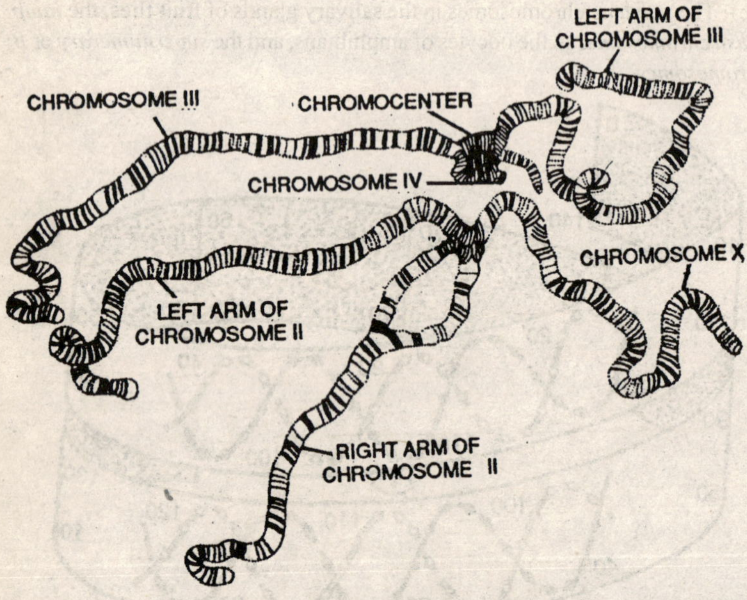

Fig. 6.15 Chromosomes
Polytene chromosomes of drosophila

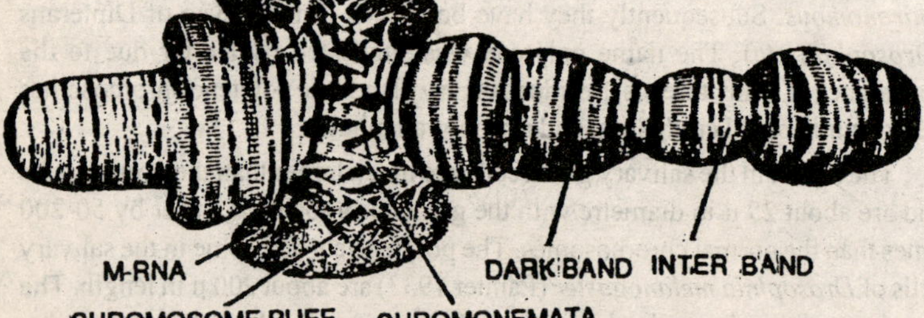

Fig. 6.16 Chromosomes
Polytene chromosomes of a Dipteran insect

The bands have chromomeres arranged at right angles to the long axis of the chromosome. The bands actually represent regions of tight coils of chromonema. Van Herwerden (1911) interpreted these bands as *gyres* of a continuous spiral. This view was later supported by Kostoff (1930). The bands have a high DNA content and absorb U.V. light at 2600Å.

The interbands stain lightly and they are negative to feulgen stain indicating a low concentration of DNA. The chromonema in the interband region are less coiled and absorb very little U.V. light.

Painter (1933) and Bridges (1936) have shown that in *Drosophila* the bands are clearly associated with the genes. Association of certain defects due to mutated genes have also been associated with the bands. Certain recent studies however have shown that together with the bands, the interband regions also have genes.

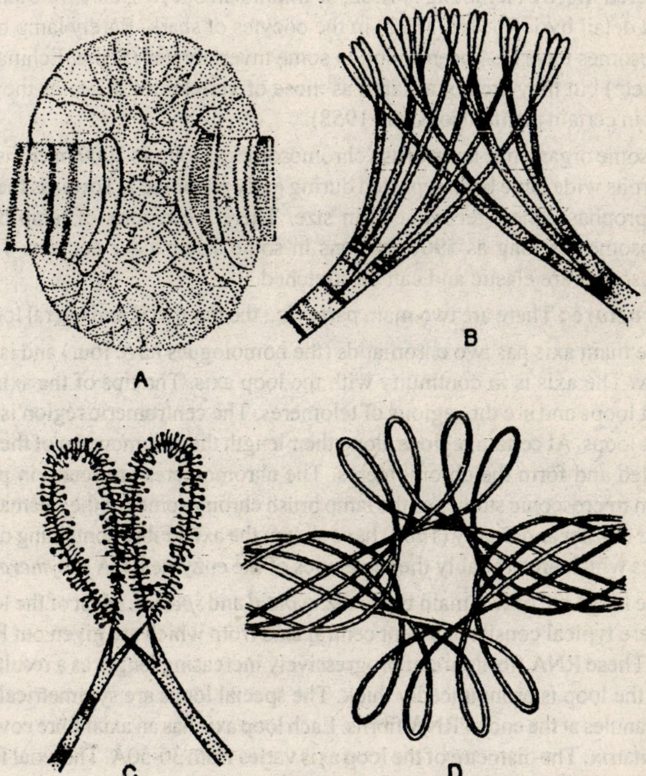

Fig. 6.17 Chromosomes
Balbiani ring in a polytene chromosome

Chromosome puffs : These are certain interesting structures associated with the bands in the giant chromosomes called *Chromosome puffs* or *Balbiani rings*. The swellings in bands at certain stages are given the name chromosome puffs. It is quite possible that these puffs are associated with the metabolic activites and represent areas of active RNA synthesis. According to Beerman and Bahr (1954), the coils in the puff region open out to form many loops. The larger chromosome puffs are called *Balbiain rings* and they show a high DNA and mRNA content.

Lamp brush chromosomes : The giant chromosomes found in the oocytes of fish, amphibians, reptiles and aves look like the brush used to clean the chimney of a kerosene lamp-hence the name *lamp brush chromosomes.* These are very large and are characterised by loops arising out of the main axis laterallv. Discovered first by Flemming is 1882, in amphibian oocytes, they were studied in great detail by J. Rucket (1892) in the oocytes of shark. Rarely lamp brush chromosomes have also been found in some invertebrates (Sepia, Echinaster, insects etc) but they are not as large as those of vertebrates. It seems they are present in certain plants also (Grun 1958).

In some organisms, lamp brush chromosomes as long as 1000 microns and 20 microns wide have been reported during early prophase I. Towards the end of the prophase, they get reduced in size. There are reports of lamp brush chromosomes as long as 5900 microns in some salamander oocytes. These chromosomes are elastic and can be stretched.

Structure : There are two main parts viz., the main axis and lateral loops.

The main axis has two chromatids (the homologues have four) and is rich in DNA. The axis is in continuity with the loop axis. The tips of the axis are without loops and are the regions of telomeres. The centromeric region is also without loops. At certain regions along their length the chromonema of the axis get coiled and form the chromomeres. The chromomeres are found in pairs. Electron microscopic studies of the lamp brush chromosomes of the salamander *Triturns* (Miller and Beatty (1969) have shown the axial Fibre containing dense granules which are probably the molecules of the enzyme RNA *polymerase.*

The loops are of two main types viz. *typical* and *special*. Most of the loops which are typical consist of a bent central axis from which are given out RNA fibrils. These RNA fibrils are of progressively increasing length as a result one side of the loop is pronouncedly thick. The special loops are symmetrical and have granules at the end of RNA fibrils. Each loop axis has an axial fibre covered with a matrix. The diametre of the loop axis varies from 30-50Å. The axial Fibre is made up of DNA, while the matrix has RNA and proteins.

Lamp brush chromosomes are involved in the synthesis of RNA and proteins. Each loop is believed to represent one long operon consisting of repetetive cistrons (structural genes). Each gene locus codes for RNA. The loop is supposed to synthesise at high rate because of repetetive gene sequence. There are also reports that the lamp brush chromosomes help in the formation of yolk material in the egg.

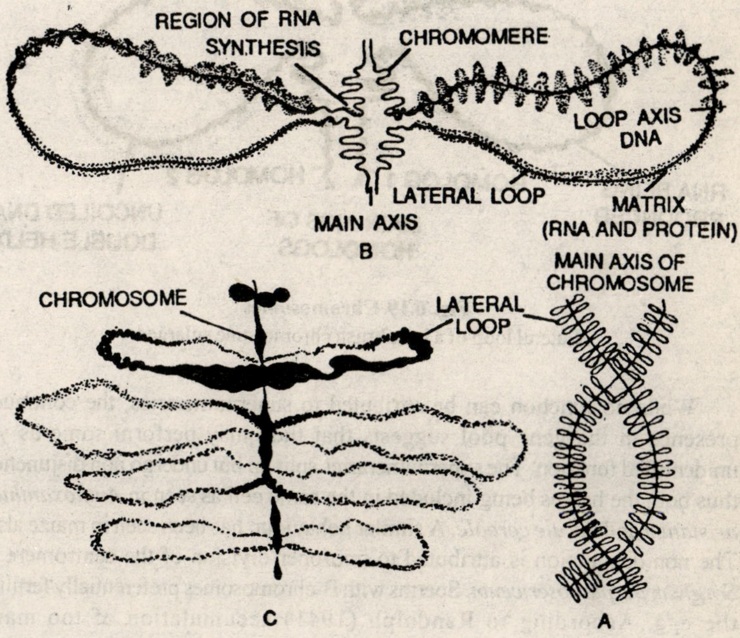

Fig. 6.18 Chromosomes
Lamp brush chromosomes, **A.** Paired homologues with two chaismata, **B.** Variation in loops, **C-A.** Chromomere with an attached loop.

Super numerary or B-chroroosomes : In many plants and animals, the cells contain in addition to the normal complement, one or more extra chromosomes called supernumerary or accessory orB- chromosomes.

These were first discovered in Hemipteran insects (Wilson 1905); since then they have been found in a number of insects and plants.

The supernumerary chromosomes are generally smaller than the others and are genetically inert hence produce little or no phenotypic expression. This suggests that these chromosomes may largely be heterochromatic which is supported by their differential staining activity. But this is not universal, for in *Tradescantia* they are entirely euchromatic, while in maize they are part euchromatic and part heterochromatic.

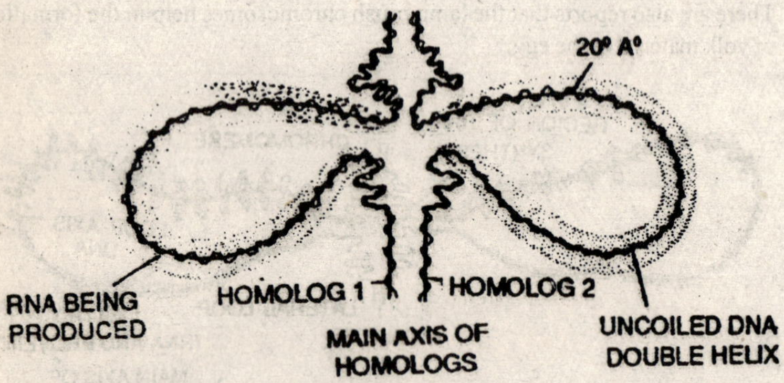

Fig. 6.19 Chromosomes
Lateral loop of a lampbrush chromosome enlarged

While no function can be attributed to supernumeraries, the continued presence in the gene pool suggests that they may perform some as yet unidentified function. The supernumeraries split up but undergo non disjunction thus both the halves being included in the same cell as seen in *Anthoxanthum aristatum* and *Secale cereale*. A similar behaviour has been seen in maize also. The non disjunction is attributed to improper division of the centromere in *Sorghum purpureosericeum*. Sperms with B-chromosomes preferentially fertilize the egg. According to Randolph (1941) accumulation of too many supernumeraries in an individual will result in loss of vigour as seen in maize. The increase in the number of supernumeraries is due to irregular fragmentation. The origin of supernumeraries in plants is unknown, while in some animals they can be traced to the Y chromosome (Wilson 1905). This is the case in *Metapodius*, where the chromosomes have a diffused centromere, hence any fragment can survive.

7

GENOME IN PROKARYOTES

The hereditary material in all organisms is remarkably similar. Having been evolved in the remote past, life has been able to maintain itself because of the ability of the hereditary material to maintain a basic uniformity in structure and function. The hereditary material in all living beings (whether it is a border line entity like a Virus or an evolved human being) is Nucleic acids without exception, even though there may be some stray instances of proteins (as prions) believed to carry out inheritance. The structure of the nucleic acids is unique; it has a basic uniformity, yet sufficient plasticity to allow for its manifestation from most primitive to the advanced organism.

In eukaryotic organisms, the genetic material is organised into large entities called chromosomes which allow for proper replication and distribution of genetic material during cell division and reproduction.

In prokaryotic organisms also,the nucleic acids constitute the chromosome, but the chromosome of prokaryotes is a naked strand of DNA (not associated with proteins) lying free in cytoplasm. The entire genetic system of each species is encoded in a single chromosome. Even in Viruses, the genome is either DNA or RNA.

The prokaryotic genome is refered to as the chromosome, centrosome, nucleoid, chromatin body or the gneophore. Some traditional cytogeneticists object to the word chromosome and prefer to use the term genophore or nucleoid. However, as Swanson (1981), points out "this is more a matter of semantics than of cytogenetics, since the prokaryotic chromosome not only has the same fundamental structure based on nucleic acid sequences, but it also carries out, the same three basic functions of its eukaryotic counter part. That is, it is the organelle which stores, replicates and transmits the coded information of biological inheritance; which is so regulated in its action that its primary products appear at appropriate times and in appropriate amounts during the life cycle of the organism; and which is capable of recombining its genetic content with other similar individuals in such a manner that the seggregating progeny of a hybrid union can have different genetic properties". Swanson (1981) therefore opines that the term "chromosome" can be applied to both eukaryotic and prokaryotic species with distnctions in structure being made at appropriate times.

The chromosome of *Escherichia coli* and *Salmonella typhimurium* are probably the most throughly mapped genomes of any cellular organism. Hundreds of identifiable genes are located in a single circular linkage group. The entire genome of a bacterium is made up of a single chromosome. Occasionally a single bacterial cell may have more than one chromosome at a given time. This should not be taken as the cell having two chromosomes. This represents a stage wherein the chromosome has replicated and formed two units but the cell is yet to divide.

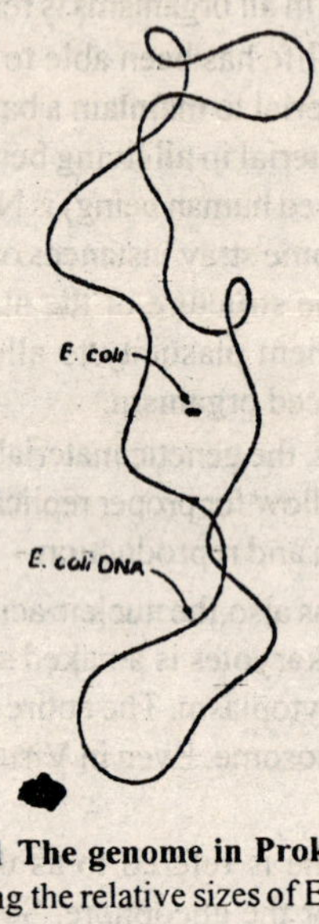

Fig. 7.1 The genome in Prokaryotes
Schematic diagram showing the relative sizes of E.coli and its DNA molecule

The chromosome of *E.coli* is a single, large double helix which is circular in outline. The DNA molecule is supercoiled. It (DNA) has no association of histones as in eykaryotic chromosomes. However, small amounts of basic proteins have been found to be associated with the isolated DNA. It is quite likely that these might prevent some sections of the chromosome from transcription thus functioning like repressor proteins. Thus it can be argued that the absence of DNA-histone association may not be such a fundamental point of difference between prokaryotic and eukaryotic DNA.

In *E.coli* the total length of the circular DNA is 1300μm, whereas cylindrical bacteria have a maximum diameter of 1 μm only. This clearly indicates that the chromosome must be highly folded in the cell.

When the DNA of *E.coli* is isolated by techniques that avoid both DNA breakage and protein denaturation, a highly compact structure called *nucleoid* can be seen. This structure contains a DNA molecule, a fixed amount of protein and variable amounts of RNA. As has been pointed out already, the proteins might play a part in repression of transcription.

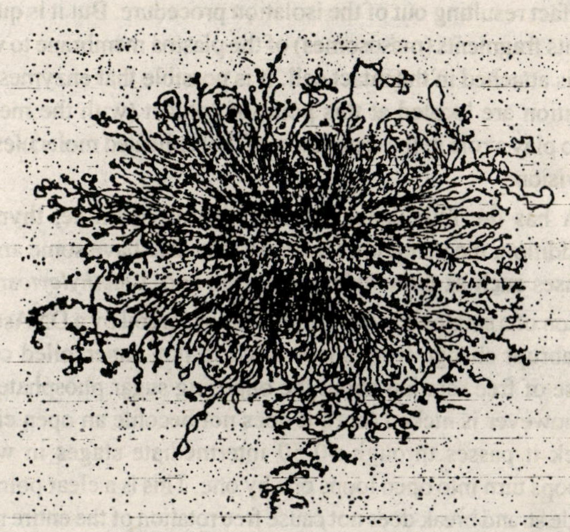

Fig. 7.2 The genome in Prokaryotes

An electron micrograph of an E.coli chromosome showing the multiple loops merging from a central region

The DNA molecule is about 1000 to 1100μm in length with a diameter of 20 Å to 40 Å. Such a molecule has more than 3.235 x 10^6 nucleotide pairs (each pairs is 3.4 Å long and there are 2941 base pairs per micrometer). The molecule has a molecular weight of 2.5 x 10^9 daltons (one dalton is equivalent to the weight of one hydrogen atom). This entire molecule is limited in the nuclear area of the cell which is no more than one micron and has no limiting boundary (such as a nuclear envelop), hence the molecule must be enormously folded.

It has been pointed above, that a small amount of RNA and basic proteins are associated with the DNA molecule. But the fact that the action of RNAse or protease does not alter the basic structure of DNA, indicates that neither RNA nor proteins are necessary for the basic circular nature of the chromosome.

Detailed Structure of the Chromosome

The chromosome (DNA) of *E.coli* on isolation appears to be a highly folded compact structure. These folds appear to be highly regular and not random. If they were to be random, replication and proper seggregation would not be possible. The chromosome obviously has a high level of organization. Two features of the chromosome are noteworthy. These are - (1) The DNA is arranged in a series of loops and (2) Each loop is supercoiled. A dense region containing membranous material is seen in the central part. Some people think it to be an artefact resulting out of the isolation procedure. But it is quite likely that it represents fragments (mesosomes) of the plasma membrane to which the chromosome is attached in the intact cell. It is possible that enzymes required for the replication are located at this point of contact (with the membrane). Mesosomes do play a role in the separation of the replicated molecules of DNA during cell division.

The DNA has the four usual bases - adenine, guanine, thymine and cytosine. In addition, the genome of bacteria may also have some amounts of methylated bases such as *6-methylaminopurine* and *5-methylcytosine.*

Introduction of a single strand break into the supercoil by a DNAse enzyme results in an abrupt change from supercoiled to non supercoiled condition. This is because of free rotation about the opposing sugar phosphate bond. If the nucleoid however is nicked (cut), it does not become an open circle. But with each nick it passes through 40-50 intermediate stages in which the supercoiled loops turn into open loops one by one. This is a clear pointer to the fact that a single strand break does not cause free rotation of the entire molecule. The DNA is assumed to be fixed to the proteins in such a way that does not allow overlapping of the individual loops.

The enzyme (DNA gyrase) that brings about DNA replication is also responsible for supercoiling. This can be proved by the addition of *coumermycin* an inhibitor of DNA gyrase, to the culture medium containing *E.coli* cells. The chromosomes of *E.coli* quickly lose supercoiling (on addition of coumerycin). In addition to DNAgyrase another enzyme *topoisomerase* I has the ability of unwinding the supercoils. Hence it is believed that the two enzymes *-DNA gyrase* and *topoisomerase* I act in a coordinated fashion and regulate the degree of coiling. *In vitro* experiments have shown that purified topoisomerase I enzyme relases supercoiling to a non supercoiled covalent circle. Mutants of *E.coli* lacking *topiosomerase* I have been seen to posses increased supercoiling to the extent of 32 percent more than the normal.

Some interesting observations have been made on these mutants lacking in topoisomerase I. In *in virto* conditions, the mutants undergo a further secondary mutation in or near the gyrase gene which seems to reduce the gyrase activity and return the supercoiling to near normal state.

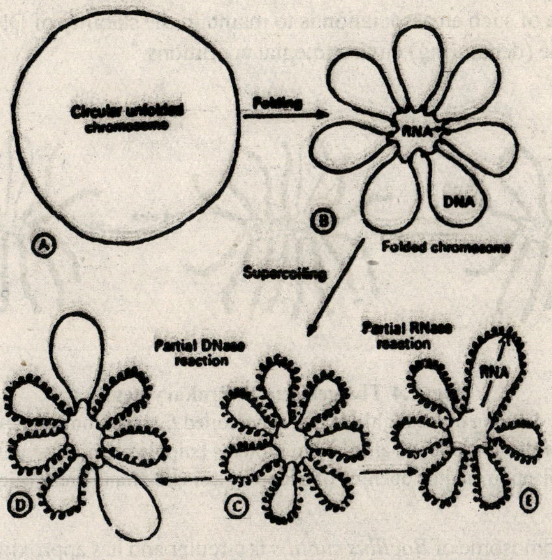

Fig. 7.3 The genome in Prokaryotes
Model of bacterial chromosome

A. Circular unfolded chromosome
B. Folded chromosome
C. Folded and supercoiled chromosome
D. Supercoiling relaxed into loops by DNAse nicks
E. RNAse cuts one RNA molecule

Other Associated Structures of Chromosomes

The isolated genome of *E.coli* has about 30 percent by weight RNA and 10 percent protein. The RNA is largely a newly transcribed mRNA, tRNA or ribosomal RNA which is yet to be released into the cell machinery. A small amount of additional RNA in this is responsible for the folded character of the genome. RNAse activity can partially unfold the genome.

Most of the proteins have been identified as RNA polymerase engaged in transcription. This is quite understandable as a metabolically active bacterial cell would be virtually transcribing throughout its life cycle. A small portion of the protein represents the mesosome.

Chromosome of Other Bacteria

The thermophilic bacterium *Thermolplasma acidophilum* possesses a chromosome that is quite unusual for a prokaryote. The genome is associated with a histone like protein which can complex with about 20% of the chromosome.

The purpose of such an association is to maintain the stability of DNA during unfavourable (denaturing) environmental conditions.

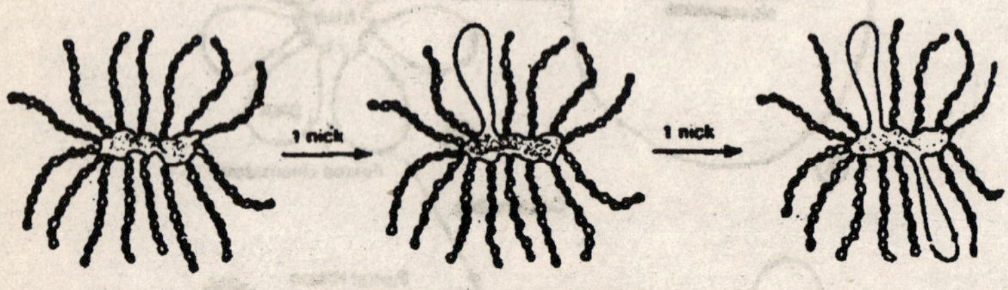

Fig. 7.4 The genome in Prokaryotes

A schematic drawing of the highly folded supercoiled *E.coli* chromosome, showing only 15 of the 40-50 loops attached to proteins (stippled region) of unknown organization, andthe opening of a loop by a single-strand break (nick)

The chromosome of *Bacillus subtilis* is circular and has approximately the same dimensions and molecular weight like that of *E.coli.* There are suggestions that the genome of *B.subtils* replicates as a linear molecule rather than as a circular molecule. *Streptomyces coelicolor* and *Salmonella typhimurium* are also known to possess circular genome with the latter acomodating 323 identified genes. Species of *M.mycoplasma* have a small circular chromosome of about 265μ in length. *Haemophilus infleuzae* the whooping cough causing bacterium, has a chromosome as long as 865μm which often appears linear with two free ends(?). Whether these ends really represent the points of a linear molecule or represent the ruptures of a circle during extraction it is difficult to say.

PLASMIDS

The bacterial cell has an additional fragment of nucleic acids in addition to its normal chromosome. This additional genetic material was given the name episome (Jacob, Sccaeffer and Woolmann, 1960). Episome can exist either independently or it can integrate itself with the bacterial chromosome. Plasmids however are always independent and never integrate with the bacterial chromosome. Plasmids control a number of traits in bacteria such as -toxin production, antibiotic resistance, pilus production etc. Some people regard that episomes and plasmids are synonymous.

The word plasmid was first used by J.Lederberg (1952). However, the term is restricted only to bacterial cells where circular DNA molecules exist independent of the main genome.

Plasmids are circular double stranded molecules of DNA and exist independently of chromosomal DNA in bacterial cells. They undergo replication during cell division and are carried to both the daughter cells. The plasmid has a right handed superhelical coil during the resting stage. There, is one super helical turn for every 400-600 base pairs. The twisted conformation is known as **covalently closed DNA (CCD).** Cleavage results in the conversion from CCD to open circular form.

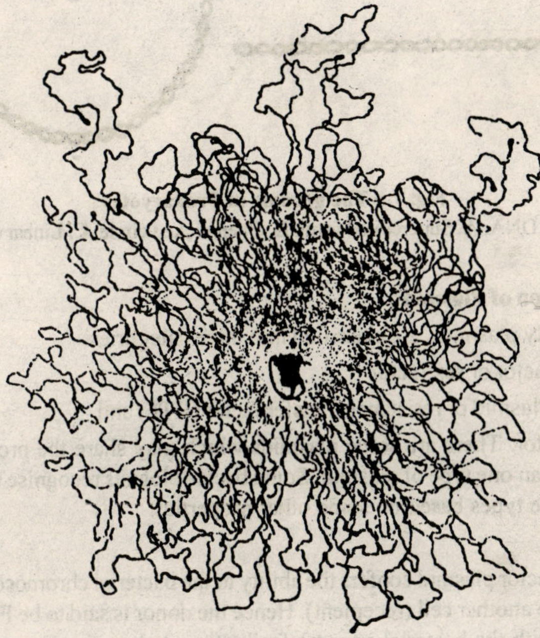

Fig. 7.5 The genome in Prokaryotes

An electron micrograph of the chromosome of the bacterium *Hemophilus influenzae.*

The following are some of the properties of the plasmids.

1. They are made up of DNA (double stranded).
2. They are capable of independent replication
3. Some plasmids control bacterial conjugation
4. Capable of reversible insertion into bacterial chromosome (only some plasmids)
5. They have the ability to get transfered from one bacterial cell to the other.

Plasmids are refered to as *conjugative* and *non conjugative* based on the ability/inability to promote their transfer during conjugation.

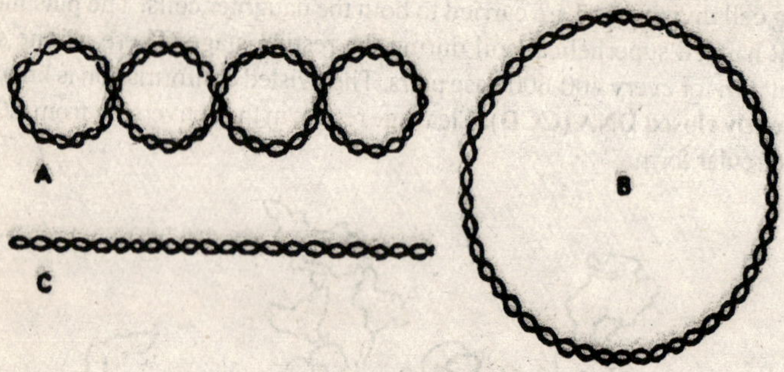

Fig. 7.6 The genome in Prokaryotes

Plasmid DNA, **A.** Supercoiled form, **B.** Open nicked circle, **C.** Linear duplex

Classification of Plasmids

Basically plasmids are classified into three categories -

1. The F factor or sex factor
2. The R Plasmid or resistance transfer factor (RTF) and
3. *Col* factor. There are some plasmids which may share the properties of more than one type of plasmid. Some bacteriologists recognise more than the three types based on some other properties.

F factor

The F factor plasmid confers the ability to the bacterial chromosome to get transfered to another cell (recepient). Hence the donor is said to be F^+. F factor integrates with the bacterial genome facilitating its transfer. Because of this integration, it is often refered to as an episome.

R Plasmid

These plasmids, when present confer on the bacterial cell resistance to several antibiotics such as streptomycin, tetracycline, chloramphenicol, sulphonamide etc. R plasmid mediated antibiotic resistance was first discovered in Japan in 1956 when *Shigella* became resistant to several antibiotics at one step. This was due to the transfer of R plasmid from one strain to the other resulting in not only antibiotic resistance but also the ability of a donor (it can donate R factor to other sensitive strains making them resistant).

R plasmid is a small extrachromosomal DNA ring. Sometimes the R plasmid has two parts - (a) Part havin drug resistant genes and (b) Part having plasmid transfer genes.

The col factor (Plasmid)

Certain bacteria like *Escherichia coli, Shigella, Salmonella* etc., produce toxins called *colicins*. These are toxic proteins and can kill other bacteria. The ability to produce *colicin* rests in the plasmid called col plasmid or *colicinogenic factor*. Col factors resemble phages since they cause death of bacteria, but they differ from phages as they are not released out during the lysis of the bacterial cell. Like the F factors col plasmids also can be transfered from one bacterial cell to the other.

The number of plasmids per bacterial cell varies. It may be *a single copy* or *multiple copies*. Multiple copy plasmids which replicate independently have been used in gene cloning experiments. A plasmid is cleaved and a desired gene is inserted into the plasmid DNA. The plasmid DNA during its replication produces multiple copies of foreign DNA. Such plasmids are called vectors.

GENOME OF CYANOBACTERIA

In cyanobacteria, the nucleoplasmic region can be identified by its low electron density when observed under electron microscope. The DNA fibres are organized into a complex helical and folded structure and are distributed uniformly throughout the centroplasm. It is quite possible that DNA is associated with histone like proteins and RNA (Fay, 1983).

The size of the genome varies widely in cyanobacteria having a molecular weight ranging between 1.6×10^9 and 8.6×10^9 daltons. Most of the unicellular cyanobacteria posses genomes of about 1.6×10^9 to 2.7×10^9 daltons. This compares favourably with similar genomes found in other prokaryotes. Some filamentous cyanobacteria however have larger genomes. The distribution of genome sizes in cyanobacteria falls into four categories - 2.2, 3.6, 5.0 and 7.4×10^9 daltons. Members with a more complex morphology obviously posses larger genomes than those with a simple structure. There is a theory that the modern day prokaryotes evolved from a primitive bacterium with a small genome size of about 1.2×10^9 daltons. Replication of this genome during the course of Evolution is supposed to have given rise to simple integer multiples seen in modern bacterial genome.

THE VIRAL GENOME

The core of the Virion is made up of nucleic acids. A virus has only DNA or RNA never both together. Within these parameters however considerable diversity exists. The nucleic acids may be double stranded, single stranded, linear or circular. Some have plus polarity; others may have minus polarity. Four types of nucleic acids are found in viruses with reference to the number of strands. These are

1. Single stranded DNA —— (ss DNA) e.g., Colliphage virus
2. Double stranded DNA (ds DNA) e.g., Herpes virus

3. Single stranded RNA (ssRNA) e.g., TMV
4. Double stranded RNA (dsRNA) e.g., Reo Virus

Single stranded DNA is found in ϕX174 Virus. It was first discovered by Sinscheimer *et al* in 1950's. ssDNA may be linea: (Paroviruses) or circular (ϕX174 Virus). The ssDNA becomes double stranded during replication and at that time it is known as the replicative form.

Double stranded DNA is found in a number of animal Viruses and bacteriophages. It has a variety of forms - linear (bacteriophages), cross linked (vaccinia Virus) or closed circular duplex as in papova Viruses.

Single stranded RNA is found in a variety of animal Viruses and icosahedral plant Viruses. The strand may be plus (infectious) as in RNA bacteriophages, togaviruses etc or minus (non infectious) as in rhabdoviruses and paramyxoviruses. Plus ssRNA acts directly as mRNA and translates proteins on the ribosomes of bacteria, whereas minus ssRNA first transcribes an mRNA and then it (mRNA) translates proteins (hence called non infectious).

Double stranded RNA is found in animal Viruses like reovirus, blue tongue Virus etc. The dsRNA has 10 or more segments.

The nuclei acid core of Viruses may be summarised as follows -

1. Plant Viruses have only RNA (ss or ds) with the exception of cauliflower mosaic Viruses (DNA virus)
2. Animal Viruses have RNA (ss or ds) and DNA (only ds no ss)
3. Bacteriophages have DNA (ss or ds) or RNA (ss or ds). However most phages or DNA Viruses.

8

CHROMOSOMAL ABERRATIONS

The chromosomes - often called vehicles of heredity are sufficiently characteristic to provide the cytologist morphological criteria of an individual that can be used for identification much in the same way as a taxonomist uses phytographic (morphological characters of organs) characters to delimit the species. The constancy of karyotype is due to the fact-as Swanson (1957) observes "at a given stage of cell division and in a given tissue each cell of an organism has a constant number of chromosomes of reasonably definite volume, length and shape........" This constancy of chromosome number, volume etc., is determined in turn by the number arrangement, and sequence of genes in a definite order.

It becomes clear from the above discussion that constancy in chromosome number and structure are very essential for the individual not only to maintain its morphological characters, but many a time even for its own survival. Occasionally however, there occur variations in structure as well as number in the chromosomes producing alterations variations etc., in the individual. Depending on the magnitude of these changes, the individual undergoing these changes either will survive with little or no change or may barely survive with great changes. In some instances however, the changes are of such a magnitude that they may be lethal to the individual. These changes are called *chromosomal aberrations.* Very often these aberrations are also called *chromosoma mutations,* as they bring about change in genetic characters of the individual. Chromosomal mutations or aberrations should not be mistaken with gene mutations as the latter are involved with single genes, while the former affect either segments of chromosomes or sometimes entire chromosomes or even the entire set of genome (the total chromosomes present in an individual).

In natural populations, the chromosomal aberrations occur spontaneously but less frequently. In grass hoppers about one in a thousand individuals is known to carry some form of chromosome rearrangement. Naturally occuring chromosomal abberrations are found in human beings also. After the initial discovery of a naturally occurmg aberration, geneticists learnt that they can induce these aberrations artificially by using mustard gas, X ray, colchicine, etc.

Of what use are the aberrations to a geneticist? Chromosomal aberrations in an individual in comparison with the normal chromosomes provide a wealth of data to geneticists to understand the structure of a chromosome and also to compare any morphological expression with a particular segment of the chromosome. If the changes brought about are not good, the geneticist may try to find a way out to overcome these aberrations. On the other hand if these aberrations produce a new desirable trait, he may learn to produce those aberrations artificially.

For a cytologist, chromosomal aberrations, particularly structural are a gold mine as he can study by camparison (with the normal chromosome) the arrangement of genes, their order, frequency etc. It helps him to map the chromosome and locate a gene in a particular segment of the chromosome.

On a broad classification, chromosomal aberrations are of two kinds- *Structaral* and *Numerical.* Structural aberrations bring about a change in the chromosome structure in terms of length, shape or sometimes in the form of altered, or loss of genes and their arrangement. When the chromosomal changes affect a large segment, the changes may even be visible morphologically. Numerical changes on the other hand do not affect the structure of the chromosome, but are only involved in alteration in the number which may be either increase or decrease when compared with the normal number. This change also has many drastic genetic influences on the individual.

STRUCTURAL ABERRATIONS

As has been pointed out already, any change in the structure and architecture of the individual chromosome comes under the perview of structural changes.

The structural aberrations are of the two following categories -

(i) **Intra chromosomal aberrations**

(ii) **Inter chromosomal aberrations.**

The alterations of the genes or gene sequences influencing only one chromosome or taking place in a chromosome are called Intrachromosomal aberrations. This should not be mistaken to mean that more than one chromosome will not undergo alteration, but it means to say that all the events leading to a particular aberration take place within a chromosome.

Inter chromosomal structural aberrations on the other hand involve at least two chromosomes with reference to an aberration. Both intra and inter chromosomal aberrations are further classified as the chart below shows.

Chromosomal aberrations

- Structural
  - Intra chromosomal
    1. Deletions
    2. Duplications
    3. Inversions.
  - Inter chromosomal
    4. Translocations
- Numerical (Details given later in the chapter)

DELETIONS

Also known as deficiencies, these involve loss of a segment or loss of a portion of the chromosome, but the entire chromosome is never lost. The deleted portion which comes out of the remainder of the chromosome will not survive if it does not have a centromere. But in cases of chromosomes with a diffused centromere the fragment or fragments that come out of the chromosome do survive and this leads to increase in the chromosome number, but no loss of genes. The portion of the chromosome with the centromere (in the case of chromosomes with a single centromere) functions as a deficient chromosome.

How does a deletion occur? A break in the chromosome at any one point results in the tearing away of a part of the chromosome. This break may occur naturally or by the influence of external agencies like chemical gas, ionising radiation, drugs etc.

Types of Deletion

Two types of deletion have been noticed in organisms. These are *Terminal deletion* and *Interstitial deletion* (Intercalary deletion).

In a terminal deletion, a break occurs in a chromosome a little away from one end and a segment comes out. For instances if a chromosome has gene loci ABCDEFGH, the deleted portion will be GH and the chromosome will now have only ABCDEF. The terminal deletion produces two raw ends-in the main chromosome. The raw end heals up, while the deleted segment is lost in the next cell division as it lacks a centromere.

In an interstitial deletion, a segment comes out of the chromosome from the middle. This is brought about by two breaks at two points in the chromosome, removal of an intercalary segment and fusion of the two broken ends in the original chromosome. For instance, in a chromosome with gene loci ABCDEFGH, there will be two nicks-one between C and D and the other between E and F, with the result a segment of the chromosome carrying gene loci DE comes out, the two ends-at C and F unite to form the deleted chromosome ABCFGH.

Between the two types of deletions, terminal deletions are generally rare as they involve the loss of a telomere. The healing end of the chromosome must be such that, it should not fuse with any other chromosome.

Deletion Heterzygote

Deletion may affect one or both of the homologous chromosomes in a diploid organism. If both the homologues lose an identical segment, it will be known as deletion homozygote or as it happens quite frequently, one of the homologues may remain normal, while the other may undergo deletion, such an individual is said to be a deletion heterozygote. Generally individuals with homozygous deletion will not survive.

Occurrence

Deletions have been reported from a wide variety of organisms both in the plant and animal kindgom maize (McClintok 1941), *Drosophila,* Grasshopper, man etc, where several phenotypic traits have been associated with deletions.

Cytological identification

A homozygous deletion (if the individual survives) is difficult to identify morphologically at the chromosome level. However if the normal chromosome has been studied previously, the deleted chromosome can be pointed out because of its reduced length and also change in shape, since a terminal deletion in a metacentric chromosome would reduce the length of one arm and produces a sub metacentric chromosome.

Heterozygous deletion on the other hand is easy to identify cytologically during meiosis, when the normal and the deficient homologues undergo pairing. The pairing homologues produce specific configurations and can be easily located. In the case of a terminal deletion, the deleted chromosome will be shorter in length, hence there is no pairing in that portion and one can see a long and short chromosome undergoing linear pairing with the terminal part of the normal chromosome left out of pairing. In the case of interstitial deficiency, the normal chromosome forms a loop in that portion (of its chromosome) where the genes are lost in the other homologue.

Deletions can be easily identified by visual observation in instances like salivary gland chromosomes of *Drosophila,* where a deletion may lead to the loss of several bands. The same thing is possible in lampbrush chromosomes also where several specific loops will be lost.

Genetic consequences of Deletion

A deletion is involved in the loss of genetic material, hence it is imperative that there will be consequences which affect not only the individual but future generations also. The magnitude of genetic effect will however depend on *the size of the deletion and the quality of the genes so lost.* In many an instance the organism survives with little or no variation or may barely survive with drastic morphological and functional alteration or as in extreme cases, it may be lethal to the individual. In general however, homozygous deletions rarely survive as both the alleles are lost.

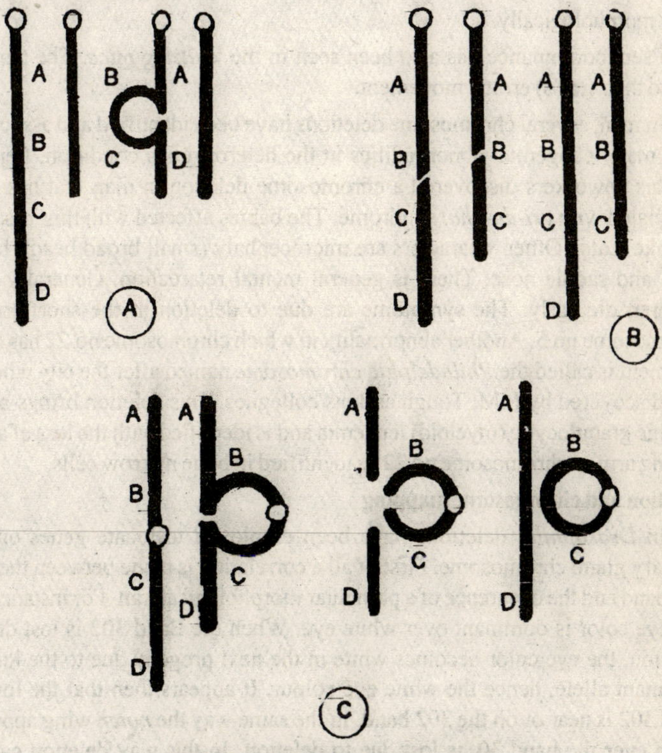

Fig. 8.1 Chromosomal Aberrations

Deletions **A.** Intercalary deletion and passing in a deletion heterozygote,

B. Terminal deletion and pairing in a deletion heterozygote,

C. Deletion and origin of ring chromosome

In *Drosophila melanogalster,* homozygous deletion involving the tip of X chromosome can survive provided they are very small characters such as yellow, scute etc, whose loss can be withstood without much problem. In *Drosophila,* several morphological traits are associated with deletions. These are blond, pale, beaded, carved, snipped and plexate. In addition to this, most of the *notch and minutte* are also known to be due to deletions.

The phenomenon of *pseudodominance* seen in some plants by Stadler is also due to deletion. In a cross between a double dominant and double recessive, the F_1 should normally be heterozygous dominant. But if a deletion affects the gene D (dominant), then the recessive allele even in the single dose will express itself morphologically.

Pseudodominance has also been seen in the *waltzing mice.* The name is due to their (rat's) erratic movement.

In man, several chromosome deletions have been identified and associated with many congenital abnormalities in the heterozygous condition. Lejeunc and his coworkers discovered a chromosome deletion in man that has been associated with *cri-du-chat* syndrome. The babies affected with this disorder cry like cats. Other characters are microcephaly (small broad head), broad face, and saddle nose. There is general mental retardation. Generally such children die early. The symptoms are due to deletion in the short arm of chromosome no.5. Another abnormality in which chromosome no.22 has lost a fragment is called the *Philadelphia chromosome* named after the city where it was discovered by L.M. Tough and his collegues. This deletion brings-about chronic granulocytic (myeloid) leukemia and is identified with the loss of a part of long arm of chromosome no 22 as identified in bone marrow cells.

Deletion and chromosome mapping

In *Drosophila,* deletions have been employed to locate genes on the salivary gland chromosome. First of all a correlation is made between the loss of a band and the occurence of a particular morphological trait. For instance the red eye color is dominant over white eye. When the Band 302 is lost due to deletion, the eye color becomes white in the next progeny due to the loss of dominant allele, hence the white eye colour. It appears then that the loss of band 302 is near or on the 302 band. In the same way the *notch* wing appears, when ever the band 30, is lost due to deletion. In this way deletion can be employed as markers to locate the genes on the chromosome.

Evolutionary importance of Deletions

It is highly unlikely that deletions have a profound evolutionary impact, since the loss generally diminishes the potentiality of the organism. But theoritically speaking, if deletion removes some genes that suppress other genes, which can then express themselves, it may lead to new and desirable phenotypic variations being prefered by natural selection. In annual herbs, the loss of chromatin material is known to lead to specialization like adaptation to a habitat, to an insect pollinator etc. In *Crepis* (Comopositae) the loss seems to be restricted to only heterochromatin material.

DUPLICATIONS

This is another kind of structural chromosomal aberration affecting a single chromosome. In the affected chromosome, a segment of the chromosome containing several gene loci duplicates itself so that the chromosome has those genes in double dose. Duplication may occur at the tip of the chromosome or in the middle. In some instances the duplicated portion may attach to the chromosome *i.e* the same sequence or in a reverse sequence. Usually terminal duplications are rare due to the presence of the telomere. The following are the types of duplications in a chromosome with a normal gene complement ofABCDEFGHI. Let us assume that the segment DEF is duplicated.

Tandem duplication

In a tandem or sequential duplication the duplicated segment is attached to the chromosome in the same locus and in the same sequence. In the present example, the chromosome with tandem duplication will have the gene sequence *ABCDEFDEFGHI.*

Reverse tandem

Here the duplicated part will attach itself to the chromosome at the same locus but in a reverse sequence. For e.g. *ABCDEFFEDGHI*

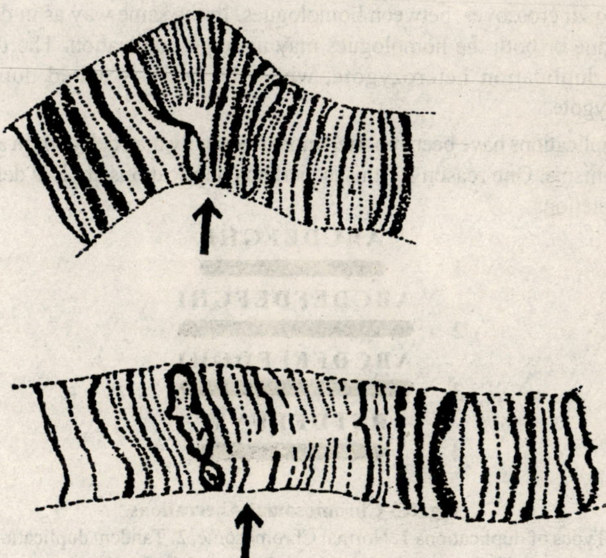

Fig. 8.2 Chromosomal Aberrations
Diagram showing loss of certain bands in the chromosome due to deletion

Displaced duplication

Here the segment DEF (duplicated portion) will attach to the same chromosome but in a different locus other than its original position. For e.g. RSTDEFUVW. Since the duplicated segment retains the sequence it is called tandem, and since it joins the chromosome in a different locus it is called *displaced tandem*. In a displaced reverse tandem duplication, the gene sequence would be RSTFEDUVW. Here the duplicated segment joins the chromosome in a different locus in the reverse order.

The displaced duplication (reverse or tandem) may take place on the same arm *(Homobrachial displacement)* or an a different arm *(Heterobrachial displacement)*. Unusually, the duplicated segment may join another non homologous chromosome, in which case it is called *transposition*. (This is different from translocation where there is no duplication of any segment).

How duplication occurs

In a tandem duplication there is a break and the duplicated part joins the point of breakage. In a displaced duplication, a break occurs in a point releasing the duplicated part and then rejoins. In another part another break occurs and the duplicated segment is accommodated. Duplication may also be produced by unequal crossover between homologues. In the same way as in deletions, either one or both the homologues may undergo duplication. The former is called duplication heterozygote, while the latter is called duplication homozygote.

Duplications have been reported more frequently than deletions in a number of organisms. One reason for this is perhaps duplications are less deleterious than deletions.

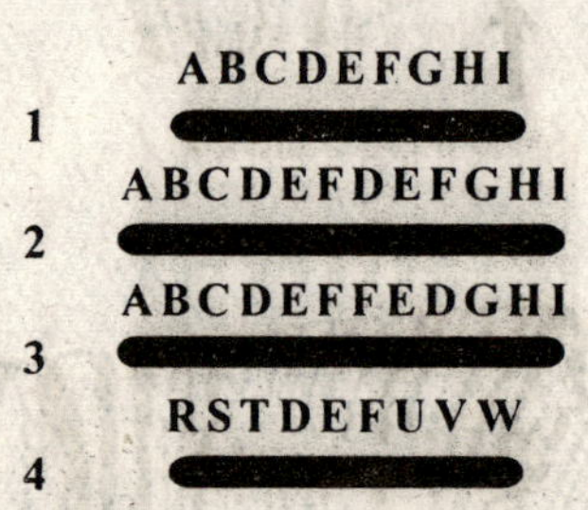

Fig. 8.3 Chromosomal Aberrations

Types of duplications **1.** Normal Chromosome, **2.** Tandem duplication, **3.** Reverse duplication, **4.** Displaced duplication

Cytological identification

The peculiar chromosome configuration observed during meiotic pairing in a duplication heterozygote provides a demonstrable visual evidence for duplication. When a normal homologous chromosome pairs with a duplicated chromosome, the duplicated fragment remains out of the synapsis in the form of loop. (In the case of deletion the normal chromosome forms a loop). Duplications are readily detected in *Drosophila* because of large size of salivary gland chromosomes, but in some plant species (haploid individuals) studies in meiosis have indicated pairing (in duplicated segments) where no pairing is expected.

Genetic effects of duplication

Generally speaking duplications are less harmful to the organism than deletions as additions are not expected to cause drastic changes. This is not true always. For instance an individual can survive a lethal gene in the heterozygous condition, but when the lethal gene is duplicated, it will be dangerous to the organism.

While deletions can be recognised genetically by the occurrence of recessive phenotypes, when they are not expected, similarly duplications can be inferred by the occurence of dominant character and total absence of recessive phenotype even in a cross between two heterozygous dominant individuals.

The phenotypic expression produced by duplication is illustrated by the attached X females in *Drosophila.* If we consider such flies which are homozygous for some reccesive, trait (located on both the X chromosomes), and these are fertilized by a male (having a *dominant gene),* the resultant individual will express the dominant character, eventhough two recessive genes are present. Evidently, the presence of dominant gene (in the same locus) in double dose on the same chromosome is sufficient to suppress the recessive allele.

In one of the recent reports published **in Cell** (July 26,1991) P.I. Patel and J.R. Lupski (1991) have observed that in many of the patients suffering from mental disorders such as Schizophrenia and Aizhiemer's disease, there are three copies of DNA (instead of two) in certain portions of Chromosomes no. 17. They believe that the duplication of DNA sequence might be the cause for mental disorders.

Position effect

A classical example of duplication and its genetic effect has been the study of *bar eye* locus in *Drosophila melanogaster* (Bridges 1919). The wild eye with the normal shape has an average of 779 ommatidia or single eyes. Genetically it is represented by two bar regions one on each X chromosome. However on a mutation in this locus a bar eye appears. As a result of mutation the bar region in one of the X chromosomes undergoes duplication, the size of the eye is reduced and it is called *bar eye* (BB,B). The individual heterozygous for bar eye has three bar regions and has 358 facets in the compound eye. In some bar individuals one more duplication may occur in the bar region (BBB, B) producing an *ultra bar* or *double bar* having totally four bar regions, each eye reduced to about 45 facets. Sturtevent and Bridges who studied these inheritance patterns of eye shape in *Drosophila* have concluded that during crossing over occuring at different levels in the chromosomes carrying bar regions, bar eyed individuals may give rise to normal individuals or even to *ultra bar*. Ultra bar is produced when crossing over joins together three bar regions. The fly having four bar regions and is homozygous bar has both the X chromosomes with two bars. Even though there are four bars, the eye will not be *ultrabar* (it has 68 facets in comparison to 45 for ultra bar), where as in heterozygous individuals with four bars, (BBB, B) there are three bar regions produced by double duplication on one X chromosome and the other normal X chromosone has a single bar locus. This individual will be *ultra bar*, because the three bar regions are located together on a single chromosome (BBB, B) while the single bar region is on another X chromosome. In the previous instance even though there are four bar regions (BB, BB) they did not produce an ultra bar, because on any one chromosome there are only two bar regions. This is due to a phenomenon called *position effect*, which is brought about by juxtaposition of bar sections (3,1) in the same chromosome having a stronger effect than the same quantity of bar regions (2,2) distrbuted on two chromosomes.

Catcheside, has found similar position effect due to duplications in *Oenothera*.

An instance of duplication and position effect in human beings is represented by the variants in haemoglobin. Haemoglobin A having 2 alpha and 2 beta chains is the most commonly found one. Haemoglobin B differs in the beta chain being replaced by delta chains. An abnormal haemoglobin (Hb-Lepore) has 2 alpha chains and one delta and one beta chain. Balgioni who studied this, reports that unequal crossing over taking place in beta and delta loci have deprived one chromosome of both the loci, while the other got both, resulting in the production of beta and delta chains.

Evolutionary significance of duplication

In contrast to deletions, duplications are certainly of some evolutionary consequence as they can produce viable and heritable morphological traits. Duplication seems to provide a feasible method for the acquisition of new genes and hence new functions. Duplications also provide the organism the survival of the original gene (in case it has any selective value) in case mutation occurs changing the original gene.

INVERSIONS

This is a kind of intrachromosomal aberration where there will be no change in quality or quantity of genes, but there will be alteration in their sequence. In order to bring about an inversion, there will be two breaks in the chromosome, with a segment getting separated from the chromosome. The segment joins back the chromosome but in a reverse sequence. For eg., in a chromosome with a gene sequence ABCDEFG, the segment BCDE is inverted, after the inverted portion rejoins the chromosome the altered chromosome would have the gene sequence AEDCBFG

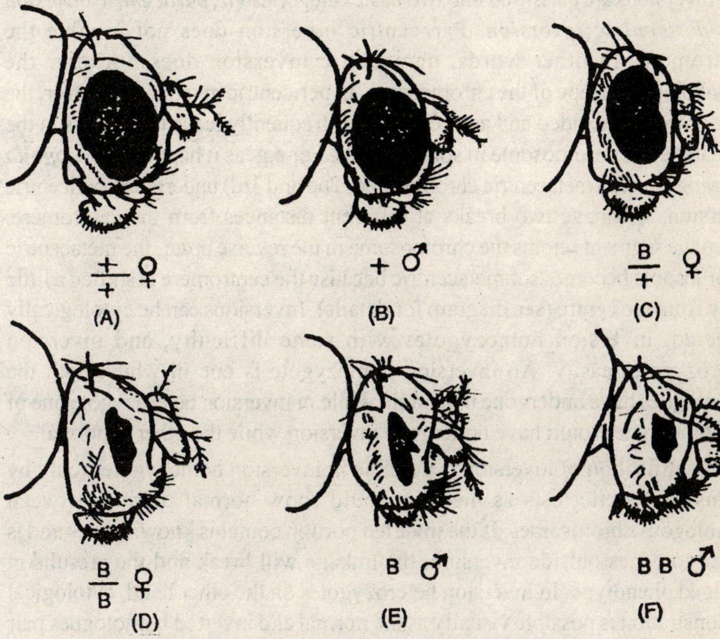

Fig. 8.4 Chromosomal Aberrations

Effect of duplication on the size in Drosophila

A. Normal female, **B.** Normal male, **C.** Normal (Heterozygous) female, **D.** Bar eyed female, **E.** Bar eyed male, **F.** Double bar male.

(Note : In D even though two bar loci are present, it is only bar eyed as the bar loci are present on different chromosome. In F, two bar loci are present on the same chromosome and the eye becomes double bar due to position effeect).

Inversions have also been reported in a wide variety of plants and animals like deletions and duplications. These perhaps have a wider distribution than the other two aberrations in natural populations. Among plants, inversions have been reported in *Paris, Tradescantia* etc. Among animal species, the favourite fruit fly, *Drosophila* exhibits quite a number of inversion types. *D.willstoni* and *D.psuedo obscura* show a variety of inversions that can be studied in great detail in salivary gland chromosomes. Several types of inversions have also been reported in maize (McClintock 1938).

Anopheles mosquito, urodeles Amphibia and many species of grasshoppers are other organisms where inversions have been reported.

Types of inversion

Inversions are classified into two basic categories viz, *paracentric inversion* and *pericentric inversion*. Paracentric inversion does not involve the centromere. In other words, paracentric inversion does not alter the morphological shape of the chromosome. In pericentric inversion however, the centromere is included and as a result quite frequently leads to changes in the appearance of chromosome in somatic cells. For e.g. as it happens *Drosophila melanogasiner,* a metacentric chromosome (2nd and 3rd) undergoing pericentric inversion, will have two breaks at different distances from the centromere. When the segment rejoins the chromosome in the reverse order, the metacentric chromosome becomes submetacentric because the centromere is shifted a little away from the centre (see diagram for details). Inversions can be cytologically detected; inversion homozygotes with some difficulty, and inversion heterozygotes easily. An inversion homozygote is one in which both the homologues have undergone inversion, while in inversion heterozygote one of the homologue would have undergone inversion while the other is normal.

Identification of inversion is possible in inversion homozygotes, only by means of genetic tests as meiosis would show normal pairing between homologous chromsomes. If the inverted portion contains known genes and is linked to genes outside inversion, the linkage will break and thus results in changed phenotype. In inversion heterozygotes on the other hand, cytological demonstration is possible visually as the normal and inverted homologues pair in a peculiar loop type configuration. While the inverted chromosome forms an overlapping loop, the normal chromosome forms a loop surrounding the overlapping loop.

Paracentric inversions : As has already been pointed out, here the centromere does not figure in the inversion. Let us assume a chromosome with gene loci *abcdefg* with the centromere between *a* and *b*. After inversion in the segment *bcde* the inverted chromosome will be *aedcbfg,* the centromere however will not be altered and it is located even now between *a* and *b*. How does pairing occur between a normal (ABCDEFG) and an inverted chromosome of this type? While the normal chromosome forms .a loop outside, the inverted chromosome will form an overlapping loop (ie one thread overlaps the other) so that all gene loci are matched. In such a configuration a cross over might take place wherein the two non sister chromatids exchange segments. In the given example let us assume a crossover occuring between C and D. What will be the type of separation and the fate of chromatids? Will all of them have same gene loci or will they be different? When the anaphasic movement begins there will be an unusual sight at the equatorial plate. Out of the four chromatids -two will move to the opposite poles, one will remain in the centre without moving to any of the poles while another will strecth between the two poles forming what is classically known as the *anaphasic bridge*. The gene loci of the above chromatids will be as follows:

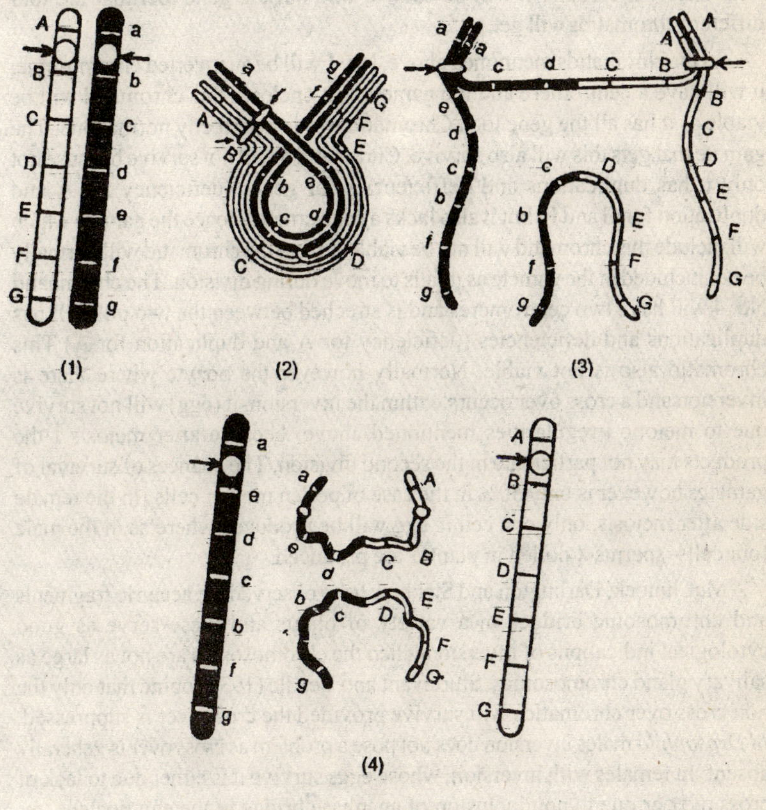

Fig. 8.5 Chromosomal Aberrations

Consequence of crossing over in a heterozygote with a paracenteric inversion

1. Homologus chromosome (Dark chromosome) shows inversion
2. Pairing and overlapping loop forming in an inversion heterozygote
3. Movement of chrosomes during anaphase (Note in the chrosome bridge formed by a dicentric chrosome and an acentric chromosome lying in the centric
4. Meiotic products showing duplications and deficiencies

Chromatids at	1 aedcbfg
Either poles	2 ABCDEFG
Chromatid at the centre	3 gfbcDEFG
Chromatid streching between poles	4 aedCBA

(If one carefully traces the diagram (at Diplotene) following the chromatid with different colours, it will be easy to find out the gene loci that the four different chromatids will get.)

In the chromatids mentioned above, No. 1 will be an inverted chromosome; it will have a centromere and the gamete that encloses this chromatid will be viable as it has all the gene loci. Chromatid two is a perfectly normal one. The gamete that gets this will also survive. Chromatid 3 will not survive because not only it has duplications and defficiencies for genes (deficiency for A and duplication for G and F) but it also lacks a centromere. Hence the gamete which will include this chromatid will not be viable. In fact the chromatid will normally be not included in the gamete as it fails to move during division. The chromnatid No. 4 will have two centromeres and is streched between the two poles. It has duplications and deficiencies (deficiency for A and duplication for A) This chromatid also is not viable. Normally however the oocyte where there is inversion and a cross over occurs within the inversion, it (egg) will not survive due to meiotic irregularities mentioned above; because after meiosis I the products may not participate in the second division. The chances of survival of gametes however is only 50% in the case of pollen mother cells.[In the female side after meiosis, only one cell *ie* egg will be produced where as in the male four cells- sperms-{ pollen in plants} are produced.

McClintock, Darlington and Stebbins have observed the acentric fragments and chromosome bridges in a variety of plants and these serve as good cytological indications of inversion when the chromosomes are not as large as salivary gland chromosomes. Sturtevant and Beadle (1936) opine that only the non cross over chromatids will survive provided the cross over is suppressed. *In Drosophila* males inversion does not pose a problem as cross over is generally absent. In females with inversion, whose eggs survive it is either due to lack of cross over or due to non inclusion of anaphase bridge in the egg nucleus.

When there are two cross overs within an inverted segment the survival will depend upon the number of chromatids involved. Double and multiple cross overs are however rare.

Pericentric inversions

The inversions that include the centromere are called pericentic inversions. Very often pericentic inversions change the morphology of the chromosome. However if the two breaks in the chromosome occur at equal distance from the centromere, there will not be any morphological change in the chromosome. While there is no estimate of natural populations where pericentric inversions have drastically altered chromosome morphology, in certain Orthoptera and species of *Drosophila,* centromeric shifts brought about by inversion have been responsible in producing new karyotypes.

Pairing in an inversion heterozygote produces loop formation in pericentric inversion also. Let us study the example of a pericentric inversion in a chromosome with the gene loci *abcdefg* with the centromere being situated between *d* and *e* .The chromosome obviously is a metacentric one with inversion taking place in the segment *bcde*, the resultant submetacentric chromosome will have gene loci *aedcbfg.* During meiosis pairing occurs in a heterozygous individual between a normal {ABCDEFG} and an inverted *{aedcbfg}* chromosome. Similar type of loop formation seen in paracentric inversion is seen here also. If a cross over takes place {see Fig. 1.90 in the inversion region between gene loci Cand D and the cross over products separate during anphase what will be the chromosome compliment of each one of the chromatids? Unlike in the case of paracentric inversion no anphase bridge or acentric fragment is produced; all the chromatids will have centromere but they {50%} suffer from duplications and deficienicies. The chromosome compliment of each of the chromatid is as follows.

	↓	
Chromatid 1	ABCDEFG	(Metacentric)
(non cross over)	↓	
Chromatid 2	ABCdea	(Submetacentric)
(cross over)	↓	
Chromatid 3	gfbcDEFG	(Submetacentric)
(cross over)	↓	
Chromatid 4	aedcbfg	(Submetacentric)
(non cross over)		

(Arrows among gene sequence indicate the position of the centromere)

In the above instance, if the inversion has occured on the male side 50% of the pollen (in plants) or 50% of the sperms (in animals) would survive. Balance would abort due to duplications and deficiencies. In the case of female however, it depends as to which of the chromatid would be included in the egg. The egg would survive if it gets chromatid 1 or 4, if it gets 2 or 3 it would not survive. In the case of embryo sacs of higher plants generally the intact chromatids (1 and 4) are so oriented that they will be included in the outer megaspores and the irregular chromatids (2 and 3) will be in the central megaspores. Consequently, the basal megaspore receives either a normal or an inverted chromosome and the gametophyte survives.

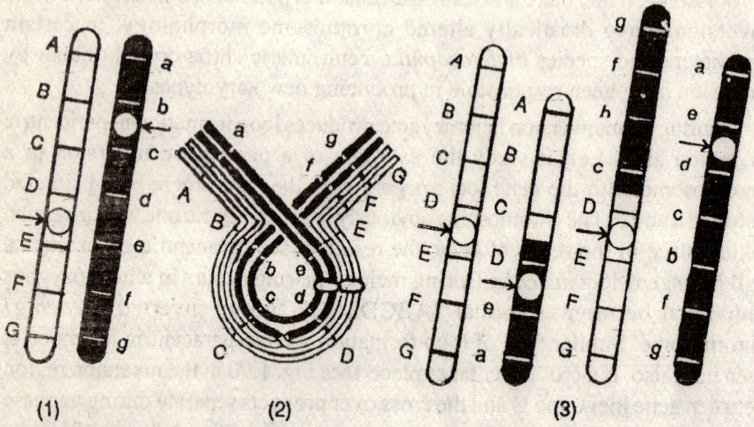

Fig. 8.6 Chromosomal Aberrations

Consequence of crossing over in a heterozygote, with pericentric inversion

1. Homologous chromosomes
2. Crossing over with loop formation
3. Meiotic products

Overlapping inversions

In some instances a second inversion may take place within the first inversion; such a type of inversion is said to be overlapping inversion. For example the normal chromosome is ABCDEFG and the inverted chromosome is AEDCBFG; a second inversion taking place within the inverted segment EDCB between B and E will result in a chromosome of the gene loci - AECDBFG.

Role of inversions in evolution : Interest in inversion having a bearing on evolution centres round paracentric inversions. Overlapping inversions studied in *Drosophila pseudoobscura* and *D.persimilis* have shown that the inversions are interrelated. An analysis of the natural populations at mountain ranges and elsewhere has shown that, populations in cool weather have a high frequency of inversions than those found elsewhere. This indicates that inversions are not only tolerated but may actually have selective value in natural populations. For the inversion to have any selective value, it must not be too long to have cross over effecting the allelic sequence but must be long enough to accumulate a genetic difference. It is possible according to Swanson (1967) that inversions can serve as foci for species divergence given sufficient time to accumulate genetic differences and the erection of barriers to prevent breeding within the population.

Inversion at the molecular level

What happens in the DNA molecule when an inversion takes place? Obviously the two stands of a DNA molecule are involved and two breaks occuring would switch the nucleotide sequence resulting in alteration. But there is one problem here due to the antiparallel nature of the helix; the segment cannot rejoin the main helix in the reverted position; it must also rotate 180 before reinsertion. Because of this rotation, there is some sort of a hybridization in both the helices in that they get a portion of the opposing helix. This will drastically alter both the helices and consequently the RNA and protein synthesis. It is this that is perhaps mainly responsible for the non viabality of the affected gametes.

TRANSLOCATIONS

This is a type of structural aberration affecting at least two chromosomes. Hence it is also known as inter chromosomal structural aberration. As the very name indicates, in *translocation* a segment of the chromosome is removed and it attaches itself to another non homologous chromosome. Let us assume that there are two non homologous chromosomes 1) ABCDEF and 2) GHIJKL; the DEF portion from the first chromsome will attach itself to the second chromosome. After traslocation, the two chromosomes would be 1) ABC and 2) GHIJKL DEF. There would be deficiency in the first chromosome, but there are no duplications, in the second chromosome. This type of translocation is theoretically possible but it will not normally take place because of the presence of telomere in the other chromosome (GHIJKL) which will not allow any attachment at the tip. Normally however two non homologuous chromosomes exchange their segments. For e.g. ABCDEF and GHIJKL exchange segments DEF and JKL. After translocation the two chromosomes would be ABCJKL and GHIDEF. In order to have this type of exchange, there will be breaks in both the chromosomes. Such a type of translocation in which two non homologous chromosomes mutually exchange segments is known as **reciprocal translocation**. The two new chromosomes thus produced will survive provided they have only one centromere. If the reunion is such that as to produce dicentric chromosomes or acentric fragments, they will generally not survive due to failure of proper seggregation during anaphase.

Like inversions, translocations may exist either in a homozygous state or in a heterozygous state. Homozygous translocations behave perfectly normal during meiosis, exhibit linear pairing except for the fact of new linkage group of genes. It they survive, they give rise to new chromosome race. These are found sporadically in many organisms, but more commonly in *Oenothera, Paeonia, Datura* etc., in plants and scorpions and roaches among animals.

Translocation heterozygotes have only one of the homologues (of 2 chromosomes) affected while the other is normal. For e.g. considering the above example the pollen mother cell or MMC (or oocyte or spermatocyte) will have the following chromosomes.

Homologue I ABCDEF and ABCJKL
Homologue II GHIJKL and GHIDEF.

Homologue I ABCDEF and ABCJKL
Homologue II GHIJKL and GHIDEF.

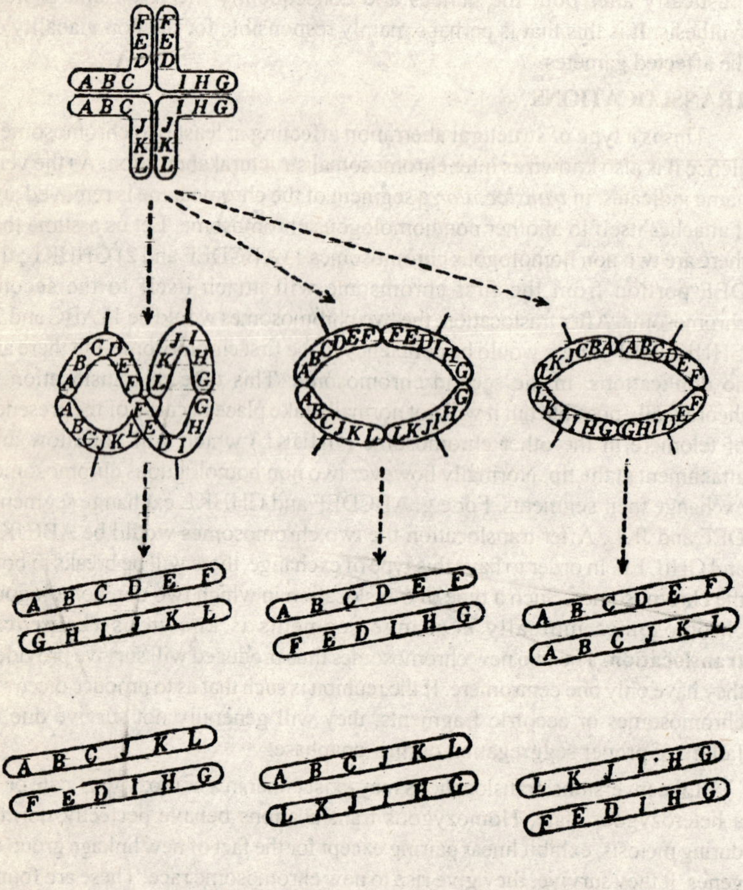

Fig. 8.7 Chromosomal Aberrations
Consequences of meiosis in a translocation heterozygote

In such a situation how can pairing take place between ABCDEF and ABCJKL; GHIJKL and GHIDEF. If there is a linear pairing roughly 50% of the length of the chromosome in both cases will remain out of synopsis. This is not conducive to the individual. Hence in order to have pairing, at all gene loci, all the four chromosomes combine and form a peculiar cross shaped or + shaped configuration at pachytene with the pairing partners being changed at the point of translocation break. In other words one half of the chromosome pairs with its homologue and the other half pairs with the allelic loci attached to a non homologous chromosome.

After pairing and cross over they have to separate out during metaphase. At that time a ring of four chromosomes is formed as the cross shaped configuration opens out. When the time of segregation comes as during metaphase and early anaphase how do they segregate to the two opposite poles?

The arrangement of the chromosomes on the metaphase plate determines the type of segregation and this has far reaching genetic consequences. There are three possible types of seggregation. *Adjacent I, Adjacent II* and *altemale* segregation. If we give the chromosomes, numbers as follow:

ABCDEF 1, GHIDEF 2
GHIJKL3 ABCJKL4.

In *adjacent segregation I,* the cross shaped configuration of prophase opens out in the form of a ring and the segregation is as follows. Chromosome 1 and 2 to one pole and chromosome 3 and 4 to another. Here the meiotic product having 1 and 2 will not survive because it has duplication for DEF but deficiency for JKL; similarly the other meiotic product receiving 3 and 4 also will not survive because it has duplication for JKL but deficiency for DEF.

In adjacent segregation II the chromosome opens out in the form of a ring; but here chromosomes 1 and 4 are adjacent and similarly are 2 and 3. Chromosomes 1, and 4 would go to one pole and 2 and 3 would go to another pole. Here also the meiotic product having 1 and 4 will not survive as there is duplication for ABC and deficiency for GHI. Similarly meiotic product enclosing 2 and 3 also will not survive because duplication for GHI and deficiency for JKL.

In both the instances mentioned above (adjacent I and adjacent II) there is 100% sterility as no viable gametes are formed.

In the third type of segretation called *alternate segregation,* the cross shaped configuration of prophase opens out in the form of number 8 (ie with two rings) in such a way that chromosomes 1 and 3 and 2 and 4 are adjacent. Meiotic product enclosing 1 and 3 and meiotic product enclosing 2 and 4 chromosomes will survive as they suffer from neither duplication nor deficiency. 1 and 3 however are normal while 2 and 4 are traslocated chromosomes.

The translocations discussed above deal with the involvement of only two non homologous chromosomes and in the ring at metaphase only four chromosomes are found. However if the arm of one of the translocated chromosomes is involved in exchange with a third non homologous chromosome, a ring of 6 chromosomes is found at the metaphase. If there is a third exchange a ring of eight chromosomes would be formed. This process can go on ultimately to involve all the chromosomes in an individual to form a *translocation complex.* This phenomenon is found in *Rheo discolor* a member of the family Commelinaceae of monocots, where a ring of 12 chromosomes are found at metaphase. This is called *chromosome ring.* (different from ring chromosome seen in some prokaryotes) and is due to the whole genome being involved in translocation. The plants *Oenothera* and *Paeonia* represent different stages (grades) of translocation complex. *Paeonia californica* with 5 pairs of chromosomes has the following combinations

(a) Ring of 4 Chromosomes and 3 bivalents
(b) Ring of 6 Chromosomes and 2 bivalents
(c) Ring of 8 Chromosomes and 1 bivalent
(d) Ring of 10 Chromosomes and no bivalent.

In *Oenolhera* also, different grades of complexes are found; while *O.hookeri* has all 7 normal bivalents, *O.lamarckiana* has all the 14 chromosomes forming a ring. (more details of *Oenothera* are discussed later)

Genetic detection of translocation

Heterozygous translocation may be detected by crossing two such individuals. The resultant progeny is of three types *viz.* Normal homozygotes, Interchange heterozygotes and Interchange homozygotes.

Translocation both in the homozygous and in the heterozygous condition affects the gene linkage. In homozygotes, the linkage is disrupted, if the translocated segment is not linked to its original group. Study of this linkage can be used to detect translocation and identify the chromosome involved. In the translocation heterozygote all the genes in the involved chromosomes are linked. This is because only the perfectly balanced gametes survive and take part in fertilization. Heterozygotes can also be detected by their semisterility as in the male side only 50% would survive. In the female side however there can be partial or complete sterility.

Evolutionary implication of translocation

The evolutionary implications of translocation are quite perplexing in that they produce new chromosome linkages. Among plants *Datura* and *Oenothera* have provided a wealth of information. In a translocation heterozygote involving two chromosomes, a ring of four is formed at the metaphase plate. The four chromosomes do not have an independent assortment. Sheer pressure of survival, forces on them alternate seggregation, resulting in two normal chromosomes forming a group and so are the two translocated chromosomes. In other words the two chromosomes which were initially independent, now are linked in spite of the fact that chromosomes exist as independent entities. As the translocation complex increases in number, the independent behaviour of the chromosomes decrease and as it happens in *Oenothera lamarckiana,* all the 14 chromosomes form one large translocation complex (a large chromosome ring is formed at metaphase involving all the 14 chromosomes). In this plant, the translocation complexes are called the **Renner complexes** named after the discoverer. Of the 14 chromosomes found at the metaphase plate, once again the chromosomes can not afford the luxury of free or independent seggregation. Survival instinct again forces them into two groups (or complexes) of 7 each. In effect there are two linkage groups with 7 chromosomes each. In a seggregation of this type there is no lethality. These two chromosome groups are called *Renner complexes.* Each ring having 14 chromosomes is actually a dual entity, because each has two complexes which may differ in genetic content. In *O.lamarckiana,* the two Renner complexes called **Gaudens** and **Velans** yield entirely different projenies when crossed with other forms. The individuals of *O.lamarckiana* are generally self pollinated and breed true and retain the structural complexity. A further refinement of the Renner complex is the *Renner effect,* when the two complexes are trasmitted in different ways ie. one *via.* egg and the other *via* sperm.

The evolutionary path in *Oenothera* is via the translocation complexes. The translocation having once arisen in the course of evolution has been stabilized in the gene pool by making it workable in the genetic machinery. The *Oenothera* is a clear example as to how a genetic irregularity deleterious to the organism to a certain degree has been incorporated into the system and made to function well. Similarly, the absence of cross pollination and retention of only self pollination, which to a certain extent is disadvantageous to the organism, is actually beneficial here as it helps in maintaining the complex, while cross pollination can break the complex by bringing in new and unknown genes into picture.

NUMERICAL ABERRATIONS

In the biological heirarchy, species form the basic genetic unit capable of surviving and maintaining its structure. This constancy (subject of course to mutational influences) of character in a species has as its basis, the chromosomal background. The number and kinds of chromosomes in a species are sufficiently constant to delimit it from others. But as the genes mutate or change, so also chromosomes are subject to variations. The process of alteration in chromosome numbers seen very often in plants and to a less extent in animals is called numerical aberrations.

Numerical aberrations in chromosomes produce two types of cells or individuals. These are 1) those whose somatic genome (chromosome complement) is the exact multiple of the basic number characteristic of the species and 2) those in which the somatic number is an irregular multiplication of the basic number. Occasionally there could be reduction in the basic number also. The first category is said to be *Euploid* and the second one is called *Aneuploid.* Euploids may be Haploid (monoploid), diploid, triploid, tetraploid and polyploid. Haploid is the basic number of the species with one set of chromosomes in the body cells, diploids have 2 sets, triploids have 3 sets, tetraploids have 4 sets and further multiplication series are refered to as polyploid.

Individuals whose genome complement is aneuploid have one or two extra chromosomes added or one or two chromosomes deleted from the normal number of diploid in the body cells. For instance a single chromosome may be missing from the diploid complement when it is called 2n -1: The following is the classification of numerical aberrations.

Numerical aberrations

- Euploidy
  - Haploidy
  - Diploidy
  - Polyploidy
- Aneuploidy
  - Hyperploidy
    - (a) Trisomy
    - (b) Tetrasomy
  - Hypoploidy
    - (a) Monosomy
    - (b) Nullisomy

ANEUPLOIDY

In aneuploidy, there is either reduction or partial increase of the chromosome number. Reduction is said to be hypoploidy, while increase is said to be hyperploidy. Hypoploidy is due to loss of one or two chromosomes. If a single chromosome is lost from a diploid complement it is said to be Monosomy (individuals are called *monosomics)* and is symbolically designated as 2n-l. If two chromosomes are lost (ie. both the homologues in a pair) it is said to be

Nullisomy (2n-2). Similarly the addition of a third chromosome to one of the bivalents is called *Trisomy* (2n + 1) and addition of 2 chromosomes to a bivalent is said to be *tetrasomy* (2n + 2).

Monosomy : In monosomic diploid individuals, (in the genome) one of the pairs of homologues would undergo a loss of one chromosome and it becomes a univalent while all others are bivalents. The diploids cannot generally withstand such a loss, while polyploids can withstand it. This is due to the fact that polyploids (see later in the same chapter) have more than two homologues for every pair. Theoretically the number of monosomics possible in an individual equals its haploid number. In common wheat where there are 21 pairs of chromosomes; there are 21 possibilities for monosomics. E.R. Sears has artificially induced these 21 monosomics in a wheat variety called *Chinese spring.* Monosomics have been induced in cotton (Endrizzi *et al)* and tobacco (Clausen and Cameron).

While diploids with monosomics do not survive, there are instances as in tomato, where monosomics could be produced. Here the chromosome number is 2n = 24. Double and triple monosomics (2n - 1 - 1) have two homologues lost from two different bivalents. During meiotic prophase, together with the normal bivalents there will be two separate univalents indicating that both these have lost their partners. Similarly in triple monosomy one homologue each is lost from three different bivalents and three univalents appear at the meiotic prophase.

Monosomy can be detected by comparing it with the normal individual and associated traits. In a cross between two monosomics, we will get normal, monosomics and nullisomics in a mixture. Nullisomics (if they survive) will not exhibit any of the morphological traits seen on the missing chromosome; there by specific traits and genes can be located on this chromosome.

Aneuploidy has been noticed in human beings also. A classical instance is the *Turner's syndrome* named after the discoverer H.H. Turner (1938). It occurs in 0.23 infants for every 1000 births. Here there is a loss of one of the X chromosomes and the females would be XO instead of XX. Adult females with Turner's syndrome have no ovaries and no secondary sexual characters and are sterile. They have abnormal jaw, hypoplasia and webbed neck. Turner's syndrome arises by the fertilization of an egg with a defective sperm (having no X chromosome)

Nullisomy : In this, an entire pair of homologous chromosomes will be missing (2n - 2). This should not be mistaken with double monosomy where 2 chromosomes are lost from two different pairs. In nullisomics, the metaphase plate at meiosis I will apparently show no abnormality and only a comparison with the normal can detect the loss of one whole pair of chromosomes. Nullisomics have been identified in wheat and other plants.

Trisomy : In trisomic individuals one of the pairs of homologues will have an additional member. Trisomic individuals exhibit a trivalent together with the normal bivalents during meiotic metaphase. These are designated as 2n + 1. There could be a double trisomy in which case two of the bivalents will have one additional member. At the metaphase of meiosis I, there will be two trivalents. The number of possible trisomy in individuals equals the number of haploid set. For eg. in barley where the haploid number is 7, seven trisomics are possible.

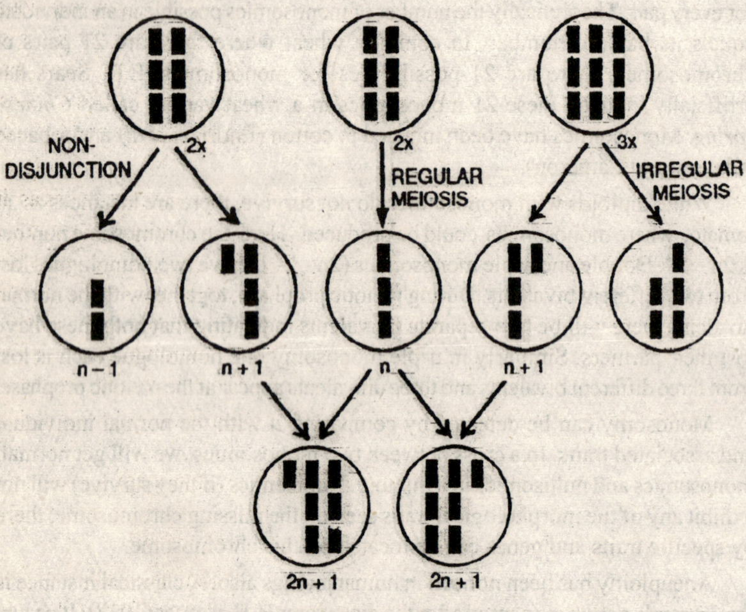

Fig. 8.8 Chromosomal Aberrations
Origin of different types of aneuploidy

Trisomics are classified into primary, secondary and tertiary based on the type of the additional chromosome. If the extra member is identical to the other two homologues, the trisomy is said to *be primary trisoinm* (there is a triplicate of a chromosome). In secondary trisomy, while two are normal chromosomes, the third member is an isochromosome (with two arms genetically identical). In tertiary trisomy, the extra chromosome is the product of translocation.

In plants, trisomy has been studied extensively *in Datura,* maize, tomato and *Nicotiana.* In animals, trisomy has been reported in *Drosophila* and others including human beings.

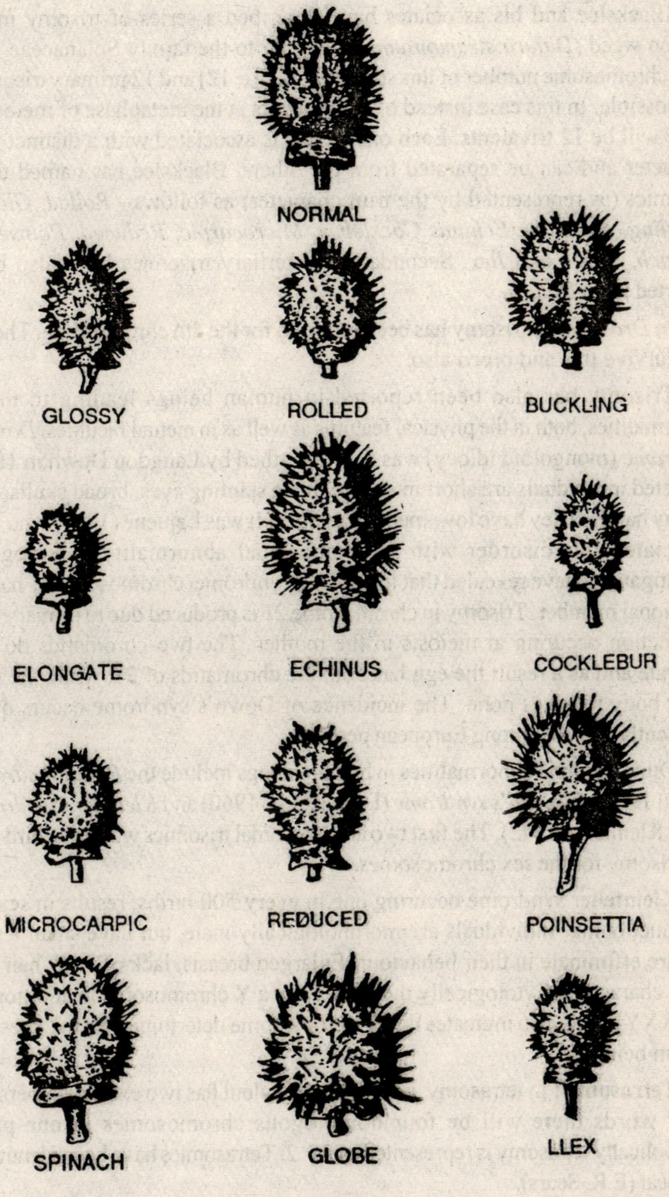

Fig. 8.9 Chromosomal Aberrations
Trisomy in Datura, resulting in different types of fruit shapes

Blackslee and his associates have described a series of trisomy in the jimson weed *(Datura stramonium)* belonging to the family Solanaceae. The base chromosome number of this species is 12 (n = 12) and 12 primary trisomics are possible. In this case instead of 12 bivalents at the metaphase of meiosis I, there will be 12 trivalents. Each one of this is associated with a distinct fruit character and can be separated from the others. Blackslee has named these trisomics (as represented by the fruit character) as follows - *Rolled, Glossy, Buckling, Elongate, Echinus Cocklebur, Microcarpic, Reduced, Poinsettia, Spinach, Globe* and *Ilex*. Secondary and tertiary trisomics have also been reported from *Datura.*

In *Drosophila,* trisomy has been reported for the 4th chromosome. The fly can survive this and breed also.

Trisomy has also been reported in human beings leading to many abnormalities, both in the physical features as well as in mental faculties. *Down's syndrome* (mongoloid idiocy) was first described by Langdon Down in 1866. Affected individuals are short in stature, have slanting eyes, broad skulls, and stubby hands. They have low mental faculties. It was Lejuene (1959) who first associated this disorder with a chromosomal abnormality. Cytological investigations have revealed that in Down's syndrome, chromosome 21 has an additional member. Trisomy in chromosome 21 is produced due to primary non disjunction occuring at meiosis in the mother. The two chromatids do not separate and as a result the egg has both the chromatids of 21, while the first polar body receives none. The incidence of Down's syndrome occurs quite frequently (1:700) among European people.

Other trisomic abnormalities in human beings include the *Patau syndrome* (Patau 1960), *Edward's syndrome* (Edward J.H. 1960) and *Kleinfeter syndrome* (H.F. Kleinfelter 1942). The first two are autosomal trisomics while the third one is a trisomy for the sex chromosomes.

Kleinfelter syndrome occuring one in every 500 births, results in sexual malfunctioning. Individuals are morphologically male, but have small testes and are effiminate in their behaviour. Enlarged breasts, lack of body hair are other characters. Cytologically the cells show a Y chromosome in addition to 2X (XXY). This also indicates that Y chromosome determines the maleness in human beings.

Tetrasomy : In tetrasomy, a particular bivalent has two extra members; in other words there will be four homologous chromosomes in one pair, Symbolically tetrasomy is represented as 2n+2. Tetrasomics have been identified in wheat (E.R. Sears).

EUPLOIDY

Euploid individuals could be haploids, diploids or polyploids and represent the multiplication of the entire genome.

Haploids : Haploid or *n* number of chromosomes in the body cells may be normal or abnormal. In lower plants and animals, haploid condition is normal in the sense, here the individuals have only one set of chromosomes in the body cells, while diploid condition is represented only in the zygote. This is of normal occurrence. Haploidy is of interest when it occurs in diploid individuals. Here normally the body cells have 2 sets of chromosomes. Reduction division takes place and haploid gametes are formed. These gametes however have no morphological expression ie. they cannot directly develop into new individuals. They fuse with another gamete resulting in the formation of a diploid individual. Rarely however haploid individuals are produced as during parthenogenesis when the egg directly develops into a new individual without fertilization. Haploids are of two kinds *euhaploids* and *aneuhaploids*. While the former are derived from euploids the latter are derived from aneuploids.

Origin and production of Haploids : In some insects haploid individuals are produced naturally due to parthenogenesis. In plants also parthenogenetic development of egg results in haploid individuals. Such haploids have been seen in cotton, tomato etc.

In rare instances, pollen tube, or microspores may develop into new individuals. Such individuals are called *androgenic haploids* as they are produced from the male tissue. Occasionally synergids, antipodals etc may also develop into haploid embryos.

Haploids can artificially be obtained by tissue culture of the anther, pollen, X ray treatment, colchicine treatment, distance hybridization etc.

Anther culture has yielded excellent haploids in *Nicotiana* and Potato. Similarly Inter specific crosses may also result in haploid individuals. According to Kasha (1970), in a cross between *Hordeum vulgare* X *H. bulbosum'*. Chromosomes *of H. bulbosum* are eliminated in early zygotic division. Embryosacs of these can be cultured to obtain haploid individuals.

Morphology of haploids : There is general reduction in size and stature of the individual. This is also reflected in their physiology and generally they are not vigorous.

Cytology of haploids : In a haploid set all the chromosomes are non homologous and hence at metaphase I, they retain as univalents. Consequently these are distributed randomly at anaphase I for e.g. in maize a haploid (n = 10) individual produces gametes whose chromosome number ranges from 0-10. As a result there will be partial or complete sterility. Restitution nucleus may be formed.

Use of Haploidy : In normal diploids, haploid individuals help us to understand the functioning of recessive genes and also the expression of other genes in the haploid state. Doubling of haploid chromosomes will also bring about a completely homozygous diploid. This is of particular interest in plant breeding as this would bring about the effect of several genĕrations of inbreeding.

POLYPLOIDS

In polyploid individuals, the body cells have more than two sets of chromosomes and consequently multivalents are formed at the metaphase I in meiosis.

There are mainly three categoreis of polyploids - *Autopolyploids, Allopolyploids* and *Autoallopolyploids.*

The following chart gives the derivation of these from three diploids with genomes AA and $B_1 B_1$ and $B_2 B_2$.

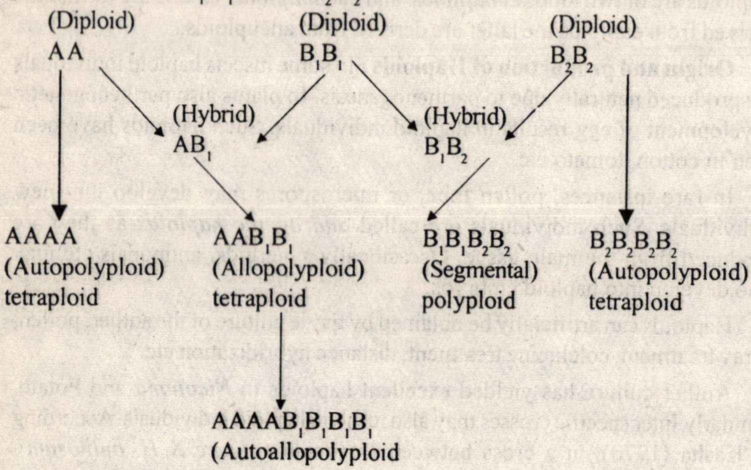

Autopolyploids : Here the same basic genome set is multiplied. For instance if the diploid genome is AA, autotriploid would be AAA, autotetraploid would be AAAA, autooctoploid - AAAAAAAA etc. An auto tetraploid would result either by doubling of somatic chromosomes or by the union of two unreduced gametes. Autotriploid can arise by a cross between a tetraploid and a diploid as shown below.

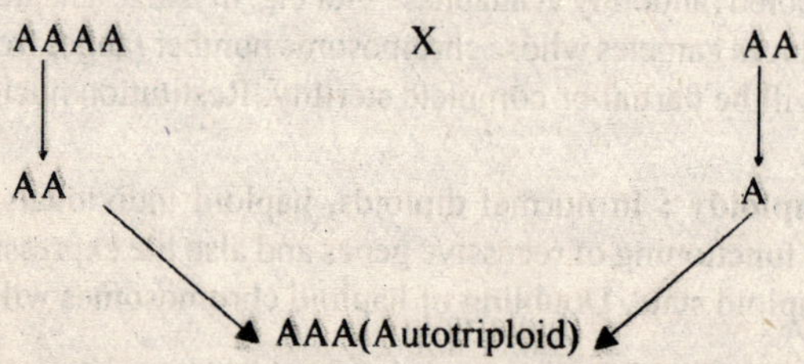

Distribution ofAutopolyploids : According to Muntzing (1936), these are widely distributed among the plants. But recent studies have shown (Clausen, Stebbins etc) that they are not as frequent as they were thought to be. Autopolyploidy has also been reported in the common Indian grass *(Cynodon dactylon)*. This is known to be an autotriploid and survives mainly due to vegetative propagation. Autotriploids are known in water melons, sugar beet, tomato etc. Similarly autotetraploids are known in rye, corn, red clover, marigolds, snapdragons, flox, grapes etc.

Autopolyploidy can be artificially induced by various treatments. These include, ionizing radiation, chemicals, mustard gas etc. Since polyploid individuals have large stature, bigger fruits, increased yield etc, various techniques have been employed to induce polyploidy. Of all the methods the use of *Colchicine* is most sought after. Colchicine is an alkaloid, obtained from the bulbs of a liliaceous plant *Colchicum autuinnale*. The drug was first isolated by Houde (1887). Doubling of chromosomes due to the treatment with Colchicine was first reported by Levan (1938). The drug however is not effective against the *Colchicum* plant due to the presence of *anticolchicine*. Colchicine treatment may be given in one of the following ways.

a) *Seed treatment* : Seeds are soaked in 0.1 to 0.5% solution.

b) *Injection* : Solution is injected into the seedlings.

c) *Bud treatment* : Cotton dipped in solution is placed on the buds.

Effect of doubling of chromosomes : Polyploids are generally larger is size, but they bring in many undesirable characters also, like lack of resistance decreased rate of cell division, slow blooming etc.

Cytology of autopolyploids : Cytologically autopolyploids produce multivalents at metaphase I. The number of multivalents is 4 for tetraploids and 3 for triploids. While there is no abnormality in the case of tetraploids as diploid gametes can be formed, the meiosis is irregular in triploids. During disjunction, the trivalents separate as 2:1, or 1:1 with one chromosome left at the centre. This depends on the type of cross over. Since there are three homologues one chromosome may have cross over with two others at different levels. This leads to irregularity in disjucntion and deficiencies in the gamete. In tetraploids, the disjunction is usually 2:1 or rarely 3:1. Hence autotetraploids may show partial sterility, while triploids are generally sterile.

Commercial use of autopolyploidy is possible as in the case of seedless fruits (Produced by Kihara in Japan). Similarly, in crop plants also polyploidy has been known to produce plants with a greater vigour.

Allopolyploids : This is produced by crossing two different species with no chromosome homology.

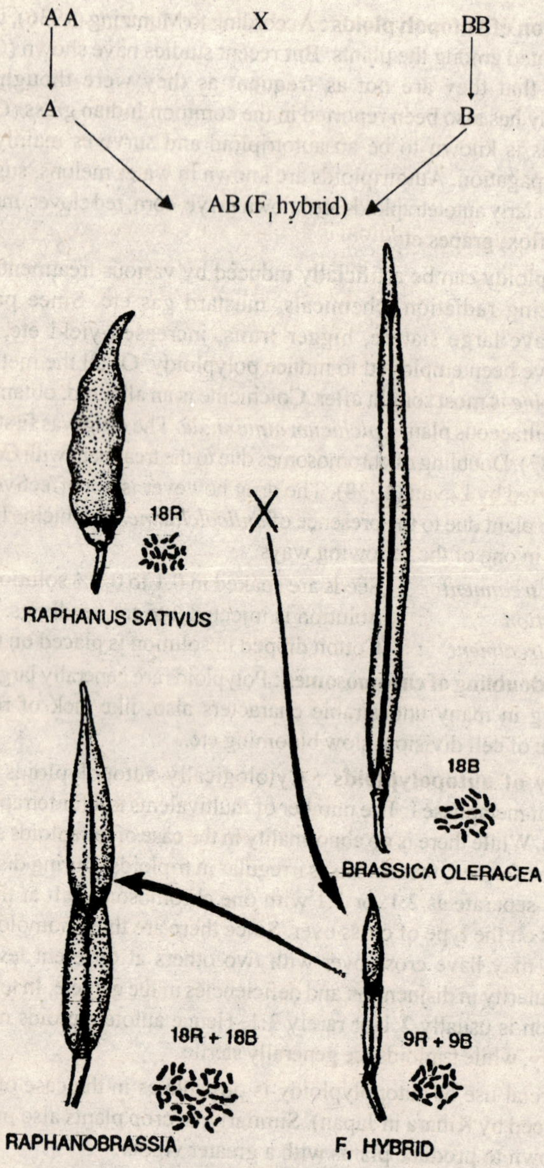

Fig. 8.10 Chromosomal Aberrations
Origin of Raphanobrassica

If one speices has AA genome and the other BB genome, the resultant F_1 will be AB. This individual is completely sterile because there is no pairing and all the chromosomes spread randomly at metaphase I and distribute irregularly at anaphase I. No gametes would survive. If the chromosomes of this F_1 hybrid (AB) are doubled, the resultant individual is called an *Allotetraploid (Allopolyploid)*. As distinct from autopolyploids, allopolyploids have multiplication of different genomes (in autopolyploids the same genome is multiplied). The Allotetraploid is fertile because the two genomes A and B will find their homologues (AA and BB) and a perfect pairing takes place Since A and B genomes are different, there is no multivalent formation (since there are only two homologues for a kind of chromosome). At metaphase only bivalents are formed. This can be easily mistaken for a diploid if one does not known the origin. It is because of this that very often Auotetraploids are called *Ainphidiploids* (tetraploids functioning like diploids).

A classical example of Allotetraploid is provided by *Raphanobrassica* reported in 1927 by the Russian scientist Karpachenko. He crossed *Raphanus sativas* (2n = 18) *and Brassica oleracea* (2n = 18) and obtained an F_1 hybrii which was completely sterile. The sterility was due to complete non homology between the genomes of *Raphanus and Brassica*. But some fertile plants were obtained which had 2n == 36, obviously due to doubling or the incorporation of all the chromosomes at metaphase into one gamete (after the division of the centromere).

There are several examples of allotetraploids artificially produced by crossing two different species and doubling the chromosome of the F_1 hybrid.

1. *Primula verticellata* (18) X *Primula floribunda* (18)
   = *Primula kewensis* (Autotetraploid) (36)

2. *Galiopsis speciosa* (16) X *Galiopsis pubescens* (16)
   = *Galiopsis tetrahedra* (Autotetraploid) (32)

3. *Spartina alternifolia* (70) X *Spartina stricta* (56)
   = *Spartina townsendii* (126)

(Numbers in parenthesis indicate the 2n chromo number)

Examples of Amphidiploidy (Allotetraploid) among cultivated plants are seen in cotton, wheat, barely etc.

Segmental allopolyploids : In certain allopolyploids, the genomes coming from different parents are not altogether different. As a result there is some degree of pairing and multivalents are formed. This means that segments of chromosomes and not entire chromosomes are homologous. Such allopolyploids are called segmental allopoyploids and they are intermediate between auto and allopolyploids. The common bread wheat is regarded as a segmental allopolyploid.

Auto allopolyploid : This is a higher series of polyploid (octoploid). It can be produced as follows. A cross between two species (AA, BB) would yield a F_1 sterile hybrid (AB); on doubling, this becomes an amphidiploid (AA BB). If there is doubling of chromosomes in an amphidiploid it results in an autoallopolyploid (AA AA BB BB). The name autoallopolyploid is due to the fact that allopolyploid genomes are doubled to give rise to a polyploid having characters of both auto and allopolyploids.

ROLE OF POLYPLOIDY IN EVOLUTION

Polyploid individuals are different from their diploid relatives in many characters; yet they retain some degree of genetic semblance (allopolyploids) with the diploids. Polyploidy influences not only the morphological attributes of the individual but also has a profound effect on the reproductive potentiality and genetic variability of the progeny. All these obviously play an important role in evolution.

Comparison of natural polyploids with their diploid relatives and artificially produced polyploids provides us an indepth knowledge into the genetic machinery of polyploids. The resynthesis of polyploids from their diploid ancestors has provided additional proof about the origin of polyploids. Natural hybridization or introgression between species and doubling of the chromosomes has contributed a great lot in the evolution of species.

Polyploidy is widely distributed among the various groups of plant kingdom, but they are relatively scarce among animals. Even though this seems to be a mystery a careful analysis of the karyotype of animals and plants will readily provide an answer for the paucity of polyploidy among animals. In majority of the animals, there is a sharp contrast of two sexes resting upon a delicate balance between autosomes and sex chromosomes. This does not permit the addition or deletion of any member of the genome as is easily done in the case of hermaphroditic plants. In animals, wherever polyploidy has been reported it is associated with parthenogenetic development. There is one exception however as in the case of the saw fly, where an authentic case of polyploidy has been reported without the accompanying parthenogenesis.

Effect of polyploidy on structure and function of the organisms

A polyploid individual arising from a diploid population can survive and stabilize itself in the population provided the genetic alterations are such that it can fit into the existing genetic pool, while still showing variations. Between allopolyploids and autopolyploids, the former have a greater chance of survival. The effect of polyploidy on the morphology and physiology of the individual to a great extent will determine, whether the individual in question will survive in the environment. One of the favourite effects of polyploidy is gigantism, but it may not be always so. The other morphological and physiological effects of polyploidy have already been discussed.

Distrubiton ofpolyploids in the plant kingdom : Polyploidy has a wide distribution in the plant kingdom except perhaps for lower plants. Among the lower plants, tetraploidy perhaps exists in baker's yeast *(Saccharomyces cereviseae)*. Tischler (1950) records a number of Algae as being polyploid. According to Manton (1952) the Horsetails, Clubmosses and the Psilotales represent the remanants of an ancient polyploid system. The Filicales also record a very high chromosome number *(Ophioglossum valgatum* has 500 chromosomes). Among the Gymnosperms polyploids are encountered in Gnetales.

Among the flowering plants however, polyploids are quite extensively distributed. According to Stebbins (1950), Tischler (1950), Darlington andJanakiammal (1945), about 30-35% of flowering plants are polyploids (allopolyploids). In grasses about 75% are polyploids. Rosaceae, Polygonaceae, Malvaceae, Crassulaceae among Dicots and Cyperaceae, juncaceae,Iridaceae and Orchidaceae among Moncots exhibit polyploid individuals.

The propensity of allopolyploids and the apparent paucity of autopolyploids in flowering plants is a clear indication that natural hybridization or Introgression and the subsequent doubling of the chromosomes have been going on in plant populations since a long time and have greatly contributed to evolution.

Polyploidy and speciation : In the evolutionary heirarchy, the lowest stable morphological unit is species. Two species are delimited not only on the basis of morphological traits, but underlying this is the chromosomal divergence. When two individuals have sufficient non homology among their chromosomes as to make a cross impossible, they are then said to have evolved into new species. If this statement is true completely; after the establishment of a species, the only factor for variation would be mutation. But evolution cannot depend on only one mechanism for its functioning. Even though species cannot be crossed generally, it does happen in nature and nature itself (or the selective forces) has found an answer to the resultant sterility in the F_1 hybrid. The chromosomes are doubled and the individual becomes fertile; has basic morphological and genetic characters sufficient enough to raise it to the status of a new species. It has happened in the case of *Primula kewensis*. Ever since then several new polyploid species have been created such as *Galeopsis tetrahedra, Spartina townsendii* etc.

Several of our cultivated crops represent a polyploid series indicating their origin from diploid ancestors. The two classical examples are those of wheat and cotton.

The wheat represents an allopolyploid series of diploid, tetraploid and hexaploid species. These three groups are called *Einkorn, Emmer* and *Vulgare* groups. The einkorn group has two diploid (2n = 14) species viz. *Triticum monococcum* and the wild *I. boeticum.* The einkorn speices are single seeded and not of much use for human consumption, because the grains are tightly held in glumes. In some parts of middle east and Europe, they are used for making dark bread.

The emmer group consists of seven species of tetraploid wheats of which the important ones are *Triticum dicoccum* and *T.durun.* The emmer wheat has arisen as a cross between an einkorn wheat and a wild grass *Aegilops* as shown below.

Triticum boeticum (2n = 14) AA X *Aegilops speltoides* (2n = 14) BB

↓

AB (Diploid sterile hybrid)

↓ Doubling

AABB

Triticum dicoccooides

(2n = 28) Fertile alloplyploid

↓ evolved

Triticum dicoccum

(2n = 28) A'A'B'B'

The vulgare group consists of five species of hexaploid wheats (2n = 42) including the familiar bread wheat *Triticum aestivum.* This is said to have been originated as a result of a cross between *Triticum dicoccum* (A'A'B'B') and another species of goat grass *viz. Aegilops squamosa* (diploid DD). The bread wheat therefore has genomes from 3 different sources. All the three wheat groups are interrelated and it is very obvious as to how polyploidy and associated chromosome doubling would have resulted in different species of wheat. But for polyploidy, the other evolutionary force (mutation) could not have produced such variety among wheat.

In cotton, the upland cotton *Gossypicum hirsutum* is a tetraploid and is a result of crossing (and subsequent chromosome doubling) of *G.herbaceum* and *G.raimondii.*

Several such polyploid series are found in *Bromus, Sanicula* etc. Among the Rosaceae the entire tribe pomoideae seems to have been arisen through poplyploidy. According to Sax (1931), the group Pomoideae with n = 17 seems to have been the result of an ancient cross between Spiraeoideae (n = 9) and Prunoideae (n = 8).

Among the polyploid series, the allotetraploid perhaps represents a stage very advantageous to the individual. Allotetraploidy combines the best of both worlds; it has the advantage of higher chromosome numbers, but the genetic and pairing behaviour of a diploid. No wonder then among the polyploids which survive, allotetraploids rank first. The higher series of polyploids however have gone too far in polyploidy and have committed themselves to a polyploid existence with its attendant advantages and disadvantages. Thus they lack the plasticity that is noticed in allotetraploids.

According to Swanson (1975), the sequence of evolution where polyploidy has been an important consideration is as follows. Gene mutation, aberrations and recombination will provide the principal raw material at the diploid level for natural selection. This results in a number of ecotypes from which arise divergent lines leading to higher taxonomic categories. In this scheme of things, autopolyploids have little role to play for they are no different genetically from their diploid parents.

Introgression and doubling of chromosomes however will lead to allopolyploidy and at once creates (evolves) a new species.

Triticale - a man made cereal : This is produced by a cross between wheat and rye. *Triticum durum* (2n = 28) *andSecalecereale* (2n = 14) are crossed producing a F_1 sterile (2n = 21). On doubling, this becomes a hexploid triticale (2n = 42). An octoploid triticale can also be produced by a cross between *Triticum aestivum* (2n = 42) and *Secale cereale* (2n = 14). The resultant F_1 hybrid (2n = 28) is sterile; on chromosome doubling this will lead to an octoploid triticale (2n =-56).

There is some acceptance for the hexaploid triticale from the point of view of grain quality and taste. These hexaploid Triticales are crossed again with wheat to bring about improvement. The products of these crosses are called *secondary Triticales* and are known to be better than *primary Triticales* (produced from wheat and rye). In producing a new species Triticale, man has just imitated the forces of nature which have brought in,an extensive array of biological diversity on earth.

9

CELL DIVISION

The unique and fundamental property of protoplasm is its power to grow and multiply by cell division. Thus new cells arise only by the division of preexisting cells in plants and animals. In unicellular organisms like bacteria, some algae, and fungi and protozoans cell division is the fundamental means of asexual reproduction. In multicellular organisms division of the single celled zygote contributes to the growth of the body. The gametes of the sexually reproducing organisms develop by means of cell division. Three types of cell division occur in living organisms. These are

1. Amitosis or direct cell division
2. Mitosis or indirect cell division
3. Meiosis or reduction division

Amitosis : This is found mainly is prokaryotic organisms like cyanobacteria, bacteria, yeasts etc., (among plants) Protozoa among animals are also known to divide by amitosis. Mostly found in unicellular organisms, amitosis is a means of reproduction. During amitosis, the nucleus elongates and a constriction appears in the centre resulting in a dumb bell shaped structure. The constriction deepens and the nucleus gets divided into two bits. There is no spindle formation and no formation of chromosomes. The nuclear division is followed by cytoplasmic division and the cell gets divided into two daughter cells. Thus amitosis is only a quantitative division.

MITOSIS

Occuring in somatic cells of multicellular organisms mitosis is the chief means of multiplication of cells contributing to the increase in size of the individual. It is the chief means of embryonic development into the adult. Thereafter the capacity for division is restricted to the cells at the tip of the stem, root tips and the cells of the cambium in flowering plants. In animals it is limited to the replacement of worn out cells like blood cells, skin, intestinal epithelium, and the germinal epithelium of the gonads. Mitotic division also occurs during the repairing of wounds in plants and animals.

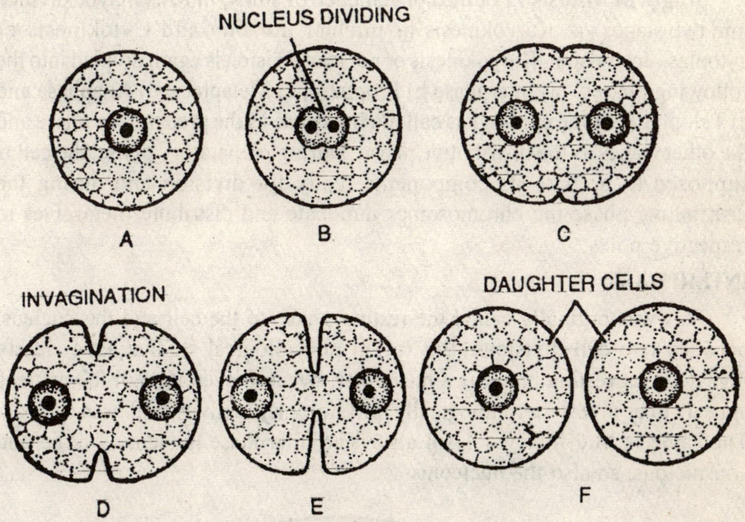

Fig. 9.1 Cell Division
Stages in Amitosis

Definition : The division of the somatic cells is generally called mitosis (Gr *mitos* = thread). It is a complex process involving series of changes leading to the formation of two equal daughter cells from a single parental cell. The term mitosis was first proposed by W.Flemming (1882). It is also called somatic cell division.

Cause of cell division : Why do cells divide? It is very difficult to obtain an answer to this question, although Kinetin a hormone has been isolated which acclerates cell division even in extremely small quantities. The possible reasons are - a) To maintain a relative volume of nucleoplasm and cytoplasm, b) To maintain the nuclear surface to nuclear volume.

Initiation of cell division : Chromosomes may release certain substances which initiates the nuclear changes and cause cytoplasmic division. Cell division may also be resulted by a periodically released hormone called cell division hormone. According to Heilbrunn and Wilson (1948), changing viscosity of the cell may initiate division, the viscosity being lowest at the beginning and gradually increasing and once again becoming low. While it is true that viscosity changes occur during division whether these changes are cause or effect is still not known.

Stages of Mitosis : For the convenience of study, mitosis maybe divided into two stages viz. Karyokinesis or nuclear division and Cytokinesis or cytoplasmic division. Karyokinesis or nuclear division is again divided into the following phases - a) Interphase b) Prophase, c) Metaphase d) Anaphase and e) Telophase. Some cytologists call the Interphae as the preparatory phase and the other stages as the distributive phase. During preparatory phase, the cell is supposed to prepare its components ready for division and during the distributive phase the chromosomes duplicate and distribute themselves to respective poles.

INTERPHASE

This was orginally called the resting phase of the cell and the nucleus, between two cell divisions. But recent physiological studies have clearly revealed that resting phase is a misnomer, because even though the nucleus appears to be at rest morphologically, physiological activity will be at its peak. The same is true for cytoplasm also. The interphase nucleus is large and conspicious, so also the nucleolus.

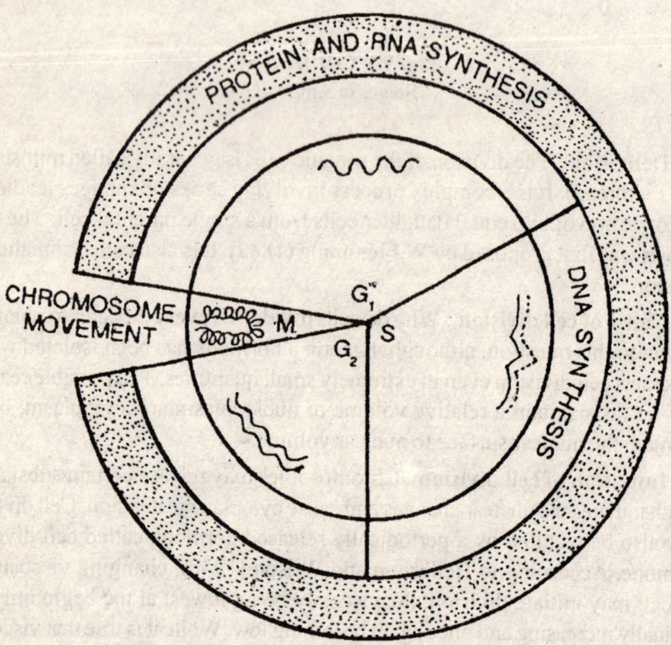

Fig. 9.2 Cell Division
Stages in the inter phase (between mitotic circle)

Three important stages are recognised in the interphase. These are G_1, phase, S phase and the G_2 phase.

The G_1 phase also known as the post mitotic gap phase occurs at the end of every cell division (at the beginning of subsequent division). During this period the daughter cells grow in size. Proteins and RNA are synthesised during this period, but there is no synthesis of DNA.

The S phase, also called the synthetic phase is the most active stage from the point of view of DNA synthesis. It is in this phase that new DNA is formed by replication. Cell division will not proceed if S phase is inhibited.

In the G_2 phase also called the premitotic gap phase, RNA and protein synthesis continues. The volume of the nucleus increases with the increased synthesis of various types of RNA. DNA synthesis however stops in this phase.

In the division cycle G_1 phase is the longest with G_2 and S phase lasting equal amount of time.

Some cytologists use the term M phase or Mitotic phase for the entire distributive phase involving prophase, metaphase, anaphase and telophase and the following cytokinesis.

PROPHASE (Gr. *pro* = before, *phase* = appearance).

This is the first stage of nuclear division. This is the longest stage in the mitotic phase lasting from one to several hours. In the case of onion root tip cells, it lasts for 71 minutes, while in grasshopper neuroblast-102 minutes and in the cells of pea endosperm about 40 minutes. The following are the important features and events taking place in prophase.

1. The cell becomes spheroid (in animals) with increase in its viscosity and refractivity.

2. Differentiation of chromosomes : Chromonemata start condensing and as aresult a long coiled net work called spireme is formed. Continued coiling of the spireme produces thick threads called chromosomes. By the end of prophase the chromosomes contract up to about 1/25 of their length. Specific number of chromosomes are formed (specific to each species).

3. Duplication of chromosomes : Each chromosome splits longitudinally into two identical chromatids connected by a centromere. Two types of coils develop in the chromatids namely somatic coils and minor coils. While the former are larger, the latter are smaller.

4. Shortening of the chromosomes : As the prophase progresses, the somatic coils increase in size but decrease in number. As a result of this,the chromosomes become thick and short.

5. Coiling of the chromatids : The two chromatids are coiled round each other and cannot be easily separated. The coiling is called plectonemic coiling unlike the paranemic coiling of meiosis.

6. Condensation of chromatids : The nuclear matrix begins to accumulate on the chromatids and the chromosomes assume a hazy outline due to irregular accumulation of nuclear matrix

7. Production of achromatic figure : The centrioles which have undergone duplication during interphase and situated above the nucleus start moving in opposite directions. Spindle fibres appear in between the two centrioles. At the same time, radiating fibres called astral rays arise from each centriole forming the aster. The spindle fibres between the two centrioles constitute the amphiaster. The amphiaster is achromatic and does not take stain. Taylor has shown that in Newts, the centrioles move at the rate of one micron per second. When the centriole is present and particpates in cell division it is said to be centric. In acentric mitosis centrioles are absent. Cell division in which aster is formed from the centroile is called astral mitosis (animals and lower plants), when aster is absent it is said to be anastral mitosis (higher plants)

8. Dissolution ofnucleolus : As the coiling continues, the pars amorpha region of the nucleolus decreases in size and finally disappers. But the nucleolonema expands and gets associated with the chromosomes. There is also increase in the RNA content of the chromosomes

9. Dissolution of nuclear envelope : Towards the end of prophase, the nuclear membrane breaks down and gets dispersed into cytoplasm to be absorbed by it. The chromosomes, now free of the nuclear envelope get collected inside the spindle fibres.

PROMETAPHASE

Some cytologists (Threadgold 1968) regard this to be the last stage of prophase, when nuclear envelope disintegrates.According to White (1963), prometaphase is the stage when the spindle is formed and the chromosomes try to reach the equatorial region of the spindle fibres.

METAPHASE

In the cell cycle the metaphase lasts only for a short duration. The following are the main events during metaphase

1. In early metaphase the highly shortened and condensed chromosomes show characteristic radial arrangement on the equatorial plane of the spindle. This pattern of orientation is known as the metaphasic plate or the equatorial plate. It is formed at right angles to the spindle axis.

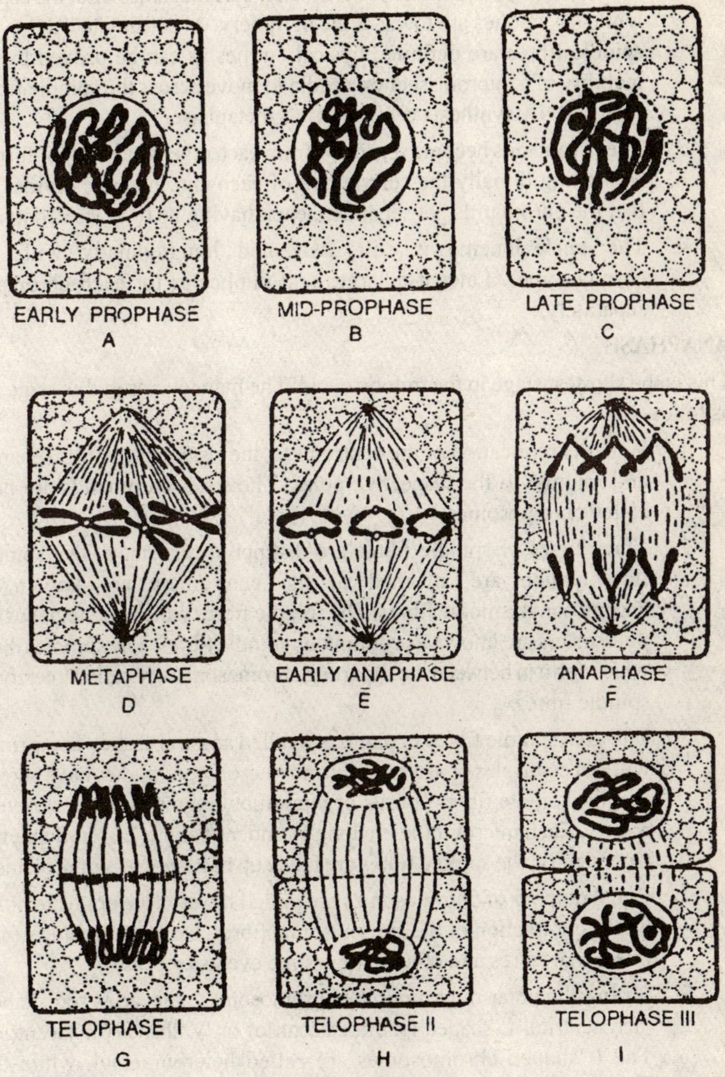

Fig. 9.3 Cell Division
Stages of mitosis in a plant cell

2. The chromosomes lie at the equator with the centroiles pointing towards the poles attached to the spindle fibres, and the arms lying freely in the cytoplasm. In plant cells, chromosomes are irregularly

scattered on the equatorial plate. Smaller chromosomes lie at the centre, while larger ones are towards the periphery. According to Taylor, the spindle fibres are definite physical entities as can be proved by the inability of a microdissection needle to move across the spindle fibres easily. RNA synthesis ceases during metaphase.

3. The chromatids become separated from each other as a result of further shortening. Finally the centromere of each chromosome divides, so that the chromatids get separated, each having its own centromere
4. The nucleolonema is still associated longitudinally with the chromosomes. Later it enlarges and duplicates for each chromatid separately.

ANAPHASE

This is the shortest stage in the mitotic cycle. The main events in this stage are as follows-

1. With the replication of the centromere, the sister chromatids separate and migrate to the respective poles. The sister chromatids are now called chromosomes
2. Three types of spindle fibres are distinct at this stage. The spindle fibres which are attached to the centromere are known as chromosomal spindle fibres. The spindle fibres which connect the two polar asters are known as continuous spindle fibres. The spindle fibres which form in between the departing chromosomes are called interzonal spindle fibres.
3. The total spindle fibres in plants are called anastral as they are formed without centrioles or asters. Electrom microscopic studies have shown that the spindle fibres consist of microtubules embedded in a protein matrix. Each microtubule is a long cylinder of about 20Å in diametre. Chemically, the spindle fibres are made up of monomers of proteins.
4. Equal number of chromosomes are pulled towards the opposite poles by the contraction of the chromosomal fibres, by the stretching of the interzonal fibres and other cytoplasmic events (see later)
5. During the polar migration, the chromosomes, appear as rod shaped (acrocentric), L shaped (sub metacentric) or 'V shaped (metacentric). The L shaped chromosomes are called heterobrachial, while the 'V'shaped ones are called isobrachial as they have arms of equal length.
6. In this manner, the genetic material is equally distributed between the two parts of the cell, which eventually become two daughter cells.
7. Since the centromere is essential for movement,those chromosomes which are without a centromere fail to move to the opposite poles. Such chromosomes are called laggards.

8. The velocity of movement of chromosomes during anaphase ranges . from 0.2 μ per minute to about 5 μ per minute. The rate of movement is independent of the size of the chromosomes.
9. Generally all the chromosomes move simultaneously except for the sex chromosomes which lag behind. Some chromosomes move very early before the group has started migrating. Such movement is said to be precocious movement.
10. End of the anaphase is marked by the appearence of clusters of chromosomes at each pole of the cell.

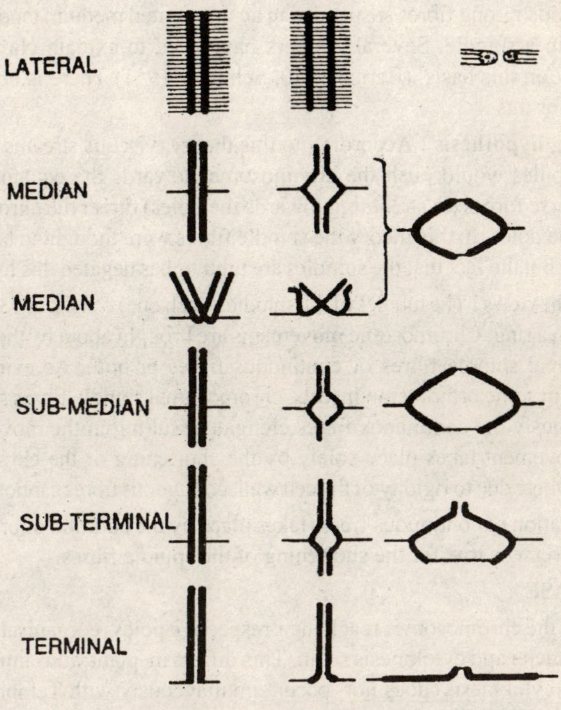

Fig. 9.4 Cell Division
Movement of Chromosomes during anaphase according to the mode of attachment

Chromosome movement during anaphase : Several theories have been proposed to account for the anaphasic movement of the chromosomes. Some of these are-

Electrostatic force : According to Lillie (1905), the chromosome movement is due to electrical charge. The cytoplasm is electronegative, while the nucleus (not chromosomes) is electropositive. Due to this difference in charge, the chromosomes move. This theory however does not explain how chromosomes having same charge as cytoplasm can move.

Hydrodynamic theory : According to this theory proposed by the physicist Bjerknes (1919), two spheres pulsating in a liquid medium set up hydrodynamic forces resembling electric or magnetic forces. In the cell, the spindle poles represent the pulsating forces and they attract the neutral spheres ie., chromosomes. this theory has not been acepted as it will not explain the formation of metaphasic plate.

Tactoids : Long fibres suspended in an unoriented medium tend to line up parallely in a spindle. Several workers have tried to explain chromosomal movement on this basis. (Bernal 1940, Schrader 1951) There is however no evidence for this.

Streaming hypothesis : According to this theory, viscous streams ernnating from the poles would push the chromosomes towards the equatorial plate, while reverse forces (ie streaming towards the poles) direct the chromosomes towards the poles. In this theory the spindle fibres were thought to be lamellar structures, but the fact that the spindles are tubular has negated this hypothesis.

Present views : The tubules of the spindle, (each one) consist of 13 filaments arranged in a ring. Chromosome movements are brought about by the action of chromosomal spindle fibres or continuous fibres or both. As evidence has indicated, in some orthopteran insects, chromosomal spindle fibres shrink and simultaneously the continuous fibres elongate resulting in the movement. In plants, movement takes place solely by the shortening of the chromosomal spindles, where due to rigidity of the cell wall, continuous fibres cannot elongate.

Elongation of continuous fibres takes place by the addition of protein unit and the reverse is true for the shortening of the spindle fibres.

TELOPHASE

When the chromosomes reach their respective poles reorganisation of the daughter nuclei and cytokinesis set in. This differs in plant and animal cells. In plants, cytokinesis does not occur simultaneously with Telophase as in animal cells. The following are the nuclear events in telophase.

1. The chromosomes begin to uncoil into their strands and become indistinct.
2. Nucleolous begins to appear as the nucleolonemal strands become thicker and accumulate.
3. The *gel* state of the spindle reverts to the sol state and the spindles disappear.

4. In animal cells, the asters lose their fibres and reconverted into centrioles. The centrioles take up their natural position outside the nucleus.
5. The nuclear membrane reappears forming a regular nucleus.

CYTOKINESIS

In plants, cell plate is formed between the two groups of chromosomes, by the accumulation of phragmoplasts at the equatorial region. The cell plate is formed at the centre, they grow on either side and join the cell wall. The cell plate formed first will have only middle lamella.

In animal cells, cytokinesis takes place by furrowing, a cleavage furrow appears at the early telophase which becomes deeper as the spindle starts disappearing. The furrows begin from either side and both join at the centre separating the two daughter cells. Various views have been put forward to explain the mechanism of furrowing. Some of these are -

1. **Contractile ring theory :** (Swann and Mitchison 1958) The ectoplasm contracts like the non motile part of amoeba resulting in the formation of a furrow.

2. **Expanding surface theory :** According to this view, some secretions from the nucleus allow the cytoplasm to enlarge at the poles resulting in their contraction at the equational region and a furrow results. But the phenomenon of nuclear secretion has been questioned by Naehtwey (1965).

3. **Spindle elongation theory :** (Dan and Dan 1947, 1958) According to this theory, spindle and astral Fibres are responsible for furrowing. The elongation of the spindle results in contraction at the centre.

4. **Astral relaxation theory :** (Wolpert 1963) According to this, the surface of the cell has uniform tension, but the tension is reduced at the poles when the asters reach the poles. However the tension (being retained) at the equator results in the contraction.

5. **Vescicle formation theory :** (Threadgold 1968) The cell elongates during anaphase causing increased electron density. With the plasma membrane also increasing its electron density, a dielectronicfibrllary plate is formed in the equator. As the furrow progresses, small membrane lined vesciles appear on either side of the plate and coalesce with one another. These seem to arise from the ER. Finally the fusing vesciles form the two daughter cells.

Thus the two daughter cells are formed from the parental cell. During division, the cell organelles like mitochondria, plastids, golgi complex, lyososomes and the cytoplasm are distributed equally to the two daughter cells. Of these organelles, the plastids and mitochondria reproduce themselves, while the behaviour of the other organelles is not known. The two daughter cells are genetically identical with each other. Soon they enter into interphase.

Mitotic apparatus : The mitotic apparatus consists of spindle, centrioles and the aster. The spindle Fibres are of three types (for details see anaphase) The centrioles lie just outside the nuclear membrane.

Frequency and Duration of mitosis : Varies according to the type of organism, tissue, nutrition, temperature and other physical and chemical forces. Bacteria divide every 20 minutes. Paramecium divides every six hours. The cells of higher plants and animals divide once or twice a day. In man about 1-2% of worn out somatic cells are replaced daily. How long does it take a cell to go through the entire process of mitotic division? This can be determined by examining a dividing cell (this is possible in cells grown under tissue culture). In human fibrocytes a duration of 18 hours is required from one interphase to another. But the actual division process from prophase to telophase requires only about 45 minutes. This means that a cell will be in prepration for cell division for over 17 hours.

In the neuroblast cells of the grass hopper embryo, the time required (in minutes) for each stage of division (at 38°C) is as follows. Prophase 102, Metaphase 13, Anaphase 9, Telophase 57, Interphase 27. In this cell, surprisingly the interphase is short compared to human cells. The duration however is dependent on temperature. Lower temperature increases the duration, while higher temperature shortens the duration, subject however to a limit.

In *Tradescantia*, the cells of the staminal hair reveal strikingly the influence of temperature on cell division. At 10°C a complete division takes about 135 minutes. Root tip cells generally take about 22 hours to complete one division at ordinary temperatures, but they can divide at 0°c also. In warm blooded animals however cell division ceases below 24°C and above 46°C.

Significance of mitosis:

1. Mitosis is an extremely regular process. It maintains the qualitative and quantitative distribution of hereditary materials to daughter cells.
2. It maintains constancy of the diploid number of chromosomes of species
3. It maintains the constancy and balance in the DNA and RNA content in the cell
4. It maintains the nuclear and cytoplasmic balance in the cell. In all the cells, the cell cannot expand indefinetly; it has to maintain a balance between the cytoplasm and nucleus called the nucleoplasmic index.
5. Mitosis balances the surface volume ratio of the cell. When the cell increases in size, the surface area in relation to increased volume becomes less. By mitotic division, cells become smaller in size and the surface/volume ratio is restored.

6. Mitosis results in the growth and development of the organism. An idea of growth brought about by mitosis can be obtained from the fact that adult human body consists of 60,000,000,000,000 cells all derived from a single cell.
7. Repair and replacement of dead cells is ensured by mitosis. In human body, dead cells of upper epidermis, gut, RBC are constantly being replaced. According to an estimate 500,000,000,000 cells are replaced daily.
8. It plays an important role in the asexual reproduction and in the formation of gametes in sexually reproducing organisms.

Role of Mitosis in cancer : The cell division in organisms is a highly controlled process and takes place at a specific rate. Usually,after every division there is a gap of time so that the cells physiologically mature, develop polarity and individuality. In other words the cells are allowed to differentiate. This differentiation is the single most important character that is responsible for the integrated and orderly growth of organs and organisms. Strictly speaking, all cells derived from a parental cell by mitosis should be alike but they will not be so due to differentiation. After two cell divisions it is not just four cells that are formed, but four cells with individual characters. If there were to be no phenomenon like differentiation, all organisms produced by zygote should have been nothing but lumps of cells.

If for some reason the mechanism of differentiation operating between cell divisions fails, cells divide at a rapid rate there being no opportunity for them to differentiate. The result will be uncontrolled, unintegrated growth thus producing a cluster of undifferentiated cells. This is called cancerous or tumorous growth. {The rate of cell division is generally uniform for a particular cell type, and cancerous cells violate this}. Also called neoplastic growth, cancerous cells bring disorder and chaos in the structure and physiology of the organ where they are produced. They consume more nutrition, more energy than is the normal case, thus depleting other parts,of the vital ingredients of life.

Mitosis is of great significance in cancer because, the latter is the result of uncontrolled division. What makes the regular rate of mitosis to alter, resulting in the hazardous growth is as yet fully not known. There are many mitotic abnormalities in cancerous cells. The chromosomes differ in their size and number. Chromatid separation is delayed resulting in multinucleate cells. There is a high quantity of DNA in the cancerous cells. The cancerous cells show loss of contact inhibition ie,, ability to grow even in contact with others indefinitely, while normal cells stop growing after they establish a contact with other cells. Much of the cytological details of cancerous cells are understood by working on a human cell culture maintained since a long time called *Hela cells*; these are cells oblained from Henrita Lacks who died of cancer.

Hypotheses on cancer : What makes mitotic division to go haywire? or why the cells become cancerous? The answer to these questions are badly needed in order to control cancer. There are many hypotheses. The following are some of the important ones.

Somatic mutation hypothesis According to this,a mutation occuring in the somatic cells (non germ ells) will alter the control mechamism or inhibit the production of repressor proteins, which in turn block the functioning of the gene.

Viral gene hypothesis : Viruses may be responsible in altering the mitotic mechanism thus producing cancerous cells. This was first discovered by Rous (1911), but people did not beleive it at that time. While there is enough evidence of Viruses causing cancer in animals, hitherto there is no concluding evidence regarding Virus induced cancer in human beings. There is however one evidence of Virus cancer relationship in Burkitt's lymphoma, a tumour occuring in certain regions of Africa.

Carcinogens : Certain compounds like coal tar, nicotine etc are known to produce cancer.

Defective immunity hypothesis : The body has its own defence mechanism or immune system which destroys cancerous cells even when they are formed. This is called immunological surveillance. If for some reason this fails, cancer cells survive and produce tumours.

In spite of the above theories, it has to be conceded that none of these satisfactorily explains what causes the cells to divide. All these merely attempt to explain the various influences (external agencies) that induce rapid cell division. But the basic question that has remained unanswered is which machinery in the cell (either at morphological or at molecular level) gets altered by mutation or immuno difficiency or whatever cause resulting in unregulated division. Possibly the ultimate answer to cancer lies in understanding the basics of interphase. It is here that the cell prepares itself for division. Even in interphase perhaps it is the S phase (as the important stage of DNA synthesis) which commits a cell for division needs to be studied in more detail to understand the rapid sequence of divisions.

MEIOSIS

In higher plants and animals, sexual reproduction takes place by the union of specialized sex cells called sperms and ova. The fusion of these sex cells that prevents the doubling of chromosomes in every generation. The answer lies in a special type of nuclear division called meiosis. It precedes the formation of gametes, so that each gamete acquires only half the number of chromosomes of the somatic cell. Thus when two gametes unite, the resulting zygote has the normal number of chromosomes. For example human body cells have 46 chromosomes in 23 pairs. But the human ovum and sperm have only 23 chromosomes, as aresult of meiosis. The reduced number of chromosomes in gametes is termed haploid, while the full complement of chromosomes in somatic cells is called diploid.

Definition of meiosis : Meiosis is a special type of division occuring in the diploid germ cells during which the chromosomes divide once, while the nucleus and cytoplasm divide twice resulting in the formation of four haploid cells. Hence meiosis is also *reduction division* as the number of chromosomes is reduced in comparison with the parental cell. These terms were coined by J.B-Farmer and J.E.Moore in 1905.

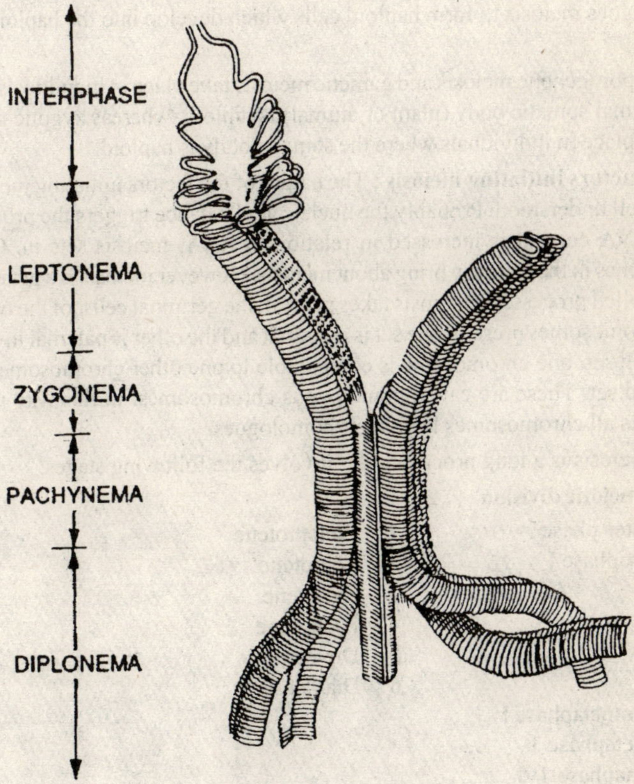

Fig. 9.5 Cell Division
Chromosomal threads during Prophase I of meiosis

The events of meiosis are uniform both in plants and animals. But depending on the time of occurrence, at different stages of life cycle the following types of meiosis may be identified.

1. **Sporogenetic meiosis :** In certain plants meiosis takes place in the sporophyte (2x) at the time of formation of spores. These spores develop into gametophyte.

2. **Gametic meiosis :** In most animals and some plants, reduction division takes place during the formation of gametes, so that haploid gametes are produced.

3. **Zygotic meiosis :** This is seen in lower plants where two haploid gametes produced by mitosis fuse to form a diploid zygote. The zygote undergoes meiosis to form haploid cells which develop into the haploid plant body.

Sporogenetic meiosis and gametic meiosis take place in individuals where the actual somatic body (plant or animal) is diploid, whereas zygotic meiosis takes place in individuals where the somatic body is haploid.

Factors initiating meiosis : The nature of the factors initiating meiosis is not well understood. Probably the nucleic acid balance triggers the process. If the DNA content is increased in relation to RNA, meiosis sets in. Certain hormones in the cell may bring about meiosis. However meiosis is a genetically controlled process. As meiosis takes place in the germinal cells, of the two sets of chromosomes present, one set is maternal and the other is paternal in origin. In each set, one chromosome is comparable to one other chromosome in the second set. These are called homologous chromosomes. In this way in both the sets all chromosomes have their homologues.

Meiosis is a long process and it involves the following stages.

First meiotic division

Inter phase	1	Preleptotene
Prophase I	2	Leptotene
	3	Zygotene
	4	Pachytene
	5	Diplotene
	6	Diakinesis

Prometaphase I
Metaphase I
Anaphase I
Telephase I

INTER KINESIS

Second meiotic division

Prophase II
Metaphase II
Anaphase II
Telophase II

Meiosis I is also called heterotypic division because here a diploid nucleus gives rise to two haploid nuclei. Meiosis II is called homeotypic division because here, the chromosome number is maintained. Meiosis II is actually nothing but mitosis.

INTERPHASE : The interphase consists of the same Gl phase, S phase and G_1 phase same as in mitosis. The essential events are as follows-

1. There is replication of RNA and synthesis of proteins during G_1 phase.
2. DNA is synthesized only in S phase and not during G_1 and G_2 phases.
3. DNA replication takes place by a semiconservative process. As a first step, an incision enzyme initiates a nick in one of the strands. Both the strands of DNA participate in the replication process under the influence of DNA polymerase. Together with DNA, histones are also synthesised. DNA is synthesised in short segments (Okazaki segments) which later join together to form large molecules.

PROPHASE I : This is the longest phase in meiosis. It has the following stages-proleptotene, leptotene, zygotene, pachytene, Diplotene and Diakinesis.

Proleptotene : Replication of DNA having already taken place in interphase, the chromosomes appear double stranded. The other events in proleptotene are-

1. Nucleus enlarges in size
2. Chromosomes are thin and hazy except perhaps for sex chromosomes

Leptotene (Leptonema) : This is also called the slender thread stage. Chromosomes appear distinct and the double strand (chromatid) nature can be seen clearly. The following are the other structural details of leptotene chromosomes.

1. Chromosomes are distinct,long and less coiled.
2. Chromosomes appear as threads with regularly placed beads or granules called chromomeres.
3. Electron microscopic observations have revealed that leptotene chromosomes have an axial filament with chromatin fibres attached to it in a series of lateral loops.
4. In certain areas the lateral loops cluster together to form chromomeres. The axial filament has two protein fibrils. These fibrils later get transformed into a part of the *synaptonemal complex*.

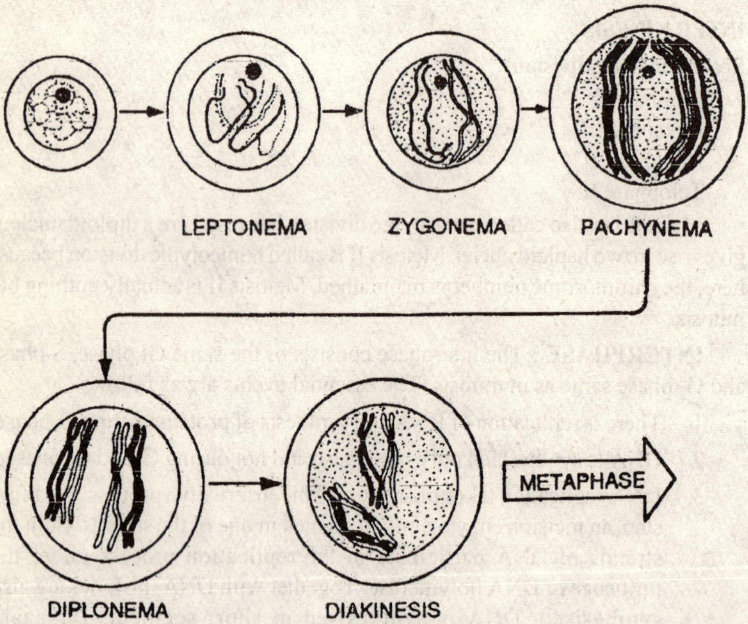

Fig. 9.6 Cell Division
Stages in Prophase I of meiosis

5. The homologous chromosomes are associated at their tips where they are attached to the nuclear membrane
6. Leptotene chromosomes may be uniformly distributed or localized into *bouquets*.
7. In some plants, chromosomes may form a tangled mass of fibres called *synizetic knot*.
8. Cytoplasm of a leptotene cell has many polyribosomes but vesicles are less in number. Nucleolus increases its size to the maximum due to increases in RNA synthesis.
9. The centriole duplicates and each daughter centriole migrates to the opposite poles of the cell. On reaching the pole the daughter centriole duplicates again. '

Zygotene (zygonema) : This is a very important stage where pairing of the homologous chromosomes takes place. The following are the important events with reference to zygotene chromosomes.

1. The chromosomes become shorter and thicker.
2. Lengthwise pairing of the homologous chromosomes begins as they are attracted towards each other.
3. Of the two homologues, one is maternal in origin and the other is paternal. These are called bivalents.

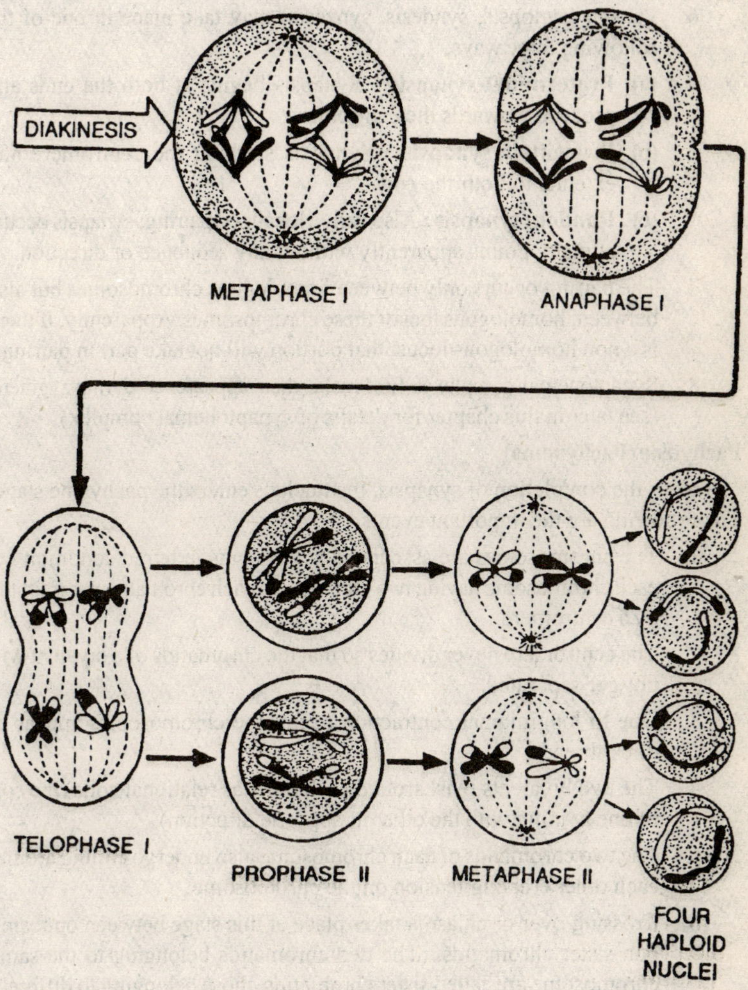

Fig. 9.7 Cell Division
Stages in meiosis (after prophase)

4. Pairing also called synopsis is precise and takes place chromomere - for chromomere. As a result,the chromosomes (homologues) align themselves parallel to each other throughout their length.
5. The bivalent has two homologous chromosomes; each homologous chromosome has two chromatids i.e. totally there will be four chromatids (tetrad).
6. Pairing (synopsis, syndesis, synzesis) may take place in one of the following three ways.
   - (a) **Proterminal synapsis :** Synapsis begins at both the ends and proceeds towards the centromere.
   - (b) **Procentric synapsis :** Synapsis starts at the centromere and extends to both the ends.
   - (c) **Random synapsis :** Also called localized pairing, synapsis occurs at many points apparently without any sequence or direction.
7. The pairing occurs only between homologous chromosomes but also between, homologous loci of these chromosomes. Apparently, if there is a non homologous locus, that portion will not take part in pairing.
8. Synaptonemal complexes first make their appearence during zygotene (see later in this chapter for details of synaptonemal complex).

Pachytene (Pachynema)

After the completion of synapsis, the nucleus enters the pachytene stage. The following are the important events.

1. The chromosomes are associated as bivalents in tetrad condition i.e. each chromosome having two chromatids; each chromatid pair is united by a centromere.
2. The centromere never divides so that the chromatids of a bivalent will not get separated.
3. Due to longitudinal contraction pachytene chromosomes appear as thick threads.
4. The two bivalents twist around each other as relational coils (the coil of one twining with the other in opposite direction).
5. The two chromatids of each chromosome also undergo coiling around each other creating tension on the chromosome.
6. Crossing over or chiasma takes place at this stage between opposing non sister chromatids. (The two chromatids belonging to the same chromosome are called sister chromatids, those belonging to different chromosome are called non sister chromatids)
7. Of the four chromatids (of the 2 bivalents), only two opposing

chromatids take part in crossing over, while the other two (which are away from each other) do not participate in crossing over.

8. Crossing over takes place because of breakage and reunion at one or two points between opposing non sister chromatids. It takes place as follows. First one or two transverse breaks occur at the same level in the two non sister chromatids opposing each other. (The breaks will never occur in both the sister chromatids) The break is followed by reunion, but their union will not join the same segments of a sister chromatid. The chromatid which breaks at one point will unite with the segment of the opposing non sister chromatid. Break and union occurs at 1, 2 or 3 points. As a result after the cross over, each chromatid has 1, 2 or 3 pieces of the other non sister chromatid. If break occurs at one point it is called single point cross over, at two points is called double point cross over etc. Due to crossing over, the chromosomes produce cross shaped configurations called chiasmata. The number of points at which cross over can take place depends on the length of the bivalents. Thus as a result of cross over in the bivalents, there will be two unbroken or original chromatids (which are away from each other) and two broken and reunited chromatids opposing each other which have exchanged their segments.
9. Exchange of genes takes place between homologues due to exchange of segments.
10. Synaptonemal complex is very well organised at this stage. It has a central element and two lateral elements, (see later for detailed explanation)
11. Nucleolus remains unaltered; it may increase in size. It is found to be associated with the nucleolar organizing region of certain chromosomes.

Diplotene (Diplonema)

The diplotene nucleus is characterised by repulsion of the homologues, while there is coupling in pachytene. The following are the important features of diplotene stage.

1. Homologues start separating (repulsion), but are held together at one or more points called chiasmata.
2. Chiasmata are very clear in diplotene than in pachytene stage because of increased condensation of chromosomes.
3. Chiasmata are found in meiosis of almost all eukaryotic organisms. However in certain Dipteran insects including *Drosophila*, there is no chiasma in males. Meiosis here is termed non cross over meiosis or

achiasmatic meiosis. Achiasmatic meiosis has also been reported in oocytes of Copepoda and Lepidoptera.

4. Chiasma may be formed at the ends (terminal chiasma) or in tshe middle (interstitial chiasma) of the chromosomes.

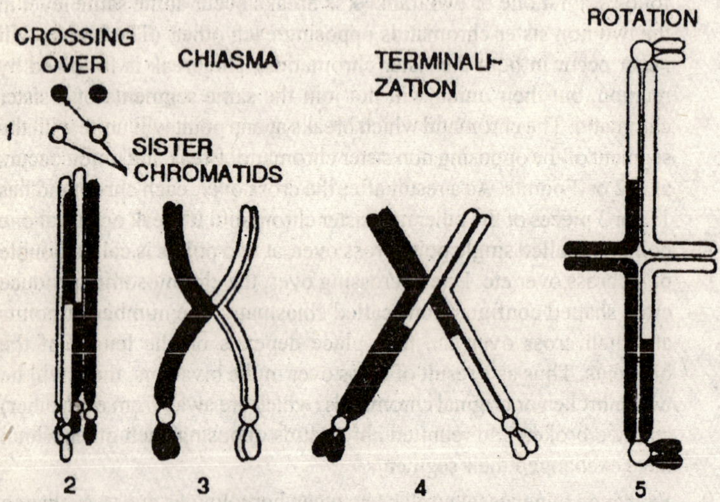

Fig. 9.8 Cell Division

5. The most important event occuring in diplotene is the teminalization of the chiasma. Terminalization or uncoupling of chiasma begins due to repulsion in homologous chromosomes. The chromatids begin to separate at the centromere and gradually progress towards the ends. As a result the terminal chiasma slip off or uncouple and progressively the chiasma towards the centromere move towards the end. When the terminalization is almost complete, the two homologues remain in contact through the terminal chiasma.

   The degree of terminalization may be expressed in the form of terminalization coefficient (T).

$$T = \frac{\text{Number of terminal Chiasma}}{\text{Total number of bivalents}}$$

   Chiasma frequency (Fq) is the average number of chiasma in bivalents of a nucleus. This may be calculated as follows

$$Fq = \frac{\text{Total number of chiasma}}{\text{Total number of bialents}}$$

During terminalization there is rotation of chromosomes; when there is a single chiasma, the chromosomes rotate through 180° and form a cross; when there are two chiasmata a loop is formed; when there are more than two, a number of loops are formed and rotation is brought about by the forces of repulsion.

6. Synaptonemal complexes usually disappear, but occasionally may persist towards the end of bivalents particularly where they are attached to the nuclear membrane.
7. There is increase in the endoplasmic vesicles.

Diakinesis

This is the Final stage of prophase 1. The structural details of this stage are -

1. Bivalent chromosomes are very thick and highly contracted.
2. Bivalents are distributed more towards the periphery of the nucleus.
3. Terminal chiasma may be retained maintaining contact between homologous chromosomes.
4. The nucleolous detaches from the chromosomes and finally disappears.

PROMETAPHASE I

1. The nuclear membrane disappears. The centrioles are joined by spindles which develop from tubules.
2. The chromosomes reach their maximum contraction.

METAPHASE I

At the end of diakinesis, the amphiaster (spindle) becomes clearly visible and it becomes more pronounced now. The bivalents arrange themselves on the equatorial plate. The centromeres of the bivalents lie towards the poles, wilile the arms lie towards the equator. The centromere is attached to the spindle fibres. These are called chromosomal fibres.

ANAPHASE I

It is at this stage, the homologous chromosomes move to the opposite poles. The following are the main features of anaphase I.

1. Each homologous chromosome of each bivalent moves towards the opposite pole. The movement is random unlike in mitosis.
2. The homologues do not separate quickly. While short chromosomes separate easily, longer ones take a little more time (due to interstitial chiasmata).
3. The homologous chromosomes migrating to the opposite poles are different from the ones that undergo pairing during prophase in the sense in each chromosome one chromatid is unaltered, while the other is a mixture of paternal and maternal segments.

4. The centromere does not divide (It divides in mitosis).
5. The chromosomes assume a V shape as they are pulled towards the opposite poles.

TELOPHASE I

The following are the important events during telophase I.

1. The chromosomes reach the respective poles. The spindles persist for sometime.
2. Chromosomes undergo despiralization, becoming indistinct.
3. Nucleolus reappears, so also the nuclear membrane. In some instances nucleolus may not appear at this stage.
4. Cell membrane is formed in animal cells generally by furrowing, and in plant cells, cell wall is laid down in the form of plate. In some of the plant cells cytokinesis does not take place at this stage. It takes place when both meiotic divisions are complete. In pollen mother cells of flowering plants cell wall is laid down after meiosis I and II is called successive and if laid down only after meiosis II is called simultaneous. After Telophase I, two cells or two nuclei are formed.

INTERKINESIS

The two daughter nuclei or daughter cells undergo a resting period. This intervening phase is called interphase or Interkinesis. This phase is of a very short duration. In some instances interkinesis is absent, the incompletely formed nuclei of telophase I may enter prophase II. This is seen in plants like *Trillium.*

MEIOSIS II

The second meiotic division is essentially a mitosis in which both the chromosomes and cell divide.

But the main difference is DNA does not duplicate unlike in the interphase of mitosis. And also (as has been pointed out already) the interphase or interkinesis is short.

PROPHASE II

This is essentially similar to the mitotic prophase. The salient features of this stage are -

1. The centrioles divide into two and two pairs of centrioles are formed. They migrate to the opposite poles.
2. The microtubules get themselves arranged at right angles to the previous plane (during meiosis I).
3. The arms of the chromosomes remain separate and there is no relational coiling.
4. Nucleolus as well as nuclear envelope disappear with the formation of the achromatic figure.

METAPHASE II

1. It is of a very short duration like in mitosis.
2. Chromosomes (dyads) with their (two) chromatids arrange themselves on the equatorial plate.
3. The centromeres lie on the equator while the arms are directed towards the poles.
4. The centromere divides, thus separating the two chromatids (monads) which eventually become separate chromosomes. At this stage they can be called daughter chromosomes.
5. The centromere is attached to the chromosomal spindle fibres in the achromatic figure.

ANAPHASE II

1. The daughter chromosomes start their migration towards the opposite poles. The movement is brought about due to the contraction of chromosomal spindle fibres and stretching of continuous spindle fibres.
2. The chromosomes are not very thick and short like in anaphase, but are like the anaphase daughter chromosomes of mitosis.

TELOPHASE II

1. The chromosomes having reached the opposite poles uncoil and become less distinct.
2. Nuclear membrane and nucleolus reappear resulting in the formation of a daughter nucleus. The nucleus gets into the interphase state.
3. The nuclei are haploid; they have half the number of chromosomes in comparison with the parental cell.

CYTOKINESIS

Wall formation begins either as a furrow or as a plate and two daughter cells are formed. Thus totally at the end of meiosis four daughter cells are formed. In some instances cell wall (in some plants) would not have been laid after meiosis I. As a result at the end of Telophase II four daughter nuclei are formed.Cell walls are laid down now resulting in the formation of four cells.

SYNAPTONEMAL COMPLEX

This is a special structure visible during meiotic prophase - specially during zygotene and pachytene. Observed first with the help of electron microscope in the spermatocytes of cray fish- **Procambams darkii** (Moses 1956) and in Pigeon, Cat, Man etc (Faweett 1956), the synaptonemal complex consists of ribbon like structures associated with the chromosome core.

As these were observed during synapsis, Mosel (1958) named them synaptonemal complex (SC) subsequent to this, SCs have been found in a wide variety of organisms like Algae, Fungi, Gymnosperms, Angiosperms Protozoans, insects, molluscs, amphibians, aves, mammals etc. Hence SCs can be said to be of universal occurrence.

Structure : These are three partite ribbon like structures situated between the homologous chromosomes. Each SC is made up of a dense central axis from which arise dense lateral filamentous structures. Each lateral element on either side of the axis is attached to the inner side of the homologous chromosomes. The space between the central axis and lateral elements are traversed by a series of transverse units or LC fibres. Each lateral unit has a width ranging from 300-500 Å and the space between the lateral elements is between 900- 1200 Å. The width of the central element is betwee 150-500 Å. The SC is attached to the nuclear membrane through the lateral elements at the ends.

Comings and Okada (1971) have reported the emergence of a serie of chromatin loops from the lateral elements, which make up the chromosome material. The central axis (central element) is formed of the fusion of a series of small loops.

Each lateral element consists of two protein fibres one for each non sister chromatid. The lateral elements and LC fibres are also made up of proteins.

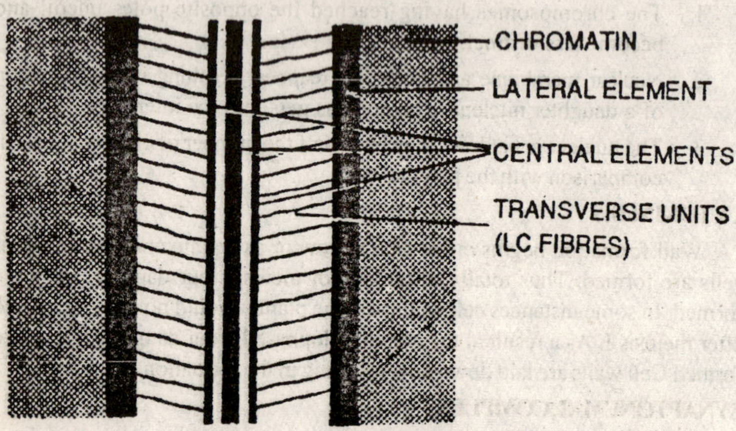

Fig. 9.9 Cell Division
Diagram of synaptonemal complex

Function of synaptonemal complex : Appearing first during zygotene, when pairing between homologous chromosomes occurs, they complete their structural development during pachytene. The SCs diasappear during diplotene, even though remnants may be seen during diakinesis. The above facts clearly attribute an important role to SCs in crossing over and exchange of segments between homologous chromosomes. According to Meyer (1964), the absence of SC in achiasmatic meiosis (as in males of dipteran insects) is proof enough of SC's role in chiasma formation. But in some instances SCs have been found in achiasmatic meiosis also.

According to Comings and Okada (1971), SCs help in chiasma not only at the morphological level but even at the molecular level also.

The SCs disintegrat gradually into cytoplasm as they disassociate from the chromosomes.

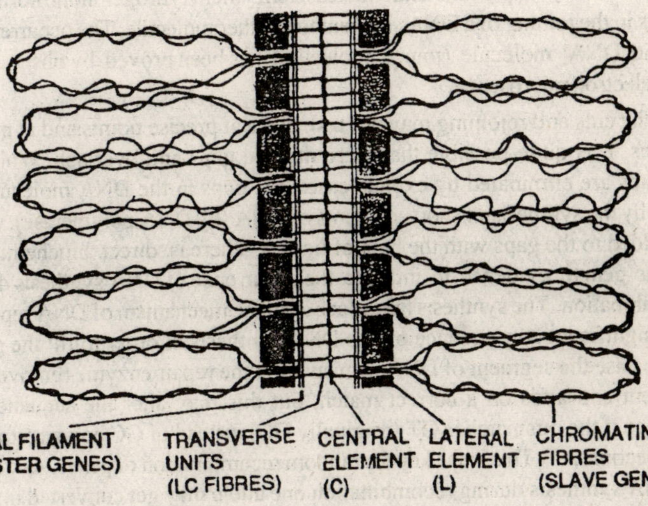

Fig. 9.10 Cell Division
Synaptonemal complex (Composite diagram showing details)

Significance of Meiosis

1. Helps to maintain constant chromosome numbers in organisms.
2. Crossing over which is the central focus in meiosis brings about recombination of genetic material leading to variation amongst individuals.
3. Meiosis in fact provides with the basic material (variation) for Evolution.
4. The random recombinations among homologous chromosomes give rise to a variety of mix up of parental characters and new characters.

Molecular mechanism of crossing over : several models have been proposed to account for recombination of DNA molecules of the homologous chromosomes. The following is the general theme of the crossing over at the molecular level.

It is generally believed that the specific interactions between two DNA molecules of homologous chromosomes leading to recombination are mediated by single stranded elements. Recombination begins probably by having an endonuclease enzyme make a 'nick' at one of the strands of the adjoining duplexes. As a result, a section of the single stranded DNA becomes displaced from that helix' and interacts with the complimentary strand of the other duplex. In order to facilitate this interaction, a second nick occurs in the neighbouring strand with the help of the endonuclease enzyme. Hydrogen bond formation assists in the joining of a DNA segment to another molecule. The occurrence of 'hybrid DNA' molecule (joined molecule) has been proved by observations with electron microscope.

The cuts and rejoining may not take place at precise points and at precise lengths. It is quite possible that there may be gaps and overlaps. While the overlaps are eliminated by exonucleases, the gaps in the DNA molecule are filled by the synthesis of short segments of DNA (by DNA polymerase), which are added to the gaps with the help of ligases. There is direct biochemical as well as genetic evidence to indicate the occurrence of DNA synthesis during recombination. The synthesis take place as in the mechanism of DNA repair. A very significant consequence of this DNA synthesis in order to fill the gap is that in case the segment of DNA is mispaired, the repair enzyme removes this segment and adds on a correct match, but this may alter the sequence for instance if the mismatch is GT (originally GC) instead of GC being restored it may become AT. This is the key for random recombination of genes. As a result of DNA synthesis during recombination one allele may get converted into the other. This may be called gene conversion and has been reported in *Neurospora*.

COMPARISON BETWEEN MITOSIS AND MEIOSIS

	MITOSIS	MEIOSIS
1.	Occurs in somatic cells	Occurs in germ cells
2.	There is one nuclear division and one cytokinesis	There is one nuclear division but two cytokinesis.
3.	Chromosome number is maintained.	Chromosome number is halved.
4.	Prophase is short and there are no substages many	Prophase I is very long and has substages

	MITOSIS	MEIOSIS
5.	The chromosomes replicate and the centromere also divides with the result, chromatids become daughter Chromosomes and they migrate to opposite poles.	The chromosomes do not replicate during meiosis I. The centromere does not divide; as a result among existing chromosomes half migrate to one pole and the other half to the other pole.
6.	No pairing and there is no association between homologous chromosomes	Chiasma takes place between homologous chromosomes resulting in exchange of genetic material
7.	Chromosomes duplicate during prophase.	Duplication of Chromosomes takes place during prophase II.
8.	Chromosomes occur as diads in prophase.	They occur as tetrads in metaphase - **I**.
9.	Centromere is directed towards the equator in the metaphase plate with the arms towards the poles.	Centromere is directed towards the poles with the arms towards the equator
10.	In anaphase the chromosomes move as monads.	Chromosomes move as dyads.
11.	During anaphase chromosomes are short and thin	During Anaphase - I Chromosomes are long and thick.
12.	Telephase always occurs.	Telephase - I is omitted sometimes.
13.	Equational division.	Reduction division.
14.	Brings about growth.	Brings about reproduction.

10

MENDELISM

The story of Mendel's life history and work is a curious mixture of luck and misfortune. Mendel was lucky because the experimental organism and the characters he chose to enunciate the laws of inheritance were admirably suited than any other organism; the misfortune is, the scientific world just ignored his epoch making discoveries. The story of success and yet a. failure to get appreciation has been there in human history since time immemorial. Mendel's is not the first and the last example. Mendel's work had to wait for nearly 34 years after he discovered them, and 16 years after bis death, the world rediscovered his theory.

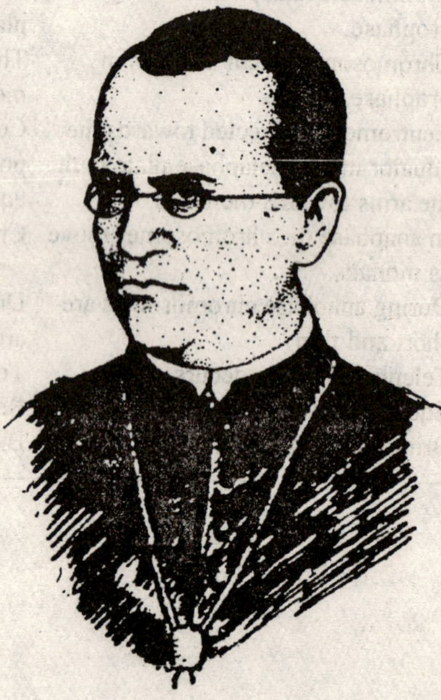

Fig. 10.1 Mendelism
John Gregor Mendel, The father of Genetics

The story of Father of Genetics began on July 22, 1822, when a boy was born to peasant parents in Moravia (then in Austria, now in Czechoslovakia). The bright boy (Johann Gregor Mendel) was sent to the upper elementary school at Leipink at the age of 11. He did well and topped the class and was sent to Troppan High School in 1934. He completed his graduation in Aug. 1840 and did a 2 years course at Olmutz philosophical Institute. In October 1843 Mendel was admitted to the Augstinian monastrey at Brunn in Moravia. After a brief assignment as a parish priest, he went to Vienna to obtain a teacher's certificate to become a school master. Mendel appeared for the teacher's certificate examination in 1850. He succeeded in passing the examination in physics, but failed in geology. However the chairman of examinations, recognising Mendel's worth, recommended his admission to the university of Vienna. Here Mendel studied zoology, systematic botany, palaeontology, physics and mathematics from 1851-1853. In 1854 Mendel joined the Brunn Modern School as a Teacher of physics and natural history. In 1856 he appeared again for a teacher's certificate, but failed again. However he continued teaching for 12 more years and then got elected to the abbot.

Mendel began his work on pea plants in 1856 and continued his work up to 1863. He conducted all his experiments in the monastery garden each summer. He read his report on pea plants in a paper entitled "Experiments on plant hybridization" at the Brunn Natural history society in 1864. The paper was published in the proceedings in 1866. The proceedings was exchanged between 120 other societies all over the world. But unfortunately none recognised the genius of Mendel, nor the originality of his work.

Pre Mendelian hybridization experiments

Gregor Mendel was not the first person to have conducted hybridization experiments on plants, but the secret of his success lies in his meticulous method of carrying out experiments and concentrating on a particular aspect.

J. Kolreuter (1733-1806) a German botanist had conducted hybridization experiments in tobacco and compared the offspring with the progeny. He demonstrated that the progeny may resemble any one of the parents or may be intermediate between them. According to him, the hybrids are more diverse than the parents. Kolereuter used' tall and dwarf varieties and found out that the hybrid offspring was of intermediate size. The hybrids in the next generation varied from tall to dwarf. But he could not explain his results properly.

Others who had worked on hybridization before Mendel include Bartner (1772-1850), Naudin (1815-1899) Kought (1799), Goss (1824) etc. The last two worked on pea plants. But none of these workers was able to rationalize and explain the results with a sure degree of repeatability.

Mendel's experiments

Mendel got interested in pea plants of the monastery garden. What attracted him to pea plants (besides luck - as will be explained later) was the immense variety of floral and vegetative characters available in the plants. The other reasons being

1. The characters are well defined - tall or dwarf, red or white, round or shrunken etc.
2. The plants could be self pollinated easily as the flowers are bisexual.
3. They are generally self fertilized.
4. Many pure breeding varieties are available
5. They can be easily hybridized and the hybrids resulting from the cross are fertile.
6. The plants are annuals and many generations could be easily studied within a short span of time.

Main reasons for Mendel's success

Unknown to Mendel at that time, it was a chance that made him select the plant and the characters (This aspect will be explained later). The single factor that was responsible for Mendel's success was his concentration on any one character during an experiment on inheritance. The failure of earlier workers was - When they selected the parents for hybridization, they regarded it as a complex of characters and studied the inheritance patterns of all characters simultaneously. They went astray because different characters have different inheritance patterns and they cannot be hypothesised in a similar manner. Mendel was aware of the failure of earlier works, that is why in every hybridization experiment his aim was specific - to follow the inheritance pattern of any one character at a time. He was not bothered about other characters. Besides this - Mendel kept accurate records in crosses and even maintained exact number of seeds or plants produced. Since the process of fertilization between a sperm and an egg was a matter of chance; in order to obtain a valid explanation he conducted large number of experiments (more than 2-3 thousand) to exclude chance factors. Mendel also used in his experiments some thing that was unusual at that time - the use of statistical and mathematical principles to obtain and compute the results properly. Above all these, perhaps it was also his genius and intution that made Mendel succeed.

Characters chosen by Mendel

Mendel selected seven pairs of contrasting characters for his study. These are

	Character	Alternatives
1.	Seed form	Round/wrinkled
2.	Cotyledon colour	Yellow/green
3.	Seed Coat colour/flower	Gray/white, red/white
4.	Pod form	Inflate/constricted
5.	Pod colour	Green/Yellow
6.	Flower position	Axial/Terminal
7.	Plant height	Tall/dwarf

Technique of crossing in pea plants

Garden peas are self fertilizing, so in instances where self crossing is to be done, the young buds are to be covered by bags. In case of cross pollination where pollen from one specific plant is to pollinate another specific plant certain measures are to be taken in order to avoid self pollination as the plants have bisexual flowers.

In the plant selected as the female parent (for cross pollination), the anthers have to be removed from flowers before maturity. This is called emasculation. Then pollen from the required parent should be dusted on the stigmatic surface and then the flower should be closed by a bag. For each of the seven characters mentioned above Mendel used one alternative as the female parent and the other as the male parent.

Mendel conducted reciprocal crosses also in that he switched the characters between male and female parents. The example below will illustrate this.

	Male parent		Female parent
Cross 1.	Red flower colour	X	White flower colour
Reciprocal cross	White flower colour	X	Red flower colour

The purpose of reciprocal cross is to ascertain whether both the parents contribute equally to the offspring.

After artificial pollination, seeds are allowed to mature. In case a seed character is the subject of experimentation it can be studied immediately. Otherwise, the seed has to be sown and allowed to grow into a plant to observe the characters. The plants raised thus constitute the first offspring or filial generation (F_1). These F_1 plants may be allowed to have self pollination, the flower buds are covered so as not to allow foreign pollen to fertilize the plant. The seeds thus produced are sown and plants are obtained. These plants represent second offspring generation or Filial generation two (F_2).

Terms used in Mendelian experiments

1. **Factor** : Unit or particle of inheritance responsible for all the characters.
2. **Gamete** : Haploid sex cell produced from a diploid parent (as in pea plant).
3. **Genotype** : Genetic character of the individual which it obtains from the parents.
4. **Phenotype** : The external appearence of the individual which is a reaction of the genotype and environment.

5. **Homozygous**	:	An individual in which the two factors for every character are identical ie. the two homologous chromosomes have the same alleles. Homozygous individual produces only one type of a gamete for every character ie. all the gametes carry identical factors.
6. **Heterozygous**	:	An individual in which the two factors responsible for a character are dissimilar. Heterozygotes produce at least two different types of gametes. The number of types of gametes produced in a heterozygote depends on the number of characters for which factors are not identical. For eg. Heterozygotes for one character, 2^1 gametes, for 2 characters 2^2 4), for 3 characters 2^3(8), for n characters2^4 etc.
7. **Pure line**	:	A character in a plant for which the plant breeds true *ie* even after repeated generations the same characters is repeated.
8. **Hybrid**	:	A plant produced by crossing two pure lines. Hybrid for one character is called monohybrid, for two characters dihybrid, for 3 characters trihybrid, for many characters polyhybird etc.
9. **Allele or Allelomorph**	:	The term used to refer to a member of a gene pair in a diploid organism responsible for a particular trait. These alleles occupy the same locus on the homologous chromosomes.
F_1 generation	:	The progeny produced as a result of cross between two parents (P_1). First filial generation.
10. **F_2 generation**	:	Progeny produced from a cross between two F_1 individuals.
11. **Parent generation**	:	The individuals used for the first cross. It is referred to P_1 generation.
12. **Dominant**	:	A character in the parent which appears in the F_1 generation suppresting the other allele.
13. **Recessive**	:	The character that is suppressed in the F_1 generation in spite of being present in the genotype.

14. Monohybrid cross : A cross in which the inheritance pattern of only one character is followed.

15. Dihybrid cross : A cross in which the inheritance pattern of two characters are followed.

16. Reciprocal cross : In this, the sexes of the crossing parents are reversed with reference to the first cross.

17. Back cross or Test cross : This is performed to find out whether the two factors (dominant and recessive) are present in the F_1 generation. This is done by crossing the F_1 progeny back with one of the parents (recessive).

Symbols used in Mendel's experiments

Mendel used several genetic symbols in order to present the results of various crosses.

In order to represent the characters Mendel used genetic symbols in the form of English alphabets. For every character he used the first letter of the word. The dominant character was given the capital letter and its recessive allele the small alphabet of the same capital letter. For eg. Tall is *'T'* dwarf ist (and not d). Two letters *TT* designate that there are two factors and are similar. *Tt* represents that the two factors are not similar. Thus *TT*, and tt are homozygous, while *Tt* is heterozygous.

Monohybrid cross : In this cross the inheritance of only one character is followed. Mendel selected for the cross in each experiment clear contrasting characters like Red or white (flower colour) or Tall or dwarf (height of the plant) etc. We shall study the inheritance pattern of red dnd white flower colour which serves as a typical example.

Mendel selected two pure breeding races of red and white (flowers) plants. He used one as the male and the other as the female. The two were crossed and seeds obtained. These seeds when sown produced the F_1 hybrid plants; all of them having red flower colour. It did not matter as to whether the red parent provided the pollen and the white parent acted as the seed bearing plant or *vice versa.* The character of white plant did not appear in the F_1 generation.

The morphological appearance of the red flower colour was exactly like that of the red parent. It was not intermediate (not pink in colour). It looked as if the white parent did not contribute anything towards the development of flower colour in the F_1 offspring. Mendel was interested to know as to what had happended to the white flower colour.

The F_1 plants were allowed to self pollinate (selfing) and seeds were sown to raise the plants. These plants are referred to as F_2 progeny. There was something surprising awaiting Mendel in the F_2 generation. There were not only red flower coloured plants but were white flower coloured plants too - pure white, exactly like grand parents (P_1 generation).

A white flower colour was produced from two apparently red flower coloured plants.Of the total number of the plants produced (Mendel did not cross only one plant, he did it for hundreds of plants to take an average) roughly there were 3 red plants for every single white plant (3:1). This was true for other characters of the pea plant also.

The above experiment may be represented as follows by genetic symbols.

	P_1 generation	
Red	X	White
RR		rr
R R		r r

Rr F_1 (Red)

	R	r
R	RR red	Rr red
r	Rr red	rr

F_2 generation

3:1 red : white
white

Of the three red plants found in the F_2 generation, Mendel found that only one of them bred true (pure line) in that, on being allowed to self pollinate it produced only red plants resembling the red plant of the P_1 generation. The other two red plants on being allowed to self pollinate, each of them behaved like the F_1 red plant in that they in turn produced progeny, in the ratio of three red plants to one white plant. The white plant bred true.

The result obtained in the case of red and white flower colour (F_1 showing only one character; F_2 showing 3:1 ratio of both the characters) was true for all other characters Mendel studied in pea plants. Mendel offered the following explanation to the above experiment.

Explanation of results ofMonohybird Cross

According to Mendel, in every sexually reproducing diploid individual, there exist two factors in the genetic material for every character. Of these one is contributed by the mother and the other by the father. These two factors are similar in a homozygous individual, but dissimilar in a heterozygous individual. In the present case, red flower colour (RR) and white flower colour (rr) breed true (on being selfed they always-repeat the character). These two parents with contrasting characters are crossed. The red flowered parent produces only one type of a gamete; all of them carry only the R factor (During gametogenesis; there will be reduction division hence the gametes carry only one factor for every character.) While the white parent also produces only one type of a gamete; all of them carry only the factor r with reference to flower colour. When these two gametes fuse to form the F_1 progeny genetically it will be Rr. This plant appears red phenotypically. According to Mendel when a pair of contrasting characters are crossed only one character makes its appearance in the FI generation and the other does not show morphologically in spite of being present in the genotype. The character appears in the FI generation is called *Dominant* and the other *recessive*. The F_1 plant is genotypically a hybrid or heteorzygote for it carries factors for both red and white. This is called *monohybird* (hybrid for one character)

When the F_1 plants are allowed to self fertilize, two types of gametes are formed both on the male and female side. Since the F_1 genotypically has Rr; during meiosis 50% of gametes would carry R and the rest carry r. During self fertilization there is random mating of these gametes. The gamete carrying R can mate with either R or r, with the result three combinations are possible RR, Rr, and rr in the ratio of three - RR, Rr, Rr (red) to one rr (white). Of the three red plants, one is pure line and the other two are hybrids. These results made Mendel to formulate the following laws.

1. **Theory of particulate inheritance :** Characters from parents to offspring are trasmitted in the form of discreet units or particles called factors (genes). These factors determine the characters in the individual. Two such factors are present in the individual's body, while gametes have only one (in diploid organisms).

2. **Law of purity of gametes :** Irrespective of the fact whether the individual is homozygous or heterozygous for a character, the gamete would always carry only one factor in the uncontaminated form. For instance when a hybrid having two different factors in its genotype forms the gametes, they carry these factors in two different gametes without any alteration.

3. **Law of Dominance :** When a pair of contrasting characters are crossed, only one character makes its appearence in the F_1 generation. This is known as the dominant character and the other, which does not show itself, inspite of being present in the genotype is called the recessive character.

   According to Mendel, all characters exist in two alternatives in diploid organisms. This is due to the fact that the two homologous chromosomes carry the two alleles. In the case of flower colour, R and r are alleles. R is the original form hence dominant and r is the mutated form hence recessive.

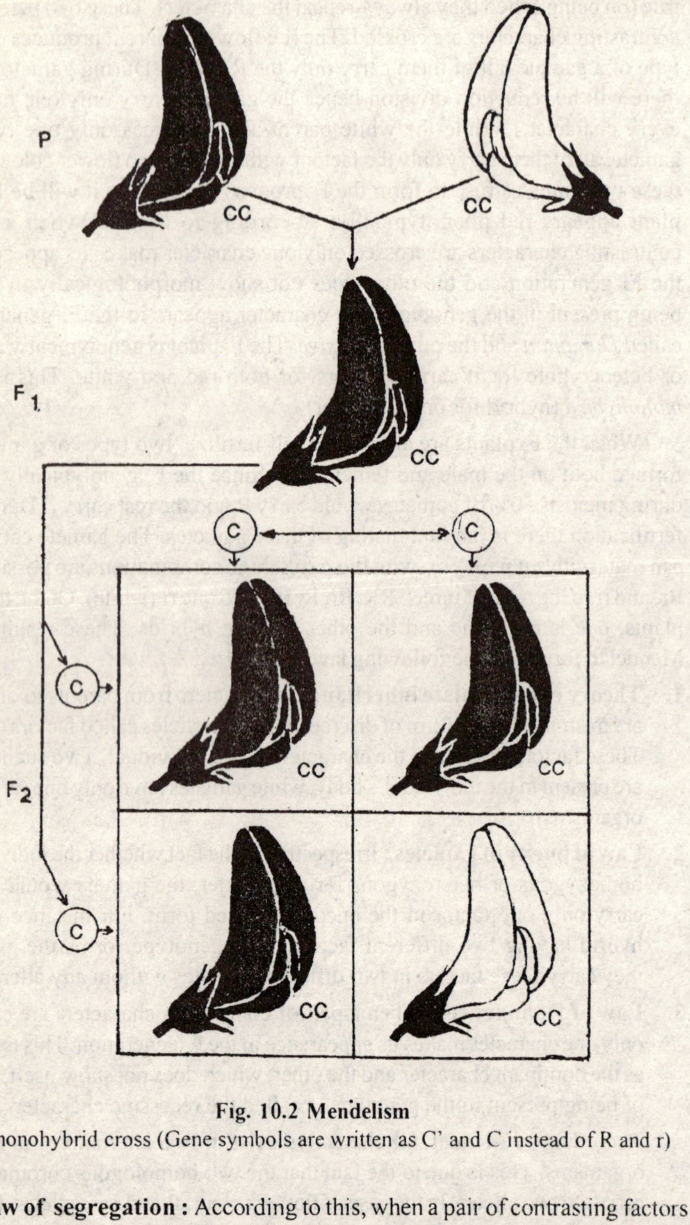

Fig. 10.2 Mendelism

The monohybrid cross (Gene symbols are written as C' and C instead of R and r)

4. **Law of segregation :** According to this, when a pair of contrasting factors are brought together as in a hybrid, in the next generation, they segregate to different gametes without undergoing any mixing or alteration or

combining. Thus when a cross of contrasting characters are made, even though it appears that the two characters are mixed; in the F_2 generation, the two of them segregate as in seen in RR and rr.

According to Mendel (in the above Cross) the two characters brought together in the F_1 hybrid did not combine, but just remained together and at the time of next reproduction (to produce F_2) they segregate. The fact that there is no mixing of red and white in the F_1 is proved by their reappearance in the F_2 in their original parental form.

The following table gives the actual number of progeny obtained in the F_2 generation for all the seven characters which Mendel studied in pea plants.

	Character	Dominant in F_2	Recessive in F_2 plants	Total No. of plants in F_2	Ratio of dominant/ Recessive
1.	Height	Tall 787	Dwarf 277	1064	2.84:1
2.	Flower position	Axial 651	Terminal 287	858	3.14:1
3.	Pod colour	Green 428	Yellow 152	580	2.82:1
4.	Pod shape	inflated 882	Constricted 299	1181	2.95:1
5.	Seed colour	Gray 705	White 224	922	3.15:1
6.	Seed form	Round 5474	Wrinkled 1850	7324	2.96:1
7.	Flower colour	Red 6022	White 2001	8023	3.01:1

Monohybrid ratio : The ratio of red and white plants obtained in the F_2 generation is called the monohybrid ratio. This is of two types.

Phenotypic ratio : For every three red flowered plants there will be one white flowered plant. This is3:1.This ratio is based on morphological appearance.

Genotypic ratio : Of the three red flowered plants, genotypically one (RR) is homozygous red, the other two (Rr, Rr) are heterozygous and one white (rr) is homozygous. The ratio is 1:2:1. This ratio is based on the genotype.

Test Cross : This is performed to test the hypothesis that the F_1 offspring has both the factors viz R and r in equal proportion. This is also called back cross because, the F_1 is crossed back with its parent. In the back cross, the F_1 is usually crossed with the double recessive parent (white) and not with the double dominant (red) parent. The reason is, if the F_1 is crossed with the dominant parent it will not be possible to assess the factors of the F_1 because the two dominant factors of the red parent will always exhibit the dominant character, irrespective of what is present in the F_1 progeny; on the other hand if the F_1 is crossed with the double recessive parent, the actual genotype of F_1 comes out, because the white parent can only contribute recessive genes which has no effect in morphological expression unless present in double dose. The test cross is as follows.

F_1	Red	X	White
	Rr	X	rr

	Rr	rr
R r	R Rr	r rr

Red and white flowered plants are produced in equal (1:1) ratio. Here, since the white parent can provide only r, the other r should have come from the F_1, thus indicating that the F_1 has both R and r in equal proportion.

Dihybrid Cross : In this cross Mendel took into consideration the inheritance pattern of two characters at a time to decide whether the two characters present together in a .parent will always remain together or can be separated also. The two characters chosen for the experiment were - Seed colour and seed shape. Each one has two alternatives.

Colour	Yellow/green
Shape	Round/wrinkled

In the seed colour yellow was dominant over green anu in shape; round was dominant over wrinkled. By careful selection, Mendel obtained two pure breeding plants of yellow round and green wrinkled. He crossed these two plants differing in two characters. The F_1 generation showed yellow and round (the other, green and wrinkled suppressed). The F_1 was allowed to self fertilize and produce the F_2. In this, (on analysis) Mendel found four different types of plants with reference to seed shape and colour. These were 1) Yellow round, 2) Yellow wrinkled, 3) Green round and 4) Green wrinkled in the ratio of 9:3:3:1. Figure along side will clearly illustrate the genotype and phenotype of these progenies.

Explanation of results of dihybrid cross : The two homozygous parents have YYRR and yyrr respectively in their genotype. These two produce each only one kind of a gamete viz. YR and yr. In the F_1 generation with the genotype of YyRr, four kinds of gametes are possible - YR, Yr, yR and yr, when seggregation takes place during meiosis. This happens when the F_1 is allowed to self pollinate. During the cross to produce F_2 the four gametes mate randomly and they have equal chance. Any one gamete can mate with any three. If all these possibilities are taken into consideration, 16 different possibilities arise. Phenotypically they belong to four categories as mentioned above. In this, the genotypes are as follows -

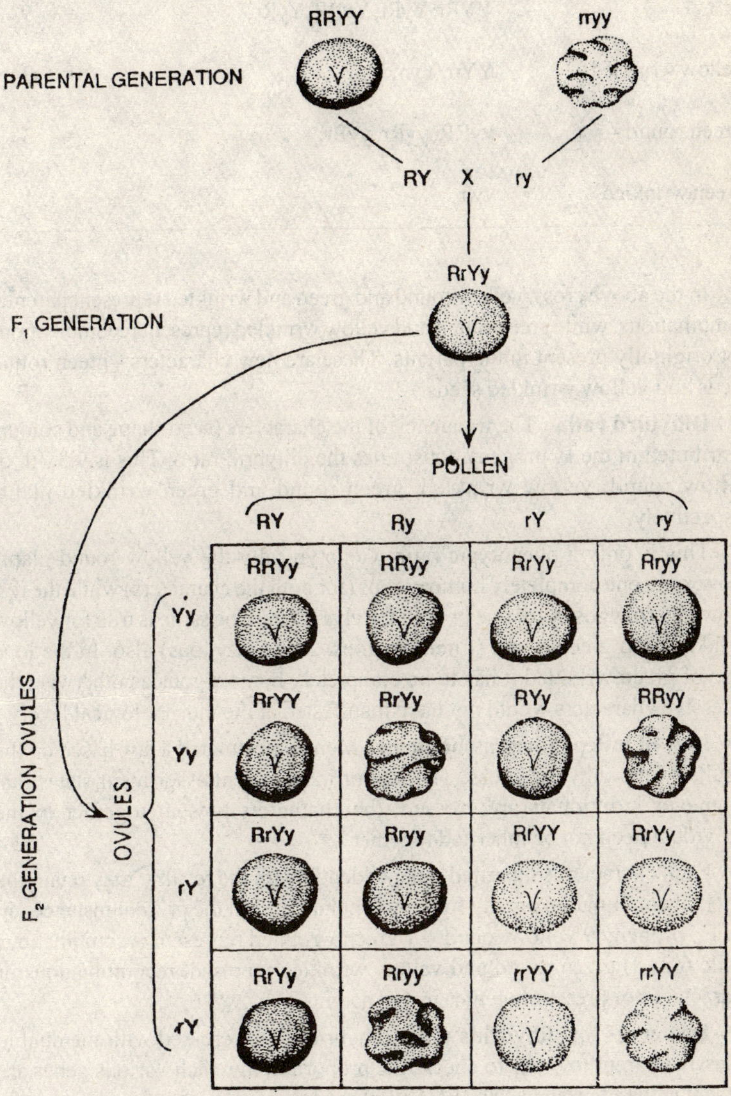

Fig. 10.3 Mendelism
Dihybrid cross

Yellow Round -	YYRR, YYRr, YyRR, YyRr, YyRr YYRr, YyRr, YyRR, YyRr	=	9
Yellow wrinkled -	YYrr, Yyrr, Yyrr	=	3
Green round -	yyRR, yyRr, yyRr,	=	3
Green wrinkled-	vwr	=	1

In the above cross, yellow round and green and wrinkled represent parental combinations, while green round and yellow wrinkled represent recombinations not originally present in the parents. These are new characters - green round seeds and yellow wrinkled seeds.

Dihybird ratio : The frequency of the characters (seed shape and colour) distributed in the F_2 progeny constitutes the dihybrid ratio. This is,9:3:3:l; of yellow round, yellow wrinkled, green round and green wrinkled plants respectively.

This is only a phenotypic ratio. Genotypically the yellow round plants show, only one completely homozygous (for both tne characters) while the rest show heterozygosity for one or both the characters. The same is true for yellow wrinkled and green round (I homozygous, 2 heterozygous) also. In the lone case of green wrinkled it has to be completely homozygous as otherwise the recessive characters would not have manifested at the morphological level.

Law of independent assortment : Mendel postulated a law based on the results of the dihybrid cross. The law of independent assortment states that whenever individuals are crossed, the characters present together in the individual need not be inherited together.

Each character is inherited independently with the result it may retain the parental combination or may form recombinations. In the present instance - in the F_2, progeny 9 yellow round + 1 green wrinkled represent recombinations while 6(3+3) green round and yellow wrinkled represent recombinations or characters not present together in the parents.

Test cross for dihybrids : The dihybrid (FI) is crossed with the double recessive parent in order to check, the proportion in which various genes are present in the FI progeny. The FI (YyRr) produces four types of gametes, while the double recessive parent, (yyrr) produces only one type of a gamete. The results of the cross are as follows.

Yy Rr X yy rr

YR Yr yR yr

	YR	Yr	yR	yr
yr	Yy Rr	Yy rr	yy Rr	yy rr
	Yellow round	Yellow wrinkled	green round	green wrinkled

The above plants are produced in the ratio of 1:1:1:1 indicating that in the F_1, the genes responsible for yellow, green, round and wrinkled are present in equal proportion.

Checker board : This is a method of representing the results in a tabular form. All the possible gametes on the male side and the female side are written at right angles to each other and each one of the female is crossed with all the male gametes to obtain the probable progeny. For e.g. in the monohybrid cross since there are two kinds of gametes on the male and two in the female the number of types in F_2 will be 2x2 = 4. In the dihybrid cross, the F_1 produces four kinds of gametes in both male and female. Hence in the F2 generation the possibilities are 4x4 == 16. Checker board method is the convenient way of representing all the probabilities in a cross.

Mendelian traits in other organisms

The type of inheritance proposed by Mendel is not limited to pea plants only. It is true for all the sexually reproducing diploid organisms. Ever since Mendel established his laws (at least after their rediscovery in 1900) inheritance pattern in hundreds of animals and plants have been checked and they are found to follow the pattern of inheritance suggested by Mendel. The characters or traits in any organism that follow the pattern suggested by Mendel are called *Mendelian traits or characters* and the inheritance is called Mendelian inheritance. Mendelian inheritance is in fact of universal occurrence.

Mendelian characters in Man : There are several human traits which follow Mendelian principles. Some of the Mendelian traits observed in man are Albinism, skin spotting, Taste blindness to PTC, brown and blue eye colours, M - N blood group etc. The study of inheritance pattern in human beings is difficult, for you cannot make any individual cross with any other as can be done in plants and animals. Data can be collected by studying family history. This is known as *Pedigree* studies, which records the data of all individuals in a family for as many generations as possible and the probability of the character in question appearing in future generations can be predicted. In the following paragraphs, we shall discuss briefly the inheritance pattern of some of the characters in man.

Albinism : This is a trait in which the pigments in skin, eye, and hair are completely or near totally absent. The trait follows the Mendelian inheritance. Albinism is a recessive trait in comparison with the coloured character. Albinos occur in all human races, but of quite frequent occurrence in cacusoid race of Europe. The skin is pale, so also the iris and the hair is .like straw. Albinism is due to a recessive allele *a* present in the homozygous condition. The wild gene for this is *A* (coloured) and it is dominant. We shall study one or two examples to know the inheritance pattern. If two normal human beings (male and female) produce an albino child, the genotype should be as follows.

Normal male		x	Normal female
Aa		x	Aa
A a			A a
AA	Aa	Aa	aa
1	2	3	4

The two parents are heterozygous for the albino gene, but phenotypically they are normal as the dominant gene suppresses the albino gene. Among the progenies however phenotypically there are two kinds - 3/4 are normal (1, 2 and 3) and 1/4 albino. Genotypically however there are 3 categories viz. Homozygous normal, Heterozygous normal and Homozygous albino in the ratio of 1:2:1. This is the typical ratio in the monohybird cross. The situation here is comparable to what happens when the F_1 is selfed in the monohybrid cross. Among the offspring who are normal 1/3 is completely normal (albino gene in absent); remaining 2/3 are normal but carriers; they carry the gene for albinism in heterozygous state.

Taste blindness to PTC : Phenylthiocarbamide or PTC is a bitter compound, but curiously, certain percentage of human population cannot find out the taste: obviously because their taste buds cannot recognise PTC. Thus we have two groups, tasters and non tasters. In the American population from where the data is available about 70% are tasters and 30% non tasters. The pedigree analysis of several families indicates that the ability or inability to taste PTC is a Mendelian character. Tasters have one or two domimant gene T and taste blindness is due to recessive allele t. Obviously the non tasters have a genotype tt. While the tasters are of two types - Homozygous TT or Heterozygous Tt. Marriage between heterozygous tasters would produce 3:1 ratio as in albinism.

Brown and blue eye colour : The colour of the iris in human beings is either black (usually brown) or blue. Pedigree studies have once again shown that the difference in eye colour is due to an allelic difference in a gene pair. Black eye colour is governed by a dominant gene B, while blue eye colour is decided by recessive gene b. Blue eyed individuals always have a genotype bb, while black eyed individuals may be homozygous BB or heterozygous Bb.

M - N blood groups : Landsteiner and Levine have discovered that in all human beings the blood group may be divided into M, N and MN (Note this is different from A, B, AB and 0 blood group which is a multiple allelic character) and they follow the typical Mendelian inheritance. These blood groups however do not cause any agglutination in human blood, so that there can be blood transfusion between these unlike in A, AB, AB and 0 groups. Then how are these blood groups M, N and MN can be identified? They are identified by the agglutination they cause in the RBC of rabbits. The red blood cells of M people carry an antigen M and these can be agglutinated by the anti M sera of the rabbit (A rabbit produces anti M sera when injected with M blood). The red cells of N people carry N antigen and it is agglutinated by N anti sera. MN people have both M and N antigenes and can be agglutinated by both M and N antisera. The genes that control these blood groups function as follows. M people will have M^m gene and N people have M^n gene. These two do not show any dominance hence the heterozygotes show MN blood groups and are genetically M"M". This can occur when M and N individuals marry among themselves. The following table gives the frequency of occurrence of blood groups in various marriages.

Blood groups of parents	**Blood groups of Children**		
M	MN	N	
M x M	9	8	1
N x N-	-	-	27
M x N	-	43	1
M x MN	183	196	-
N x MN	-	156	167
MN x MN	71	141	63

(Adopted from Wiener)

In the marriage between MN and MN which is similar to the selfing of F_1, in monohybird cross that roughly M, MN and N give a genotypic ratio of 1:2:1.

Deviations from Mendelism : Mendel believed that the characters in individuals exist either as dominant or as recessive alleles only. He did not visualise any intermediate behaviour. This is a deviation from Mendelian postulate and is called incomplete dominance.

The phenomenon of incomplete dominance has been seen in snapdragons *(Antirrhinum majus)*, four o clock plants *(Mirabilis jalapa)*, Andalusian fowls etc.

We shall study the example of 4 Oclock plants. In 4^0 clock plants also just as in pea plants, the flower colour is controlled by a pair of alleles. Red flower colour is RR and white flower colour is rr genotypically. The two are crossed as follows:

Red	X	White
(4o'clock plant)		(4 o'clock plant)
RR	X	rr
R		r
	Rr	F_1 pink flowers
	selfing	

	R	r
R	RR Red	Rr Pink
r	Rr Pink	rr White

When a red flowered plant is crossed with a white flowered one (both are pure breeding) the F_1 heterozygote progeny will be pink in colour. (it is red in the case of a Mendelian cross) It appears as if the red and white are blended to produce the pink colour. When the F_2 is raised by selfing the F_1 not only red and pink flower colours appear but the white colour also appears in the ratio of 1:2:1 of red, pink and white respectively.

Explanation of the results : While the inheritance pattern in 4^0 clock plants is basically Mendelian there is a slight deviation, in that R is incompletely dominant over r. Thus the F_1 produces an entirely new phenotype not seen in the parents. Hence in 4^0 clock plants the heterozygous condition is always pink, while the homozygous individuals are either red or white. Another significant feature in incomplete dominance is that the phenotype and genotype are always same as there is no dominance. All characters (red, white) except pink can express themselves morphologically only in the homozygous condition. Hence the ratio of the *2* progeny is always 1:2:1.

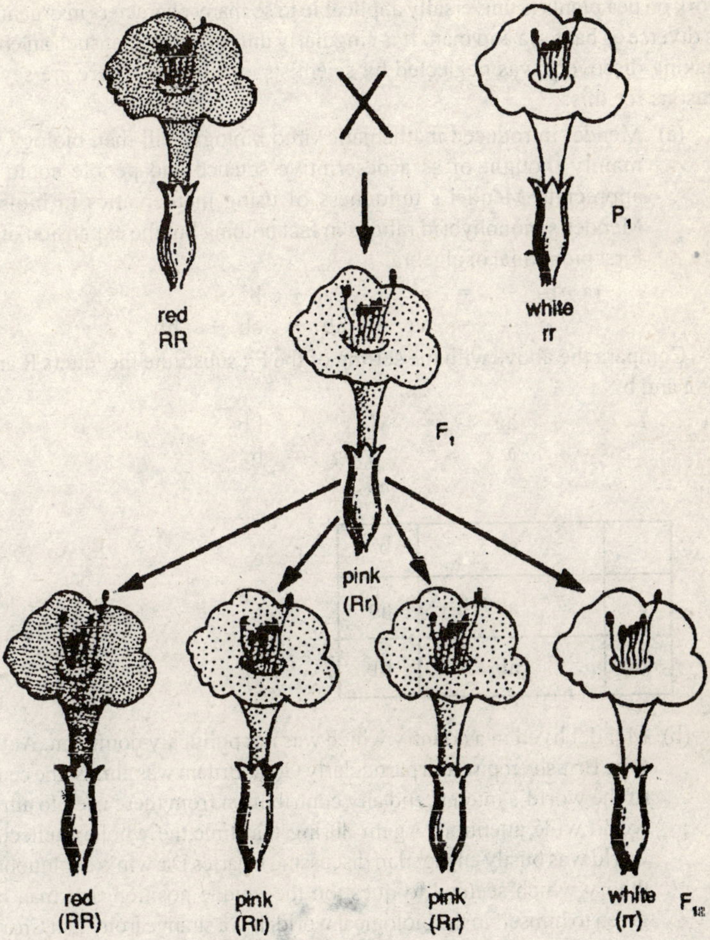

Fig. 10.4 Mendelism

Incomplete domonance in mirabilis jalapa

Significance of Mendel's Work : Mendel's work actually was far ahead of his times and the scientific world at that time was not in a position to appreciate the fundamental nature of his contribution. In fact it is not an exaggeration to say the science of genetics got a firm foundation from his work. It was Mendel who thought of a physical basis for inheritance. It was he again, who proposed that inheritance of characters from parents to offspring is brought about by discreet units or particles called factors. These were later named genes. Mendel's work on pea plants is universally applicable to so many characters in organisms as diverse as bacteria and man. It is singularly unfourtunate that such an epoch making discovery was neglected by scientists of his time. There are several reasons for this.

(a) Mendel introduced mathematics into biology. Till then biology was mainly thought of as a descriptive science and people could not appreciate Mendel's uniquness of using mathematics in biology. Mendel's monohybrid ratio is in fact nothing but the expansion of the First bionomial of algebra.

$$(a + b)^2 = a^2 + 2ab + b^2$$
$$= aa + ab + ab + bb$$

Compare the above with the selfing of the F_1; substitute the letters R and r for a and b

aa X bb

a b

ab

	a	b
a	aa	ab
b	ab	bb

(b) Mendel lived in a country which was not politicaly dominant. At that time British empire and particularly Great Britain was almost the centre of the world's interest and any contribution from there used to attract world wide attention. Again during that time,the whole intellectual world was busily engaged in discussing Charles Darwin's evolutionary theory which seemed to question the unique position that man had given to himself in the biological world. It is a strange irony that Charles Darwin was not aware of the existence of Mendel much less of his work. Had only Darwin knew about Mendel's work, he (Darwin) would have greatly modified his théory on evolutionary mechanism. The uniqueness of Mendel's work not only lies in propounding the law of inheritance but also in providing an explanation for the origin of heritable variations. Darwin evaded the most fundamental aspect in the mechanism of evolution namely the origin of heritable variations. Mendel provided an answer in the form of producing new heritable variations from the existing ones. The basic variation however has to be brought about by mutation. Mendel explained the means , whereby variations present in different individuals get distributed, undergo various permutation combinations thus producing new traits. What Mendel did with the pea plants ie. hybridization, has been going on in nature ever since life began, to produce myriads of forms and expressions of life.

Is Mendelism an exception or rule in Genetics

The classical genetical work that Mendel did no doubt established the science of Genetics. There is also no doubt that Mendelian principles of inheritance hold good for majority of the characters in almost all organisms. But except for the basic principles of inheritance, the whole of modern Genetics is an exception to Mendelism. It (Modern Genetics) seems to defy if not question the universality of Mendelian inheritance. We will briefly analyse a few of these aspects -

(a) Mendel believed that one gene governs one character ie. one gene one character hypothesis. There are many exceptions to this. Several genes control the development of one character as in comb pattern in fowls, flower colour in Indian corn, coat colour in mice etc.

(b) Mendel believed that the inheritance of one gene is not influenced by the other and genes assort themselves independently. Linkage of genes, where characters present in one individual always are inherited together (maize) shows that Mendel's laws are not universal.

c) In governing a character a gene will not be influenced by the other according to Mendel. There are several instances of qualitative (flower colour in some plants, plumage colours in fowls etc) and quantitative (skin colour in man, aleurone colour in wheat etc) interactions of genes; again an exception to Mendelism.

d) Mendel opined that there are only two alleles for every gene and the characters are always contrasting. This is not true as proved by the existence of multiple alleles and by the intergradation of characters as in quantitative inheritance.

e) Characters are either always dominartt or recessive - Mendel. This need not be so. There are instances of incomplete dominance or a non allelic dominant gene suppressing another dominant gene (Epistasis).

f) Mendelism is based on chromosomal or nuclear inheritance. But there are several instances of inheritance of characters through cytoplasm.

The facts mentioned above reveal, that every one. of the Mendelian hypothesis has been questioned as to its/applicability to the entire biological world which was once believed to be true. Indeed in modern Genetics Mendelism is something of an exception than of a rule. The pattern of inheritance is not as simple as Mendel thought it to be. Mendel however was lucky in choosing pea plant and the characters. Every one of the characters he chose (the genes responsible for them) was present on a different chromosome and there was no linkage. If he were to choose linked characters, he could not have enunciated the law of independent assortment. Having said this, it must be conceded, that these discoveries of modern Genetics have not made Mendelism either obsolete or irrelevant. The rules of inheritance propounded by Mendel though not universally applicable, still hold good for quite a majority of traits, and they (rules of inheritance) remain for ever, the corner stone on which is founded the science of Genetics.

11

INTERACTION OF GENES

The rediscovery of Mendelian laws in 1900 by three scientists independently added a new vigour and enthusiasm for genetic studies. Geneticists and plant breeders began hybridization experiments in a variety of plants and animals in order to establish the pattern of inheritance and produce new varieties. But much to the dismay of many breeders, the results obtained in several crosses, seemed to negate instead of supporting Mendelian hypothesis. As deviations in inheritance pattern began to accumulate it became clear that a vast majority of organisms follow a different heriditary mechanism and that Mendelian principles are not universal. Indeed in some instances, the results obtained even questioned the very basis ofMendelism. Some of the characters of parents seemed to blend in the offspring questioning the particulate inheritance. The Mendelian ratios of 3:1 and 9:3:3:1 appeared in but few crosses. One of the basic postulates, that was seriously doubted was whether every character is always controlled by a single gene or could there be more than one gene responsible for a character. Do the genes function in isolation or several genes function in co-ordination to influence a particular phenotype?

A careful study of the many crosses which apparently violated the Mendelian rules revealed, that confusion in many instances could be clarified, by assuming the involvement of more than one gene in delimiting a character. Very often the phenotypic expression in an individual is the result of interaction between these genes. The phenotypic ratio in a F_2 cross depends upon the type of interaction, while the fundamental laws of inheritance remain the same. During the earlier part of this century many studies were conducted to analyse these apparently aberrant phenomena. Studies have revealed that in many instances two, three or even many pairs of genes control the expression of a character. For instance in *Drosophila* the eye pigmentation is controlled by several pairs of factors. This phenomenon witnessed in several organisms is called **interaction of factors, Genic interaction or factorial interaction.**

Genic interaction is of two types - qualitative and quantitative or cumulative. In, the qualitative interaction, the interaction produces any one of the contrasting characters, but not different degrees or shades of the same character. The parameters for the characters are fixed. For instance if the dominant gene produces a character, its intensity will not change irrespective of the fact whether the dominant gene is in the homozygous condition or in the heterozygous condition. On the other hand in cumulative inheritance, the character varies in quantity or intensity depending on the number of genes involved and in the process produces a range of quantitative variations between the two extremes. In this chapter we shall study some examples of qualitative interaction of factors. Broadly categorizing, the various genic interactions fall into two categories viz. modifications of monohybrid ratio and modifications of dihybrid ratio. Modifications in the 3:1 ratio (in the F_2 generation) due to the involvement of lethal genes is discussed below.

Lethal genes : Some of the genes are known to be harmful to the organism to the extent of being the cause of death. Such genes are called lethal genes. Luckily most of the lethal genes are recessive and the individuals possessing them can survive provided they are heterozygous. Heterozygous individuals possess a dominant gene and its allele the recessive lethal gene. The lethal genes besides causing lethality in the homozygous condition are also known to control many phenotypic traits.

Lethal genes vary in time at which they bring about lethality. Some bring about death as early as in the zygote; others have a delayed effect allowing the organism to survive for quite sometime.

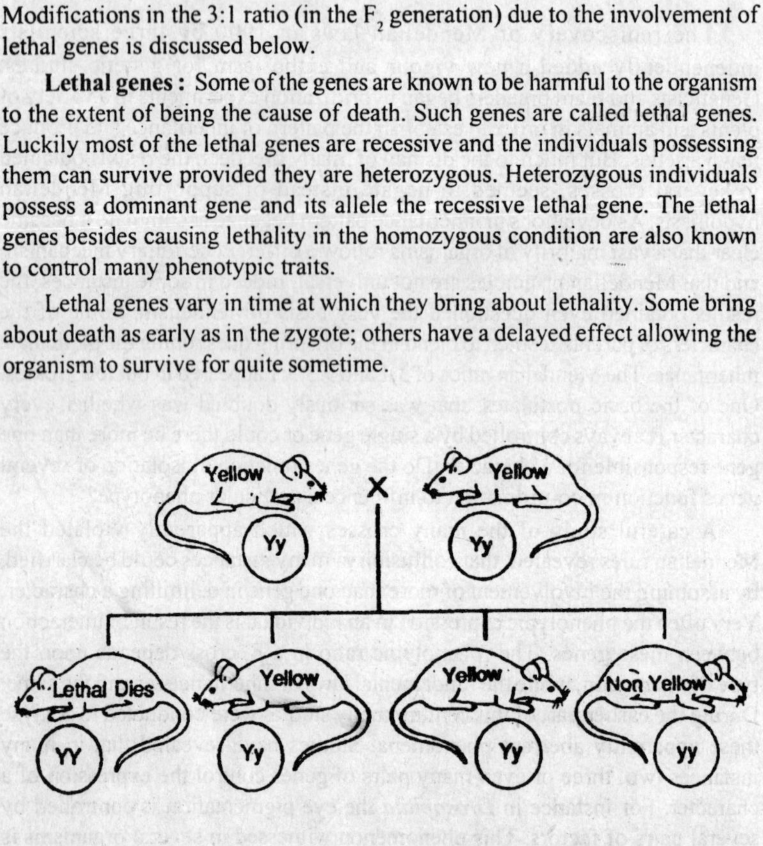

Fig 11.1 Interaction of Genes
Inheritance of lethal genes in mice (2:1 ratio)

The presence of dominant lethal is visualised, but it cannot be analysed because individuals possessing dominant lethals die immediately. Their presence can be assumed when a dominant gene expression is assumed but fails to figure among the progeny.

A typical example of recessive lethal gene is that of yellow mice discovered by Stiegleder (1971). In some earlier experiments Cuenot has reported in yellow mice that the breeding is not true in the sense, in cross between, two yellow mice, always yellow and brown are obtained in the ratio of 2:1 respectively. But Stiegleder analysed this and found out that 1/4 of the yellow mice die in the embryonic condition due to lethal gene and only the dominant heterozygotes live. Let us assume that the lethal gene is *L* and its recessive allele is / responsible for the brow colour. Due to lethality the mice with genotype LL cannot survive. Heterozygous individuals can survive according to Cuenot, because the gene L has multiple effects, while it is dominant with reference to bod colour (Ll produces yellow colour) it is recessive with reference to lethality that is the reason why double dominants will not survive. The mice crossed by Cuenot are obviously heterozygous yellow. The cross is as follows.

Ll X Ll

L 1 L 1

	L	.1
L	LL 1	Ll 2
1	Ll 3	11 4

1. Does not survive due to double lethal genes. 2 and 3 yellow coloured survive since the genotype is heterozygous. 4. Brown colour (lives)

The ratio would be 2:1 yellow and brown respectively.

There are several other examples also of lethal dominant genes like the creeper legs. Obviously here also the gene has different functions, while it is dominant for creeper legs, it is recessive for lethality. The inheritance pattern is same as in yellow mice.

An instance of lethal gene in human beings is *brachyphalangy* (short fingers - having two joints) with the same inheritance pattern mentioned above.

Modification of Dihybrid ratio : In the examples listed below the normal Mendelian dihybrid ratio of 9:3:3:1 is variously modified due to different types of interaction among the genes. We shall study five such examples. In some examples the ratio remains same but more than one pair of genes interact.

1. Combs in fowls (9:3:3:1)
2. Flower colour in sweet pea *(Lathrums)* (9:7)
3. Coat colour in mice (9:3:4)
4. Plumage in poultry (15:1)
5. Duplicate genes in *Capsella* (15:l)

COMBS IN FOWLS (Collaborative genes)

In this example, while the final dihybird ratio is not altered, the manner in which the character in question is controlled is a clear indication of involvement of more than one pair of genes. Worked out in terms of genetic analysis by Bateson and Punnett, four types of comb patterns are found in fowls. These are - *rose comb* found in *Wyandotte* breed, *pea comb* in *Brahma* breed, *single comb in. Leghorn* breed, and *Walnut comb* found *in Malay* breed of fowls. The first three types were known to be related to each other while the fourth one was thought to be unrelated to the other three. Each of the types mentioned above breed true (they can exist in the homozygous condition).

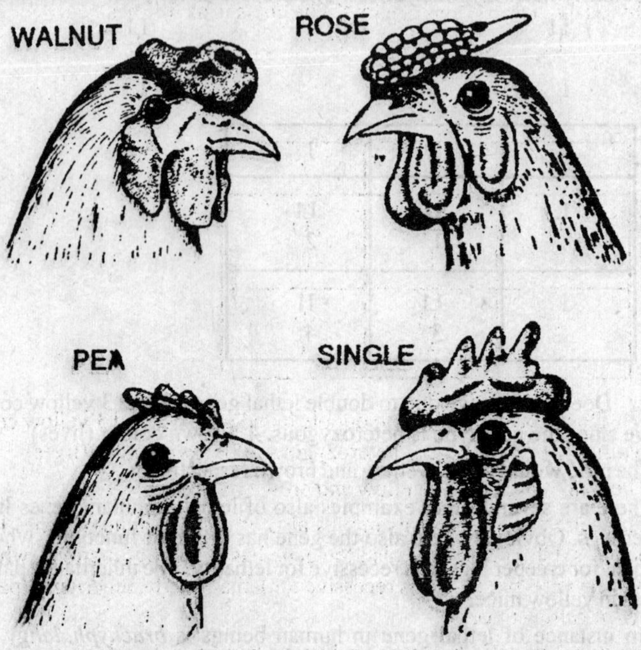

Fig 11.2 Interaction of Genes
Comb shapes in fowls, **A.** Pea, **B.** Rose, **C.** Single, **D.** Walnut

A cross between rose and single combed birds showed that, the latter was recessive to the former and in the F_2, they seggregate into typical 3:1 ratio. Similarly in a cross between pea comb and single comb, the latter again acts as recessive to the former with a typical 3:1 ratio in the F_2 generation. When the rose combed birds were crossed with pea combed, however an interesting result was obtained. The F_1 was Walnut, previously thought unrelated to any other three types of combs. When F_1 Walnuts were bred in between them, the F_2 generation showed (see the checker board) walnut (9), rose (3) pea (3) and single (1) comb in the ratio of 9:3:3:1.

Explanation for the experiment : The fact that single comb acts as recessive to both *pea* and *rose* indicates that it (single) must be having recessive alleles for both rose and pea. Again, rose and pea must have dominant alleles, and these alleles must be having something common between them as otherwise they could not cross with single. The fact that single has recessive alleles for both rose and pea indicates that it must have more than one pair of alleles controlling the comb shape. The fact that rose and pea both are dominant to single is an indication that in them, the dominant genes present must exist together with recessive genes. The production of walnut in F_1 is a clear indication that the dominant alleles of both (rose and pea) have interacted. This clearly illustrates the operation of two pairs of genes. In the present case rose comb is produced by R gene together with pp gene (the genotype can be RRpp or Rrpp), the pea comb is controlled by P gene together with recessive rr (the genotype can be rrPP or rrPp) genes. Single comb is produced by both gene pair P and R in their recessive state (rrpp). Both P and R present together will, produce the walnut comb by their interaction (the genotype can be RRPP, RrPP, RRPp or RrPp). What is important to produce walnut comb is the presence of P and R either in homozygous or heterozygous state. The following checker board will give the results of this cross.

Pea comb (pure) X Rose comb (pure)

rrPP X RRpp

↓

rP → ← Rp

RrPp (F_1 di hybrid)

(Walnut)

FI produces 4 kinds of gametes RP, Rp, rP and rp. Self breeding of *FI* produces offspring as follows.

	RP	Rp	rP	rP
RP	RR PP 1	RR Pp2	Rr PP3	Rr Pp4
Rp	RR Pp 5	RR pp6	Rr Pp7	Rr pp8
rP	Rr PP	Rr Pp 10	rr PP 11	rr Pp 12
rP	Rr Pp 13	Rr pp 14	rr pP 15	rr pp 16

In the above checker board, giving 16 probable types of progenies when the mating between four types of gametes is random - the phenotypes of progenies are - 1, 2, 3, 4, 5, 7, 9, 12, 13 are *walnut,* 6, 8, 14 are *rose,* II, 12 and 15 *are pea* and 16 is *single* giving a ratio of 9:3:3:1 respectively.

The basic mode of inheritance of the genes in reality does not differ from the Mendelian pattern. The main difference being the F_1 does not resemble either parent and new character appears in the F_2 in the form of single. Obviously the walnut is the result of interaction between two independently inherited dominant genes, the recessive alleles of both producing the single comb. The single comb produced in F_2 is double homozygous recessive as can be proved by the fact that on self breeding it produces only single comb. This type of genetic interaction is due to the action of *collaborative genes.* These may be defined as two different non allelic genes present on separate loci, but influence the same trait and interact to produce a new trait that neither of them could produce alone.

Flower colour in sweet pea (Complementary genes)

In sweet peas *(Lathrus odoratus)* the flower colour is of two types - purple and white. Bateson and Punett conducted several crosses and obtained two strains of white races which bred true. But when these two races are crossed with each other, the F_1 progeny had purple coloured flowers. The F_1 on self pollination produced in the F_2 generation both purple and white flowers in the ratio of 9:7 as against the Mendelian ratio of 9:3:3:1.

According to Bateson and Punnett, the development of the purple colour is dependent on the presence of two independent dominant genes C and P; both of which interact to produce the anthocyanin pigmentation. Gene C is responsible for the formation of the colourless compound *chrortlogen.* This produces an enzyme that catalyzes the formation of raw materials necessary for the formation of anthocyanin. Gene P controls the conversion of the raw material 7into anthocyanin. Hence both C and P are necessary for purple colour. If there is no C the first step is blocked and pigment is not formed, and if there is no p the second step is blocked and the raw material does not get converted into anthocyanin. In a way C and P act as complementary to each other's functions. In order to produce the colour, they should be present either in the homozygous condition CC or PP or in the heterozygous condition (Cc or Pp). The fact that the two pure breeding white races produce a purple colour is because each of them have either C or P and not both. In the F_1 C and P come together to produce colour. Since two independent non allelic genes are involved, it goes without saying that the recessive alleles of either C or P must be present in white flowered plants together with one of the dominant genes (either C or P). The cross is as follows.

White X White
CCpp ccPP
↓ ↓
Cp → CcPp ← cP

F_1 hybrid (purple)

gametes

CP, Cp, cP, cp

	CP	Cp	cP	cp
CP	CC PP 1	CC pp 2	Cc PP 3	Cc Pp 4
Cp	CC Pp 5	CC pp 6	Cc Pp 7	Cc pp 8
cP	Cc PP 9	Cc Pp 10	cc PP 11	cc Pp 12
cp	Cc Pp 13	Cc pp 14	cc Pp 15	cc pp 16

The FI hybrid (purple) forms four different types of gametes which on random mating produce 16 possible types of offspring. In the above checker board wherever both C and P are present together, either in the homozygous or in the heterozygous condition the flower colour is purple. In the checker board, the 16th, which has all the recessive genes is also white, for there is no question of colour in the absence of both C and P.

Parental generation Pea Comb X Rose Comb

Genotype of the parents **PPrr** **ppRR**

Gametes formed **Pr** **pR**

F_1 *Hybrid generation* **PpRr** (WALNUT COMB)

Crossing the F_1 *hybrids* **PpRr** **X** **PpRr**

Gametes formed by the hybrids **PR; Pr; pR; pr** **PR; pR; pr**

F_2 *generation*

	PR	Pr	pR	pr
PR	**PPRR** WALNUT (Double dominant)	**PPRr** WALNUT	**PpRR** WALNUT	**PpRr** WALNUT
Pr	**PPRr** WALNUT	**PPrr** PEA COMB	**PpRr** WALNUT	**Pprr** PEA COMB
pR	**PpRR** WALNUT	**PpRr** WALNUT	**ppRR** ROSECOMB	**ppRr** ROSECOMB
pr	**PpRr** WALNUT	**Pprr** PEACOMB	**ppRr** ROSECOMB	**pprr** SINGLE

Dihybrid ratio : – *Genotype*

9	*Walnuts*	–	**PPRR; PPRr; PpRR; PpRr**
3	*Pea Comb*	–	**PPrr; Pprr**
3	*Rose Comb*	–	**ppRR; ppRr**
1	*Single*	–	**pprr**

Fig 11.3 Interaction of Genes

Inheritance of comb shapes in poultry (9:3:3:1 ratio)

In the checker board - 1, 2, 3, 4, 5, 7, 9, 10, and 13 are purple, while 6, 8, 11, 12, 14, 15 and 16 are white in the ratio of 9:7 respectively.

The genes C and P here are called complementary genes. They can be defined as two or more separate (non allelic) dominant genes present on different loci interacting to produce a phenotypic trait, neither of which can produce the trait alone.

A similar example of complementary genes has been reported in Indian Corn where the grains or either white or red in colour. In order to produce red colour both R and C are required. The absence of both or any on dominant allele, the grain will be white in colour. When a homozygous red is crossed with homozygous white the F_1 progeny is red as expected in a Mendelian ratio, but when the F_1 is selfed to produce F_2 a 9:7 ratio of red and white grained plants are produced. The cross takes place as follows:

Red	X	White
RRCC		rrcc
RC		re
	Rr Cc	FI hybrid - Red

The FI dihybrid produces four different kinds of gametes - RC, Rc, rC and rc. These mate .at random to produce the following progeny.

	RC	Rc	rC	rc
RC	RR CC 1	RR Cc 2	Rr CC 3	Rr Cc 4
Rc	RR Cc 5	RR cc 6	Rr Cc 7	Rr cc 8
rC	Rr CC 9	Rr Cc 10	rr CC 11	rr Cc 12
rc	Rr Cc	Rr cc 14	rr Cc 15	rr cc 16

In the above checker board, 1, 2, 3, 4, 5, 7, 9, 10 and 13 are red and 6, 8, 11, 12, 14, 15 and 16 are white in the ratio of 9:7.

Coat colour in mice (supplementary genes)

In the common house mouse, there are several variations in the skin (coat) colour like Agouti, black, albino etc. The agouti colour is a mixture of red and grey and has two pigments in the fur. This coat colour is found in wild rodents such as Norway rat, meadow vole, guinea pig, grey squirrel etc. From this wild or agouti colour, several variations have arisen in domestic rats. The most common variation is the albino.

In albinos the coat colour is white with pink eyes. Albinos breed true and are recessive to all other colour variations. Another variation in coat colour is black. This is produced by the removal of grey pigment from the coat. Black is recessive to agouti but dominant over albino. The black mice breed true.

When a pure breeding black mice is crossed with albino, the Fi will be agouti. When the F_1 agouti hybrids are crossed among themselves in the F_2 generation, the following varieties are produced. Agouti 9/16, Black 3/16 and 4/16 albinos. This is a modification of the 9:3:3:1 ratio in that the last two categories have joined to form the third category of albinos. The results can be explained by assuming that the coat colour is due to two independent dominant genes namely C and A. The gene C by itself either in the homozygous condition (CC) or heterozygous condition (Cc) can produce black colour provided A is absent. However when both C and A are present they interact to produce agouti colour. When there is no C, irrespective of the fact whether there is dominant A gene or not, the coat colour will be albino. C gene is necessary to produce colour. The following gives the details of the cross.

Black	x	Albino
CC aa		cc AA
Ca		cA
	Cc Aa	Fl hybrid - Agouti

The Fi agouti produces four kinds of gametes:
CA, Ca, cA, and ca.

	CA	Ca	cA	ca
CA	CC AA 1	CC Aa 2	Cc AA 3	Cc Aa 4
Ca	CC Aa 5	CC aa 6	Cc Aa 7	Cc aa 8
cA	Cc AA 9	Cc Aa 10	cc AA 11	cc Aa 12
ca	Cc Aa 13	Cc aa 14	cc Aa 15	cc aa 16

In the above checker board 1, 2, 3, 4, 5, 7, 9, 10 and 13 are agouti 6, 8 and 14 are black, while 11, 12, 15 and 16 are albinos.

Supplementary genes may be defined as two independent pairs of genes one of which is capable of producing a phenotypic trait, provided the second gene is absent. When both the dominant genes are present together they interact and produce a different trait.

In the above cross, C will produce black colour, but when supplemented (supported) by A the colour agouti is produced.

Plumage colour in poultry (Epistasis) : In some of the poultry birds, the plumage is either coloured or white and it seems to have a peculiar type of inheritance. The white plumage of white Leghorn birds is dominant over the black plumage of barred and other coloured varieties. However there are other birds with white plumage such as the Wyondettes or Plymouth rocks which are recessive to the coloured plumage. Obviously the white plumage colour in Leghorns and Wyandottes is controlled by different genes. In order to Find the genotypes of the coloured plumage and white plumage of both leghorns and wyandottes, a cross can be made between the two varieties of white birds *viz.*, Leghorns and Wyandottes. The pure lines of such birds when crossed produce an F_1 with a white plumage with dark flecks (resembling an F_1 from a cross between white Leghorns and black birds). An interesting result awaits when these F_1 birds are bred together. Both white and coloured plumage appears in the F_2 in the ratio of 13:3. The white birds resemble the F_1 bird.

Explanation : It is assumed that the white Leghorns contain a colour gene C, but also an inhibitor gene I. Which does not allow C to function and produce colouration. Then the Leghorns are genetically coloured birds but have two dominant genes one of which suppresses the expression of the other. It is because of this, that Leghorns are dominant over both black and white Wyandotte birds. The white Wyandotte birds on the other hand are genetically white in the sense that they do not have a coloured gene. What is the effect of the inhibitor gene I in the absence of the coloured gene C? none, because there is no gene to be suppressed by it. The plumage colour in this instance will be white because there is no coloured gene (C). This is a peculiar pheonomenon where two dominant non allelic genes interact but the interaction is not co-ordination, complementary or supplementary. One dominant gene (C) by itself can bring out a morphological trait and the sole function of the other (I) is to suppress it whenever it is present. The gene I does not seem to have any function in the absence of C. This phenomenon is called *Epistasis.* Epistasis may be defined as a phenomenon in which one non allelic dominant gene suppresses the action of another dominant gene. The two genes are situated on different loci. The gene that suppresses another gene is called *Epistatic* (I) and the dominant gene that is suppressed (C) is called hypostatic.

In the above cross the genes may be designated as follows.

I epistatic gene, i = recessive allele

C hypostatic gene, c = recessive allele

The following is the checker board representation of the cross.

White leghorn	x	White wyandotte
IICC		iicc
IC		ic
	Ii Cc	F_1 hybird - White

This produces four kinds of gametes - IC, Ic, iC and ic. They mate randomly to produce the following 16 types.

	IC	Ic	iC	ic
IC	II CC 1	II Cc 2	Ii CC 3	Ii Cc 4
Ic	II Cc 5	Ic cc 6	Ii Cc 7	Ii cc 8
iC	Ii CC 9	Ii Cc 10	Ii CC 11	Ii Cc 12
ic	Ii Cc 13	Ii cc 14	ii Cc 15	ii cc 16

In the above checker board, 1, 2, 3, 4, 5, 6, 7, 8, 9, 10, 13, 14 and 16 are white, while II, 12 and 15 are coloured in the ratio of 13:3.

Polymeric genes (Additive genes)

In some of the plants like *Cucurbita pepo* the fruit shape or of different types in different varieties. The fruit shapes may be long, spherical or discoid. The shape of the fruit seems to be governed by two pairs of interacting factors. When two individuals with spherical fruits are crossed only discoid fruits are produced in all the progeny. On the selfing of the F_1, in the F_2 progeny discoid, spherical and long types of fruits are produced in the ratio of 9:6:1. As has been pointed already two pairs genes are responsible for the fruit shape. When both the gene pairs are dominant the fruit shape is discoid; when both gene pairs are recessive the fruits are long. If one pair of genes is dominant and the other recessive spherical fruits are produced (in a gene pair even if one gene is dominant the recessive gene is suppressed. In otherwords one gene pair is dominant means atleast one of the genes is dominant in the pair). The genes involved in this are called polymeric genes and the phenomenon is known as polymerism. The following checker board will give the details of the above explanation.

P_1	Spherical	X	Spherical
	$S_1S_1s_2s_2$		$s_1s_1S_2S_2$
P_1	↓ S_1s_2		↓ S_1s_2
		↓	
F_1		Discoid $S_1s_1S_2s_2$	

F_1 gamets→ ↓	S_1S_2	S_1s_2	s_1S_2	s_1s_2
S_1S_2	$S_1S_1S_2S_2$ Discoid	$S_1s_1S_2s_2$ Discoid	$S_1s_1S_2S_2$ Discoid	$S_1s_1S_2s_2$ Discoid
S_1s_2	$S_1S_1S_2s_2$ Discoid	$S_1S_1s_2s_2$ Spherical	$S_1s_1S_2s_2$ Discoid	$S_1s_1s_2s_2$ Discoid
F_2 s_1S_2	$S_1s_1S_2S_2$ Discoid	$S_1s_1S_2s_2$ Discoid	$s_1s_1S_2S_2$ Spherical	$s_1s_1S_2s_2$ Spherical
s_1s_2	$S_1s_1S_2s_2$ Discoid	$S_1s_1s_2s_2$ Spherical	$s_1s_1S_2s_2$ Spherical	$s_1s_1s_2s_2$ Long

Duplicate genes : In some of the poultry and plants *(Capsella bursa pastoris)* more than one pair of genes seem to affect a single trait. These are non allelic but to produce a particular trait both the dominant genes should be present or atleast one of them should be present either in the homozygous condition or in the heterozygous condition. We can take an example in poultry to illustrate this.

Certain breeds (Langshans) in poultry have feathers on their shanks, while others (buff rocks) have clean shanks (no feathers). Feathered shanks are dominant over clean shanks. When two birds - one feathered and the other clean (both pure line) are crossed, the F_1 bird is feathered. When these F_1 feathered birds are self bred, in the F_2 progeny 15 birds will be feathered and one bird will have clean shanks in the ratio of 15:1.

In the above checker board, 1, 2, 3, 4, 5, 6, 7, 8, 9, 10, 13, 14 and 16 are white, while II, 12 and 15 are coloured in the ratio of 13:3.

Duplicate genes : In some of the poultry and plants *(Capsella bursa pastoris)* more than one pair of genes seem to affect a single trait. These are non allelic but to produce a particular trait both the dominant genes should be present or atleast one of them should be present either in the homozygous condition or in the heterozygous condition. We can take an example in poultry to illustrate this.

Certain breeds (Langshans) in poultry have feathers on their shanks, while others (buff rocks) have clean shanks (no feathers). Feathered shanks are dominant over clean shanks. When two birds - one feathered and the other clean (both pure line) are crossed, the F_1 bird is feathered. When these F_1 feathered birds are self bred, in the F_2 progeny 15 birds will be feathered and one bird will have clean shanks in the ratio of 15:1. The cross is as follows.

Feathered	x	Clean
FFSS		ffss
FS		fs
	FsSs	F_1 hybrid - feathered
	Ff Ss	PI hybrid - feathered

This produces four kinds of gametes FS, Fs, fS and fs.

	FS	Fs	fS	fs
FS	FF SS 1	FF Ss 2	Ff SS 3	Ff Ss 4
Fs	FF Ss 5	FF ss 6	Ff Ss 7	Ff ss 8
fS	Ff SS 9	Ff Ss 10	ff Ss 11	ff Ss 12
fs	Ff Ss 13	Ff ss 14	ff Ss 15	ff ss 16

In the F_2 generation I to 15 are feathered while the 16th one is cicair in the ratio of 15:1.

12

MULTIPLE FACTOR INHERITANCE

Mendelian inheritance deals with characters which are contrasting and which have only two states of existence ie. dominant or recessive being controlled by a single pair of genes. In pea plants, the characters chosen by Mendel were clear cut representing two extremes without any intermediary or intergradation stages. These variations are called discontinuous variations and represent a qualitative difference between the two genes. Even in Mendel's experiments some minor quantitative differences did appear which he ignored on a statistical basis. However Mendel was able to formulate his laws, because by and large the characters he studied (luckily for him) represented the simplest pattern of inheritance.

Not all characters in organisms can be analysed by a qualitative assessement. Certain characters like height, weight, size, yield etc. are on a quantitative dimension and cannot be explained on the basis of Mendelian pattern which is wholly qualitative. These characters do not fall into two clear cut extremes and hence lead to confusion if one uses Mendelian tools to assess them. Characters such as these, seem to intergrade and indeed there is not one, but many intermediaries linking both the extremes. Consequently these characters seem to blend instead of seggregating into separate classes or entities, characters which vary within a range and represent all intergrading steps. One such typical example of inheritance of intergrading characters is that of height in *Nicotiana* unsuccessfully studied by Joseph Kolreuter, the pre Mendelian plant breeder. He reported that when tall and dwarf plants were crossed, the F_1 was intermediate and the F_2 progeny showed all grades in between tall and dwarf. He was not able to explain his results.

The answer to the apparent failure of Kolreuter in rationalizing the confusion, depends on the fact that continuously varying quantitative characters are controlled by not one pair but many pairs of genes. The number of pairs of genes involved decide the number of intergradations. Each of these genes cumulatively affect the phenotypic trait, whether it is skin colour in man, yield of milk in cows, aleurone colour in wheat or size of the fruit in squashes etc. The inheritance of such characters controlled by many pairs of genes which interact producing various grades is called multiple factor inheritance or polygenic inheritance or quantitative inheritance. This inheritance which represents yet another exception to the monogenic inheritance of Mendel is different from the qualitative interaction of genes. While the genes (more than one pair) in qualitative interaction produce clear cut characters (e.g. rose or pea, purple or white), cumulative interaction produces grades like white, whitish, purplish, purple etc., if it were to be a quantitative character. Further, in qualitative inheritance the genes are non allelic independent genes. In quantitative inheritance, the genes involved are duplicates or replicas of the same gene. (e.g. $R_1 R_1 R_2 R_2$ - $P_1 P_1 P_2 P_2$ etc). There is also one more difference between genes that affect quality and quantity. The quantitative genes (characters) largely depend on the environment for their expression. For instance, a cow may be genotypically suited to produce five liters of milk per day, but it may increase or decrease this, depending on its health, nutrition age etc. Qualitative characters however are not largely influenced by the environment.

The riddle of blending of characters and the problem of rationalizing the quantitative inheritance was first taken up by Swedish geneticist Nillsson Ehle (1908) and American geneticist East (1910, 1916). These two scientists unravelled the secret of apparent blending inheritance by proposing that continuously varying traits are controlled by the cumulative action of many genes each of which contributes in a limited measure towards that trait. English scientist Mather has evolved statistical methods for the analysis of the multiple genes.

Polygenic inheritance may be defined as the inheritance in which several duplicates of genes cumulatively affect the quantity of a character.

Salient features of polygenic inheritance : The following are some of the important features.

1. Seggregation occurs at may loci and not at any one level.
2. Polygenes have pleiotropic effects; they influence more than on trait.
3. The genes are generally bound in blocks in inversion heterozygotes which avoid crossing over at the inverted loci. In the case of inversion homozygotes however, crossing over may seggregate them.
4. Environmental factors play a pivotal role in the expression of polygenes.
5. Polygenes can be subjected to statistical analysis to assess their number in concerning a particular trait.
6. They represent instances of continuous variations and exhibit a spectrum of that trait.

In this chapter we shall study some examples of polygenic inheritance in both plants and animals.

Grain colour in wheat : It was Swedish scientist Nilsson - Ehle (1909) who first studied the inheritance pattern of the colour of the grain in wheat. In some types, the kernel colour is red (aleurone colour) and in others white and in still others which may be regarded as intermediates different, shades of red appear in the kernel colour.

Nilsson - Ehle crossed a variety of wheat having dark red kernel with the one having white kernel. The red colour is incompletely dominant over white hence the F_1 hybrid had a kernel which was intermediate between red and white. These F_1 hybrids were bred among themselves to get the F_2 generation. In the F_2 progeny the kernel colour ranged from dark red, to white, between them there were atleast three grades of colour. These shades of colour can be graded as follows.

Red, Reddish, Intermdediate (pink), light and white.

According to the law of probability, it can be assumed, that two paris of seggregating genes are responsible for the colour variation in the wheat kernel. The red kernel wheat has two pairs of genes (two pairs of alleles) both of which contribute some quantity of redness to the grain. These genes are duplicates of each other ($R_1 R_1 R_2 R_2$). The white kernel wheat had recessive alleles of both these pairs (Q R_1) and does not contribute any thing to red colouration. The F_1 possesses two dominant genes ($R_1 r_1 R_2 r_2$) hence it is intermediate between red and white. In the F_2 generation the colour varies depending on the number of dominant genes the offspring gets ie. 4, 3, 2, I or zero. The details of the cross are given below.

Red X White

kernel wheat kernel wheat

$R_1 R_1 R_2 R_2$ $r_1 r_1 r_2 r_2$

↓ ↓

$R_1 R_2$ $r_1 r_2$

$R_1 r_1 R_2 r_2$ f_1 hybrid (Intermediate)

	$R_1 R_2$	$R_1 r_1$	$r_1 R_2$	$r_1 r_2$
$R_1 R_2$	$R_1 R_1$ 1 $R_2 R_2$	$R_1 R_1$ 2 $R_1 r_2$	$R_1 r_1$ 3 $R_2 R_2$	$R_1 r_1$ 4 $R_1 r_2$
$R_1 r_2$	$R_1 R_1$ 5 $R_2 R_2$	$R_1 R_1$ 6 $r_2 r_2$	$R_1 r_1$ 7 $R_2 r_2$	$R_1 r_1$ 8 $r_2 r_2$
$r_1 R_2$	$R_1 r_1$ 9 $R_2 R_2$	$R_1 r_1$ 10 $R_2 r_2$	$r_1 r_1$ 11 $R_2 R_2$	$r_1 r_1$ 12 $R_2 r_2$
$r_1 r_2$	$R_1 r_1$ 13 $R_2 r_2$	$R_1 r_1$ 14 $r_2 r_2$	$r_1 r_1$ 15 $R_2 r_2$	$r_1 r_1$ 16 $r_2 r_2$

In the above checker board, of the possible 16 types the following will be the phenotype according to the number of dominant genes possessed by them

Red	–	All dominant genes ($R_1R_1R_2R_2$)
Reddish	–	3 dominant genes ($R_1R_1R_2r_2$ or $R_1r_1R_2R_2$)
Intermediate	–	One dominant gene ($R_1r_1r_2r_2$ or $r_1r_1r_2R_2$)
White	–	No dominant gene ($r_1r_1r_2r_2$)

As per the above categorization, in the checker board, number I is red, 2, 3, 5, and 9 are reddish, 4, 5, 6, 10, 11 and 13 are intermediate, 8, 12, 14 and 15 are light and 16 is white. The ratio is 1:4:6:4:1. In many instances this ratio is also represented as 15:1, since excepet for the last one all others have some shades of red.Nilsson-Ehle found in certain other crosses of wheat concerning the kernel colour, in the F_2 progeny only one in every 4 was white, with at least 5 intergrades between red and white. He proposed that in this instance there were three pairs of genes (R_1R_1 R_2R_2 R_3R_3) responsible for the kernel colour.

Skin colour in human beings : The interpretation regarding the skin colour in Negroes and caucusoid whites was bit of a problem to interpret from the point of view of genic inheritance. Davenport (1913) first successfully explained the skin colour inheritance in terms of polygenes. He studied skin colour of several people in Jamica and Muda. In these regions intermarriages between Negroes and whites was quite frequent and the children were called Mulattoes. He hypothesised that Negroes of central and Western Africa differ from whites in having two pairs oi dominant alleles ($P_1P_1P_2P_2$) which are incompletely dominant over the genotype $p_1p_1p_2p_2$ of whites. In a cross between a negro and a white, the F_1 called mulattoe is heterozygous to both P_1 and P_2 with the result the skin colour is intermediate. Just as in kernel colour in wheat, here also the skin colour depends on the number of dominant alleles. It is as follows - Negro - all lhe four dominant genes and white all the four recessive genes. Mulattoes - Two dominant genes. When two mulattoes marry among themselves (a mulattoe man and a mulattoe woman) in the F_2 generation 16 possible types could be found among children. Assuming that mulattoes are hybrids for both the colour genes (P_1 and P_2) there genotype should be $P_1p_1P_2p_2$; while they get dominant allele from the Negro parent, the recessive alleles are obtained from the white parent. Theoretically mulattoes both male and female produce four types of gametes which on random combination would give 16 types. In the F_2 progeny the skin colour would be black (4 dominant genes), dark (3 dominant genes), Mulattoe (2 dominant genes), Fair (one dominant gene) and white (no dominant gene).

The above cross can be represented in the form of cheker board as follows.

Negro X White

$P_1P_1P_2P_2$ ↓ P_1P_2

$p_1p_1p_2p_2$ ↓ p_1p_2

$P_1p_1P_2p_2$ Mulattoe (F_1 hybrid)

	P_1P_2	P_1p_2	p_1P_2	p_1p_2
P_1P_2	P_1P_1 1 P_2P_2	P_1P_1 2 P_1p_2	p_1p_1 3 P_2P_2	p_1p_1 4 P_1p_2
P_1p_2	P_1P_1 5 P_2p_2	P_1P_1 6 p_1p_2	P_1p_1 7 P_2P_2	$P_1.p_1$ 8 P_1p_2
P_2P_2	P_1p_1 9 P_2P_2	P_1p_1 10 P_2p_2	p_1p_1 11 P_2P_2	p_1p_1 12 P_2p_2
p_1p_2	p_1p_1 13 P_2p_2	P_1p_1 14 p_2p_2	p_1p_1 15 P_2p_2	p_1p_1 16 p_2p_2

In the above cross, the phenotype and genotype can be classified as follows

Negro - All dominant ($P_1P_1P_2P_2$)

Dark - 3 dominant genes ($P_1P_1P_1p_2$ or $P_1P_1P_2P_2$)

Mulatto - 2 dominant genes ($P_1p_1P_2p_2$)

Fair - One dominant gene ($P_1p_1p_2p_2$ or $p_1p_1P_2p_2$)

White - No dominant gene ($p_1p_1p_2p_2$)

In the checker board given above 1 is negro (black); 2, 3, 5 and 9 are dark; 4, 5, 5, 10, 11 and 13 are mulattoes; 8, 12, 14 and 15 are fair and 16 is white. The ratio would be 1:4:6:4:1 or could be 15:1 as only one is white and the rest (15) are coloured to some or the other extent.

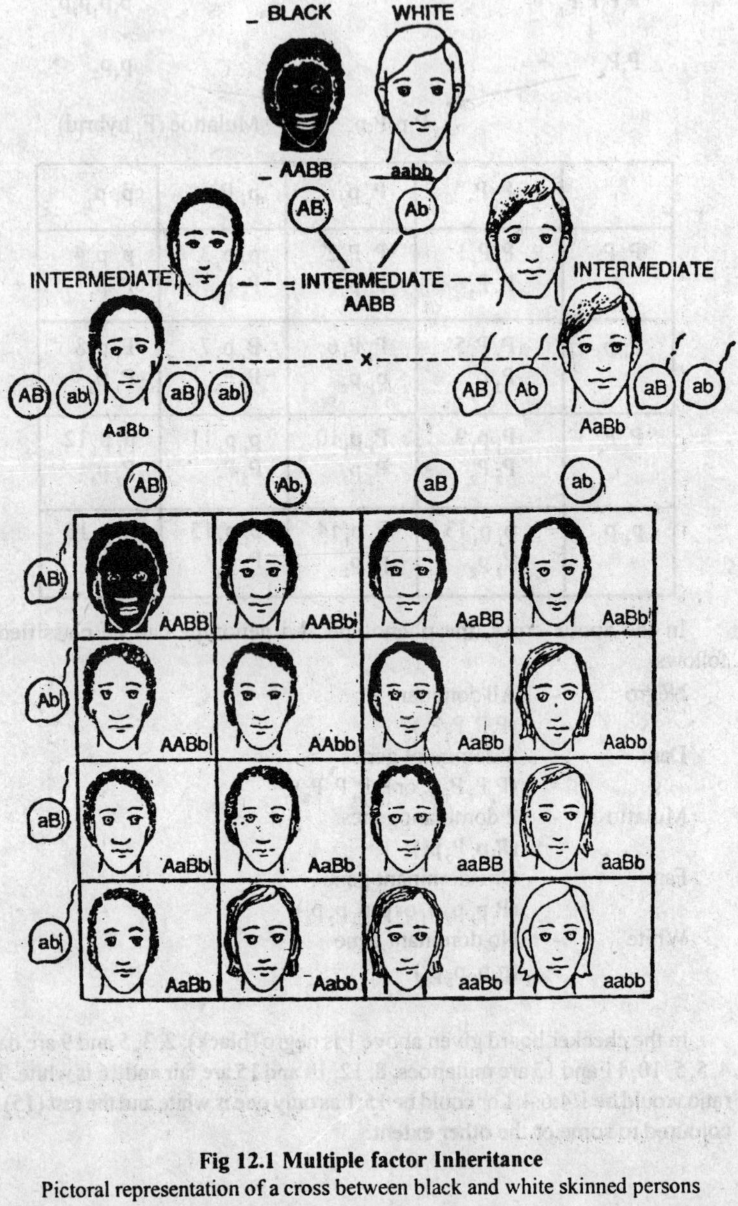

Fig 12.1 Multiple factor Inheritance

Pictoral representation of a cross between black and white skinned persons

Physiologically the skin colour in human beings depends upon the amount of melanin (a pigment) deposited on the skin. The amount of melanin depends upon the genes and its development depends upon the amount of sun light received by the skin. According to Curt Stern, the human skin colour depends on gene loci located at four to several different loci.

Height of man : The height of the body in man is another typical example ofpolygenic inheritance. The functioning of these genes however greatly depends on environmental factors. The genes control the functioning of the pituitory thus controlling growth. An under secretion of the pituitory under the influence of a 'dwarf gene' would retard the growth.

Ear length in maize : Emerson and East, the pioneers in the study of polygenic inheritance, observed many quantitative variations in ear size in maize. They worked on two varieties of maize - long eared black mexican sweet corn and short eared Tom thumb popcorn - The first variety ranges in ear length from 12 - 21 cms. with an average of 16.8 cms. The second variety has ears ranging in length from 5 - 8 cms, averaging to 6.6 cms. When these two varieties were crossed, the ear length in the F_1 progeny ranged from 9 - 15 cms averaging to 12.1 cms. Selling the F_1 progeny, F_2 was obtained much in the same way as in inheritance of kernel colour in wheat.

Ray size in flower heads of Compositae : A possible occurrence of Polygenic system operating in the ray development has been reported by the author (Sundara Rajan.) in the plant *Bidens pilosa* of Compositae. Here there are two extremes. In the one represented by a normal plant, the rays in the heterogamous heads are of normal size *ie*. they are formed by the fusion of three petals and the other 3 are reduced resulting in zygomorphy of the ray floret. In the other extreme which is a recessive mutant, the rays are completely reduced, with the result all the five petals of the ray floret are equal in size like the discfloret. The floret becomes actinomorphic. Between these, there are at least three intergradations representing cumulative interaction of these genes. The fully developed rays represent all the dominant genes. While the reduced rays represent all the recessive alleles. Work is going on to hybridize the various grades to arrive at the possible number of cumulative genes involved in the ray development.

Mechanism of gene action in a polygenic system : The mechanism of gene action as to how a cumulative effect is brought about regarding the phenotypic expression of a trait is not wholly understood in all instances. In the case of wheat however, the mechanism of kernel colour development is traceable to polyploid series. The common bread wheat which is hexaploid has six chromosomes of a particular type and hence three pairs of genes in the corresponding loci for a particular trait.The cumulative effect of these six genes produces the kernel colour. Further, the varying combinations of these during seggregation is responsible for a whole range of variation in the intensity of the kernel colour.

Modifier genes : There are certain types of genes in a polygenic system, which when present have the effect of modifying the functioning of other genes, thus bringing about change in the phenotype. Differences in size in plants and animals are particularly influenced by modifier genes. Some of the modifier genes act as enhancers, while others act as inhibitors, the final result of expression in a polygenic system is thus an average of all these effects. According to Mather, who devised a statistical analysis of the polygenes pointed that they are present in the heterochromatin. Another geneticist Milkman however opined (based on his studies on the development of cross veins in the wings of *Drosophila melanogaster)* that the polygenes are located in the euchromatin.

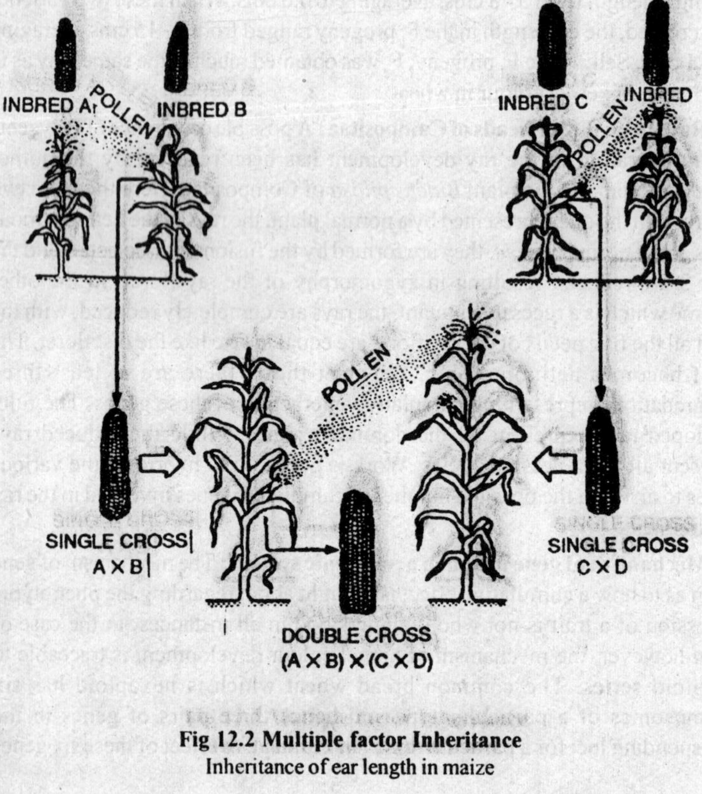

Fig 12.2 Multiple factor Inheritance
Inheritance of ear length in maize

Transgressive Variations : One of the basic characters of a functioning multigene system is that the F_2 generation of a cross between two individuals would exhibit a continuous variation forming a spectrum. But in some instances, F_2 individuals of a polygenic system vary in their behaviour in that they do not resemble any of their parents are grand parents. In some instances the characters of F_2 exceed the parameters of the P_1 generation, which is normally maintained in the F_2. In other words - suppose the parents differ in length between 2 - 6 cm, any spectrum exhibited by F_2 must be within this parametre. Instances where such variations occur trasgressing the limits are called transgressive variations. Punnet and Bailey have reported some instances of transgressive variations in poultry birds. In a cross between a large golden hamburg chicken and small sebright bantam variety, the F_1 progeny was intermediate between the two parents as could be expected in a polygene system. But surprisingly in the F_2 generation (obtained by a cross between F_1 individuals) some of the birds were either larger than the golden hamburg parent or (some) were smaller than the sebright bantam parent. This was explained as due to the fact that the either of the parents did not have all the dominant or all the recessive alleles with the result they did not set the parameters. In the F_2 generation, there is a possibility of some of the birds getting all the domiant or all the recessive genes, thus causing them to transgress the so called limits set by the parents. The genotype here is controlled by 3 pairs of genes with the golden hamburg having AABBCC and sebright bantam having aabbccDD.

Regressive variations : This is another form of variation in polygenes in which, the phenotype of the offspring tend to exhibit the mean of the Ponulation rather than that of the parents. For instance, the height in human beings is one such trait subject to regressive variations. The children of two tall parents are sometimes shorter than either of them because their height tends to-approach the mean height of the population, rather than mean height of the parents. In some cases short parents have tall children for the same reason.

13

MULTIPLE ALLELES

Hereditary characters are transmitted from parents to offspring through discreet units called genes which were called factors by Mendel. Even though it may not be possible to see a gene, its presence as a discreet seggregating particle has been proved both in the plant and animal world in a large majority of cases. Seggregation of characters is possible when large variations exist in a character. For instance if all pea plants had green seeds or only yellow seeds, it would not be possible to visualize the seggregation much less speculate on the existence of different genes. According to Mendel, in all sexually reproducing diploid organisms there are a set of factors for every character; meaning that red flower colour is controlled by two genes, white flower colour by two genes, green seed colour by two genes, yellow seed colour by two genes etc. Red flower colour and white flower colour are not two characters really; similarly the yellow and the green seed colour also. Flower colour is a character and the red and white are the two variants; similarly seed colour is a character and green and yellow are two variants. Why is it red flower colour and white flower colour are not regarded as two different characters but variations of the same trait? Because the genes responsible for these two colours (red and white) can interact producing either red or white depending on whichever character is dominant. Then what about the genes that produce these characters, are they same or are they different? The answer would be they are neither totally same nor are they totally different. They represent a pair of genes which are related to each other. They have arisen from the same source,but due to mutation one gene has become slightly different from the other. Since they are basically same, they occupy the same locus on the choromosome and control the-same character. In the case of pea plant, red flower colour is supposed to be the original colour as it is dominant. This means that originally all pea plants used to produce only red flowers and subsequently the red gene mutated and the mutated form became the white gene. The genes for white and red flower colour are variants of the same gene, that is why they can control the variants of a single character. Such genes are said to be alleles. Alleles maybe defined as alternative state of existence of the same gene occupying same loci on homologous chromosomes. According to Mendel, a character can exist only in two states -dominant and recessive and hence for every character or every gene there are only two alleles (allelomorphs).

All Mendelian characters have only two alternate expressions or have only two alleles. But this may not be true (having only two alleles) in all cases, for a gene, once having undergone mutation, may mutate again to give one more altered form or allele and in their case, there will be three alleles. Theoritically a gene 'a' may mutate any number of times leading to the formation of many variants or multiple alleles. A multiple allelic series of a gene represents a series of gene mutations in the same locus leading to a variety of phenotypic expressions seggregated in different organisms. Multiple alleles may be defined as a series of gene mutations from wild to a number of mutated forms all of them affecting the same trait. Dawson and Whitehouse have used the term *panalleles* to denote multiple alleles. Multiple alleles should not be mistaken with multiple factors where non allelic genes present in different loci affect a trait; further many pairs of genes are involved in each individual to delimit a character. In multiple alleles, the genes occupy the same locus on the chromosome in different organisms producing variants of a trait due to sequential mutations. In multiple alleles only one pair of genes is involved in each individual to delimit a character. Multiple alleles are different from the diallelic series of Mendel in that the former produce many variants, while the latter produce only two variants.

Salient features of Multiple alleles.

1. They occupy the same gene locus on the chromosome
2. In diploid organisms, as there are only two homologous chromosomes, there will be only two allelic states of the multiple series.
3. In haploid gametes multiple allelic series is represented by a single allelic state.
4. No crossing over is known to occur between multiple alleles as they occupy the same level of the homologous chromosomes. In a cross between two alleles, the F_2 generation reveals the same combination of alleles.
5. A single multiple allelic series affects only one trait - eye colour, shape, skin colour etc.,
6. Suppose there is a series of five genes in the multiple allelic series- starting with the wild A, A^b, A^c, A^d, A^e, etc., the last one representing the last mutation (A^e) on the gene series, the wild gene (A) is dominant over all others and the last mutation (A^e) is recessive to all others. In the series starting with A, all genes are recessive to their previous allele while dominant over the subsequent allele (A^b, A^c, A^d, A^e).

The fact that A is wild can be proved because it is dominant over all others and the fact that A^c is the last mutant can be proved by its being recessive to all others.

In a cross between two representatives of the allelic series, that which is dominant is old and that which is recessive is recent (from the point of view of mutation)

Gene Symbols for Multiple Alleles

The wild gene is described first and is given the symbol of a capital letter (A,B,C etc) the next in the series has the same capital letter but is superscribed on top with a suitable small letter. This small letter is the identifying mark for the allele. The series of alleles have the same capital letter but with different small letters on top. We shall study some examples of multiple allelic series both in plants and animals. The following traits have been proved to be multiple alleles in different organisms-

1. Coat colour in Rabbits
2. Eye colour in Drosophila
3. Sexual incompatibility in *Nicotiana*
4. Blood groups in Man

Coat colour in rabbits

In rabbits a series of skin colours are seen. These are -

Full Colour : (Wild) The skin colour of the ordinary rabbit is refered to as full colour with banded strips of yellow and grey with a brown or black tip.

Chinchilla : In certain rabbits the skin lacks the yellow pigment only the mixture of black and grey giving a silvery appearance.

Himalayan albino : These rabbits have pink eyes and their fur is white except for the tips of feet, tail, nose, ear etc which are either dark or brown. Such a type of pigmentation only at the extremities is known as acromelanism (Serra 1965)

Albino : In these rabbits there is total absence of pigmentation. The eyes however are pink in colour.

The above series of skin colour is known to represent a multiple allelic series as revealed by crosses.

An albino crossed to a wild (full colour) rabbit produces in the F_1 all wild rabbits. Self breeding the F_1 results in 3/4 wild and 1/4 albino in the F_2 generations indicating the colour gene and the albino genes are alleles. When the Himalayan albinos are crossed with wild ones, the F_1 shows all wild, but in the F_2 generation 3/4 wild and 1/4 Himalayan albinos are produced indicating again that colour gene and Himalayan albino genes are alleles. The most interesting cross now would be a cross between albino and Himalayan albino. If albino and Himalayan

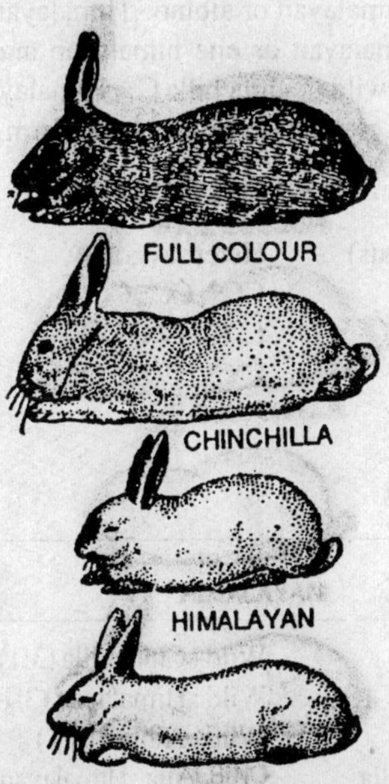

Fig. 13.1 Multiple Alleles
Coat colour in rabbits

are due to two different genes there must be a dominant allele in each of the two resulting in the appearence of full colour in the F_1 progeny. In a cross between Himalayan and albino, the F_1 are all Himalayan and the F_2 has Himalayan and albino in the ratio of 3:1. Reversion to full colour does not occur. This is due to the fact that a gamete never carries Himalayan and albino genes together. It has only one of the genes, similarly coloured animal in the heterozygous condition will carry either Himalayan or albino but never both. This clearly reveals that the Himalayan gene, colour gene and the albino gene are located on the same locus on the homologous chromosome (any two in the any one only in the gamete); that is why they do not seggregate. It is obvious then that these are allelic representing the variants of the same gene. Himalayan and albino are allelic to eath other and both are allelic to full colour. Full colour is dominant over both Himalayan and albino, while Himalayan is recessive to full colour and dominant over albino. Albino is recessive to both Himalayan and full colour. The other variant of skin colour, Chinchilla is less intense in colour. It is dominant to all others except to full colour. The genes for all these represent a multiple allelic series starting with the wild and ending up with albino. The series will be as follows in the order of decreasing dominance.

Wild -Chinchilla -Himalayan Albino -Albino.

These represent a series of mutations occuring in the same locus starting with wild gene. Genotypically each one could be either totally homozygous or heterozygous except for albino. In albino, since the allele is completely recessive it has to be homozygous to produce the trait. In other cases each dominant allele can have the recessive alleles. For eg. wild type may have in addition to a dominant allele an allele either of chinchilla, Himalayan albino or albino. Three types of heterozygous genotypes are possible for the wild type. Chinchilla may have both dominant alleles of its own in the homozygous condition one of its dominant allele and the other either Himalayan or albino. Himalayan will have two genotypes; both alleles of Himalayan or one himalayan and one albino. The genes for various colours are - wild C, chinchilla C^{ch}, Himalayan C^{h} and albino C^{a}. The .various genotypes are given below in a tabular form.

Phenotype of the organism	Genotype (Homozygous)	Genotype Heterozygous)
Wild (full colour)	CC	CC^{ch}, CC^{h}, CC^{a}
Chinchilla	$C^{ch}C^{ch}$	$C^{Ch}C^{h}$,$C^{ch}C^{a}$
Himalayan albino	$C^{h}C^{h}$	$C^{h}C^{a}$
Albino		

Results of Cross between various colours

	F_1	F_2
1. Wild x Chinchilla	Wild	Wild : Chinchilla (3:1)
2. Wild x Himalayan	Wild	Wild : Himalayan (3:1)
3. Wild x Albino	Wild	Wild : Albino (3:1)
4. Chinchilla x Himalayan	Chinchilla	Chinchilla : Himalayan (3:1)
5. Chinchilla x Albino	Chinchilla	Chinchilla : Albino (3:1)
6. Himalayan x Albino	Himalayan	Himalayan : Albino
7. Albino x Albino	Albino	All Albino

Albinism in other Organisms

Allelic series of genes bringing about albinism have been found in many other animals like mouse, rat,guinea pig, cat- etc., In the domesticated cat one of the alleles in the albino series gives a colour called Siamese colour favoured by many. In human beings also an allele of albinism is there leading to loss of pigmentation in skin and hair. Albinos have all recessive alleles of the lowest order in the series and can exist only in the homozygous condition, sequential mutation from C to C^{a} has occurred in almost all mammals. But this trait has not been encountered quite frequently in the wild state as they can not compete with the normal ones. They survive only in the domesticated state.

Eye colour in Drosophila : T.H.Morgan (1909) a geneticist, discovered a mutant white eyed fly among a population of red eyed flies of *Drosophila melanogaster*. This colour originated as a mutant in the X chromosome. Subsequently several mutations have been identified in the same locus all affecting the eye colour. To date, between the wild red eye and the mutant white eye about 10 variants have been reported. These are sequential mutations, with the individual gene becoming more and more recessive with every mutation. The table below gives these series of mutations in the decreasing order of dominance.

Colour of eye	Gene symbol	Colour eye	Gene symbol
Red R	R	Honey	R^h
Coral	R^{co}	Buff	R^b
Blood	R^{bl}	Tinged	R^+
Eosin	R^{eo}	Pearl	R^p
Cherry	R^{ch}	Ivory	R^i
Apricot	R^a	White	r

The wild allele (R) is dominant over all others and the mutant of the lowest order (r) is recessive to all others.

Wing size in Drosophila : This is another multiple allelic trait in *Drosophila.* The normal wings are long in *Drosophila.* But there are two more variations at this, in the form of vestigial wing and antlered wing. These two traits arise as a result of mutation in the same locus. Having arisen in the same locus, the vestigial wing and antlered wing are alleles of each *other* and also of the normal long wing. These three form a series in the order of decreasing dominance. Normal → Vestige → antlered. These three may be represented as follows - Genetically wild gene is represented as + +, and the others by the letters representing that particular mutation.

Normal wing	+/+,	+/vg,	$+vg^a$
Vestigial wing	vg/vg,	vg/vg^a	(Intermediate)
Antlered wing	vg^a/vg^a		

Results of Cross between various colours

	F_1	F_2
1. Normal x vestigial	Normal	Normal : vestigial (3:1)
2. Normal x Antlered	Normal	Normal : antlered (3:1)
3. Vestigial x Antlered	Intermediate,	Vestigial : Intermediate : Antlered (1:2:1)

The last (3rd) cross mentioned above needs some clarification. While normal wing is dominant over both vestigial and antlered, the two mutant alleles do not show dominance or recessiveness between them, with the result a cross between them results in an intermediate wing (vg/vg^a) in the F_1. Interbreeding of the F_1

produces in the F_2 vestige, intermediate and antlered in the ratio of 1:2:1. When two alleles interact without showing dominance or recessiveness they are called *allelic compound*

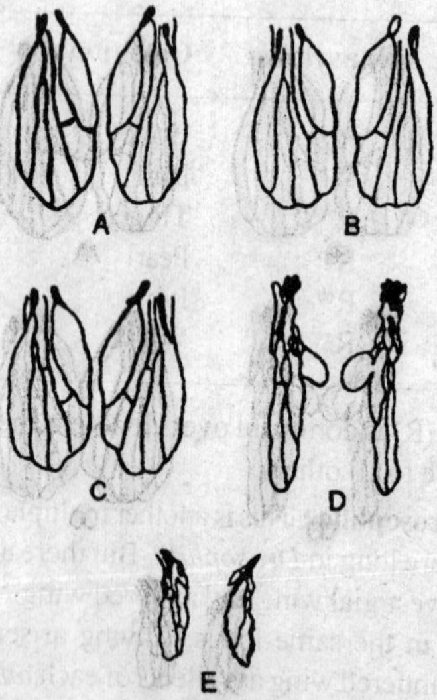

Fig. 13.2 Multiple Alleles
Types of wings in Drosophila, **A-B.** Normal, **C.** Intermediate, **D.** Antlered, **E.** Vestigial

In this instance the intermediate wing is a compound

Sexual Incompatibility in Nicotiana : In bisexual flowers, self pollination is more likely than cross pollination as both male and female gametes are in the vicinity. But in many instances, even though the gametes (male and female) produced by"the plants are both functional, fertilization failsi to take place either due to failure of pollen to germinate on the stigma or the pollen tube growth is extremely slow. Such a condition where the gametes of the same flower fail to fuse is known as self incompatibility or self sterility.

Nicotiana, a member of the family Solanaceae is a typical example of self incompatibility.

Two types of self incompatibility have been noticed in flowering plants. These are Gametophytic self incompatibility (GSI) and Sporophytic self incompatibility (SSI). GSI has been reported in families like Liliaceae, Gramineae, Solanaceae etc., while SSI is found in families Cruciferae, Cempositae etc.,

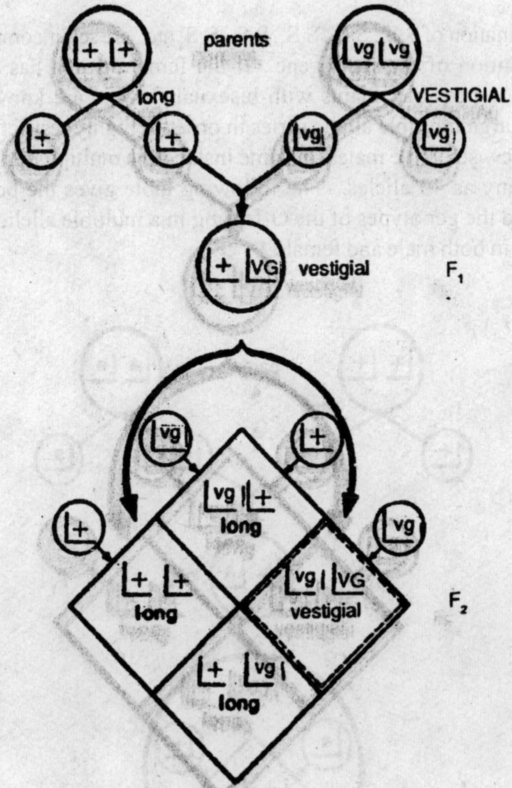

Fig. 13.3 Multiple Alleles
Cross between normal (long) winged and vestigial winged Drosophila

East observed that multiple alleles are responsible for self incomptibility. He and Manglesdorf (1925) explained the genetic basis of self incompatiblity. According to them the wild gene for self incompatibility can be designated as S gene, which has undergone a series of mutations producing the allelic series S_1, S_2, S_3, S_4, S_5 etc., In GSI suppose a plant is of the S_1S_2 genotype its pollen will have either S_1 or S_2 gene. Hence it would not germinate on a pistil with S_1 or S_2 beceause similarity of genes would bring about incompatibility. Fertilization would take place if the pollen grain carrying either S_1 or S_2 gene falls on SD_3 S_4 pistil. In the cases of SSI the pollen should not carry even a single gene that is similar to the female parent. If the male parent has the Genotype S_1S_2, the pollen carrying this can only pollinate a stigma where both S_1S_2 should be absent. For eg., a combination of S_1S_2, S_1S_3. S_2S_3, S_1S_4, S_2S_4 etc., are self incompaticle because of the repetition of the same gene. If the female parent has S_3S_4, S_3S_5 etc. pollination is possible. Plants with bisexual flowers are known to have an extremely large multiple allelic series in order to highly restrict mating and to have very few selective mates. In some instances a multiple series is known to have as many as 40 alleles. The following table gives the possible mating chances and the genotypes of the Offspring in a multiple allelic series having S_1S_2 and S_3 in both male and female.

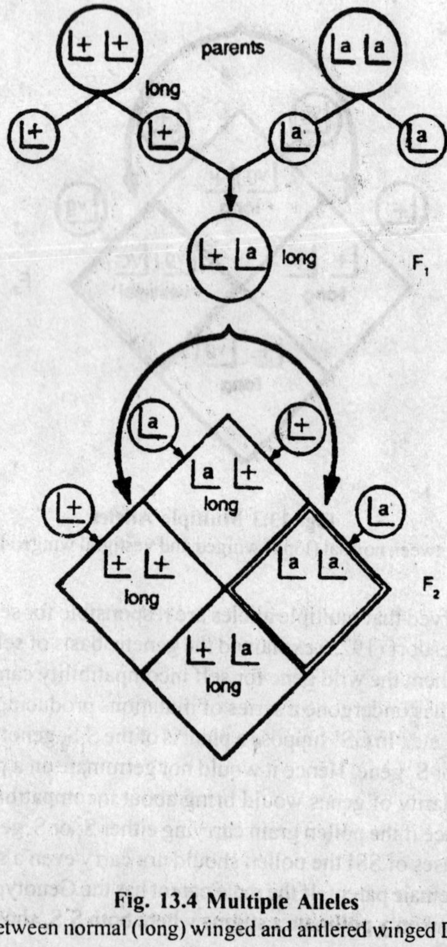

Fig. 13.4 Multiple Alleles
Cross between normal (long) winged and antlered winged Drosophila

Table showing successful mating of genotypes in self incompatible plants

Female / Male	S_1S_2	S_1S_2	S_2S_3
S_1S_2	–	S_2S_3	S_1S_2, S_2S_3 S1S3
S_1S_3	S_2S_3	–	S_1S_2 S_1S_3, S_2S_3
S_2S_3	S_1S_3	S_1S $2S_2S_3$, S_1S_3	–

Multiple allelism in maize (Mosaic dominance)

In some organisms as in maize, the multiple allelic series may influence different combinations of traits in different parts of the body. Stadler who worked on a multiple series of gene (R) affecting the purple colouration of the plant in seed as well as in the stem and leaves found that an allele may affect various parts variously. For eg., if a particular allele produces colour in the seed, it may or may not produce colour in the stem or leaves. The following four combinations of phenotypic traits have been shown by Stadler –

1. R^R Purple seed, purple plant
2. r^r White seed, Purple plant
3. R_g Purple seed, green plant
4. r^g white seed, green plant

In this instance the gene R" acts as though it is a compound gene having two parts -R controlling the seed colour and r controlling the plant colour. When mutation occurs it may occur in only one component resulting in the change of the components of the compound gene. As a result, the two components of the gene may cause various combination of traits like purple seed-green plant, white seed-purple plant etc.. Here the purple seed colour and purple plant are dominant over white seed and green plant. As a result of the mutational change there may be mixture of dominant and recesive characters in a plant (controlled by the same allele). This is called mosaic dominance. There may be a question as to why these two components of a gene should not be regarded as seperate genes, if they can undergo mutation separately. However since these two are located so close they cannot be separated by cross over hence they have to be regarded as components of the same gene. Stadler further noticed in maize that the R' gene in various strains distributes the pigment in various ways. These may be possible due to sub alleles. which may be defined as variations of the components of a compound gene.

Blood Groups in Man

Blood can be transfused from one individual to the other in case of emergency. Blood transfusions were tried as early as 18th century in England and France. But some cases were successful and in some instances the receipient died soon after transfusion. On testing it was noticed that the blood had coagulated or clumped. However this did not happen in all instances. In some instances the blood of two individuals mixed smoothly. It was Karl Landsteiner who in 1900 found the reason behind clumping or smooth mixing. He noticed that the plasma and red blood cells (RBC) of a person when recombined after separation mixed smoothly so also blood from some persons. But in certain other instances the plasma and the RBC did not mix, the RBC clumped. Landsteiner worked in detail on this and came to the conclusion that the mixing or clumping depends on the antigen and antibody reaction present in the blood. He discovered that there are two antigens in the blood. A and B and two serum antibodies that clump or agglutinate them. Correspondingly the blood of all human beings could be classified into four types based on the antigen present in the RBC.

These are

1. Antigen A – Blood group A
2. Antigen B – Blood group B
3. Both Antigen A and B – Blood group AB
4. No Antigen – Blood group O

Before we proceed on further discussion we will try to understand what is meant by antigen - antibody reaction.

[Blood is a connective tissue in fluid form. It has two main parts - cells and plasma. The cells are RBC, WBC, and platelets.The plasma consists of protein, fibrinogen and the serum.

When the serum is injected into the blood stream of another organism, a substance is produced in the blood which reacts with the serum protein and neutralizes it. The substance produced by the blood cell is known as antibody and the protein in the serum which causes the production of antibody is called antigen. Antibody is also-called *Agglutinin* (because it agglutinates) and antigen is also called *Agglutinogen* (because it causes agglutination). The reaction between antibody and antigen is very specific and is often compared to the lock and key mechanism.

Landsteiner discovered A,B and O blood groups. His students Von Decastello and Sturii discovered the AB groups. Besides these, scientific investigations have also proved the existence of two other blood groups -Viz MN blood groups andRh factor. In this chapter we will discuss the A,B,OMood groups and the Rh factors. 'MN blood groups have already been discussed in the Chapter on Mendelism. It (MN) is controlled by a single gene)

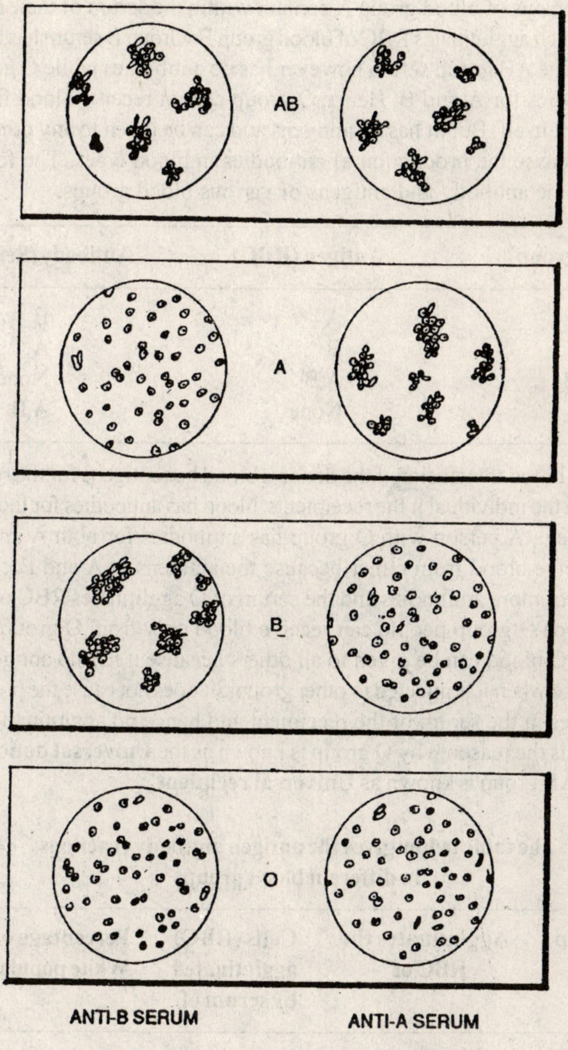

Fig. 13.5 Multiple Alleles
Appearance of erythrocytes in four blood groups (A, B, AB and O) when tested with anti B serum (from A left) and anti A serum (from right)

A, B, AB and O groups : In these blood groups, some of them contain natural antibodies against certain others. It has been pointed out already, there are two antigens **(agglutinogen)** A and B and there are two antibodies **(agglitinin)**

A and B. Persons of blood group A contain within the serum of their blood an antibody which agglutinates RBC of blood group B. Group B serum has antibody against A. The AB group serum however has no antibodies while O group has both antibodies for A and B. Hence O group cannot receive blood from any group except itself. But .it has no antigens and can be given to any other group it does not cause the production of antibodies in blood types. The following table gives the antibody and antigens of various blood groups.

Blood group	Antigen (RBC)	Antibody (Serum)
A	A	B
B	B	A
AB	A,B	None
O	None	A,B

During blood transfusion if the donor's blood has antigens for the recipient, it will. harm the individual it the receipients blood has antibodies for the donor's blood. For eg., A person with O group has antibodies for both A and B and cannot receive blood from either because the antigens in A and B cause the production of more antibodies and the serum of O agglitinates RBC of both A and B. Hence O group people can receive blood only from O group. On the other hand O blood can be given to all others because it has no antigen for A and B. Hence when it is injected to other groups, it does not cause the production of antibodies in the serum of the receipient and hence no agglutination takes place. This is the reason why O group is known as the **Universal donor**. In the same way AB group is known as **Universal recipient**.

The table below gives the antigen antibody reactions in different blood groups

Blood group	Agglutinates the RBC of	Cells (RBC) agglutinated by serum of	Percentage of White population
A	B, AB	O,B	3.7
B	A, AB	O,A	13.4
AB	None	O,A,B	5.7
O	A,B,AB	None	37.3

Genetic basis of A,B,O Blood groups

It is believed by many that O is the original gene, and two dominant mutations from this have given rise to A and B blood groups. The blood groups are determined by a series of three allelic genes viz., I^A, I^B and i (Bernstein 1925). The genotypes of different blood groups are given in the following table.

Blood group	Genotype Homozygous	Genotype Heterozygous
A	I^AI^A	I^Ai
B	I^BI^B	I^Bi
AB	–	I^AI^B
O	ii	–

In the above table, alleles I^A and I^B are dominant over i allele. But when they are together, they behave as an intermediate or compound producing the AB blood group. This is an example of codominance where both the genes have equal expression. It will be interesting to observe the possible genotypes of offspring and their phenotype (blood group). When marriage occurs between people belonging to different blood groups. The following table gives the genotypes and phenotypes of parents and ofspring in different combinations.

Genotypes of Parents	Blood groups of Parents	Blood groups of Offspring	Genotype of Offspring
1. I^AI^A x I^AI^A	A x A	A	I^AI^A
2. I^AI^A x I^A i	A x A	A	I^AI^A, I^Ai
3. I^Ai x I^Ai	A x A	A, O	I^Ai, ii
4. I^BI^B x I^BI^B	B x B	B	I^BI^B
5. I^BI^B x I^Bi	B x B	B	I^BI^B, I^Bi
6. I^B x I^Bi	B x B	B, O	I^BI^B, ii
7. I^AI^B x I^AI^A	AB x AB	A, AB, B	I^AI^A,I^BI^B,I^AI^B
8. I^AI^B x I^AI^A	AB x A	A, AB	I^AI^A, I^AI^B
9. I^AI^B x I^Ai	AB x A	A, B AB	I^AI^A, I^AI^B, I^Ai, I^Bi
10. I^AI^B x ii	AB x O	A, B	I^Ai, I^Bi
11. I^AI^B x I^BI^B	AB x B	A, B	I^Ai, I^Bi
12. I^AI^B x I^Bi	AB x B	AB, B	I^AI^B, I^BI^B
13. I^AI^A x I^BI^B	A x B	AB	I^AI^B
14. I^AI^A x I^Bi	A x B	AB, A	I^AI^B,I^Ai
15. I^A x I^BIB	A x B	AB, B	I^AI^B, I^Bi
16. I^Ai x I^Bi	A x B	AB, A, O	I^AI^B, I^Ai, ii
17. I^AI^A x ii	A x O	A	I^Ai
18. I^Ai x ii	A x O	A, O	I^Ai, ii
19. ii x I^BI^B	O x B	B	I^Bi
20. ii x I^Bi	O x B	B, O	I^Bi, ii

Sub divisions of A, AB and B

The A group RBCs are divided into two sub groups namely A_1 and A_2. The latter is not very common and is found in about 20% of the group. There is no agglutination reaction between A_1 RBC and A_2 serum and *vice versa.* But both A_1 and A_2 are agglutinated by B and O serum. The B group has two types of antibodies. The A_1 antibody agglutinates both A_1 and A_2 corpuscles and the other A_2 stongly agglutinates only A_1, but agglutination against A_2 is very weak. Similarly the AB group is also known to have two to four sub groups, A B, A_2 B, A_3B, A_4B etc.,

Blood group inheritance and parentage : In cases of disputed parentage when blood groups of parents and children are known it can be easily decided (see table) whether a given child is born to particular parents or not. When the parent's blood groups are known, their genotype can be worked out and the child's genotype and blood group can be blood group of mother, child and the unlikely blood group.of father ie., if the blood group of mother and child is of a particular type, the disputed father cannot have the genotype given in the table in that he is not the father. It should be noted however that in instances when both the babies and families are of the same group it will not be possible to decide (if the disputed father also has the matching blood group) parentage on the basis of blood group.

Blood Group of Child	Blood Group of Mother	Blood Group of unlikely Father
O	O	AB
O	A	AB
O	B	AB
A	O	O, B
A	B	O, B
B	O	O, A
B	O	O, A
AB	A	O, A
AB	B	O, B
AB	AB	O

Rh factor

Landsteiner and Wiener (1940) discovered one more type of antigen (agglutinogen) in the RBC's ..of human beings. It is named after the Rhesus Monkey *(Macaca rhesus)* and called the Rh factor or Rh antigen. It is present in about 95% of Indians (about 85% of whites also have it). However the serum does not have the corresponding antibody in the human beings. When blood of rhesus monkey is injected into the rabbit, the rabbit produces antibodies against it. When this antiserum (serum with antibody) is tested against human blood, agglutination takes place in about cases. In about 15% no agglutination takes place. Persons whose blod agglutinates with Rh serum of monkey are called Rh positive and where no agglutination takes place they are called Rh negative. Six groups of Rh factors have been identified in human beings C , c, D , d, E and e. Out of these D and d are commonest. D is a Mendelian gene hence is dominant over d. Almost all human beings (85%) who are Rh positive belong to D group while Rh negative people belong to d group.

The importance of Rh factors can be ascertained from the following examples.

A. Assume that a Rh negative individual gets a blood transfusion from a Rh positive individual. At the first instance nothing will happen as there are no natural antibodies in the serum of Rh negative individual. But the presence of Rh blood will induce antibody production. Nothing will happen however as there are no sufficient antibodies. Should the same Rh negative individual require another transfusion from Rh positive blood the donor blood will show agglutination due to the antibodies already present. This may be harmful to the recipient.

B. A Rh negative woman marries a Rh positive man. The child of this couple obviously belongs to Rh positive as the gene D is dominant over d. In the first pregnancy however the child is not harmed eventhough the maternal blood and the child's blood mix. Once again the mother's Rh negative blood will not produce enough antibodies to haemolyse the child's blood. But with each succeding conception the antibodies in the mother's blood accumulate, sometimes the third or even the second child itself may have its blood (Rh positive) haemolysed leading to erythroblasts from the bone marrow enter the blood (to compensate for the haemolysed RBC) This condition is called *Erythroblastosis foetalis.* Such a baby is generally still born or even when born highly anaemic. It can be saved with total transfusion of Rh negative blood.

Pseudoalleles

The alleles are so called because they occupy the same locus virtually permitting no cross over. But in some instances different genes may be so closely linked that there is no cross over even though they are not alleles. such genes which are basically different but because of occupying almost the same locus behave as alleles are called pseudoalleles. (Lewis 1951) There is some, controversy regarding the exact identity of the pseudoallele. While Lewis (1955) and Green (1963) regard pseudoalleles as two different genes with their own function, Pontecorvo (1958) believes them to be different functional sites within a same gene. The functional part is called cistron, while the recombinant part is called the recon.

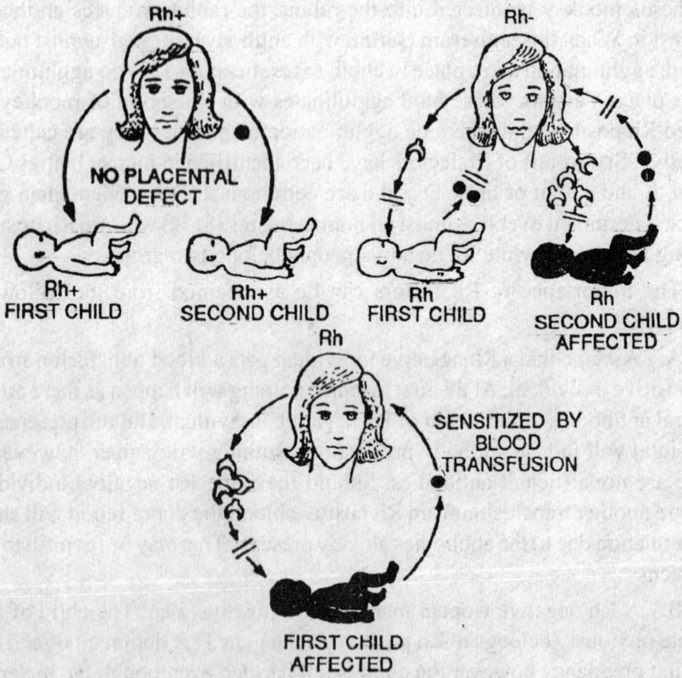

Fig. 13.6 Multiple Alleles

Pseudoallelism has been observed in the sex linked genes for eye colour in *Drosophila.* The eye colour varies from white to red with a range of eye colours between. All these allies are located,at about 1.5 on the X-chromosome map. Lewis (1951) in one.ot his experiments reported in a cross between apricot and white eye.the F_1 had intermediat eye. In the F_2 instead of the white and apricot seggregating he found the wild type also, showing the two genes are actually non allelic. But if they are non allelic they should be two different genes. But apricot and white are known to be allelic as seen by other experiments, but they behave as non allelic. Lewis called such genes as pseudoalleles.

Significance of allelism

The study of allelism is significant in that it proves that a gene can mutate several times, that a gene can suppress other genes to different degrees and a gene can be a compound gene with its sub units mutating in diverse directions.

14

LINKAGE AND CROSSING OVER

Mendel, while enunciating ,his law of independent assortment, ascertained that two or more elements, that constitute a hybrid, undergo independent seggregation without being influenced by the other. Mendel's principles of independent assortment apply not only to genes but to chromosomes as well, so that paternal and maternal hromosomes are seggregated to separate gametes during meiosis. It is for this reason that genes carried on different chromosomes undergo complete seggregation. Fortunately for Mendel, all the seven charcters that he chose for study were on different chromosomes (there are seven pairs of chromosomes in pea plants).

There are hundreds of characters in organisms and if there is a gene for every character as Mendel visualised (which is a fact also) there must be hundreds and indeed thousands of genes, and if genes are situated on the chromosomes there must be hundreds or thousands of chromosomes. But this is not so; while there could be thousands of genes, the number of chromosomes in most of the individuals hardly exceeds hundred, in fact it is much less. In *Drosophila*, where hundreds of characters have been studied there are only four pairs of chromosomes. In human beings with thousands of characters, there are only 23 pairs of chromosomes. If genes are situated on the chromosomes, it means then several genes responsible for so many characters must be situated on a single chromosome. When this is so, genes or characters on a single chromosome cannot segregate. They cannot be assorted independently instead they tend to be inherited together.

It was Sutton (1903) who first pointed out the anomalous situation in beleiving total independent assortment for all the characters, when the number of chromosomes are far less than the number of genes. For eg: if we identify two genes located on a chromosome and perform a dihybrid cross, the chances are the two genes will tend to go together, instead of being assorted independently. The two traits controlled by these will appear together in an individual, instead of seggregating to two individuals. In a dihybrid cross of this type, Mendel's

9:3:3:1 ratio will be modified. This phenomenon of genes (present on a single chromosome) showing the tendency to be inherited together is called linkage. However until Morgan's work in 1910, Genetics did not have a satisfactory explanation for the tendency of the genes to assort together in the offspring. We shall consider some of the hypotheses concerning the above mentioned behaviour of genes.

Sutton's view : As has been pointed out already, Sutton (1903) opined that several genes are present on the chromosome and they tend to be inherited together. However he did not visualise the concept of linkage. Instead he said that there are groups of genes, and these groups in an individual correspond to the number of chromosomes. Sutton did not experimentally confirm his views.

Coupling and repulsion hypothesis : This hypothesis was put forward by Bateson and Punnett (1906), who observed in a variety of sweet pea the 'violation' of the law of independent assortment. The experiment involved flower colour (purple/red) and pollen shape (long/round). When two varieties of sweet pea were crossed-one purple and long and the other red and round, the F_1 plant was purple and long. On selfing, the F_2 progeny should have exhibited the 9:3:3:1 ratio. But this did not happen so. Instead the purple long and red round plants appeared in large numbers ie., more frequently than what was expected in a dihybrid cross assuming independent assortment. These are the parental combinations ie., characters present together in one individual. The new combinations ie., purple round and red long did appear in the F_2 but in a lesser frequency. Here parental combinations are more than new combinations or recombinations. The following example illustrates this phenomenon.

Purple long X Red round
PPLL ppll
↓ ↓
PL → Pp Ll ← pl (Purple long) F_1 hybrid
selfing

F_2 Progeny	Purple long	Purple round	Red long	Red round
Expected	1199	400	400	133
Observed	1528	106	117	381

Data from K.B. Ahluwalia, Genetics, 1985

The experiment was repeated by Bateson and Punnett in a different way. This time they selected a new combination of characters in the parents. The parents were Purple round and Red long. the F_1 showed the dominant purple long characters. In the F_2. generation again parentalcharacters (Purple round and Red long) were more than the recombined characters (Purple long and Red round). This experiment also showed the tendency of the parental genes to remain together instead of seggregating.

Test Cross : Bateson and Punnet also performed a double cross. They crossed the F_1 dihybrid - Purple long (PpLI) with the double recessive parent (red round - (rrll). In a Mendelian inheritence, the result would be 1:1:1:1 of Purple long, purple round, Red round and red long. But Bateson and Punnett obtained a ratio of 7:1:1:7 of Purple long, purple round, red long and red round respectively.

Bateson and Punnett explained this deviation as the phenomenon of coupling of the characters coming from a single parent to remain together. Similarly the tendency of the characters belonging to two different parents to remain seperate is called **repulsion.** The coupling and repulsion hypothesis of Bateson Punnett did not visualise the actual reason for the coupled genes to remain together.

Bateson pointed out an explanation to coupling and repulsion hypothesis as due to "differential multiplication of cells containing different combination of characters of genes". The combination of genes seggregate before gametes are formed. After seggregation and gamete formation one set of gametes multiply at a faster pace than the other. This takes part in fertilization in large numbers than the other kind of gamete, hence the modification in the ratio of a typical dihybrid cross.

Morgan's concept of Linkage : The explanation of Bateson for coupling and repulsion was not very satisfactory. It was T.H. Morgan (1910), who was working on *Drosophila* together with his associates A.H. Sturtevant, H.J. Muller and C.B. Bridges, offered a plausible reason for the phenomenon of coupling and repulsion. According to Morgan, coupling and repulsion are but two facets of the same phenomenon. He further stated that pairs of genes from homozygous parents tend to enter the same gamete, while the same genes from heterozygous parents tend to enter different gametes and remain apart. The tendency of the genes to retain their original combination is due to their location on the same chromosome. Another significant aspect of linkage underscored by Morgan was that the strength of linkage (tendency to go together) depends on the distance between the linked genes, on the chromosome. The closer the genes, the stronger will be the linkage, and the farther the genes, the weaker will be the linkage. Tendency to remain together will be more if the linkage is stronger and the tendency to seggregate more will be there if the linkage is weak. Morgan and Castle formulated the chromosome theory of linkage.

The main features of this theory are-

1. Genes showing linkage are on the same chromosome.
2. Genes are arranged on the chromosome in a linear fashion. Linkage of genes is also linear.
3. The distance between the genes determines the strength of the linkage. Strong linkage indicates proximity of the genes, while weak linkage indicates that they are farther apart.
4. Linked genes will remian together during inheritance.

Cytological studies have given the physical proof of linkage. Linkage of genes as observed by the inheritance of traits has helped cytologists to map the chromosomes (for details see later in the chapter).

Arrangement of the linked genes : In a heterozygous individual with two pairs of linked genes, the linkage can be of any one of the following types.

(a) The dominant alleles of both characters are on one chromosome and similarly, the recessive alleles are on another chromosome. For example if the gene paris are Aa and Bb, A and B are on one chromosome and a and b are on another chromosome (AB/ab). This arrangement is called *cis* arrangement and the heterozygous individual is said to be a cis heterozygote.

(b) This arrangement is *vice-versa* of the *cis* type. Here, of the two pairs of genes one chromosome has dominant allele of one and the recessive allele of the other (Ab); like wise the other chromosome has recessive allele of the fyst pair and the dominant allele of the second pair (aB). This arrangement (Ab/aB) is called the *trans* arrangement in which a chromosome has one dominant and one recessive allele. The heterozygotes are said to be *trans heterozygotes*. According to Singleton (1967), *cis* arrangement exhibits the coupling phase, while the *trans* arrangement denotes the repulsive phase.

We shall now study a few examples of linkage in plants and animals.

Linkage in Maize : The phenomenon of linkage can be easily demonstrated in maize, as recombination also can be seen and traits in the seeds can be easily observed. Each ear having hundreds of seeds makes the observation easy. Hutchison has demonstrated linkage in two varieties of maize. One had coloured and full seeds, while the other had colourless shrunken seeds. The gene for colour is *C* and *f* is dominant over the colourless condition *c*. Similarly the full seed *F* is dominant over shrunken condition. The genotypes of the parents which represent the pure line is *CCFF* and *ccff*. In a cross between the two, as expected the F_1 is coloured and full. The genotype is *CcFf*. The genotype however is written as *CF/cf* to indicate C & *F* and *c* & *f* are linked. The gene combinations are written in the manner in which they enter the zygote. If the genotype is- written as *CcFf,* it is indicative of independent assortment.

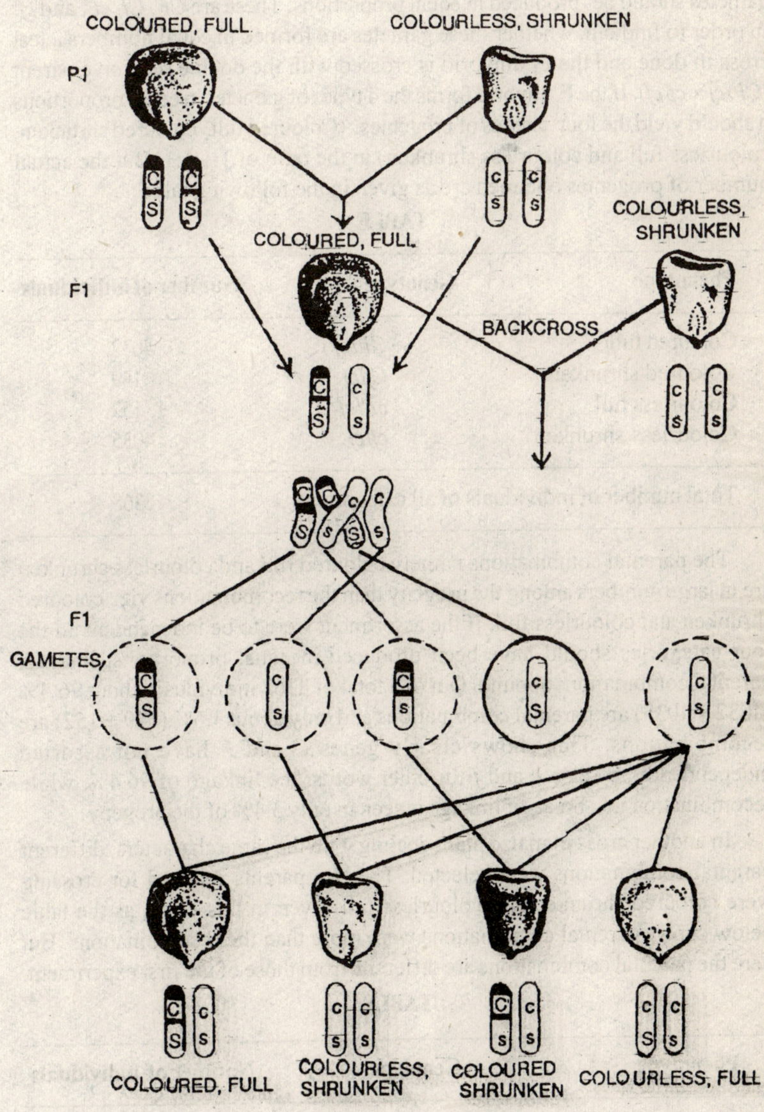

Fig. 14.1 Linkage and Crossing over

If the F_1 follows the Mendelian pattern of seggregation, four kinds of gametes should be -produced in equal proportions. These are *CF, Cf, cF,* and *cf.* In order to find out, whether these gametes are formed in equal numbers a test cross in done and the F_1 dihybrid is crossed with the double recessive parent *(CF/cf* x *cf/cf).* If the F_1 ihybrid forms the 4 types of gametes in equal proportions it should yield the four classes of progenies. (Coloured full, coloured shrunken, colourless full and colourless shrunken) in the ratio of 1:1:1:1. But the actual number of progenies obtained are as given in the following table.

TABLE

Phenotype	Genotype	Number of individuals
Coloured full	*CF/cf*	4032
Coloured shrunken	*Cf/cf*	149
Colourless full	*cF/cf*	152
Colourless shrunken	*cf/cf*	4035
Total number of individuals of all categories =		8368

The parental combinations namely coloured full and colourless shrunken are in large numbers among the progeny than the recombinations viz., coloured shrunken and colourless full. If the assortment were to be independent all the four categories should have been produced in equal proportions. Instead, parental combinations abound. Out of a total of 8368 individuals about 96.4% (4032 + 4035) are parental combinations and only about 3.6% (149 + 152) are recombinations. This shows clearly genes *C* and *F* have not assorted independently, so also *c* and *f.* In other words, the linkage of 96.4%, while recombination i.e., break of linkage is seen in only 3.4% of the progeny.

In another cross in maize plant dealing with the same characters, different parental combinations were selected. The two parents selected for crossing were coloured shrunken and colourless full. Even in this cross, as the table below shows parental combinations were more than the recombinations. But here the parental combinations are different from those of the first experiment.

TABLE

Phenotype	Genotype	Number of individuals
Coloured full	CF/cf	639
Coloured shrunken	Cf/cf	21379
Colourless full	cF/cf	21906
Colourless shrunken	cf/cf	672

Total number of progenies	=	44595
Parental combinations		97.06%
Recombinations		2.94%

(Tables adopted from Principles of Genetics, Sinnott Dunn and Dobzansky, 1958)

This experiment shows clearly, that whatever parental characters are there, they tend to be inherited together and not assorted independently. This example in maize, however is not an example of complete linkage, because at least in some instances recombinations are seen indicating the break in linkage. While it is true linkage is there in 96.4% and 97.06% cases in the above two experiments, it is also true that the genes have assorted independently in at least 3.6% and 2.94% cases. Thus the type of linkage seen in maize is called **Incomplete linkage.** In a complete linkage, parental combinations are retained in 100%, there are just no recombinations.

Linkage in Drosophila : Genes for body colour and wing shape are known to be linked in *Drosophila*. Morgan and his associate Bridges (1910) experimented with grey body and long winged fly. They were able to obtain by mutation another stock of fly which had black body and vestigial wings. These mutations were located on the same chromosome. The normal allele can be indicated by + and the recessive allele for body shape (*b*) and vestigial wing (*v*). When a pure line grey bodied long winged fly was crossed with another pure line black and vestige (++/++ X *bv/bv),* the offspring has grey body and long wing (+ +/*bv*). If Mendelian independent assortment takes place, the F_1 individual should produce gametes of all types in equal proportions. The four gametes are + +, +*v*, +*b*, and *bv*. When a F_1 female was crossed with a recessive male *(bv/bv),* four kinds of offspring are produced not in equal proportion but in the ratio given below. In the genotype of the offspring, the male contributes to each only the recessive genes *bv*, rest coming from the female *parent*.

1.	Grey wing	+/*bv*	41%
2.	Black vestigial	*bv*/*bv*	41%
3.	Grey vestigial	+*v*/*bv*	9%
4.	Black long	*b*+/*bv*	9%

In the above, 1 and 2 accounting for about 82% of the progeny are parental combinations, while 3 and 4 accounting for about 18% are recombinations. The strength of linkage is 82% and of cross over is 18%. In another experiment the two characters body colour and wing shape were taken in different combinations. A black long fly (b+/bv) was crossed with another grey vestigial (+*v*/*bv*). Among the four classes of progeny obtained, once again the parental combinations were more. In this experiment, the parental combinations are - black long and grey vestigial.

1. Grey vestigial $+v/bv$ 41%
2. Black long $b+/bv$ 41%
3. Grey long $++/bv$ 9%
4. Black vestigial bv/bv 9%

Again here parental combinations are 82% and recombinations are 18%. Morgan pointed out that the two genes *B* and + and *b* and *v* are linked to each other (*B* to + and *b* to *v*). This is because they ae situated on the same chromosome. In the case of *Drosophila* males, complete linkage between genes is observed as there is no cross over. Consequently the characters always appear together. When a grey long male is mated with black long double recessive female, the progeny has grey long and black vestigial.

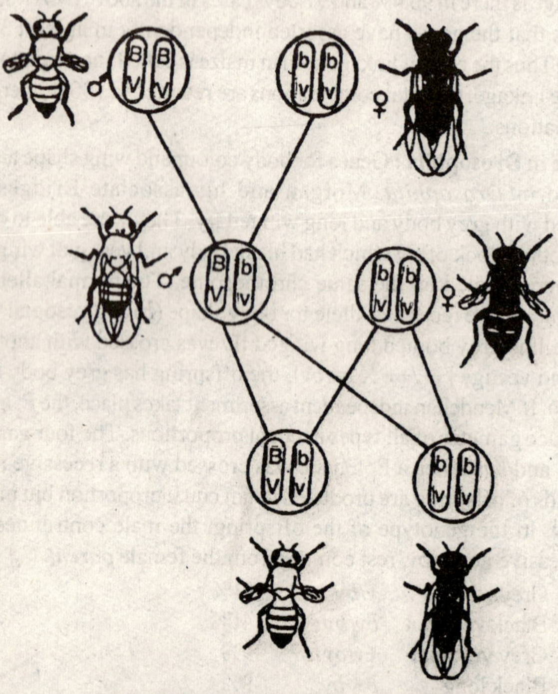

Fig. 14.2 Linkage and Crossing over
Cross in Drosophila showing complete linkage

Linkage in mammals : In several mammals linkage groups have been identified and they have been identified with their phenotypic traits. In rabbits out of 22 pairs of chromosomes, about six linkage groups have been identified. In guinea pig one linkage group has been found in human beings, but generally

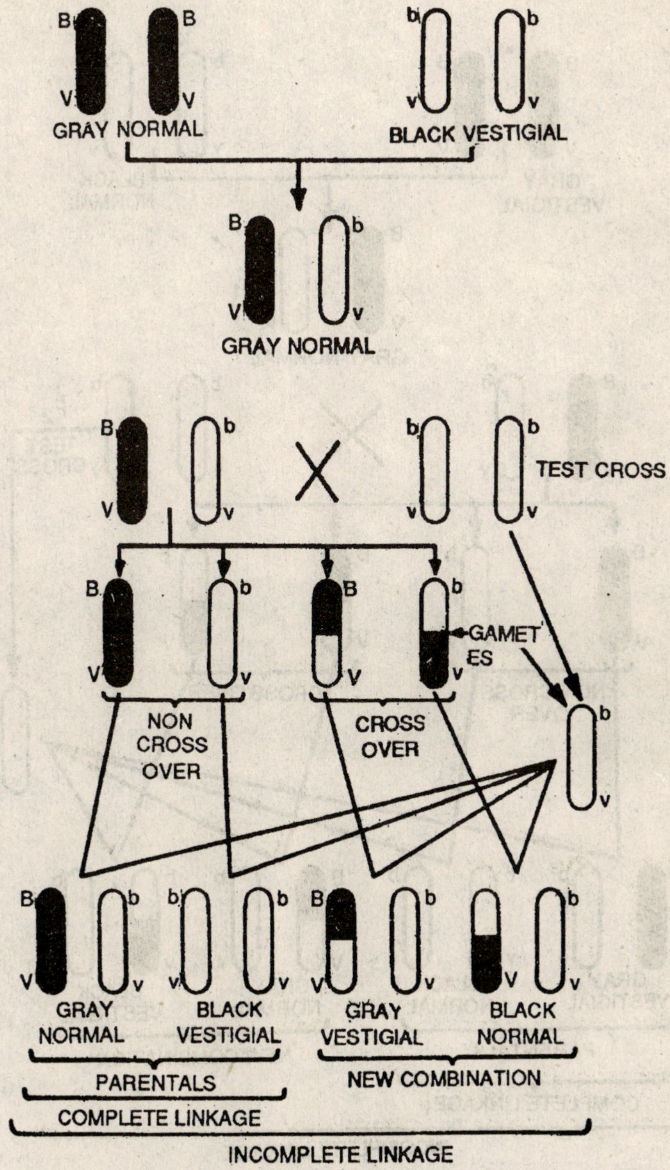

Fig. 14.3 Linkage and Crossing over
Linkage in Drosophila showing coupling

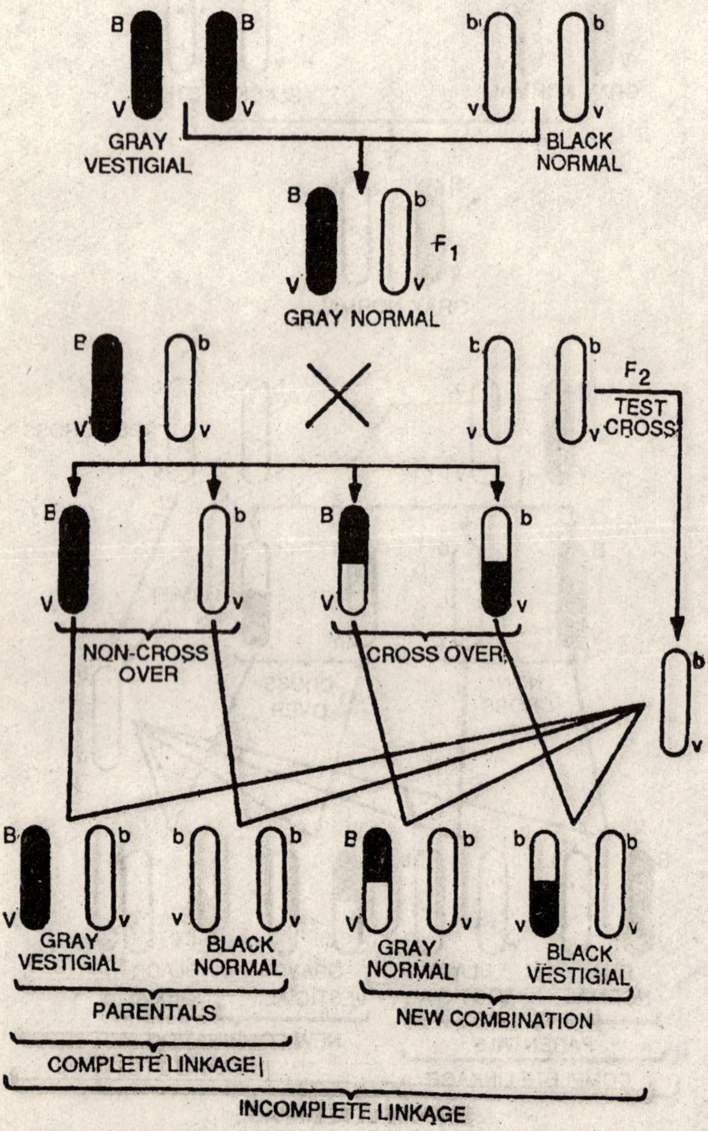

Fig. 14.4 Linkage and Crossing over
Linkage in Drosophila showing repulsion

it is difficult to study linkage or any genetic phenomenon in man as one cannot have the desired type of crosses or test crosses. Pedigree studies or family history studies will reveal some amount of information, where linked characters passed down together in several generations can be studied. Genes on sex chromosomes can be easily studied than those on the automosomes. Some amount of linkage has been seen between deutan colour blindness and haemophila as reported by Haldane. In a study of 34 individuals Haldane reported that the two genes have a recombination value of 11.4%. Similarly the gene for the absence of the enzyme G6PD (Glucose 6 Phosphate dehydrogenase) in RBC is known to have a cross over value of 6.5. The data about linked genes in human autosomes is very difficult to obtain. One study reports linkage between the gene for ABO blood group is linked with the gene for nail patella syndrome with 10% cross over value. The gene for Rh factor and the gene for ciliptocytosis are also known to linked with a recombination value of 30%. Similarly the gene for dufty blood antigen and the gene for dominant cataract of the eye are linked; so also the genes for hemoglobin B and hemoglobin S, but the cross over value for these genes is not known.

Linkage in Bacteria : In haploid organisms like bacteria, where there is no homologue, it is not possible to study linkage strength by means of cross over value. Geneticists however worked out a method by which the sequence of genes is established on the bacterial chromosome. This is assessed and calculated during bacterial reproduction, when certain genes are transfered from one cell to the other. This transfer is calculated against time, and reproduction or conjugation is stoped mid way. The genes that are transfered are then found out. The procedure is as follows. A male strain (Hfr) of *Escherichia coli* which has some marker genes is allowed to conjugate with the female strain (F.) which does not have these marker genes (genes whose phenotypic trait has not been established). The circular chromosome of male enters into the recipient cell. The conjugation is stopped at different time intervals - 5,10,15, minutes etc., The receipient cell is analysed as to its acquisition of new genes, by culturing it on various media. The gene acquired by the recipient strain after 5 minutes is located first, the second one after 10 minutes etc., In this way the distance and location of the genes can be calculated. Some of the genes transfered from Hfr to female against particular time interval are as follows. Conjugation in the first five minutes will result in transfer *oiarg* D gene, after 10 minutes *-pho* gene, after 16 minutes *gal* A gene and after 24 minutes *try* C gene are transfered from male to female.

Linkage groups : The total number of groups of the linked genes present in an individual constitute the linkage groups. Broadly speaking all genes located on a chromosome are linked to some or other degree. The strength of linkage varies. The closer they are, the chances are less of their seperation. The total linkage groups in an individual equals the number of chromosomes. If there are 7 chromosomes, there are 7 linkage groups. *Dorsophila* with four chromosomes has four linkage groups, Maize with 10 Chrosomes has 10 linkage groups etc. Sometimes in exceptional cases as in the *Gaudens* and *Valens* varities of *Oenothera* all chromosomes may form one single large linkage group. This however is a special situation brought about by translocation.

Classification of linkage : There are two types, complete and incomplete. In complete linkage, there is virtually no recombination. The same characters appear in unison for several generations. This type of linkage however is rare in nature and occurs due to absence of cross over. Male individuals of *Drosophila* and certain other insects show complete linkage. In incomplete linkage which is quite prevalent in biological world, the linked genes get seperated due to crossing over during meiosis. The extent of seperation of the linked genes depends upon the distance between the two genes.

In addition to this, interchromosomal linkage or false linkage as Longley (1945) calls it is brought about due to cytological irregularities like translocation.

Measurement of linkage : The easiest method to obtain linkage in terms of percentage value is to cross two individuals differing in two pairs of genes. The F_1 is back crossed to the double recesssive parent to obtian the parental and recombinations. The percentage of parental combinations in the total progeny gives the strength or percentage linkage between the two genes responsible for the characters.

A higher percentage of parental combinations indicates a strong linkage between the two genes and a higher percentage of recombination is indicative of weak linkage. The strength of linkage between any two pairs of genes is inversely proportional to the distance between them, lesser the distance stronger is the linkage and longer the distance, weaker is linkage.

Factors affecting the strength of linkage : There is no doubt that the distance between the two genes is the single most important factor governing the strength of the linkage. Besides this, there are several other physiological and environmental factors influencing the strength of linkage - these are

1. **Age of the organism :** Generally, increase in age decreases the chance of recombination thus strengthening the bonds of linkage. In *Drosophila melanogaster* the amount of recombination becomes smaller with increasing age.
2. **Temperature :** Initially increase in temperature increases the cross over value, hence it reduces the linkage.
3. **Radiation :** Organisms subject to ionising radiation show reduced linkage strength among the linked genes.

4. **Chemicals :** Chemicals and food consisting of various types of chemicals are also known to affect the strength of linkage.

Importance of linkage : Linked genes particularly of the desired trait play a great role in hybridization programme. As linkage helps to hold the parental characters together, selection of an individual for breeding program is based on the combination of characters which the breeder wants to remain together.

Another significance of linkage among genes in terms of evolution is that they tend to retain the identity and individuality of species by the clustering of characters.

Crossing over : It is an established fact that the genes are located on the chromosome and they (genes) tend to follow the inheritance of the chromosome on which they are situated. This means that the morphological traits whose genes are situated on a chromosome must always be inherited together. In other words in generation after generation, parental characters must repeat and the genetic composition of the chromosome must remain unaltered. But contarary to this expectation, it has been observed in almost all cases, linked genes do not always stay together even though they are on the same chromosome. This is particularly true in case of genes which are situated farther apart on a chromosome. The disruption of the linked genes has been traced to a phenomenon that generally occurs during meiotic cell division, where homologous chromosomes exchange the segments in a reciprocal fashion. This reciprocal exchange of parts of chromosomes between homologous chromosomes is called Crossing over (Morghan) and is primarily responsible for genetic variation between the individuals of the same species. It is as a result of crossing over that in the progeny, recombinations occur together with the parental combination of characters.

Crossing over may be defined as *'reciprocal exchange of segments between homologous chromosomes (generally occuring during meiosis, bringing the recombination of the linked genes particularly of those which are not very closely situated.*

There are two types of cross over depending on the type of cell where it occurs. The first type called **germinal or meiotic** cross over is of universal occurrence and is primarily responsible for variation among the individuals of a species. This type of cross over occurs, when the reproductive cells undergo meiosis during gametogenesis.

The second type of cross over which is of rare occurrence is the somatic or mitotic cross over taking place in the somatic cells during mitotic cell division. This is of no significance from the point of view of inheritance. Somatic crossing over has been observed *Drosophila* (Stern), *Aspergillus nidulans* (Pontecorvo) etc. After a somatic cross over, chromosomes will have unequal chromatids and in about 50% of the cases identical alleles go to the same pole. In the rest non identical alleles reach the same pole and if the genes involved are recessive, the cell (or its products) can be morphologically recognised.

Crossing over (meiotic) is of universal occurrence in all sexually reproducing organisms. The instances of incomplete linkage in *Drosophila* and maize also serve as illustrations of meiotic cross over.

Recombination in maize : As has already been pointed out under linkage, in a cross between coloured full and colourless shrunken a coloured full (heterozygoos) individual is produced. This F_1 hybrid when crossed with the double recessive parent the following progenies are produced.

1.	Coloured full	48.2%
2.	Colourless shrunken	48.2%
3.	Coloured shrunken	1.8%
4.	Colourless full	1.8%

Of the above 1 and 2 represent parental combinations while 3 and 4 represent recombination. The two recombinations have arisen as a result of exchange of gene loci for colour and shape between the homologous chromosomes. In this example 96% is linkage and 3.6 is cross over value. Similarly cross over value can be demonstrated in *Drosophila* also, when a grey vestigial fly is crossed with a Black long fly. (For details see linkage).

Meiotic cross over : In the meiotic cross over there are four steps. These are - a) Synapsis, b) Duplication of chromosomes c) Crossing over and d) Terminalization of chiasma.

(a) Synapsis : The homologous chromosomes present in the germinal cells come closer and pair longitudinally. This process called pairing or synapsis takes place during the zygotene of prophase 1. This is very important from the point of view of exchange of segments. The pairing is very specific and allelic loci in each homologue only undergo pairing. The paired chromosomes are called bivalents. Synapsis, which begins during zygotene continues up to pachytene, when chromosomes maintain physical contact at one or more points called chiasmata. Mutual attraction brought about by allelic gene loci is believed to be responsible for synapsis. The force of attraction is called the synaptic force. In order to account for the synaptic force Darlington has proposed a theory. The theory is known as the precocity theory.

Precocity theory : This theory proposed by Darlington C.D. (1937) assumes, that the chromosomes, to have an independent behaviour during division, must possess two chromatids. In other words they must replicate as it happens during mitosis. However, during early prophase the chromosomes do not replicate and they have only one chromatid which represents an unbalanced or unsaturated state. As a result, the chromosomes seek their partners and pair. During pachytene, when the chromosomes start exhibiting the double chromatids, their pairing need is satisfied and the chromosomes move apart. Darlington opines that synapsis is due to the precocious movement of the chromosomes.

Recent studies at the molecular level of the synaptic phenomenon have indeed supported the precocious movement theory of Darlington. The studies of Hotta, I to and Stern (1966) have indicated that, some amount of DNA (about 0.3%) is actually synthesised during zygotene and pachytene in the pollen mother cells of *Lilium.* The bulk of the DNA however is synthesized during premeiotic interphase. This shortage of DNA (0.3%) according lo Stern in responsible for pairing. The studies of Bogadnov *et al* (1968) is *Glyclus domesticalis* have also revealed a similar synthesis of DNA during meiotic division.

Synaptonemal complex : The appearence of a complex anastamaose of filamentous structures during the process of pairing has been reported in a number of organisms. This structure called synaptonemal complex is thought to function as a promoter of synapsis (For details see cell division).

(b) Duplication of chromosomes : The bivalents undergo duplication during pachytene. Each chromosome now consists of two chromatids (but the centromere will not divide); thus there will be four chromatids (tetrad).

(c) Crossing over : This takes place at the tetrad or the four strand stage. At the time of cross over the two opposing non sister chromatids (chromatids belonging to two different chromosomes), have a break at identical points. This is brought about due to the action of the enzyme endonuclease. The two chromatids exchange an identical length of the genome. After exchange the segments fuse with the chromatids due to the action of the enzyme called ligase (Stem and Hotta, 1969). There is some synthesis of DNA during this stage, as it is necessary to repair the broken points of the chromosome. The crossing over is physically demonstrable in the form of **chiasma.**

(d) Terminalization : After the exchange of segments, the two chromosomes start moving away from each other as the synaptic force lapses. The separation begins from the centromere and moves towards the ends of the chromosomes. It is this uncoupling of chiasma that is called terminalization. During diakinesis the homologous chromosomes get separated except at their ends.

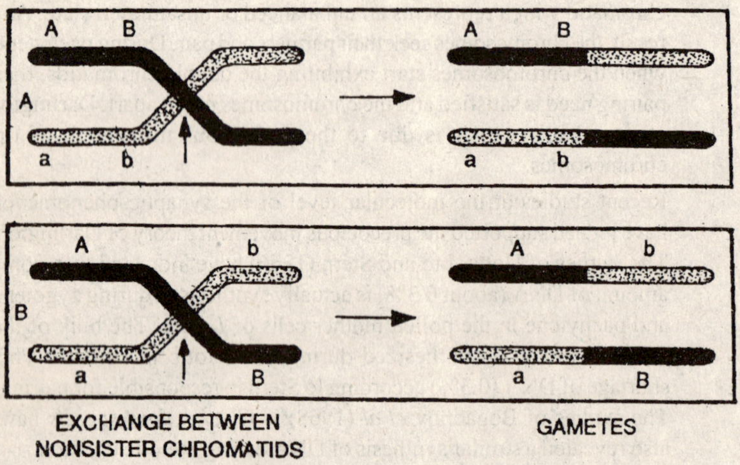

Fig. 14.5 Linkage and Crossing over

Mechanism of crossing over

Salient features of crossing over

1. Crossing over always takes place at the tetrad stage of bivalents.
2. Out of four chromatids only the two opposing chromatids participate in cross over.
3. Cross over always takes place between non sister chromatids; never between the two chromatids of the same chromosome.
4. The number of chiasmata (ie. points of contact between chromosomes) depends upon the length of the chromosome - longer chromosomes will have more number of chiasmata.
5. Linked genes get seperated particularly those which are not very close.

Chiasma : The process of chiasma development was first studied and explained by the Belgian cytologist Jaussens (1909) who showed the formation of a cross shaped configuration during chiasma. Subsequently a number of cytologists have studied chiasma formation, of whom the name of C.D. Darlington (1937) merits a mention. The exchange of segments is a highly sophisticatd and precise proces, where the two segments exchanged are of identical length, so that the participating chromatids neither lose nor gain genes. But even today, the precise mechanism which causes the breakage in the chromosome is still a matter of speculation. The position of chiasma on a chromosome is never fixed. The number of chiasma per chromosome varies from one to eight.

Relationship betwen crossing over and chiasma : There are several views to explain the relationship between the crossing over and chiasma formation. The following are some of them.

Disassociaton and Reassociation of chromatids : According to this theory, the two sister chromatids disassociate from each other and reassociate. During reassociation, they may do so with the non sister chromatid of the homologous chromosome.

Breakage and reunion theory : As per this theory, the break occurs first in the chromatids and only then they cross over forming the chiasma. According to this, it is the chiasma that brings the cross over and not *vice-versa*. In other words the chromosomes twist around each other (chiasma) and at the points of contact exchange of segments (cross over) takes place.

Partial chiasmatype theory: This theory was first proposed by Jaussen (1909). According to this, of the tetrad of chromatids, only two take part in chiasma. Thus chiasma is partial as two chromatids are left out of chiasma.

Mechanism of crosssing over : As has already been pointed out, the precise mechanism, which brings about breakage and reunion at specific points on the chromosome is not fully understood. Several theories have been put forward to account for the mechanism of crossing over. The following are some of them.

1. **Classical theory :** This view proposed by Karl Sax in 1932 states that, chiasma is formed due to alternate opening out between sister and non sister chromatids. At the points of overlap breakage and reunion occur resulting in cross over.
2. **Duplication theory :** When the chromosomes duplicate, longitudinal splitting occurs and the two non sister chromatids, which are close to each other may over lap, leading to break, exchange and reunion.
3. **Breakage and exchange theory :** Stern and Hotta (1969) have described the involvement of two enzymes viz. endonuclease and ligase in the break and reunion respectively of the chromatids.
4. **Breakage theory :** This theory proposed by Muller argues that there is a mechanical break in non sister chromatids first, leading to the exchange and then reunion. No cross over would have taken place before breakage.
5. **Copy choice theory :** This theory was first proposed by Belling (1932). Belling opines that the mechanism of crossing over involves two steps. First step is the duplication of chromatids resulting in the formation of new genes. Second step relates to the new connections between genes and chromosomes. When DNA synthesis takes place during

pachytene, the portion of the new helix synthesized may copy a non sister helix rather than a sister helix thus bringing about recombination. This is called the copy choice. The main objection to this theory is that it asssumes DNA duplication after synapsis, while it is known that, duplication would have taken place much earlier to synapsis. According to the copy choice theory, the recombination of the chromatids is entirely due to the DNA synthesised anew. It beleives that when the chromosomes duplicate, the new chromatid will use the chromatid of one parent as a template and then switches on to the chromatid of another parent; as a result the newly formed chromatid is a recombined product.

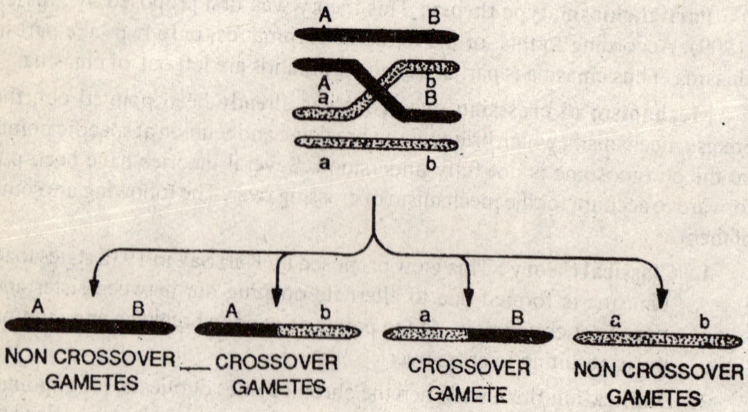

Fig. 14.6 Linkage and Crossing over
Crossing over between non sister chromatids

There is one basic difference between the breakage reunion theory and copy choice theory. The latter assumes the recombined chromatid to be a newly synthesised one while the former beleives that recombination is due to the break and exchange of existing genetic material. The copy choice mechanism however cannot be supported in view of the semi conservative nature ofDNA duplication. Meselson (1964) has shown in lambda bacteriophages, recombinant chromosomes have resulted from the mutual exchange of segments between unreplicaled DNA.

6. **Strain theory of Darlington :** According to Darlington, the specific relational coiling in the chromatids is responsible for breakage and reunion. The homologous chromosomes are rationally coiled around each other in zygotene; with the sister chromatids of each chromosome also being coiled, but in opposite direction to that of the coiling of the chromosomes. When chromosomes pair and seperate, the unravelling of the chromosomes and chromatids apparently takes place in opposite directions, thus exerting a strain on the latter resulting in breakage.

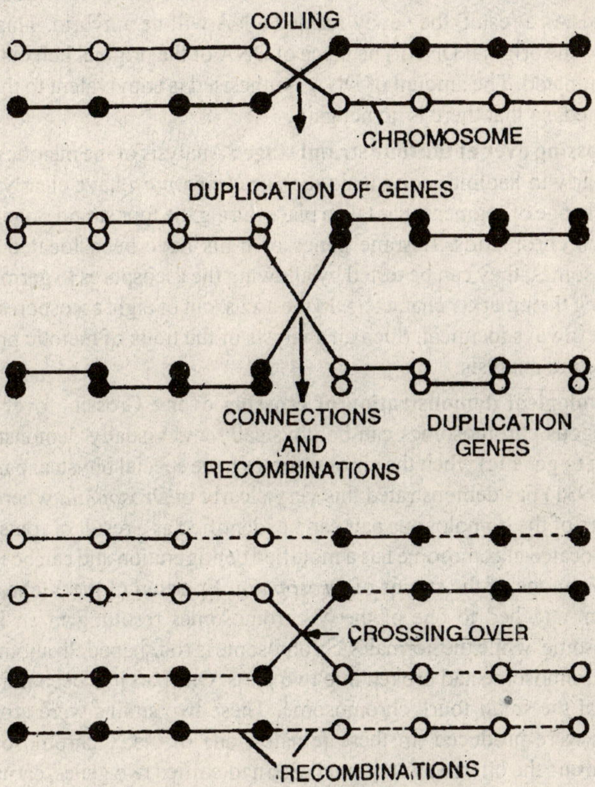

Fig. 14.7 Linkage and Crossing over
Copy choice theory of Belling

7. **Contact theory :** According to this theory, the homologous chromosomes touch each other first and as a result cross over. Breakage and reunion take place as a consequence of contact.

Molecular model for crossing over : Whitehouse and Hastings (1965) have proposed a molecular model of the crossing over phenomenon. According to them, DNA replication is practically completed prior to crossing over. When the chromosomes synapse, along their length, breakage is possible at several sites. Usually breakage occurs in one of the chains of the double helix induced by the endonuclease enzyme (Good enough and Levine 1974). The free end of the DNA unwinds from its original helix. The gap is now filled by the newly formed DNA which however uses the DNA of the non sister chromatid as a template. As a result, the newly formed DNA will be a hybrid. This attaches firmly to the original DNA. The piece of DNA of the original helix is removed and eliminated. The amount of DNA synthesised is equvivalent to the amount eliminated, so that there is no net gain.

Crossing over at the four strand stage : Analysis of the meiotic products, particularly in haploid individuals such as *Neurospora* have clearly revealed that exchange of segments has taken place during the four strand stage affecting only two chromatids. If some genes or traits have been located on these chromosomes, they can be tested by allowing the ascospores to germinate and observing their marker characters. In the ascus, out of eight ascospores adjacent ones are always identical. Such an analysis of the traits of meiotic products is called tetrad analysis

Cytological demonstration of crossing over : Crossing over between homologous chromosomes can be physically and visually demonstrated (in addition to genetic) when the chromosomes have special physical parameters. Stern (1931) has demonstrated this very clearly in *Drosophila* where the two members of the homologous pair can be identified as a result of translocation. A translocated chromosome has a modified configuration and can be identified visually. In one of the strains of *Drosophila,* a portion of the Y chromosome had been attached to one of the X chromosomes resulting in an L shaped chromosome, while the normal X chromosome is rod shaped. In another strain, the X chromosome had broken into two parts. One part had been translocated to one of the small fourh chromosome. These two strains were crossed and females were produced. In these females, one of the X chromosomes was Lshaped and the other was very small.Stern identified two genes, carnation eye (recessive mutant) and bar locus in the short X chromosome while the normal alleles were present on the L shaped X chromosome. Such a fly has red and bar eye. When such a fly was crossed with a male having carnation and bar gene located on its X chromosome, four classes of offspring were produced. Among the females of the offspring, there were two cross and two non cross over categories.

Cross over category	Carnation and normal shape red with bar shape.

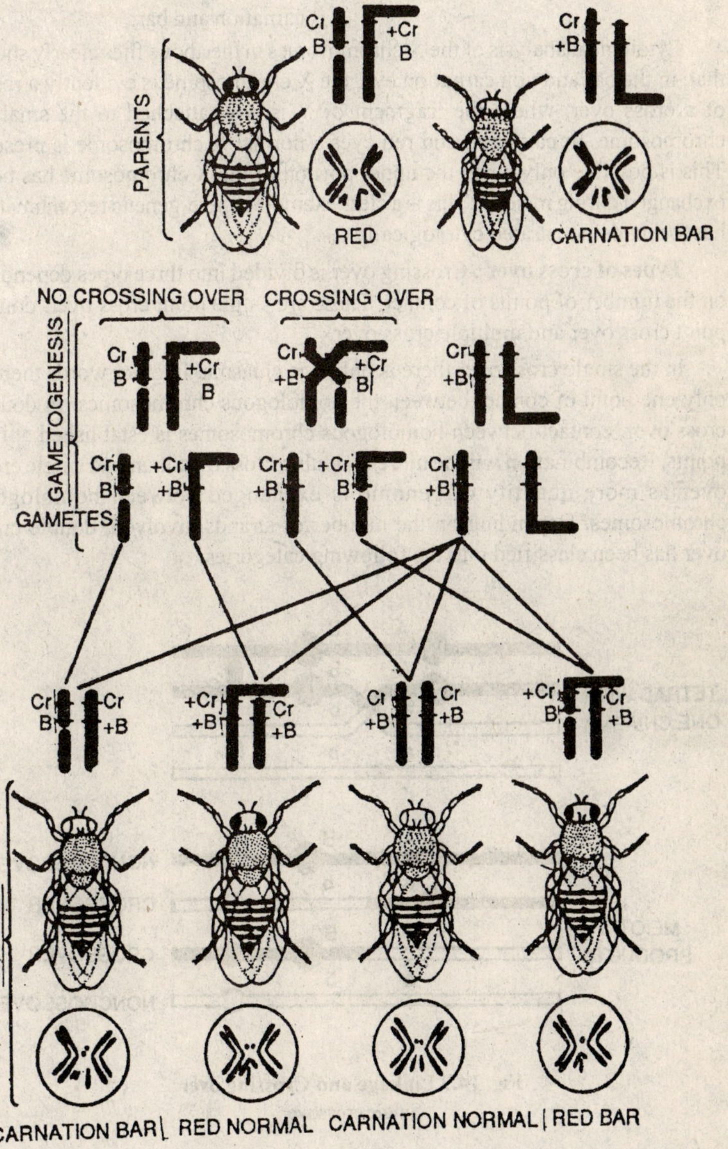

Fig. 14.8 Linkage and Crossing over
Stern's Experiment with attached chromosomes

Non cross over category — Carnation and normal shape carnation and bar.

Cytological analysis of the X chromosomes in the above flies clearly shows that, in the bar and non carnation eye, the X chromosome is evidently a result of a cross over, where the fragment of Y is now attached to the small X chromosome. In carnation and red eyes a normal X chromosome is present. This is possible only when the upper portion of the X chromosome has been exchanged during meiosis. This is a clear example where genetic recombination has been demonstrated cytologically.

Types of cross over : Crossing over is divided into three types depending on the number of points of contact. These are single point cross over, double point cross over and multiple cross over.

In the single cross over there is only one chiasma. In other words there is only one point of contact between the homologous chromosomes. In double cross over, contact between homologous chromosomes is established at two points. Recombination will be more in double cross over than in a single cross over as more quantity of genome is exchanged between homologous chromosomes. Depending on the number of strands involved, double cross over has been classified into the following categories.

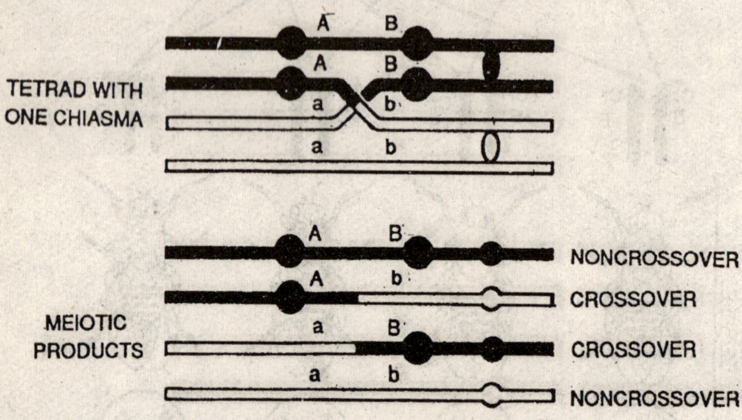

Fig. 14.9 Linkage and Crossing over
Single crossover

(a) **Two strand cross over :** In this type of double cross over, the same (two) non sister chromatids are involved in the cross over at both the points. As a result, two chromatids are cross over chromatids and the other two non cross over chromatids.

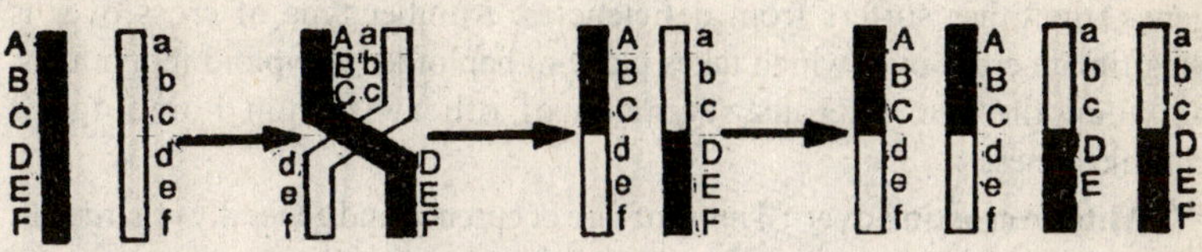

Fig. 14.10 Linkage and Crossing over
Two strand cross over

(b) **Three strand cross over :** In this case, one of the points of contact is between the two chromatids while the second contact is between one of the chromatids of first contact and another non sister chromatid. In this way three chromalids are involved in cross over, while only one will be a non cross over chromatid.

(c) **Four strand** ***cross over*** **:** In this type of cross over, all the four chromatids are involved in the cross over. First chiasma involves two chromatids, while the second chiasma involves the other two chromatids of the tetrad with the result there is no non cross over chromatid. Such chiasmata are called **complementary chiasmata.**

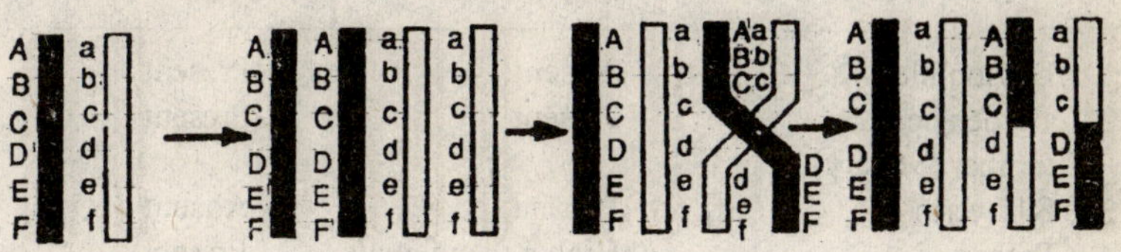

Fig. 14.11 Linkage and Crossing over
Four strand cross over

Multiple point cross over : When there are more than two points of contact between homologous chromosomes, the cross over is said to be multiple. But usually multiple cross overs are rare as there will be interference.

The cross over is also said to be **regressive** in the case of two strand cross over, **digressive** if four strands are involved and **progressive** when three strands are involved.

Certain special types of cross over have been reported in some organisms. According to Sturtevant (1952) who has reported them in *Drosophila*, an unequal cross over produces two chromatids which are unequal in the sense the exchange is not fair. While one of the chromatids has duplication of some genes, the other suffers from deficiencies. Another type of cross over is illegitimate cross over which takes place in haploidor polyploid individuals, between the homologous segments of otherwise non homologous chromosomes.

Mitotic crossing over : This is of rare occurence and generally regarded as an abnormality - This has been reported in the somatic cells of certain strains of *Drosophila* (Stern 1936). Stern observed actual pairing and cross over in some somatic cells during the course of development. Such a cell may multiply and produce a patch of a tissue. Such a patch of cross over tissue may form a mosaic among the non cross over tissues in the body.

Factors affecting crossing over. : The frequency of cross between genes is basically dependent upon the distance between the two, but a number of other genetic, environmental and physiological factors are known to affect the frequency of cross over. The following are some of them.

1. **Sex of the organism :** In certain individuals, cross over may be reduced, suppressed or even totally eliminated altogether. The following table gives a comparison between the male and female individuals of a species with regard to the frequency of cross over.

	Organisms	Male	Female
1.	Drosophila	Absent	Present
2.	Garden pea (anther & ovary)	Present	Present
3.	Silk worm	Present	Absent
4.	Pigeon	Higher than female	Present
5.	Mouse	Present	Higher than male

The table given above clearly illustrates the role of sex in influencing the frequency of cross over. Among the instances cited above we-will discuss in some detail the situation in *Drosophila* male as it has been extensively studied. When a cross is made between gray bodied vestigial winged fly with a black bodied long winged one, the F_1 hybrid will be gray and long. Here gray body colour *G* is dominant over black body colour *b* and normal wing *V* dominant over vestigial wing *v*. When the F males of the above phenotype are crosseed with double recessive females (black vestige), only two kinds of progeny are produced. Gray vestigial and black long. The recombinants namely gray long and black vestigial do not appear at all. However if an F_1 female is crossed with a double recessive (black vestige) male all the four classes of progeny (black vestige, black long, gray vestige, and gray long) appear with 83% parental combinations and 17% recombinations. The percentage of recombination is quite high indicating that the genes for wing and body colour are situated quite far apart. Hence the non occurrence of recombinants in a cross between F_1 male and double recessive female is not due to the closeness of the genes but due to the absence of cross over in males during spermatogenesis.

2. **Mutation :** The studies of Growen (1933) have indicated that in some strains of *Drosophila,* mutation has resulted in complete suppression of cross over.

3. **Age of the organism :** Bridges (1917) in his studies on *Drosophila* has shown that with the increasing age in the flies, the frequency of cross over particularly of those genes close to centromere would be substantially reduced.

4. **Temperature :** The rate of cross over will be fairly normal at a temperature range between 17 to 29 (Plough 1917). Any alteration in this range,either decrease or increase will correspondingly decrease or increase the frequency of cross over. This is however subject to certain limit.

5. **Decreased Hydration :** Lowering of water content in the surroundings is known to reduce the frequency of chiasma. It may even result in complete suppression of cross over in extreme dehydrated conditions (Sybenga 1972)

6. **Distance between the genes :** This is perhaps the most important factor influencing the frequency of cross over between two gene loci. As has been repeatedly pointed out, proximity between genes reduces the chances of cross over while distance increases the rate of cross over.

7. **Ionizing radiation :** Organisms subject to the effect of ionizing radiations show increased cross over frequency as seen in the case of *Drosophila.* One of the reports (Sybenga 1972) indicate that even in *Drosophila* males, crossing over may be induced by radiation. Work on *Lilium* and *Chlamydomonas* (Lawrence 1965) have indicated radiation effects on chiasma frequency.

8. **Chemicals :** Certain chemicals which induce chromosomal aberrations are also known to induce or suppress crossing over. Ethyl methane sulphonate is known to induce somatic cross over. Colchicine also prevents cross over by preventing pairing between chromosomes. High dose of selenium will also reduce crossing over frequency.

9. **Chromosomal aberrations :** Inversion in chromosomes alters the gene sequence and thus reduces pairing and crossing over. This is particularly true in inversion heterozygotes, when any cross over in the inverted portion would result in duplications and deficiencies in the meiotic products.

In addition to the above, some of the cytoplasmic factors are also known to have an influence on the frequency of cross over.

Significance of crossing over : The following are some of the significant features of cross over which make it a unique phenomenon in providing variation within a parameter among the individuals of a species.

1. Intraspecific variation among individuals is due to crossing over. Crossing over produces new grouping of genes and thus produces new phenotypic traits. Hence it is of great significance in breeding programme.
2. Crossing over provides physical proof for the linear arrangement of genes on the chromosomes.
3. Gene mapping on a chromosome is made possible by assessing the cross over value. The percentage of cross over is a function of distance between two gene loci.
4. Crossing over provides a new definition for the gene. According to this "Gene is the smallest section of the chromosome within which no cross over can take place.

CHROMOSOME MAPPING OR GENE MAPPING

One of the most useful aspects of the study of the phenomenon of linkage and crossing over is the help it provides in locating different genes on the chromosome. This is made possible by observing the products of a cross as to their phenotypic traits. The inheritance pattern of two gene loci and their corresponding phenotypic trait provides a clue as to the distance between them. A comparison between the parental combination and recombination among the progeny provides an understanding of the possible distance between the two genes in question. A higher parental combination with a relatively low recombination suggests that the two genes are very close, while an increased recombination value indicates that the genes are apart. The following are some of the salient features which are to be borne in mind as a preparation for the construction of linkage maps of chromosomes.

1. The number of genes far exceeds the number of chromosomes. Hence many genes are present on any single chromosome.
2. Genes are arranged in a linear fashion on the chromosome and they follow the chromosome during inheritance.
3. Generally speaking, all the genes on a chromosome behave as a single large linkage group and are inherited together. The number of linkage groups corresponds to the number of chromosomes.

4. Linked genes however may be assorted separately due to cross over taking place between their loci. The extent of separation is an index of the distance between two genes in question.
5. The strength of linkage is inversely proportional to the distance between two genes.
6. Each gene in a linkage group has a definite sequence or order as the cross over value between any two genes is always constant.

It was Sturtevant (1913), who thought that the constant value of cross over between any two genes can be exploited successfully to determine their location and relative distance on the chromosome. One can also determine the order of genes in a large linkage group. The first map of a chromosome was constructed for the X chromosome of *Drosophila* by Sturtevant and Morghan. They plotted the position of five genes.

Chromosome map may be defined as the graphic representation of genes in a linear fashion, with the distances between them (genes) being decided by cross over values.

Construction of linkage map The construction of linkage map involves several steps. At the first instance, several variants of the organism in question have to be studied and a pure breeding stock has to be obtained. Several breeding experiments are to be conducted in order to establish the linkage groups. The next step would be to identify the number of genes in the linkage group. The relative distance between these genes can be established by analysing the frequency of recombinations between these genes. The following is a detailed stepwise analysis of the construction of a linkage map.

1. **Determination of linkage groups :** Cross breeding should be conducted between two variants of a species involving at least three characters. The results of these crosses are to be analysed as to whether there is independent assortment or parental combinations far exceed the recombinations. When the parental combinations far out number recombinations, such traits or genes are said to form a linkage group.
2. **Determination of relative positions of genes :** Breeding experiments are to be conducted in such a way as to ascertain the value of recombination between one gene and the rest. For instance there are three genes A,B,and C. Cross over value for A and B and A and C has to be established first and then between B and C also has to be studied. Assuming the genes A,B,and C are linked in the same sequence, the cross over value between A and B will be less than A and C indicating, that the genes A andB are closer to each other than A and C. When the value of A and C is known, the value between B and C will help us to locate the gene in its exact position between A and C. If we assume the percentage cross over is 2% between A and B, then the distance between A and B is 2 units of map distance or 2 map unit morgan or 2 **centimorgan.**

If the F_1 hybrid (AB/ab) in a cross with the double recessive produces 16% of cross over individuals (Ab,aB) then the distance between A and B is 16 centimorgan. Each chiasma produces 50% of cross over products. 50% cross over is said to be equivalent to 50 centimorgans. If the mean number of chiasma are known for a pair of bivalents, the total length of the map may be predicted as follows.

Total length = mean number of chiasma x 50

Two point test cross : In a two point test, cross over is known to occur at two points between two gene loci A and B. For example if an F_1 individual (AB/ab) is test crossed with the double recessive (ab/ab), among the progeny (F_2) we obtain 37% dominant genes (*AB*), 37% double recessive *ab/ab*, 13% first locus dominant second one recessive Ab/ab and 13% first gene recessive and second one dominant aB/ab. The last two Ab and aB are cross over gametes totalling to about 26%. Hence the distance between A and B is 26 centimorgan. Double cross over does not occur between genes less than 5 centimorgans. In order to asses the genes situated closer than this distance, a three point test cross is adopted.

Three point test cross : A three point test cross helps us not only to understand the relative distance between these genes, but also to analyse the linear order in which the genes are placed. Let us take an example in which three hypothetical genes are involved - A,B and C. These three are linked genes and they could be arranged in any one of the following sequences ABC, BAC or ACB. In the first sequence, B is in the middle, while in the second and third A and C are in the middle position.

Therefore in finding out the sequences the middle gene has to be found out first in order to locate the other two. Let us study the results of the following cross in order to understand the gene sequence from the cross over value. Pure line parents with the genotype AABBCC and aabbcc are crossed to produce F_1 hybrid with the genotype ABC/abc. When this F_1 individual is crossed with the double recessive parent abc/abc the following progenies are produced with the hypothetical frequencies given against them.

	State of cross over	Genotype	Phenotype	Supposed Frequency
1.	Non cross over	ABC/abc	ABC	36% - a
2.	Non cross over	abc/abc	abc	36% - b
3.	cross over (A - B)	Abc/abc	Abc	9% - c
4.	Cross over (A - B)	aBC/abc	aBC	9% - d
5.	Cross over (B - C)	ABc/abc	ABc	4% - e

6.	Cross over (B - C)	ABc/abc	ABc	4% - f
7.	Cross over A - B and B - C	abC/abc	abC	1% - g
8.	Cross over A - B and B - C	aBc/abc	aBc	1% - h
				Total 100 - T

If we assume, that the cross over value between A and B = X and that of B and C = Y and that of A and C = Z, it can be calculated as follows.

1. Cross over between A - B (both double and single cross overs)

$$X = \frac{c+d+g+h}{T} \times 100$$

$$X = \frac{9+9+1+1}{T} \times 100$$

= 20 centimorgan (distance between A and B)

2. Cross over between B - C

$$Y = \frac{e+f+g+h}{T} \times 100$$

$$Y = \frac{4+4+1+1}{T} \times 100$$

= 10 centimorgan (distance between and B and C)

3. Cross over between A - C

$$Z = \frac{c+d+e+f}{T} \times 100$$

$$Z = \frac{9+9+4+4}{T} \times 100$$

= 30 centimorgan (distance between A and C)

To summarise the distance are as follows :

A - B = 20
B - C = 10
A - C = 30

Determining the gene sequence : To mark these genes on the chromosome in their proper order, let us suppose, gene A is in the middle -

I

B 20 A 30 C

B 10 C

(Actual distance)

In the above example if we assume A is in between B and C, since the distance between B and C is known to be only 10 and the distance now works to be 20 + 30 (B + A and A + C) = 50. This assumption is not correct. A cannot be in the middle.

II Let us assume that gene C is in the centre (ACB)

A 30 C 10 B

A 20 B

In this instance, the distance between A and B works out to 30 + 10 (A + C, + C + B), while the actual distance is 20. Hence C cannot be placed in the middle.

III Let assume that gene **B** is in the middle.

A 20 B 10 C

A 30 C

The above sequence of location of genes A-B-C is correct since the value of A + B and B + C (20 + 10) equals the actual value between A anc C (30). Hence the genes A, B, C are in the order in which they are noted below.

A B C

Linkage map in maize : We shall study one more example of linkage map with an illustration from maize, using a three point test cross. Three characters are chosen, all dealing with the endosperm.

1. Coloured aleurone (C) and colourless alleurone (c)
2. Full endosperm (Sh) and shrunken endosperm (sh)
3. Non waxy endosperm (Wx) and waxy endosperm (wx)

When a pure breeding coloured shrunken non waxy (C sh Wx / C sh Wx) is crossed with another pure breeding colourless full waxy individual (c Sh wx / c Sh wx) the F_1 will be coloured full and non waxy with the genotype C Sh Wx / c Sh wx. When this F_1 hybrid is crossed with the double recessive individual (c sh wx/c sh wx) the following kinds of progeny are obtained in F_2 generation. The data given below are those of Hutchinson (1922).

		Gametes C sh wx	**Number of individuals in F_2**
No cross over	C sh Wx	Csh Wx/c sh wx (coloured, shrunken non waxy)	5246

	c Sh wx	c Sh wx/c sh wx (colourless, full waxy)	
Single cross over	C Sh wx C sh Wx	C Sh Wx/c sh wx (coloured, full waxy) c sh Wx/c sh Wx/c sh wx (colourless, shrunken non waxy)	229
Single cross over sh - Wx	C sh wx c Sh Wx	Csh wx/c sh wx (coloured, shrunken waxy) C Sh wx/c sh wx (colourless, full waxy)	1227
Double cross over C - sh - and sh - Wx	C Sh Wx c sh wx	C Sh Wx/c sh wx (coloured, full non waxy) c sh wx/c sh wx (colourless, shrunken waxy)	6

As has been shown in the previous example involving hypothetical genes ABC, the cross over values for C - Sh, Sh - Wx and C - Wx can be worked out in order to find the linear distance between C, Sh and Wx.

1. Cross over value for C -sh $= \dfrac{229+6}{6708} \times 100 = 3.5\%$

2. Cross over value for Sh - Wx $= \dfrac{1227+6}{6708} \times 100 = 18..4\%$

3. Cross over value for C - Wx $= \dfrac{229+6}{6708} \times 100 = 21.7\%$

Here the cross over value C - Wx (21.7%) is approximately equal to the total value of C - Sh and Sh - Wx x (21.9%).

Hence Sh should be located between and C and Wx as follows.

C 3.5 Sh 18.4 Wx

The slight difference 0.2% (21.9 - 21.7) is due to the fact that double cross overs are not included in the C - wx cross over value.

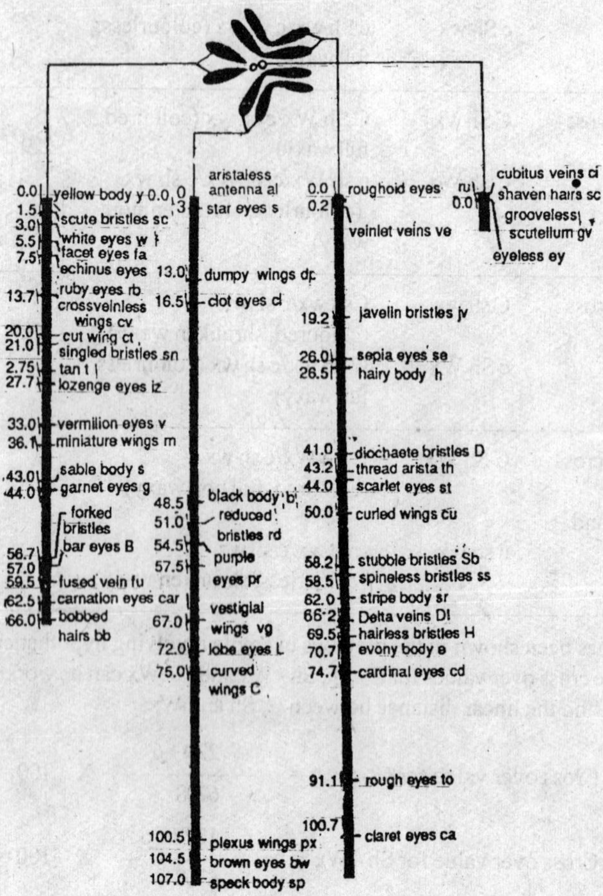

Fig. 14.12 Linkage and Crossing over

Interference and coincidence : When the genes are located in the order A, B & C and recombination values of a -b and b - c are independent of each other, one should be able to get the double cross over value between a -c by simply multiplying individual values of a -b and b - c. For example if a-b is 10% and b-c is 20%, then the double cross over would be 10% of 20% or 2%. However in practice, the value of double cross over obtained is always less than the expected value. This is due to the fact that crossing over at any one point interferes with any other cross over near by. This phenomenon is called

Interference. It is because of interference cross overs between close gene loci is not possible. In *Drosophila,* interference prevents double cross over in genes less than 10 units apart.

The degree of interference varies in different regions, and is inversely proportional to the percentage of crossing over. If the double cross overs are totally absent, then the interference is said to be 100%. When the frequency of double cross over is according to the expected Figure, then there is no interference - Muller (1911) first discovered this phenomenon and opined that interference may also serve as an index of the distance between the genes.

As has been pointed out already, the degree of interference varies from chromosome to chromosome and within a chromosome also between different regions. Generally interference is maximum near the centromere and at the two tips of the chromosome. In the mapping of the chromosome, interference has to be taken into consideration in order to locate the genes exactly.

Coincidence is a term used to express the phenomenon of interference in terms of ratio of the expected cross over and actual cross. This is indicated as coefficient of coincidence as follows.

$$\text{Coefficient of coincidence} = \frac{\%\ \text{actual cross over}}{\%\ \text{expected cross over}}$$

In the example mentioned above expected cross over is 2% and if the observed value is 1% then the coefficient of coincidence is 0.5%. or 50% coincidence, when the coincidence is greater, interference will be less and *vice versa.*

Positive and negative interference : The instance mentioned above, where cross over in any one region suppresses the cross over in the adjacent region is called Positive interference. This is found in higher organisms. In some lower organisms like some fungi *(Aspergillus),* bacteriophages etc, there is what is known as negative interference, ie., cross over in a given region enhances the chances of cross over in the adjacent regions. This maybe due to the peculiar modes of reproduction seen in them. It is opined that in these organisms, effective pairing sites exist in the genome to enhance the frequencies of recombination.

Linkage maps of some organisms : The study of linkage groups in organisms has led to the construction of linkage or genetic maps of chromosomes. Detailed linkage maps have been prepared for *Drosophila* and Maize.

Chromosome map of Drosopliila : Sturtevant (1911) constructed the first two chromosome maps in *Drosophila melanogaster.* Later Bridges and others constructed the maps for the remaining chromosomes. There are four linkage groups in *Drosophila* corresponding to four pairs of chromosomes. In terms of cross over frequencies the unit length of the X chromosome has 66 units, second chromosme 107.3 units, third chromosome has 106.2 umts and the fourth has only 0.2 units. These frequencies correspond fairly well with the observed length of the chromosomes.

Linkage maps in Maize : Among the plants,the chromosomes of Maize are quite extensively mapped. The pioneering works of Emerson, McClintock are worth mentioning in this regard. There are 10 linkage groups in maize corresponding to 10 chromosmes. Chromosome maps in man: A detailed map of all the chromosomes is highly desireable and perhaps will go a long way in combating genetic disorders and improving the health of man. But the construction of genetic maps of human beings is a very arduous task and is beset with many difficulties. This is not only because of a large number of genes (estimated to be about I lakh) involved but also due to many sociological constraints. It is not possible to choose mates for any desired experiment. Hence pedigree studies have to be made and results have to be computed. Sex chromosomes have been studied and tentative maps have been prepared. Recently attempts have been made by an international group of scientists to map the autosomes of human beings.

15

SEX DETERMINATION

In a large majority of higher organisms (specially among animals), the most striking difference between the individuals of same species from the point of view of reproduction is sex. The individuals differ in their mode of producing gametes. Some individuals produce less number of generally non motile gametes (egg) while others produce a large number of motile gametes (sperm). Thus the individuals are classified into male and female. In a large majority of animals the male and female individuals are differentiated from each other by a number of secondary sexual characters in addition to the primary difference. Hence in animals there is generally sexual dimorphism (between male and female individuals). In plants however, the sexes are seperate no doubt, but both the sex organs are borne on the same individual. Such individuals in which both the sexes are found on the same individual are called Hermaphrodite or monoecious. In some of the plants *(Vallisnaria),* however the male and female individuals are different dioecious in that the sexes are separated on two individuals. There will be a male plant and female plant. But it has to be pointed out however that unlike in the case of animals, there are no secondary sexual characters in plants to distinguish between the individuals. Except for sex organs, both individuals look alike. The basis of dioeciousness is one of the most interesting problems in biology. What constitutes the basis of difference between male and female individuals, is it structural or physiological or both? What constitutes the additional differences between males and females in addition to sex? The attempt to find out answers to these questions is discussed in this chapter. The problem of sex determination has been engaging the attention of biologists since a long time. Ancient scientists, philosophers etc have given their valued opinions on the subject. The following is a brief history of sex determination.

Brief History : Ancient men emphasized on the extraneous factors as deciding the sex of the new born rather than any inherent potentiality of the individual. According to Conway Zirkle (1951) the most distinguished genetic historian, there were three fantastic beliefs among ancient people regarding sex determination. According to this, the two testicles of man are more than a coincidence in that one helps in the production of male while the semen from the other produces female. And quite justifiably of course, the right testicle produced the dominant sex male and the left the female. This was the idea of sex determination among ancient Hebrews.

Another funny notion regarding sex determination was that the sex of the new born depended upon the aggressive sexual behaviour of one of the parents. Accordingly an effiminate man produces only daughters. The third and the funniest notion among the three is that of the role played by the direction of the wind at the time of mating. Males would be produced when north wind blew and females would be engendered if south wind blew. Even the great Aristotle beleived in this view.

Some of the ancient philosophers like Hippocrates beleived that the sex of the offspring depended upon the ripeness of the ovum at the time of fertilization. If an egg is fertilized soon after ovulation, the individual would be female, on the other hand if the egg remains in the oviduct for sometime before 'fertilization, the resultant individual would be male. Galen beleived that the ovary of the right side produced males while the left ovary produced females. Schenk an Austrian scientist beleived that high dose of nutrition to the pregnant mother produced male individuals, while reduced nutrition to the would be mother resulted in female individual.

The theories and opinions mentioned above are only of historic interest and do not have any scientific basis.

Discovery of sex chromosomes : Even after the chromosomes were discovered and identified as vehicles of heredity, nobody bothered to attribute a role to them in the determination of sex. It was beleived that physiological and environmental parameters are decisive in the sex determination of the offspring. The X chromosome was first observed by the German biologist Henking (1891) during spermatogenesis in male bugs. He called it X body. But he did not speculate on the function of the X body. Mc Clung (1902) described the chromosome numbers in the male and female grasshoppers; the male had 23 chromosomes, while the female had 24 chromosomes. Wilson and Stevenes (1905) followed the path of the X bodies during oogenesis and spermatogenesis in *Protenor* (a genus of insects). They came to the realization that the so called X body is the X chromosome which influences the sex. Wilson and Stevens further pointed out, that the females had two identical X chromosomes while the males had one X and another smaller chromosome Y. The X and Y chromosomes may be identified both cytologically as well as genetically. The discovery of sex chromosomes made many geneticists to think in terms of the chromosomal basis of sex determination. However our present knowledge of sex determination clearly reveals that besides the chromosomes, several other factors also govern the functioning of the sex. In the paragraphs below we shall discuss, some of the mechanisms of sex determination.

Theories of sex determination : These are as follows.

1. Genetic sex determining mechanism.
2. Metabolic sex determining mechanism.
3. Hormone controlled sex determination.
4. Environment controlled sex determination.

Genetic determination of sex : The male and female individuals possess different structural attributes in terms of chromosomes to decide the sex of the new born. Genetic determination of sex is based on the chromosomes deciding the sex of the offspring. In these individuals the chromosomes are of two categories - **Autosomes** and **sex chromosomes**. Autosomes are responsible for all the somatic characters, while the sex chromosomes decide the sex besides carrying genes for some somatic characters also. In sexually dimorphic individuals (including man) there is a pair of chromosomes meant to govern the sex, these are called X and Y or Z and W chromosomes. Whatever may be their nomenclature their role is same. The chromosomal mechanism of sex determination varies in different individuals, although essentially in all these cases, sex chromosomes decide the sex of the offspring. The following table summarises the variations in chromosomal determination of sex.

Adopted *horn Principles of Genetics* - Sinnott, Dunn and Dobzhansky

Variations in chromosomal sex determination

Organisms	**Heterogametic Sex**	**Gametes**		**Zygotes**	
		Sperms	**Eggs**	**Females**	**Males**
Drosophila, man etc	Male	x, y	All x	xx	xy
Protenor, grasshopper etc.	Male	x - o (nil)	All x	xx	xo
Birds moths etc.	Female	All x	x, y	xy	xx
Fumea (a moth)	Female	All x	x, o (nil)	xo (nil)	xx

[Note : In the above table 'o' indicates the absence of the sex chromosome, xo means only one sex chromosome]

Structure of the sex chromosome : The X and Y sex chromosomes exhibit certain structural differences as revealed by cytological studies. In most of the organisms the X chromosome is straight, rod like and larger than the Y chromosome. The Y chromosome is smaller in size with one end slightly hooked or curved as in *Drosophila.* In man however no such curve is found in the Y chromosome. X chromosomes have a large euchromatic area and hence carry many sex linked somatic characters. The Y chromosome has less of euchromatic region and carries but few sex linked somatic characters.

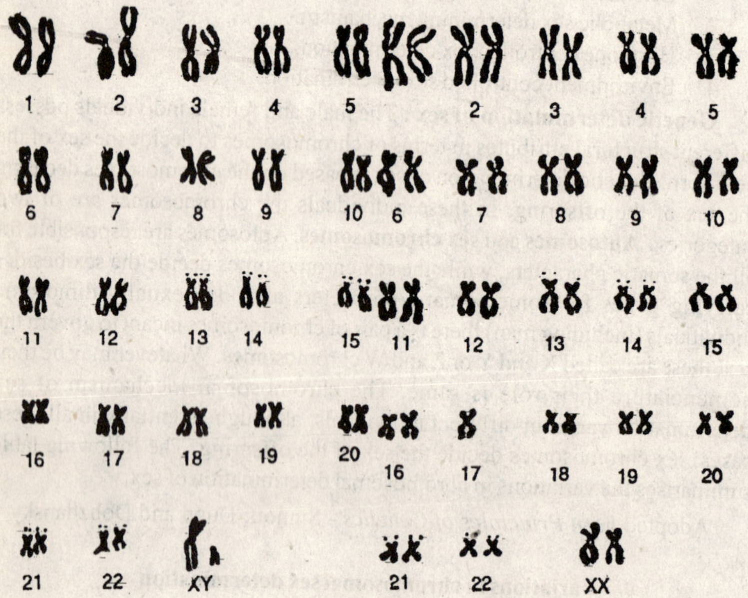

Fig. 15.1 Sex Determination
Human chromosomes at metaphase, Male (left) and female (right)

In dioecious organisms chromosomal sex determination is of basically two categories - Heterogametic males and Heterogametic females.

Heterogametic males : The male individual produces two types of sperms. 50% of the sperms carry one type of sex chromosome (X) and the rest carry another type (Y) of sex chromosome. All the females carry only one type of sex chromosome (X). Hence the females are said to be homogametic. The sex of the new born depends upon the type of sperm fertilizing the egg. The female gamete has no role in deciding the sex in the sense it always carries only one type of a chromosome. Sex determination in heterogametic males belongs to any one of the following types.

1. XX - XY type : In man, *Drosophila* etc, where male is the heterogametic sex, the male and female have the following types of sex chromosomes (this type was first studied in milkweed bug *Lygaeus turcicus*, hence it is also called as the **Lygaeus type**).

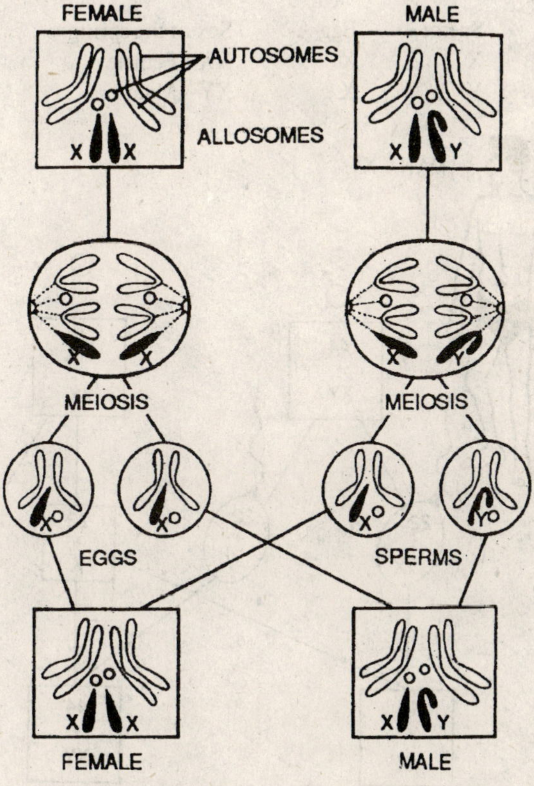

Fig. 15.2 Sex Determination
Sex determination in Drosophila (XX, Xy type)

	Organism	Sex	Autosomes	Sex chromosomes
1.	*Drosophila*	Male	3 pairs	xy
2.	*Drosophila*	Female	3 pairs	xx
3.	Human being	Male	22 pairs	xy
4.	Human being	Female	22 pairs	xx

In the XX - XY type, the male produces two types of sperms. 50% sperms would carry X chromosome and the rest carry Y chromosome. All the eggs are of only one type in that all of them carry a single X chromosome. The sex of the new born depends on the type of sperm (carrying X or Y) fertilizing the egg. It is as follows.

Sperm	Egg	Sex of the spring
X	X	XX – Female
Y	X	XY – Male

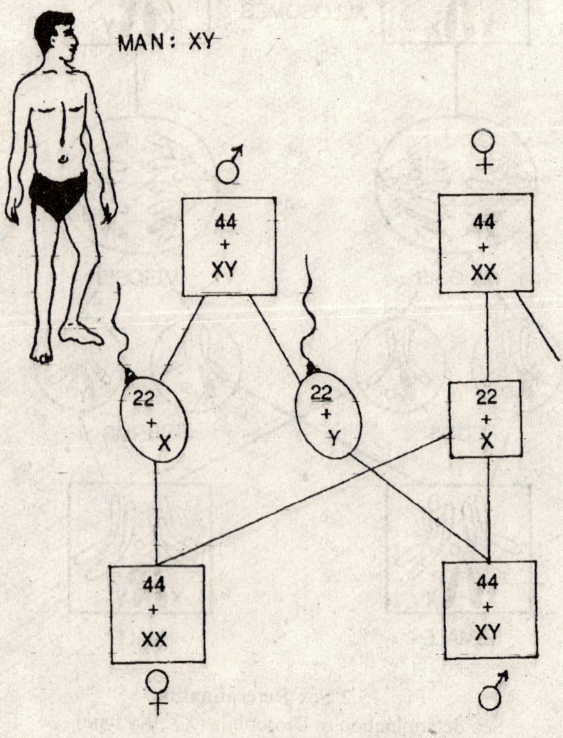

Fig. 15.3 Sex Determination
Sex determination in human beings

2. **XX - XO type :** In certain types of insects, specially those belonging to Hemiptera and orthoptera, the female has two X chromosomes, while the male has only one X chromosome and thus refered to ås XO (O refers to the absence of another sex chromosome). Here the male produces two type of sperms.

Male– 50% sperms - Autosomes + X chromosome.
Male– 50% sperms - Autosomes + no sex chromosomes.
Female 100% eggs - Autosomes + X chromosome.

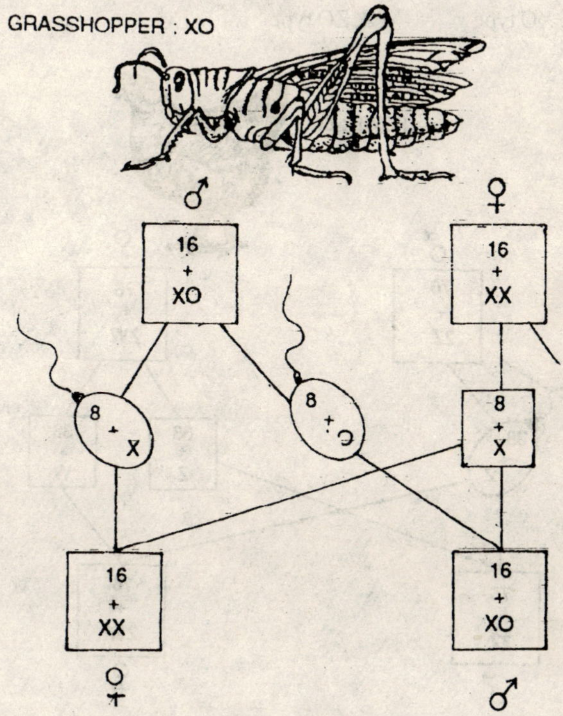

Fig. 15.4 Sex Determination
Sex determination in grasshopper (XX–XO type)

If a sperm carrying X chromosome fertilizes the egg (X) the resultant individual will be XX and female. If on the other hand, a sperm carrying only autosomes but no sex chromosome fertilizes the egg, the resultant individual is XO and male.

Heterogametic females : In a large group of animals such as butterflies, moths, birds and some Fish, another method of sex determination is found which is just the reverse XX and XY type. Here it is the female which is heterogametic producing two types of eggs. X and Y or X and O (O means sex chromosome is absent, the egg carrying only autosomes). The males have two X chromosomes and the sperms are all of the same type in that they carry one X chromosome. The sex of the individual depends upon the type of egg fertilized by the sperm. This is also of two types as explained above. XX, XY and XX, XO type. In order to distinguish this from the conventional XX, XY type new symbols are used- X = Z and Y = W.

XX, XY type = ZZ, ZW type

XX, XO type = ZZ, ZO type.

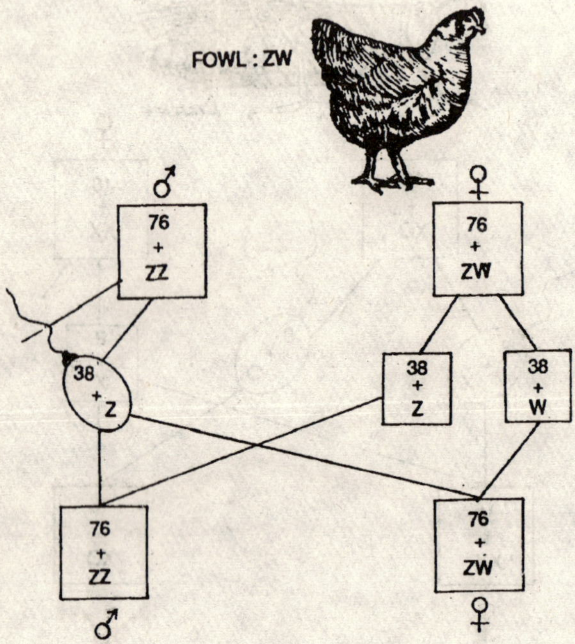

Fig. 15.5 Sex Determination
Sex determination in birds

The mechanism of sex determination in ZZ, ZW type is same as in XX, XY type except that the female is heterogametic.

Sperm	Egg	Sex of offspring
Z	Z	ZZ Male
Z	W	ZW – Female

In the ZZ, ZO type the female produces two types of eggs. 50% would carry Z chromosome and the other 50% would carry no sex chromosome (O).

Female	50% eggs	–	Autosomes +	Z chromosome
Female	50% eggs	–	Autosomes +	no sex chromosome
Male	100% sperms	–	Autosomes +	Z chromosome

Sperm	Egg	Sex of offspring
Z	Z	ZZ Female
Z	O	ZO Male (no sex chromosome)

Haploid Diploid type : In wasps, honey bee and a few other hymenopteran insects the males are usually haploid (16 chromosomes), while the females are diploid (32 chromosomes). In females, meiosis occurs during oogenesis, so that the eggs are haploid: Meiosis does not take place during spermatogenesis. After fertilization (16 +16) the zygote develops into female because it (zygote) is diploid. How are males produced then? In some cases, the eggs (16 chromosomes) develop parthenogenetically (without fertilization) into males.

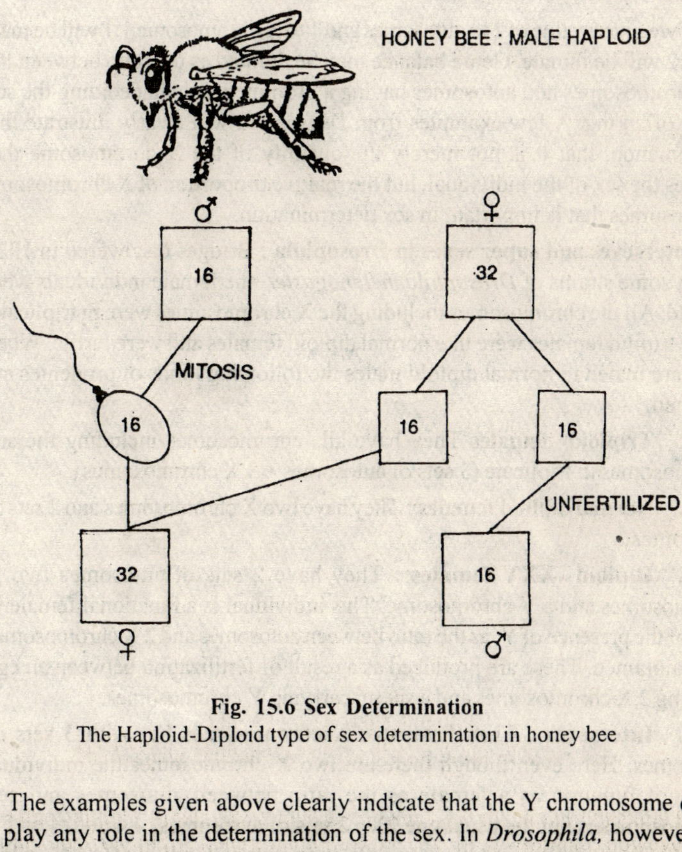

Fig. 15.6 Sex Determination
The Haploid-Diploid type of sex determination in honey bee

The examples given above clearly indicate that the Y chromosome does not play any role in the determination of the sex. In *Drosophila,* however, Y chromosome is necessary for the fertility of the male sex.

GENIC BALANCE THEORY : This theory was put forward by Bridges who opined that in *Drosophila* and other organisms, the Y chromosome is practically inert as far as the determination of sex was concerned. He opined that the sex of the individual actually depends on a delicate balance between the sex chromosomes and autosomes. According to him the X chromosome consists of genes for femaleness, while the autosomes carry the genes for maleness. Any increase in the dose of the X chromosome (XX) will result in femaleness, while any reduction will produce maleness. The development of an individual either into male or into female depends on the ratio or balance between X chromosome and autosomes.

Male	X : 3	pairs of autosomes
Female	XX : 3	pairs of autosomes

If we give a value of 1 to autosomes and 1 to X chromosome 1:1 will be male and 1:2 will be female. Genie balance may be defined as the ratio between the sex chromosomes and autosomes having a prominent role in deciding the sex of the offspring. A few examples from *Drosophila* will clearly illustrate this phenomenon, that it is not merely the quantity of the X chromosome that decides the sex of the individual, but the relative proportion of X chromosome to autosomes that is important in sex determination.

Intersexes and super sexes in Drosophila : Bridges discovered in 1922 that in some strains of *Drosophila melanogaster,* the female individuals were triploid. All the chromosomes including the X chromosomes were in triplicate. These tripilid females were like normal diploid females and were fertile. When these are mated to normal diploid males the following kinds of progenies are obtained.

1. **Triploid females** They have all chromosomes including the sex chromosomes in triplicate (3 sets of autosomes + 3 X chromosomes)

2. **Normal diploid females :** They haye two X chromosomes and 2 sets of autosomes.

3. **Diploid XXY females :** They have 2 sets of autosomes two X chromosomes and a Y chromosome. This individual is a functional female in spite of the presence of Y, as the ratio between autosomes and 2 X chromosomes are maintained. These are produced as a result of fertilization between an egg carrying 2 X chromosomes and a sperm carrying Y chromosomes.

4. **Intersexes :** They have two X chromosomes but with 3 sets of autosomes; Here even though there are two X chromosomes the individual does not function as a female as the ratio between autosomes and sex chromosomes is not the usual one 2X : 2 sets of autosomes.

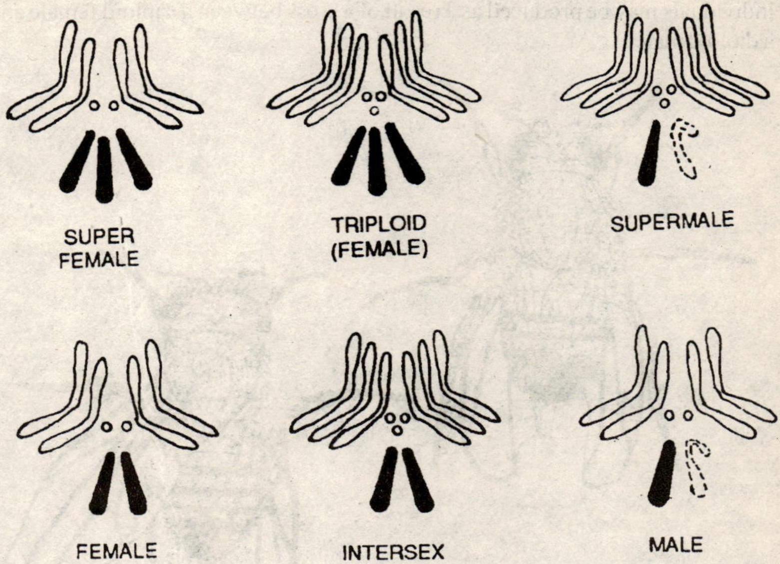

Fig. 15.7 Sex Determination
Genic balance and sex determination in Drosophila

5. Intersexes : They are morphologically indistinguishable from the above category (4), but genetically they have two X chromosomes, one Y chromosome and 3 sets of autosomes.

6. Normal males : They have one X, one Y chromosome and two sets of autosomes.

7. Superfemales : They have three X chromosomes, and two sets of autosomes. Here again, the ratio between autosomes and X chromosome is disturbed. An excess of X chromosome without an increase in autosomes will result in superfemales.

8. Super males : These have one X, one Y and three sets of autosomes. Here there is increase in autosomes (which are supposed to carry genes for maleness) without increase in X chromosomes, hence the individual will be super male.

Intersexes are sterile individuals as theycannot function either as male or as female. This is due to the disturbance of the normal ratio of one or two X chromosomes with 2 sets of autosomes. Supermales and superfemales are also sterile individuals. The following table shows how the ab›ve 8 types of individuals may be produced as a result of a cross between a triploid female and a dioloid male.

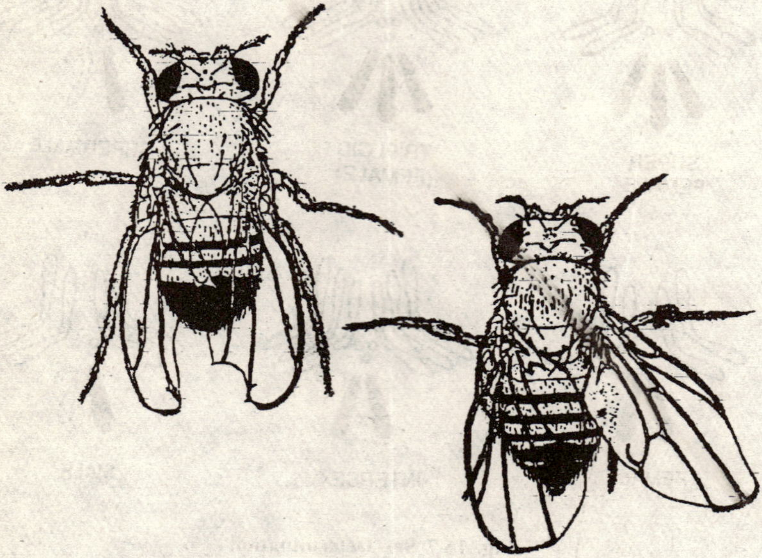

Fig. 15.8 Sex Determination
Male and female intersexes in Drosophila

TRIPLOID FEMALE	X	DIPLOID MALE
3A + XXX		2A + XY

Gametes (Females)	Gametes Male	
	A + X	A + Y
2A + XX	3A + XXX Triploid female	3A + XXY Triploid intersex
A + X	2A + XX Diploid female	2A + XY Diploid male
2A + X	3A + XX Triploid intersex	3A + XY Super male
A + XX	2A + XXX Super female	2A + XXY Diploid female

In the above table, it is clearly illustrated as to how any increase or decrease in the ratio of autosomes and sex chromosomes disturbs the normal functioning of sex. If we give a ratio of 1.0 (2 X chromosomes and 2 sets of autosomes) for female and 0.5 (one X chromosome and 2 sets of autosomes) for male, any deviation between this would alter the sexual behaviour. For instance a ratio between 1 and 0.5 would be intersexes, a ratio above 1.0 would be superfemales and a ratio below 0.5 would be supermales. The following table gives the genic ratio and the control of sex in *Drosophia melanogaster*

X/A ratio	Sex
>1.0	Super females
1.0	Females
1.0 to 0.5	Inter sexes
0.5	Male
>0.5	Supermale

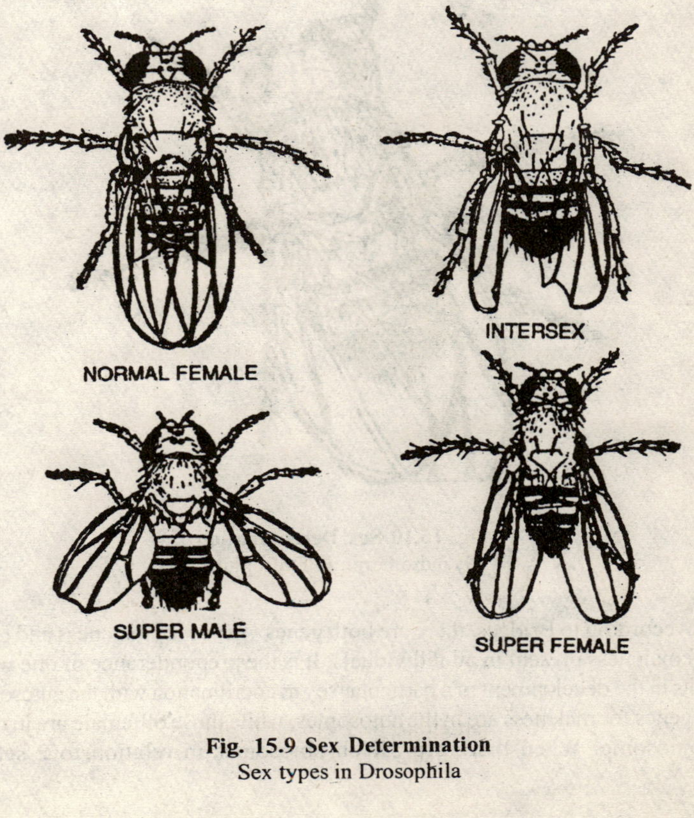

Fig. 15.9 Sex Determination
Sex types in Drosophila

Bridge's explanation to the genic balance theory

The following explanation in Bridge's own words sums up nicely the relative functioning of autosomes and sex chromosomes in the control of sex. "The intersexes and 3n (triploid) types lead to the conclusion that sex in *Drosophila melanogaster* is determined by the autosomes as well as the X chromosomes, the ratio of autosomes to X's being the significant relation. The old formulation of 2X = female is at once seen to be inadequate; for here we have individuals with 2X chromosomes and yet they are not females. They are shifted out of the female class by the presence of an extra set of autosomes and thereby the autosomes are proved to play a positive role in the production of sex. Since the intersexes differ from females by the assumption of certain male characters, this effect of the autosomes- is due to an internal preponderance of male tendency genes".

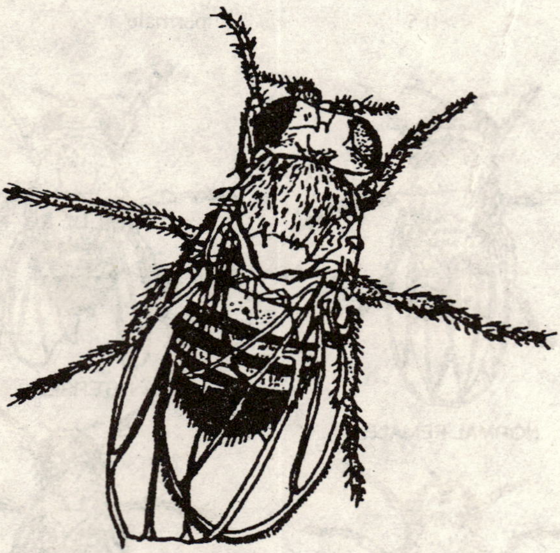

Fig. 15.10 Sex Determination
Gyandromorph in Drosophila

According to Bridges, there are both genes - genes for maleness and genes for femaleness present in all individuals. It is the preponderance of one which results in the development of a particular sex in coordination with the autosomes. The genes for maleness are in the autosomes, while those of female are in the X chromosome. When there are 2X chromosomes in relation to 2 sets of autosomes, the female tendency genes outweigh the male tendency genes and the individual would be female. On the 'other hand if one X chromosome is removed, some quantity of the female genes are eliminated, resulting in the tilt towards male genes and the individual would be male.

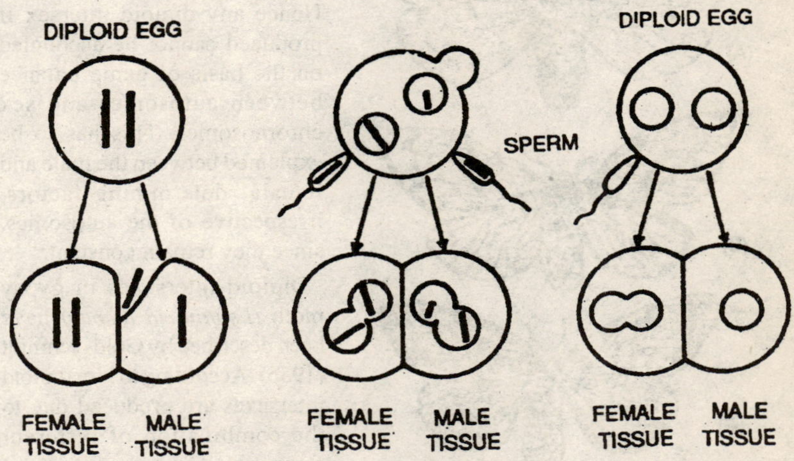

Fig. 15.11 Sex Determination
Origin of Gyandromorph

Gynandromorphs : These are individuals in which one half of the body is male and the other: female. These should not be mistaken with intersexes. Intersexes are neither males nor females. Morgan and Bridge's (1919) explained the' basis underlying the developments of gynandromorphs in *Drosophila.* Gynandromorphs arise from zygotes with 2X chromosomes and should normally develop into females. But during early cleavages of the zygote, due to misdivision, one of the of the X chromosomes is lost in one cell. The product of this cell will have only one X chromosome and hence develop male body into parts; the cells that have two X chromosomes develop into female body parts. The individual will have a mix of male cells and female cells.

Goldschmidt and Katsuki have described a different mechanism for the origin of gynandromorphs in the silkworm moth. Some of the eggs have two nuclei instead of one. In such a case the two egg nuclei may be fertilized by different sperms. One nucleus fertilized by a Y sperm develops into male parts of the body, while another fertilized by a X sperm develops into the female parts of the body.

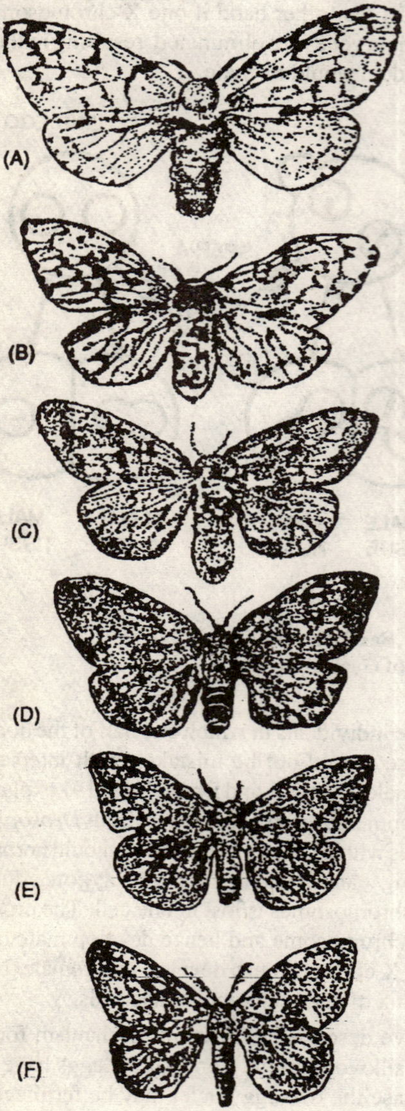

Fig. 15.12 Sex Determination
Intersexes in Gypsy moth

Diploid intersexes in gypsy moth : In *Drosophila,* diploids cannot be intersexes; they have to be triploid or polyploid. Hence any diploid intersex if produced cannot be accounted on the basis of genie balance between autosomes and sex chromosomes. This has to be explained between the male and female determining factors, irrespective of the autosomes, since they remain constant.

Diploid intersexes in gypsy moth *(Lymantria dispar)* have been described by Gold- schmidt (1955). According to him diploid intersexes are produced due to the combination of different strength of sex different geographical areas carry sex factors of varying potency. Consequently a cross between moths of different geographical regions would produce hybrids which are intersexes. The following cross involving a European race and Japanese race will clearly illustrate this phenomenon.

In gypsy moth, the female is heterogametic and male is homogametic. One of the European races were found to be weak. The females of this race were given the genotype Fw Mw and the males Mw Mw. The cross between male and female would produce perfect males and females. Similarly a strong Japanese race was found in the moths and the females of this race had the genotype Fs Ms and males Ms Ms. Here also the cross of individuals of the same race would produce normal progeny. However when a weak European female (Fw Ms) was crossed with a strong Japanese male (Ms Ms), the resultant individual (Fw Ms) would be intersex because the female tendency of the Fw gene cannot over come completely the male effects of Ms gene. In a reciprocal cross a Japanese female crossed to a European male (Fs Ms x Mw Mw) no intersexes are obtained. The genotypes of the offspring would be 1) Fs Mw and 2) Ms Mw. The First one is female because the female factors of Japanese origin can suppress the European male factors. The second one would be normal male because, the Japanese male factors and European male factors interact to produce maleness.

Metabolic differentiation of sex : According to Crew (1927), Shull (1921) Whitney (1923) etc., the rate of metabolism has a profound effect on the determination of sex in the new born. Shull showed that in rotifers, increased metabolism leads to the production of only males. In pigeons also it is known that a low rate of metabolism leads to the birth of female individuals, while the increased rate leads to male offspring.

Hormonal theory of sex differentiation : In animals hormones secreted by the endocrine glands produce a wide range of body reactions. These however do not determine the sex but rather influence in the proper functioning of sex. For instance lack of proper hormones may render an individual sterile even though the individual may be structurally either male or female. Hormones control the secondary sexual characters (sex differentiation or functioning of the sex) rather than the primary sexual characters (structural sex). Chromosomes determine whether an individual should be male or female structurally, while hormones decide whether the individual should function as male or female. In other words chromosomes decide the development of either ovary or testis, while the hormones control their function as effective male and female reproductive organs. The hormones produced by the gonads (male and female) are distributed all over the body inducing the secondary sexual characters. The influence of hormones as secondary sexual characters may be studied with the help of examples like partial sex reversals. In partial sex reversal, a male or female individual may be made to develop a few characters of the opposite sex by injecting appropriate hormones.

In Salamander, grafting between male(upper part) and female (lower part) would produce the individual with suppressed ovaries. The male hormone coming from medulla suppresses the ovaries.

Walker, in his experiments with poultry has shown that a testicular extract from a rooster, when injected into a hen would make her (hen) produce a comb.

It has also been observed that generally egg laying hen, when they grow old begin to show characters of male and may even develop comb and start crowing.

Free martin cattle : When twin calves belonging to opposite sex are born to cattle, it has been observed, that the female calf is generally abnormal and sterile. Such a calf is said to be a free martin. The detailed studies of Frank Lillie on twin embryos in cattle have revealed the secret behind the free martin calf. Frank Lillie found that the two calves - male and female have common blood vessel junction in the uterus. As a result hormones can easily pass from one calf to the other through blood circulation. Since the male hormones develop early in development they exert their influence on the female calf. As a result a partial sex reversal is noticed in the female calf.

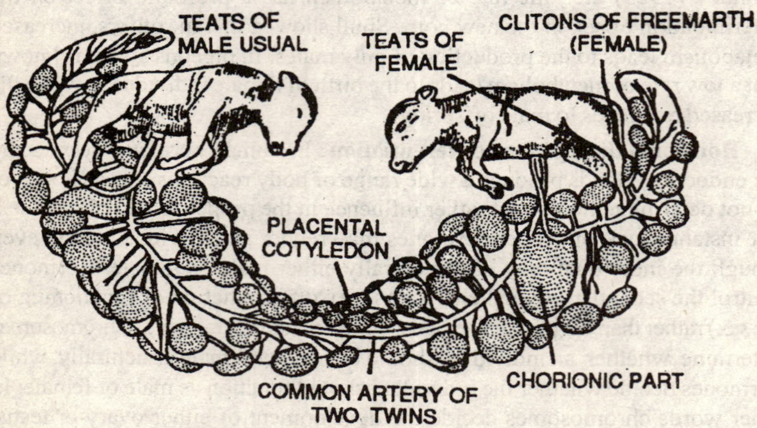

Fig. 15.13 Sex Determination
Free martin cattle

Environmental determination of sex : In certain cases environmental factors rather than chromosomes are known to influence sex as is seen in marine worm *Bonellia,* molluscs *(Crepidula),* daphnids,rotifers, aphids etc. The mechanism of sex determination in *Bonellia* has been studied by Baltzer. The male and female individuals are strikingly dimorphic. The female worm is leaf like and several centimeters long. There is a long probosis extending from the anterior part of the body. The ovaries are distended. The male individual is an extremely minute creature which lives in the reproductive tract of the female. The only function of the male is to fertilize the eggs produced in the ovaries of the female.

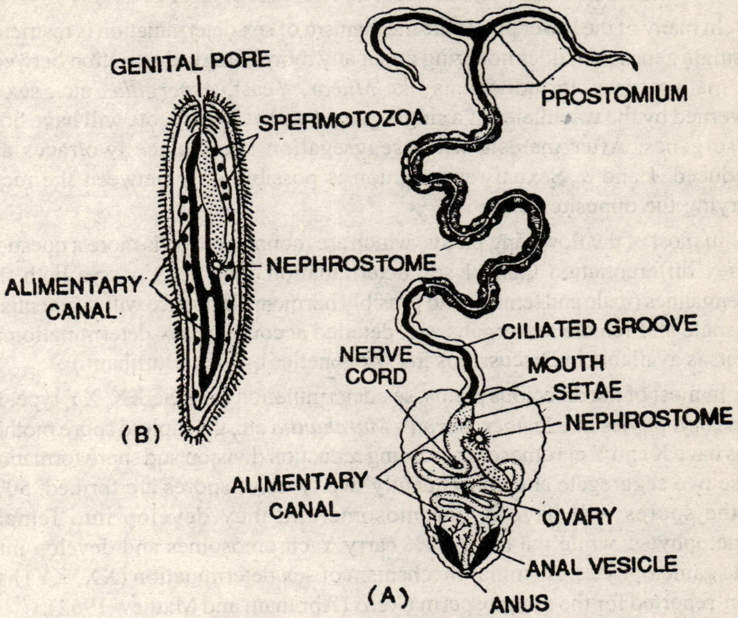

Fig. 15.14 Sex Determination
Mechanism of environmental sex determination in Bonellia

Baltzer discovered that, if a single worm is reared seperately from others, it invariably develops into female, while the worms patched together and released into water containing mature females tend to develop into both male and female worms. Some of the young ones attach themselves to the probosis of the female and obtain nourishment. These become male worms and eventually migrate down to the oviducts. It is assumed that some hormonal secretion at the probosis region in the female transforms the attached young ones into male.

In the marine gastropod *Crepidula plana,* Gould (1912) and Coe (1943) have described environmental influence on sex determination. Young ones reared in isolation tend to develop into females, while those reared in groups in close contact with adults develop into males. This is also traceable to some chemical influence from the adult organisms. Whitney and Shull have reported that in rotifers, by changing oxygen level and nutrition supply, sex changes may be induced. In daphnids, crowded development tends to influence the formation of male individuals as reported by Banta.

MECHANISM OF SEX DETERMINATION IN PLANTS

In many of the lower plants the mechanism of sex determination is restricted to single gene and it does not bring about any morphological variation between the mating types. In individuals like *Mucor*, Yeast, *Aspergillus* etc., sex is governed by the two alleles of a single gene *A* and *a*. The zygote will have both these genes. After meiosis when seggregation takes place two/races are produced *A* and *a*. Sexual reproduction is possible only between the races carrying the opposite genes.

In most of the flowering plants, which are monoecious, it is more a question of sex differentiation than of sex determination. The cells posses both the potentialities (male and female) and possibly hormonal influence will differentiate the male and female sex organs. (A detailed account of sex determination in plants is available in Discussions in Cytogenetics by C.R. Burnham.)

In most of the dioecious plants, sex determination is of the XX, XY type. In some bryophytes like *Sphaerocarpus, Marchantia* etc, the diploid spore mother cells have X and Y chromosomes. During reduction division and spore formation these two seggregate and consequently two types of spores are formed. 50% of the spores will have X chromosome and they develop into female gametophytes, while the other 50% carry Y chromosomes and develop into male gametophytes. A similar mechanism of sex determination (XX, XY) has been-reported for the gymnosperm *Cycas* (Abraham and Mathew 1962).

In the pteridophytic member *Equisetum,* there is a controversey aş to whether the gametophytes are monoecious or dioecious. While Walker (1921) beleives the prothalli to be monoecious, Kashyap (1917) opines that crowded prothalli (growing in a limited area) tend to be dioecious. Joyet Lavergne (1931) has proposed a theory of cytoplasmic sexualization with reference to the sexual behaviour of the spores in *Equisetum.* According to him, the spores of *Equisetum* are morphologically alike, while physiologically different. Spores which have lower oxidising power, and possessing a fat which reduces osmic acid develop into gsmetophytes which form only archegonia (female), while spores with high oxidising power and lacking the fat will tend to develop into gametophytes that from only antheridia (male).

Sex determination in maize : The maize plant is monoecious with both staminate inflorescence (tassel) and pistillate (ear) inflorescence located on the same plant. Many genes which are sex promoting are distributed throughout the ten chromosomes maintaining a balance, so that the tassel produces the pollen and the ear produces the seed.

Many mutants in the sex genes in maize have been identified (Singleton and Jones, 1930). A male sterile gene has been identified on chromosome 6 with the result, the tassel does not produce pollen. Another male sterile gene induces silk (pistil) formation in tassel. These genes render the plants effectively female.

Another gene 'silkless' acts in the opposite direction preventing pistil formation, thus the plant will be staminate.

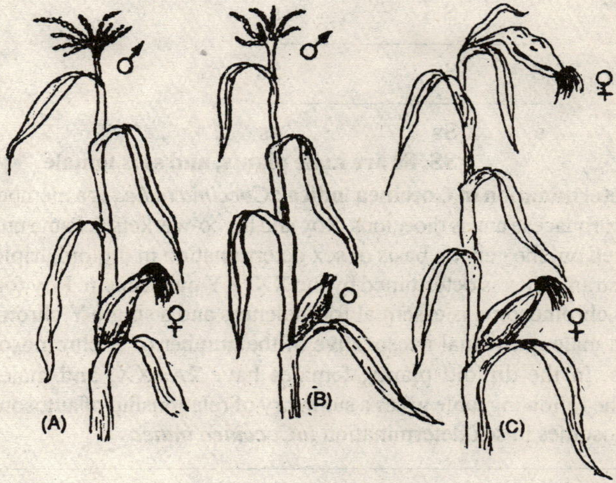

Fig. 15.15 Sex Determination
Genic sex determination in maize

Jones(1930) by genetic analysis came to the conclusion that the sex determination in mutants of maize is due to a single gene. The fertile silk gene (+) mutates and forms a barren gene, sk. The gene in the homozygous condition renders the plant male, by eliminating the ears. On the other hand another gene (recessive) ts, in the homozygous condition transforms the tassel into a functional pistillate structure. The genotype ++, ts ts, would be pistillate, while, sk sk.ts ts would be staminate.

Monogenic sex determination in Asparagus : *Asparagus* is a dioecious plant, with staminate and pistillate plants occuring in equal numbers. In some rare instances, female flowers bear rudimentary anthers and staminate flowers bear rudimentary pistils. Very rarely the pistils of staminate flowers may produce seeds (Rick and Hanna). When these seeds are raised into plants there was a ratio of 3:1 male and female plants respectively. When the male plants raised thus are used to pollinate pistillate flowers on female plants, one third produced only male plants and two thirds showed seggregation into male and female indicating the control of a single gene. The genetic explanation is as follows. Sex is controlled by a pair of alleles S and s. S gene produces maleness and apparently all male plants are heterozygous (S/s), while female plants are homozygous recessive (ss).

Ss (Rare male plant)
Selfing

	S	s
S	SS	Ss
s	Ss	ss

SS, Ss are male plants, and ss is female

Sex determination in Coccinea indica : *Coccinia indica* is a member of the family Cucurbitaceae and is dioecious. Roy and his co-workers at Patna university have worked out the genetic basis of sex determination in diploid, triploid and tetraploid strains. Sex is determined by the XX, XY mechanism. Roy found out that, the Y chromosome is essential for maleness and a single Y chromosome results in a male individual irrespective of the number of X chromosomes or autosomes. In the diploid plants, females have 2A+XX, and males have 2A+XY.The following table gives a summary of relationship of autosomes and sex chromosomes in sex determination *inCoccinea indica.*

Genome Constitution	Sex	Ratio of sex chromosomes to autosomes.
Diploid		
2A + XX	Female	**1.00**
2A + XY	Male	**0.50**
2a + xxy	Male	**0.50**
Triploid		
3A + XXY	Male	**0.67**
3A + XXX	Female	**1.00**
Tetraploid		
4A + XXXX	Female	**1.00**
4A + XXYY	Male	**0.75**

Sex determination in Melandrium : The mechanism - of Sex determination in *Melandrium album* has been studied by Warmke (1946). Here also irrespective of the number of X chromosomes and autosomes, one or more Y chromosomes would render the individual male, and in the absence of Y chromosome, the individual becomes female. Only when the ratio between X and Y reaches 4:7, some effects of femaleness could be discerned inspite of the presence of Y. The number of autosomes do not seem to have an effect on the expression of sex. Like *coccinea*, in *Melandrium* also, individuals are either diploid, triploid or tetraploid. The following table gives the details of sex expression with different numbers of X chromosomes and autosome sets.

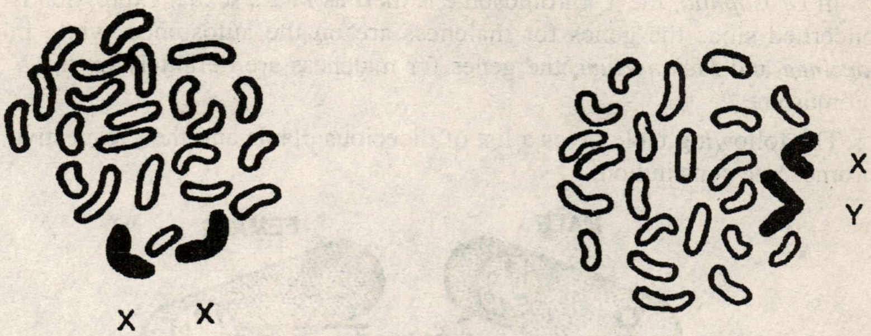

Fig. 15.16 Sex Determination
Chromosmal sex determination in Melandrium

Genome Constitution	Sex	Ratio of X/A
Diploid		
2A + XX	Female	**1.00**
2A + XY	Male	**0.50**
2A + XXY	Male	**1.00**
Triploid		
3A + XXY	Male	**0.67**
Tetraploid		
4A + XY	Male	**0.50**
4A + XY	Male	**0.25**
4A + XXXY	Male, occasional bisexual	**0.75**
4A + XXXXY	Hermaphrodite (occasionally male)	**1.00**

The details of geneic control in *Melandrium* as shown by Warmke indicate that the Y chromosome is longer than the X chromosome. Plants in which the X and Y chromosomes were fragmented were studied and as a result it was found out that both the chromosomes had five different segments. These segments are known to control the different stages of development of sex organs. Segment IV is common between X and Y chromosomes and it is this that helps in pairing and regular disjunction during meiosis. The other segments on Y chromosome supress femaleness and initiate and control anther development. The X chromosome has a segment V promoting femaleness.

In *Drosophila,* the Y chromosome is inert as far as sexual expression is concerned since the genes for maleness are on the autosomes, while in *Coccinea* and *Melandrium*, the genes for maleness are definitely on the Y chromosome.

The following table gives a list of dioecious plants and their respective chromosome constitution.

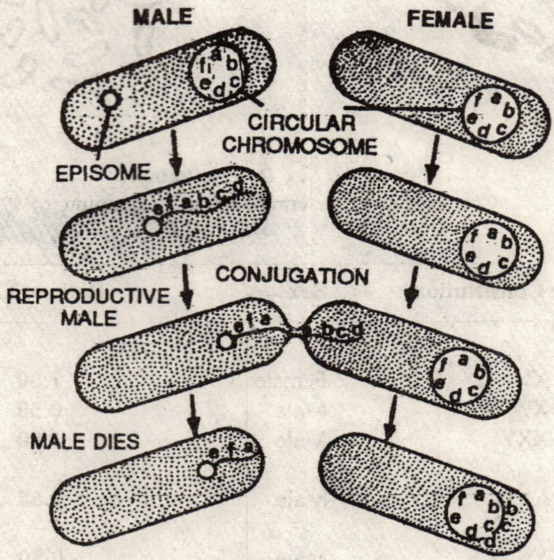

Fig. 15.17 Sex Determination
Mechanism of sex determination in bacteria

	Plants	Mechanism of sex
1.	*Humulus lupulus*	Male heterogametic
	Melandrium album	(XX, XY)
	Rumex angiocarpus	
2.	*Populus spp Salix* spp,	Male heterogametic
	Smilax spp	(nor confirmed)
3.	*Vallisneria spiralis*	Male heterogametic
	Dioscorea sinuata	(XO – male, XX female)
4.	*Phoradendron flavescens*	Male heterogametic
	Phoradendron villosum	(male has an extra chromosome)

	Plants	Mechanism of sex
5.	*Fragaria elatior*	Female heterogametic (male XX, female XY)
6.	*Rumex acetosa*	Compound chromosomes
	Humulus japonicus	(male $Y_1 XY_2$, female XX)
7.	*Spinacia oleracea*	
	Ribes alpinum	
	Vitis cinerea	
	Vitis rupestris	Not sex chromosomes are found, Autosomal genes control sex.
	Vitis vinifera	
	Carica papaya	
	Asparagus officinalis	
	Bryonia indica	

Sex determination in Bacteria : During conjugation one of the bacterial cells acts as male and the other female. A portion of the chromosome from male is passed on to the female. In all the male bacteria, there is a structure called episome, which is abseat in females. Male cells arise by division of the pre existing ones, or when the episome gets into a female cell.

16

SEX LINKED INHERITANCE

The laws of inheritance as propounded by Mendel indicate that reciprocal crosses always yield the same result in hermaphrodite individuals. In other words in a cross between tall and dwarf plants the resultant offspring would be tall irrespective of the fact whether tall parent is male or female. This means that tallness or dwarfness are inherited irrespective of the sex of the individual and obviously the genes responsible for these characters must be situated on the autosomes. On the other hand there are certain characters which seem to be associated with a particular sex or sex chromosome and such characters are not inherited in the same pattern in reciprocal classes.

The genes (characters) in individuals then may be classified under two categories - these are a) characters which do not show any difference in inheritance pattern in reciprocal classes and b) characters which are inherited differently in reciprocal crosses. The characters of the first category are on the autosomes, while those of the second category are on the sex chromosomes. Such characters which are located on the sex chromosomes are called sex linked characters (sex linked genes) and the inheritance is called **sex linked inheritance.** In sex linked inheritance a particular character always follows a particular sex chromosome as the gene for the former is located on the latter.

Discovery of sex linked characters : The name of TH. Morgan (1910) ranks first among the pioneers who have studied the inheritance pattern of sex linked genes. One of the earliest known sex linked characters is hemophilia which appeared only in the males of Royal family of Spain. In hemophilia, the blood fails to clot on exposure to air (it should normally clot). But it was not known that hemophilia is a sex linked character. It was just thought to be a heriditary character. Morgan who was working on sex linked characters in *Drosophila melanogaster* like the red and white eye, opined that hemophilia is also a sex linked character.

Chromosomes and sex linked characters : In order to understand the pattern of inheritance of sex linked characters, one should understand the inheritance pattern of sex chromosomes themselves. Among organisms exhibiting sex linked characters there are two sex chromosomes X and Y. They are genetically identical only partially. When males are the heterogametic sex they have XY and the females XX and when females are heterogametic they have XY (ZW) and the male XX (ZZ). At the time of gametogenesis (meiosis) when pairing takes place between X and Y, crossing over is restricted to genetically identical regions only. The genes located in such regions may get exchanged and they do no seem to follow a particular chromosome. Such genes are said to be partially sex linked. Whereas the genes which are located on the non homologous regions of X and Y chromosomes do not get exchanged and they always follow a particular chromosome. These are said to be of the following types.

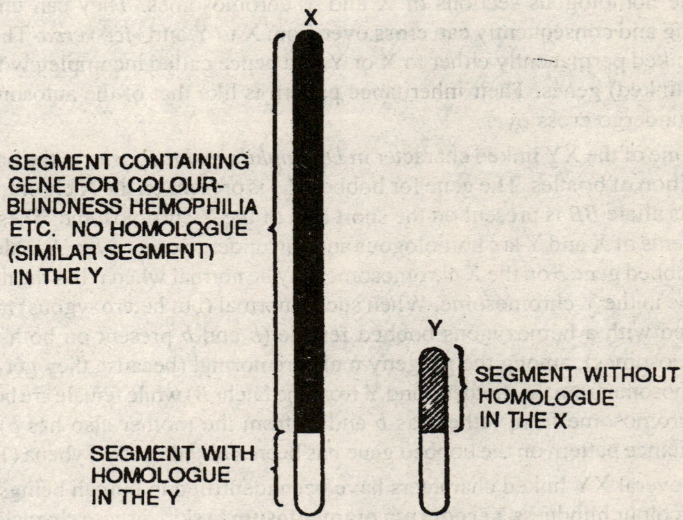

Fig. 16.1 Sex Linked Inheritance
Sex Chromosomes

1. **Holandric genes :** The genes situated on the differential region of the Y chromosome which do not participate in any cross over with the X chromosome are called holandric genes. Holandric genes are exclusive to males as they do not have their counterparts on the X chromosome These are inherited directly from male to male (Father to Son). The Y linkedcharacters in man are hypertrichosis (hair on the ear pinna), Ichthyosis hystrix etc and are known to be exclusive to males (Burns 1969).

X linked genes : The genes located on the differential euchromatic region of the X, which do not have their alleles on the corresponding region on the Y chromosome are called X linked or sex linked genes. They are not limited to one sex unlike the holandric genes. They are present in both male and females, following the particular X chromosome. Sex linked or X linked genes are many and they are much more wide spread than the holandric genes.

Sex linkage may be classified into the following categories, depending upon which chromosome carries the genes. They are -

1. XY linked characters (genes)
2. Y linked characters (genes)
3. X linked characters (genes)

Inheritance of XY linked genes : The genes which are XY linked are present on the homologous sections of X and Y chromosomes. They can undergo pairing and consequently can cross over from X to Y and *vice versa.* They are not linked permanently either to X or Y and hence called incompletely linked (XY linked) genes. Their inheritance pattern is like that of the autosomes as they undergo cross over.

One of the XY linked character in *Drosophila melanogaster* is the **bobbed** condition of bristles. The gene for bobbed, *bb* is present on the X chromosome and its allele *BB* is present on the short arm of the Y chromosome. These two segments of X and Y are homologous and can undergo cross over. A male with the bobbed gene *b* on the X chromosome may be normal when it has the normal *B* gene in the Y chromosome. When such a normal (but heterozygous) male is crossed with a homozygous bobbed female (*b* and *b* present on both the X chromosomes), among the progeny male are normal (because they get the X chromosome from the mother *b* and Y from the fatehr *B*) while female are bobbed (X chromosome from father has *b* and X from the mother also has *b*). The inheritance pattern on the bobbed gene has been worked out by Sybena (1972).

Several XY linked characters have been identified in human beings also. Total colour blindness **Xeroderma pigmentosum** (a skin disease characterised by dry patches on the skin upon exposure of light). **Epidermalysis bullosa, Retinitis pigmentosa** (a progressive degeneration of retina, accompanied by pigment deposition in the eye) certain forms of nephritis, spastic paraplegia etc., are known to the XY linked genes.

Inheritance of Y linked Characters : As has already been pointed out, some genes are exclusively linked to Y chromosome. A few instance of these in man are -(a) **porcupine man** in whom the entire surface of the skin will be warty and coarse (Ichthyosis hystrix), (b) **hypertrichosis** hair on the lobes of the ear, (c) **Kerotoma dissipatum** skin disorder affecting the hand and feet (d) Occurrence of Webbed toes in some individuals etc.

In plants, the Y chromosome contains genes for maleness and its absence induces sterelity. Unfortunately not much detail is available on the Y linked somatic characters in plants.

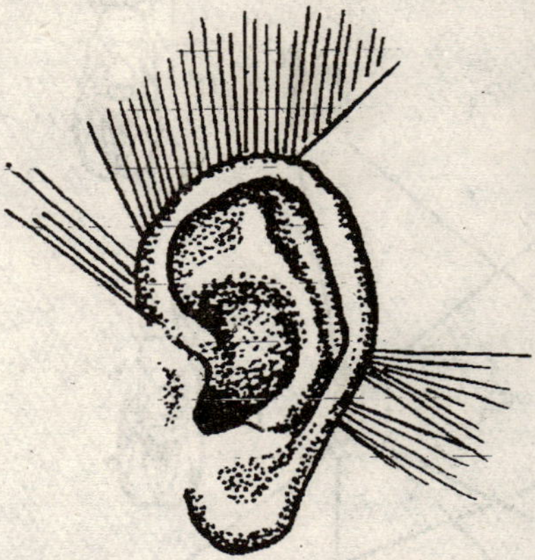

Fig. 16.2 Sex Linked Inheritance
Hypertrichosis on human ear pinna

Inheritance of sex linked or X linked genes : The genes or characters linked to the X chromosome are generally termed sex linked as they are the most prevalent sex linked characters. In order to understand the pattern of inheritance of X linked characters one should understand the inheritance pattern of the X chromosome.

In female individuals (which are homogametic) there will be two X chromosomes, while the males (which are heterogametic) have only one X chromosome in the body cells. During reproduction the eggs wll have only one X chromosome where as the sperms will be 50% X and 50% Y. When an egg is fertilized by an X sperm the resultant female (XX) individual will have one X from the mother and the other X from the father. When a Y sperm fertilizes the egg the resultant male offspring will get its X chromosome from the mother and Y from the father. In other words the X chromosome of male offspring always goes to the daughter. In the next generation the X chromosome of the male individual again goes to the female (daughter). In this way an X chromosome and the genes linked with it will alternatively go to male and to female. The following chart summarises, the above explanation.

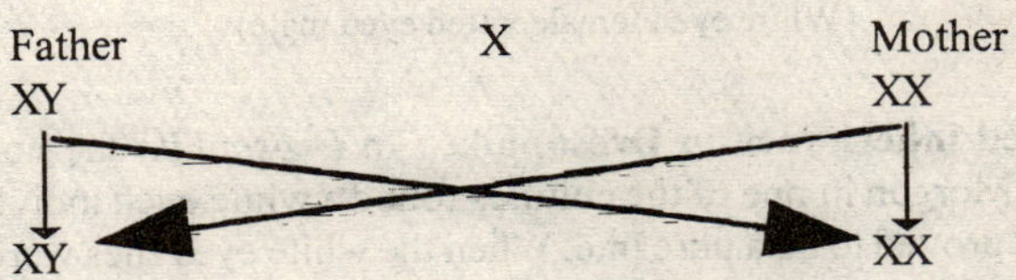

This type of inheritance of X chromosome which alternatively finds place in the male and female generations is called the **criss cross inheritance.** We shall study a few examples of this type of inheritance in *Drosophila,* cats, poultry and man.

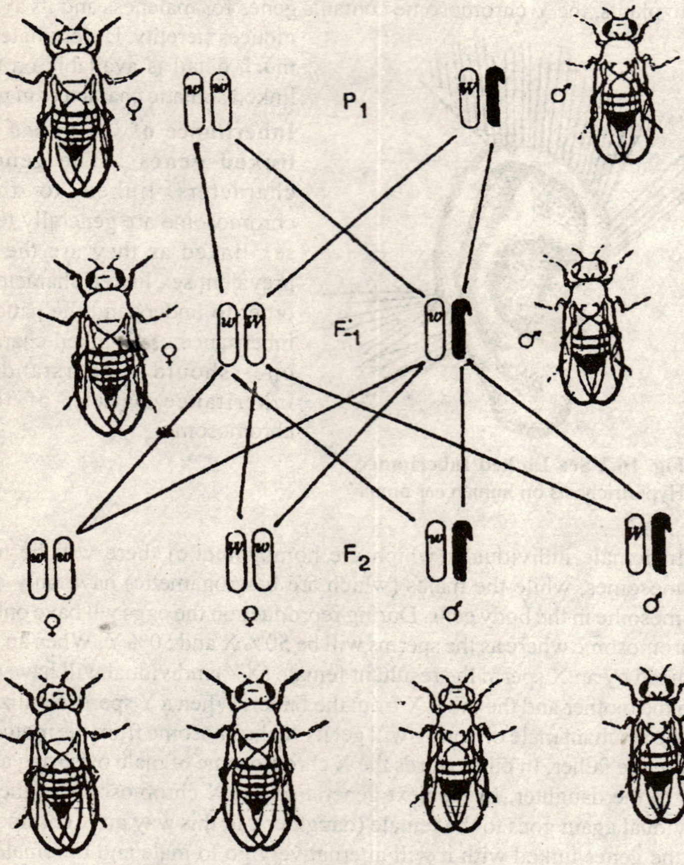

Fig. 16.3 Sex Linked Inheritance
Mechanism of Sex linked Inheritance in Drosophila
(White eyed female x Red eyed male)

Sex linked inheritance in Drosophila : In *Drosophila* the normal eye colour is red. Morgan in one of the cultures found a white eyed individual. On breeding, this proved to be a pure line. When the white eyed flies were crossed over with the wild (red) type, the results of reciprocal crosses were different i.e. white male x red female; white female x red male. The result seemed to be dependent on the sex of the parent through which the trait was introduced into the cross rather than following the Mendelian pattern. Morgan assumed this to be due to the sex linked character of the gene for eye colour. The gene for normal eye colour (red) W is present on the X chromosome. White eye colour is a recessive gene occupying the same locus (w). Hence for white eye colour to appear in the females the genes should be double homozygous (should be present on both the X chromosomes). In the heterozygous condition in femele (Ww) one X carries the W (red) gene, while the other X carries the w (white) gene. Phenotypically the heterozygous females are red eyed, but they are called **carriers** as they carry the recessive gene. The males however can not be carriers, for the gene for red or white being present on the only one X chromosome they have, their genotype and phenotype are one and the same. Even a single dose of the recessive gene (w) is enough to produce the white eye colour. This can be understood by the reciprocal crosses as follows.

1. Red eyed male X White eyed female : When a red eyed male *(Wo)* is crossed to a white eyed female *(ww)*, in the F_1 generation all the females would be red eyed and all the male individuals are white eyed. This is because the white eyed recessive gene is present on both the X chromosomes in the female parent. The F_1 male offspring gets its X *(w)* from the mother and Y from the father. Since Y chromosome does not carry the gene for eye colour the individual would be white eyed. The female offspring (F_1) having got one X (W) from the father and one X (w) from the mother would be heterozygous (Ww) genetifcally, but phenotypically show red eye colour. When the F_1 heterozygous female is crossed with the white eyed F_1 male, in the F_2 generation both red and white eyed (1:1) individuals are found in the female individuals, while in the male progeny also-red and white eyed individuals appear in equal proportion.

Red eyed female X White eyed male

When a pure red eyed female (WW) is crossed with a white eyed male *(wo)*, the F_1 offspring will have both females and males red eyed. The females however are carriers (heterozygous) as they have both *Ww* genes on their two X chromosomes. When these two F_1 individuals are crossed (heterozygous red eyed female x white eyed male), among the female (F_2) progeny (1) 50% will be red eyed (heterozygous) (2)50% will be white eyed (homozygous double recessive). Among the male progeny (3) 50% will be red eyed and (4) 50% white eyed. The genotype of these flies will be as follows.

(1) Red eyed female *(Ww)*
(2) White eyed female (*ww*)
(3) Red eyed male *(Wo* indicates Y chromosome which has no gene for eye colour)
(4) White eyed male *(wo)*

Sex linked lethal in Drosophila : Several crosses have indicated the presence of a lethal gene on the X chromosome of *Drosophila.* This recessive lethal can be tolerated in the female in the heterozygous condition, but the males with the lethal gene do not survive. When a female heterozygous for lethal *(Li)* is crossed to a normal male *(Lo)*, among the F_1 progeny of females and males, all females survive (50% females are completely normal and 50% heterozygous). Among the male progeny however 50% are normal *(Lo)* and survive, while the other 50% *(lo)* getting their X (*l*) chromosome from the mother die. Hence the ratio would be 3:1 females to males.

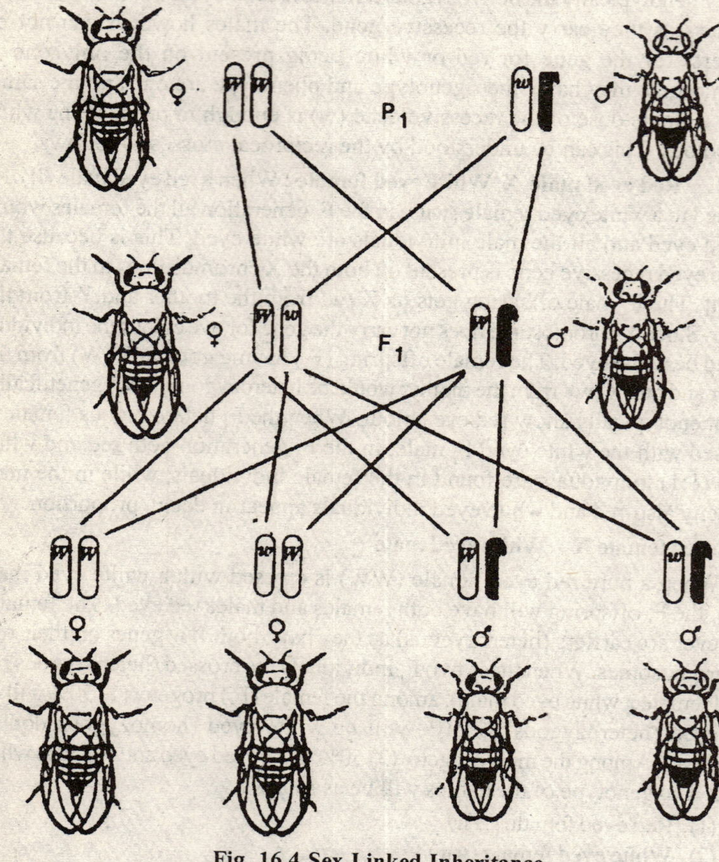

Fig. 16.4 Sex Linked Inheritance
Mechanism of Sex Linked Inheritance in Drosophila
(Red eyed female x White eyed male)

Morgan has indicated that at least about 140 characters in *Drosophila* may be sex linked, whose, genes are to be found on the X chromosome.

Sex linked inheritance in cats : The coat colour inheritance in tortoise shell cats is known to be sex linked. The tortoise shell coat colour is found only in females and is characterised by the presence of patches of black, yellow and white pigments in the skin. Tortoise shell cats maybe produced by crossing black homozygous female *(BB)*, with yellow male cats *(bo)*, the F_1 progeny will be heterozygous *(Bb)* and has tortoise shell coat. Here the gene for black *(B)* is not completely dominant over yellow (b). In a reciprocal cross also involving a yellow female *(bb)* and a black male *(Bo)*, the F_1 progeny females have tortoise shell coat *(Bb)*. Occasionally male cats are also found to have tortoise shell coat. But these males are sterile and they apparently have two X chromosomes and one Y chromosome (XXY = *Bbo)*. The presence of two. X chromosomes may be explained on the basis of non disjunction of X chromosomes during division. As a result an egg carries one set of autosomes and two X chromosomes.

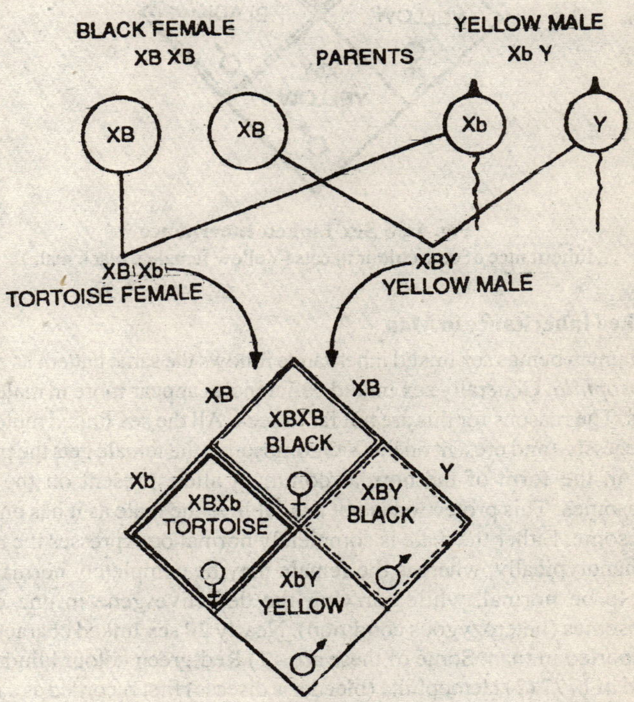

Fig. 16.5 Sex Linked Inheritance
Inheritance of coat colour in cats (Black female x yellow male)

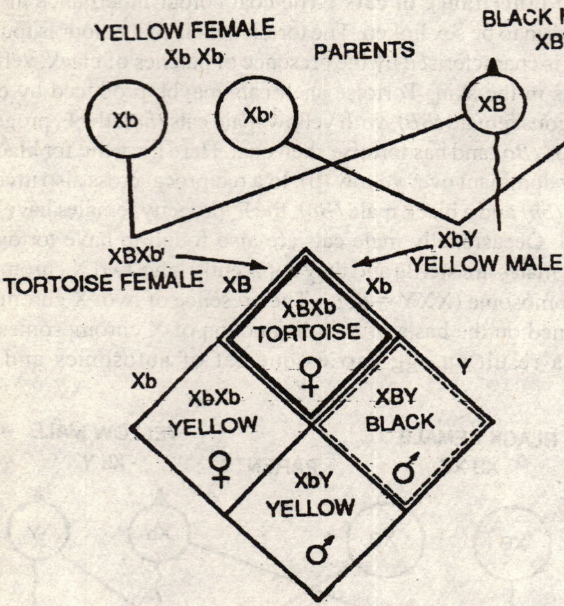

Fig. 16.6 Sex Linked Inheritance
Inheritance of coat colour in cats (Yellow female x black male)

Sex linked inheritance in Man

In human beings sex linked inheritance follows the same pattern as explained for *Drosophila.* Generally sex linked deficiencies appear more in males than in females. The reasons for this are not far to seek. All the sex linked mutant genes being recessive and present on the X chromosome, the female gets the protection readily in the form of the normal dominant allele present on the other X chromosomes. This protection is not available to the male as it has only one X chromosome. Either the male is completely normal or expresses the recessive gene phenotypically, whereas the female may be completely normal or may appear to be normal, while carrying the defective gene in one of the X chromosomes (heterozygous condition). Nearly 20 sex linked characters have been reported in man. Some of these are - 1) Red-green colour blindness first reported in 1777 (2) Hemophilia (bleeder's disease) first recorded as a heritable character in 1793 (3) Optic atrophy (degenerating disease of the optic nerve). (4) Juvenile glaucoma (hardening of the eye ball) (5) Myopia (short sight) (6) Defective iris (7) Juvenile muscular dystrophy (degenerating disease of muscles)

(8) Distichiasis (double eye lashes) (9) Mitral stenosis (Abnormal mitral valve of the heart (10) Mystagmus (involuntary oscillation of the eye ball (II) baldness and (12) Epidermal cysts. We shall study the inheritance pattern of a few of these traits.

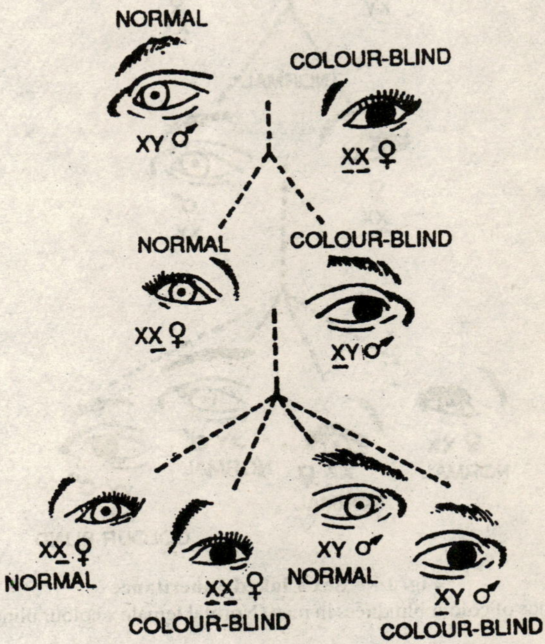

Fig. 16.7 Sex Linked Inheritance
Inheritance of colour blindness in man (Normal male x colour blind female)

Inheritance of Hemophilia : Commonly called bleeder's disease, this refers to a condition, where blood on exposure to air will not clot, as a result hemophilic individuals may bleed to death even at the slightest injury. Hemophilia is a sex linked trait offen associated with males, females being very rare, (but genetically possible). The failure of the blood to clot is due to the absence of a protein antihemophilia globulin, which is normally present in the blood of man. Hemophilic individuals lack this, as a result bleeding, when occurs may prolong for 1/2 hour to 20 hrs., leading to the death of the individual if proper measures are not taken. The production of the coagulating substance is governed by a gene present on the X chromosome. In Hemophilics, this wild gene would have undergone mutation resulting in a hemophilic gene.

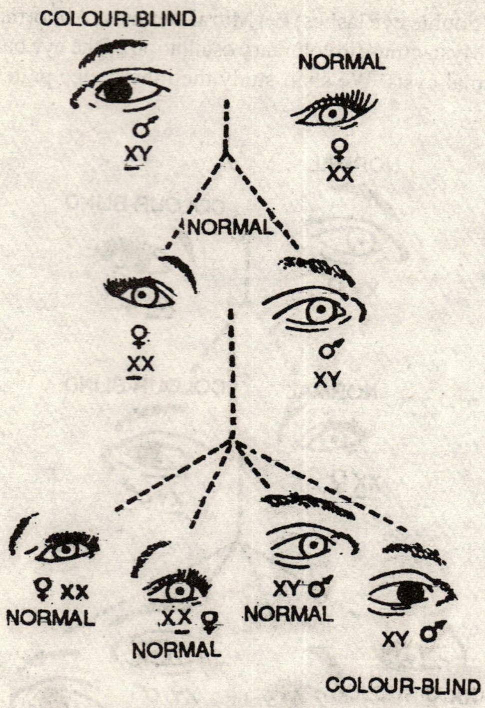

Fig. 16.8 Sex Linked Inheritance
Inheritance of colour blindness in man (Normal female x colour blind male)

Hemophilia gained some notoriety in the past as the Royal disease, as some members of British royalty were hemophilics. One of the well known victims of the disease was the great grandson of queen Victoria who died due to an injury and subsequent non stop bleeding.

As has already been pointed out, hemophilia is found predominantly in males, but the inheritance is criss cross-from father to daughter to grandson. The interesting feature is the females generally do not suffer, but they will be carriers. Hemophilia can manifest in females only in double recessive condition. Such an individual dies before adolscence. The chances of random mating producing a hemophilic are extremely rare (in males it is about 1 in 10,000); it is estimated that if all the hemophilic males survive and undergo random mating, the mathematical probability of a homozygous female would be equal to the square of 10,000 or 1 in 1,00,00,000. The genetic manifestation of hemophilic gene is as follows.

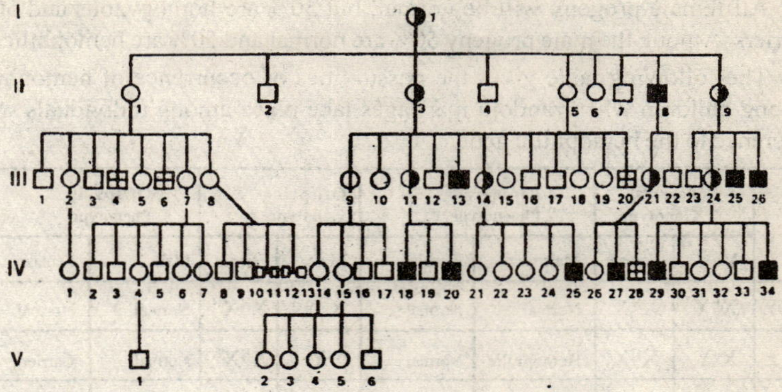

Fig. 16.9 Sex Linked Inheritance
Pedigree of haemophilics in the descendants of Queen Victoria

The hemophilic gene is a recessive allele of the wild gene situated on the X chromosome only. There is no allele for this on the Y chromosome. Hence no cross over is possible between XY for hemophilia. If we denote the normal gene as H and hemophilic gene as h, the genetic constitution of different individuals will be as follows

	Normal	**Hemophilic**	**Carriers (Heterozygous)**
Male	X^HY	X^hY	
Female	X^H, X^H	X^h, Xh	X^H, X^h

Let us study the inheritance pattern by studying a hypothetical example. When a hemophilic man marries a completely normal woman, the following are the progenies produced.

Normal Woman X Hemophilic Man

X^HX^H X^h, Y

X^HX^h, (Female) X^HY (Male)

All the progeny will be normal but the females are carriers. When these two progenies marry among themselves, the further progeny will be as follows.

X^HX^H, X^HX^h, X^HY, X^hY

Female Male

All female progeny will be normal; but 50% are homogyzous and 50% carriers. Among the male progeny 50% are normal and 50% are hemophilics.

The following table gives the possibilities of occurrence of hemophilia among children when random marriages take place among individuals with reference to the hemophilic gene.

	Parents Genotype		Parents Pheenotype		Offspring Genotype		Offspring Phenotype	
	Male	Female	Male	Female	Male	Female	Male	Female
1.	X^HY	X^HX^H	Normal	Normal	X^HY^H	X^HX^H	Normal	Normal
2.	X^hY	X^HX^H	Hemophilic	Normal	X^HY	X^HX^h	Normal	Carrier
3.	X^HY	X^HXh	Normal	Carrier	X^HY	XHX^H	Normal	Normal
4.	X^hY	X^hXh	Hemophilic	Carrier	X^HY	X^HXh	Normal	Carrier
5.	X^HY	X^hX^h	Normal	Hemophilic	X^hY	X^HX^h	Hemophilic	
6.	X^hY	X^hX^h	Hemophilic	Hemophilic	X^hY	X^hX^h	Hemophilic	Hemophilic

Note

1. X denotes X chromosome; Y denotes Y chromosome
2. X^H denotes normal dominant gene on X chromosome

   X^h denotes hemophilic gene on X chromosome
3. Normal female means homozygous

   Carrier means heterozygous; normal phenotypically
4. Homozygous hemophilic female individuals do not survive beyond adolscence. Crosses involving them (5 and 6) are only hypothetical.

Colour blindness in Human beings : The red and green colour blindness is another sex linked recessive trait in man. Individuals suffering from this defect will not be able to distinguish between various shades of red and green and hence are colour blind.

Individually red colour blindness is called **Protanopia** and green colour blindness is called **Deuteranopia.** Ishihara has designed a colour chart to identify these defects. It has been shown that the gene for colour blindness is a recessive allele of normal vision and is situated on the X chromosome. Like any sex linked defect, colour blindness also is more prevalent among males than among females. The Y chromosome does not carry any allele for vision.

A survey for colour blindness has not been conducted in our country, but the data available from USA give a figure of 8% for male and 0.5% for female in the total population. The following chart gives all the possible mating types and the possible progeny for colour blindness among human beings.

	Parents Genotype		Parents Phenotype		Offspring Genotype		Offspring Phenotype		Total Offspring	
	Female	Male	Female	Male	Female	Male	Female	Male	Female	Male
1.	X^NX^N	X^NY	Normal	Normal	X^NX^N	X^NY	Normal	Normal	50	50
2.	X^NX^N	X^nY	Normal	Colour blind	X^NX^n	X^nY	Carrier	Normal	50	50
3.	X^NX^n	X^nY	Carrier	Normal	X^NX^n X^NX^N	X^NY X^nY	Normal Carrier	Normal Colour blind	25 25	25 25
4.	X^NX^n	X^nY	Carrier	Colour blind	X^NX^n X^nX^n	X^NY X^nY	Carrier Colour blind	Normal Colour blind	25 25	25 25
5.	X^nX^n	X^NY	Colour blind	Normal	X^NX^n	X^n Y	Carrier	Colour blind	50	50
6.	X^nX^n	X^nY	Colour blind	Colour blind	X^nX^n	X^nY	Colour blind	Colour blind	50	50

Note

1. X denotes X chromosome and Y denotes Y chromosome
2. X^N denotes normal dominant gene on the X chromosome
   X^n denotes recessive allele (colour blind gene) on X chromosome
3. Normal female is homozygous. Carrier female is heterozygous.

In all individuals where sex determining mechanism follows that of man or *Drosophilia* (male being heterogametic and sex linked, recessive gene being located only on the X chromosome) the following are the salient features of its manifestation.

1. Sex linked recessive traits are phenotypically expressed more often in males than in females.
2. The trait appears among the female progeny only when it is found in the male parent.
3. The trait seldom is found both in father and son. It may be the case, when mother is hmozygous.
4. The inheritance of the sex linked recessive gene is from father to daughter to grand son.

Dominant sex linked character in Man : These characters are very few. One of the dominant sex linked genes producing a defective enamel of the teeth has been found in man. The gene for this is also located on the X chromosome.

Sex linked characters in Poultry

In birds (including poultry), moths, butterflies and certain other animals where (females are the heterogametic sex, a different kind of sex linkage exists. The mechanism is exactly opposite to what is seen in *Drosophila,* Man etc., where male is the heterogametic sex.

The inheritance of barred plumage in poultry birds is a classical example of sex linked inheritance where males are heterogametic. In poultry birds, females have only one X chromosome (XO -O indicates absence of another X chromosome), whereas males have 2 X chromosomes.

The barred plumage feathers are banded with, bars of black on a white background. The gene for barred character is a dominant allele and is dominant over black or non barred plumage. Let us study the results of reciprocal crosses (Barred male X Black female and Barred female X black male).

Barred male X Black female

When a barred male (BB) is crossed with a black female (bo), the F_1 progeny will have only barred individuals both male and female. The males however are heterozygous for barred condition (Bb) and the females have only one barred gene as they have one X chromosome Bo). When these two F_1 birds are crossed among themselves the following progeny are obtained.

1. Barred male (Homozygous BB)
2. Barred male (Heterozygous Bb)
3. Barred female (Bo)
4. Black female (bo)

Among the male progeny all are barred, however 50% of them are homozygous and the rest heterozygous. Among the female progeny 50% are barred and 50% black.

Barred female x Black male

When a black homozygous male bird (bb) is crossed with a barred female (Bo), among the F_1 progeny, the males are barred (heterozygous Bb), while the females are black as they get their only X chromosome from the male parent which is black (b). When these F_1 birds are bred among themselves, the following gametes are obtained. The barred male F_1 produces two types of sperms B and b, while the F_1 female also produces two types of eggs - one carrying the lone X chromosome carrying the b gene and the other carrying no sex chromsome *(o)*.

On random mating the progenies shown below are obtained.

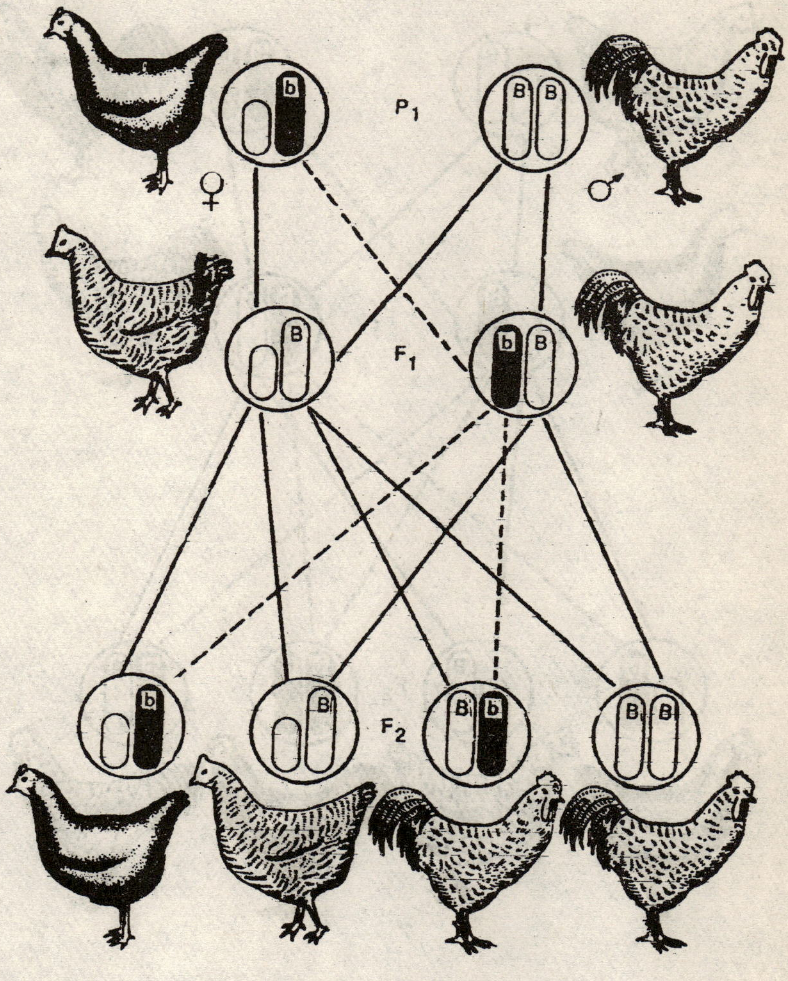

Fig. 16.10 Sex Linked Inheritance

Inheritance of plumage in poultry (Barred male x black female)

1. Barred male (Heterozygous Bb)
2. Black male (Homozygous bb)
3. Barred female (Bo)
4. Black female (bo)

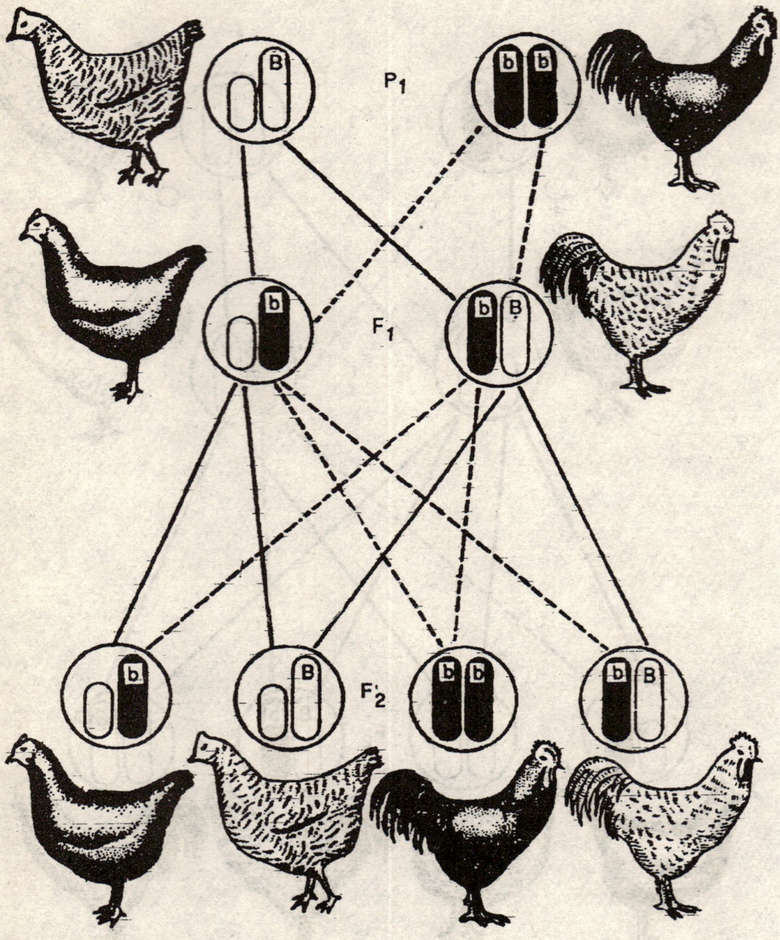

Fig. 16.11 Sex Linked Inheritance
Inheritance of plumage in poultry (Barred female x black male)

Among the F_2 progeny 50% males are barred, and 50% black and among the females of F_2 50% barred and 50% black.

Salient features of barred plumage inheritance

1. Unlike in *Drosophila,* man etc. the female is the heterogametic sex, but it does not have XY but only X, designated as XO.

2. The barred gene is domimant and is not a recessive mutant of the normal as is the case in most of the sex linked traits in *Drosophila.*

3. Male is a carrier for the barred gene (heterozygous) while the female has to phenotypically express whether a barred or black gene as it has only one X chromosome.

Significance of sex linked characters in birds : When the phenotype and genotype of the parents are known, the sex of the newly hatched can be determined by looking at their plumage pattern.

Sex influenced genes (traits)

A particular type of baldness called **pattern baldness** is quite common among human males. Here the hair is removed from the centre of the head, while the hair growth is normal on the sides. This was first thought to be a sex linked recessive character as males are more prone to this, while pattern baldness in females is extremely rare. But investigations showed clearly that the pattern of inheritance of baldness does not follow the sex linked pattern, for often a son can inherit pattern baldness from the father. The gene for pattern baldness is not situated on the X chromosome but on the autosomes. *However the same gene behaves as recessive in females, but as dominant in males.* Hence while only one gene is enough to produce baldness in males, two such genes are required for bladness in females. It seems a single gene can function only in the presence of the male hormone. In females, the absence of the male hormone suppresses the single gene from functioning. However when two genes are there they find the phenotypic expression. Such genes, which find expression only in one sex, but not linked to the sex chromosomes are called **sex influenced genes** (traits). Sex influenced genes should not bemistaken with sex linked genes for they are not situated on the X chromosome. They are also not holandric (situated on the Y chromosome) even though they are expressed predominatly in males. They are autosomal genes, whose phenotypic expression is aided by the male hormone. The genotype and phenotype of males and females with reference to pattern baldness is as follows.

Normal male	H^NH^N
Bald male	H^NH^n, H^nH^n
Normal female	H^NH^N, H^NH^n
Bald female	H^nH^n

Note

In both males and females, there are two alleles for the gene for hair growth. N-normal, n - bald gene. The genes are not sex linked.

An interesting case of pattern baldness in man being influenced by male hormone is that of an under sexed man, who took injections of male hormones to regain masculinity, but lost his hair. Evidently this man was heterozygous for the bald gene. In the-under sexed condition, the single gene could not express itself in the absence of enough quantity of male hormone. With the injection of the male hormone, the man regained his masculinity, but the single bald gene found phenotypic expression in the new environment and he lost his hair.

Another instance of sex influenced gene in man is that of length of the index finger. In normal cases the index finger is as long or longer than the fourth (ring) finger. But in some cases the index Finger is shorter than the forth Finger. This is due to amutant gene, which again is dominant in male and recessive in female.

Sex limited genes : They are genes responsible for the production of traits in any one sex; which are apparently secondary sexual characters. They are different from sex linked characters, because they are found on the autosomes and not on the sex chromosomes. They are aslo different from sex influenced characters in that, they (sex limited) are found'in. only one sex (either male or female), and there is no genetic possibility of finding expression in both the sexes. Sex influenced characters on the other hand can find expression in both the sexes under suitable genetic conditions (homozygous in females; homozygous or heterozygous in males) even though they are predominantly found in one sex. Sex limited characters are exclusively limited to one sex (male or female). The antlers in deer is a typical example of sex limited character. Females do not have the antlers. We shall study some well known examples of sex limited characters. Development of beard in males, breast development in females are typical examples of sex limited characters in man. A woman normally does not have a beard but genes for beard growth must be present, because a man can inherit these and can get facial hair. In rare instances, abnormalities in hormone secretion may influence these genes to express themselves. But here again, these are different from sex influenced genes, because in the latter, if suitable genes are present in female, even though there is no hormonal abnormality sex influenced character may appear. In sex limited characters even though genes are present, only a hormonal abnormality can produce an abnormal secondary sexual character (facial hair in women and breasts in man).

Another well known example of sex limited character is the high milk producing trait in cattle. Investigations have shown that the bull also carries genes for high milk production just like the cattle, but it does not find expression. This can be tested by a cross in which the same cow is bred with two bulls. The offspring in one case had a high yielding capacity, while in the other it was less. In these two cases, the mother was same, but the fathers were different indicating that they also carry genes for milk production. But the genes for milk production find expression only in female.

Sex limited genes in invertebrates : Colour pattern in male and female butterflies is an example of sex limited genes. In clover butterfly, the males are always yellow, but the females may be either yellow or white. The gene for white is dominant, but it can express itself only in females. The females are YY or Yy (white homozygous or heterozygous) when white and yy when yellow. However all the three genotypes are yellow in males.

Sex limited genes in birds : Sex limited traits produce a variety *of* sexual dimorphism in birds, so much so they can be distinguished merely on their morphology. In the male pheasant or pea cock, the plumage is brilliantly coloured, as a contrast to the drab plumage of females. In some domestic fowls, the female plumage pattern may be exhibited in the male when the gene combination for male plumage is absent. The dominant gene H produces the female pattern plumage in males, while the male's plumage is due to two recessive alleles hh. In females however irrespective of the genotype H or h, female plumage is produced. A female feathered cock (Hh) can be produced by crossing a male (hh) with a heterozygous (Hh) female.

Non disjunction of sex chromosomes

During gametogenesis in diploid organisms haploid gametes are produced and consequently the male gametes have one set of autosomes and one X or Y (1 A + X, 1 A+ Y) and the female gametes ie., the eggs have 1 set of autosomes and one X chromosome. During oogenesis, of the 2 X chromosomes of the mother cell, the egg receieves only one the 2 X chromosomes separate after pairing and move to opposite poles. But in some rare instances the two X chromosomes fail to separate during meiosis-I so that an egg will carry 1 set of autosomes and 2 X chromosomes instead of one. This phenomenon in which the two X chromomomes fail to separate during meiosis is called non disjunction.

In individuals showing non disjunction of X chromosomes 3 kinds of eggs are formed. These are -

(a) One set of autosomes + one X chromosome (Normal)
(b) One set of autosomes + two X chromosomes (non disjunction)
(c) One set of autosomes + no X chromosome.

The phenomenon of non disjunction was first observed in *Drosophila melanogaster* by Bridges (1916) when he was studying sex linked characters viz. red and white eye colour. When red eyed males were crossed with white eyed females, he observed that the expected, white eyed males and red eyed females did not appear in the F_1. Instead there were white eyed males, red eyed males, white eyed females etc., produced in different proportions. Bridges explained the results on the basis of non disjunction of X chromosome. Non disjunction of X chromosome is of two types **Primary non disjunction** and **Secondary non disjunction**. When the two X chromosomes in a normal female fail to separate it is called primary non disjunction; on the other hand, if the two X chromosomes fail to separate in an exceptional female (XXY)it is called secondary non disjunction.

Primary non disjunction : When a white eyed (homozygous) female is crossed with a red eyed male, the progeny will be as follows, if there is non disjunction of X chromosome in some flies.

	White eyed Female X^wX^w	X	Red eyed Male X^WY

Gametes : Male – two kinds X^W and Y

Female produces three kinds due to non disjunction in some eggs. These are

(1) X^w, (2) X^wX^w (3) O means no X chromosome autosomes only are present in the egg.

If there is random mating the following progeny are produced as shown in the cheker board.

	Females gametes		(no sex chromosome)
Male gametes	X^w	X^wX^w	O
X^W	X^WX^w Red eyed female	$X^WX^wX^w$ Super female (dies)	X^WO Red eyed male
Y	X^wY White eyed male	X^wX^wY white eyed female	YO super male (dies)

Among the progeny that survive both male and female will have 50% red *eye* and 50% white eye. But 50% of the males are exceptional in that they do not have the Y chromosome and 50% of the females have 2 X and one Y chromosome.

Secondary non disjunction : The exceptional females obtained in the previous cross are used as the female parent and crossed with a normal red eyed male. The cross and the progeny are as follows.

White eyed female (exceptional) X^WX^WY	X	Red eyed male X^WY

Gametes : Male – Two kinds X^W and Y

Female : Produces four kinds of gametes

(1) X^w, (2) X^wY, (3) X^wX^w, (4) Y

In the four kinds of gametes mentioned above, the First two kinds are produced during meiosis-I when the X would go to one pole and XY go to another pole. During meiosis-II, in the case of XY dyad after duplication XX go to one pole and Y goes to another pole, as a result the third and the fourth kind of gametes are produced. When these mate with the normal male gametes the following progeny are obtained.

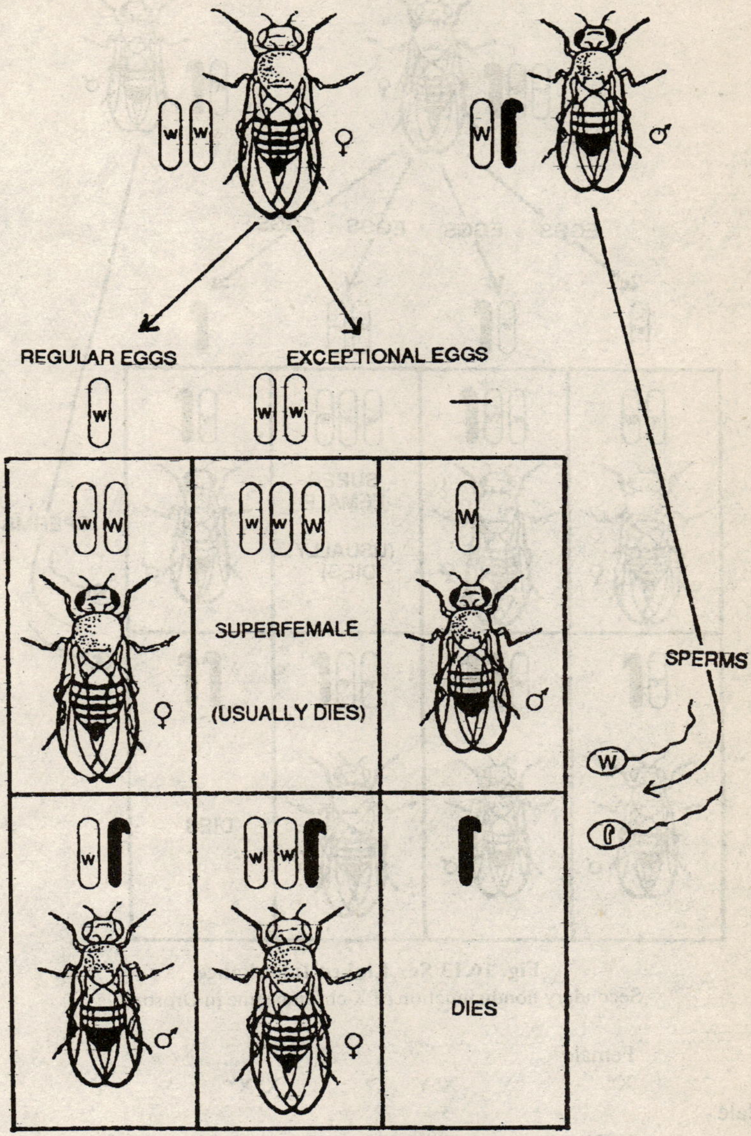

Fig. 16.12 Sex Linked Inheritance
Primary nondisjunction of X chromosome in Drosophila

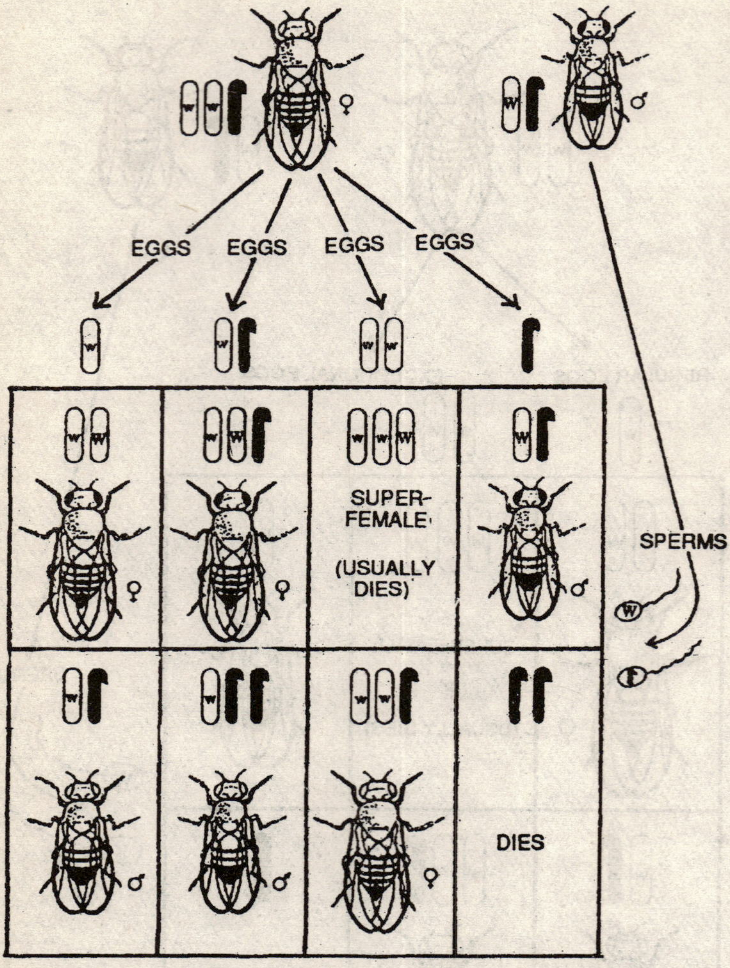

Fig. 16.13 Sex Linked Inheritance
Secondary nondisjunction of X chromosome in Drosophila

	Female			
	X^w	X^wY	X^wX^w	Y
Male				
X^W	X^WX^w Red eyed female	X^WX^wY Red eyed female	$X^WX^wX^w$ Super female(dies)	X^WY Red eyed male

Y	X^wY White eyed male	X^wYY white eyed male	X^wX^wY white eyed female	YY male (?) dies

Non disjunction of chromosomes in Man

Non disjunction of automsomes as well as sex chromosomes have also been reported in man causing various types of phenotypic abnormalities. Many of the abnormalities in human beings both sexual and other characteristics have been now known to be due to non disjunction of chromosomes, when gametes are formed during meiosis. For some reason or other with respect to one or more chromosome pairs, the gametes may be unreduced *ie.* they carry both the complements of the homologous chromosomes. When such gametes are fertilized by other normal gametes, the resultant offspring will have trisomy (three complements for a particular homologous pair) leading to abnormalities.

One of the best known trisomy of an autosome in man is the one causing the Down's syndrome or Mongolism.

The causes of non disjunction of the chromosomes during meiotic division is not known. However exposure to X radiation in *Drosophila* might bring about non disjunction (Mayor).

Sex linked characters and chromosome theory of inheritance

Although chromosomes were thought to be vehicles of genes much before the discovery of sex linked characters, the identification of a gene or a trait following the inheritance pattern of a particular chromosome provided conclusive evidence for the theory of inheritance through chromosomes. From this point of view sex linked characters are very significant.

17

CYTOPLASMIC INHERITANCE

Inheritance of characters from parents to offspring is primarily dependant on the nucleus. Oscar, Hertwig etc., had established in 1870 itself the importance of nucleus in the heriditary transmission of characters. The discoveries of Mendel further provided the genetic evidence for nucleus being the seat of all heriditary characters. The nucleus forms specific number of chromosomes during cell division and these duplicate, maintaining their number in future cell generations. Chromosomal aberrations, both structural and numerical leading to phenotypic abnormalities provided further proof for chromosomes albeit nucleus to be the only organelle concerned with the transmission of characters. The discovery of sex linked characters gave further impetus for the chromosome theory of inheritance as it was firmly established that a particular trait followed a particular chromosome. An additional proof for chromosomes being the only link between one generation and the other is the fact the gametes, atleast the male gamete consists of mainly the nucleus and very little amount of cytoplasm. With all these overwhelming evidences in favour of nuclear inheritance it was but natural for geneticists to beleive that nucleus is the only seat where all the genetic potentialities are located. But there are several instances of a peculiar type of transmission of characters both in the animal and plant kingdom which seemed to defy every known genetic law assuming the whole of inheritance to be through the nucleus. The inheritance of flower colour in 4° Clock plants, Kappa particles in *Paramecium* etc, can not be explained on the basis of nuclear inheritance. What then is the secret of their .inheritance pattern? Scientists started looking for other cell organelles which could perhaps play a role in inheritance. The gametes have some amount of cytoplasm surrounding the nucleus. The amount of cytoplasm is more in the case of female gametes, than in the male gametes. Geneticists started investigating, whether the cytoplasm also could help in the transmission of hereditary characters. If inheritance could be brought about by cytoplasm, there should be more chances of female or maternal inheritance as the egg contributes more amount of cytoplasm than the male gamete to the offspring. Further, one of the important requirements of a transmission system (if it exists in cytoplasm) is the capacity of self reproduction and it should have the basic molecules of inheritance viz. nucleic acids - particularly DNA. Further investigations did provide enough evidence of the existence of transmission systems in the cytoplasm (other than the nucleus). Plastids, mitochondria, ribosomes etc., have DNA of their own and many evidences have indicated that they replicate on their own, independent of the replication of nuclear DNA. These evidences clearly indicated a nuclear independent transmission machinery in cytoplasm and geneticists were able to explain the mechanism of inheritance in some apparently paradoxical instances in both plant and animal kingdom. Some of these are inheritance of flower colour in 4° clock plants, inheritance of killer particles (Kappa) in *Paramecium* etc. These were explained on the basis of cytoplasmic inheritance. Even though there are many organelles in cytoplasm possessing DNA, only the role of plastids in inheritance has been proved in plants. In animals, kappa particles and other traits seem to rest in cytoplasm but not in any definite organelle. The salient features of cytoplasmic inheritance are.

1. Certain somatic characters do not follow the Mendelian pattern, nor are they following the chromosomes in inheritance.
2. The genes or heriditary particles often called plasmagenes are located in cytoplasm.
3. In some instances, plasmagenes may be traced to definite organelles like plastids.
4. The most salient feature of cytoplasmic inheritance is female dominance. Since the egg contributes more amount of cytoplasm, offspring are more likely to get the maternal characters than the paternal. This has been established by reciprocal crosses.
5. Characters dependent on cytoplasm for transmission are never located on the chromosome. Hence the inheritance is also known as extra chromosomal inheritance.

In this chapter we shall study a few examples of cytoplasmic inheritance from both plant and animal kingdom.

Plastid inheritance in Mirabilis

Mirabilis jalapa, of the family Nyctaginaceae is popularly called the 4° clock plant, as the flowers bloom in the evening. The plant is unique in several respects. 1. The leaves are variegated or some times completely green. 2. The branches are of three types deep green, pale green and variegated. 3. The flowers are of various colours on the same plant in different branches they are either pink, yellow, or white with pink dots. The mechanism of inheritance in this plant was worked out by Correns, who opined that the flower and branch colour inheritance is not through the nucleus, but through the plastids. The phenotype of the progeny depends from which part of the plant the seed is obtained. If a seed is obtained from a flower on a green branch, the progeny would alway produce a green branch. Again a seed obtained from the same plant, but from a variegated branch would produce offspring with a variegatci green and pale branches. The same is true for flowers also. In thes inheritances, the source of the pollen does not seem to have any effect on the phenotype of the progeny.

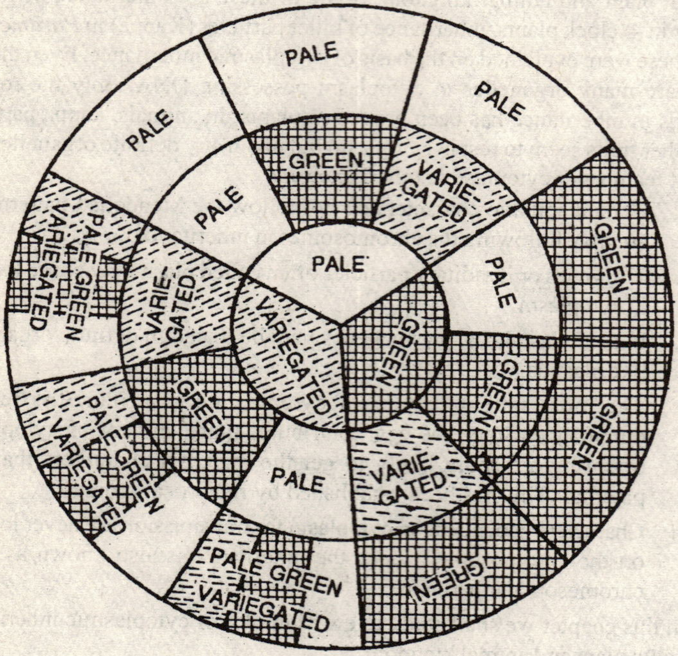

Fig. 17.1 Cytoplasmic Inheritance
Mechanism of plastid (Diagrammatic representation) inheritance

The mechanism of inheritance is as follows- The colour of the branch and flowers depend on specific plastids. The female gamete from a particular source has one or more types of plastids. The pollen carries no plastids at all as it has a limited cytoplasmic boundary. When the zygote divides, the plastids are distributed irregularly. Some cells may get plastids for green, some may get plastids for pink etc. These cells develop into branches, leaves flowers etc.

Hence the colour of the branch and flower depends on what types of plastids they have received during development.

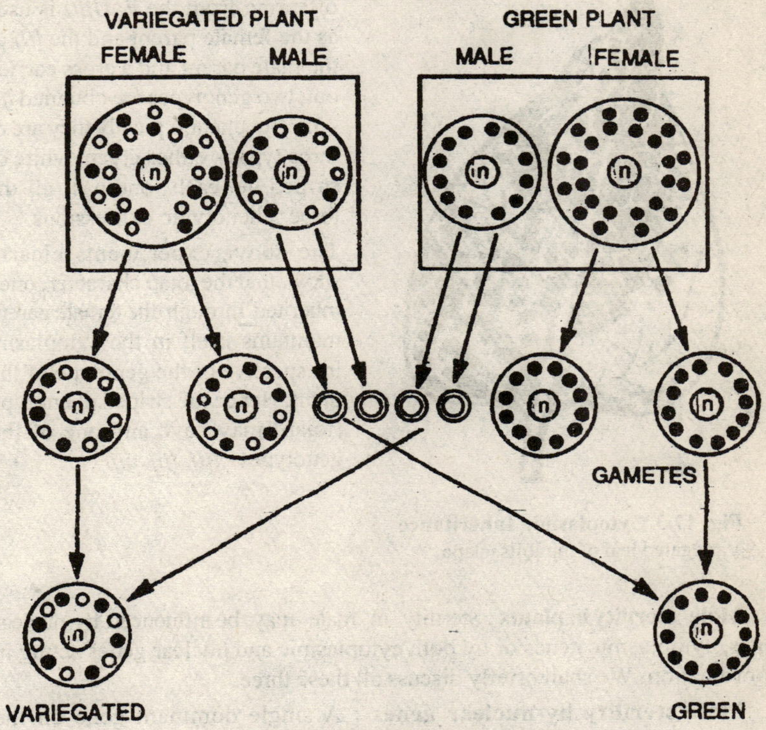

Fig. 17.2 Cytoplasmic Inheritance
Origin of variegated and green branches through distribution of plastids

Plastid Inheritance in Maize

In certain maize strains, the leaves have peculiar type of striping of green and white on the leaves. Rhodes made a study of these characters and came to the conclusion, that the **iojap** (striped) character is controlled by a gene located on chromosome number 7. The dominant gene *Ij* would produce green plastids, and its recessive allele *ij* would produce the iojap striping, *IjIj* is green and *ijij* is striped. The *ijij* plants would carry both green as well as abnormal white plastids in their cytoplasm, while *IjIj* plants would carry only the green plastids. In a cross between iojap and normal plant, if iojap parent is used as female, the female gametes carry either only green plastids, only white plastids or both green and white plastids. Consequently when iojap is the female parent and *IjIj* is the male parent, the offspring could be either green, variegated or white. The white seedlings die. If a striped offspring from the F_1 *(Ijij)* is used as the female parent and the *IjIj* as the male parent and a cross carried out, two genotypes are obtained *IjIj - ijij*. But phenotypically they are of three types - either green, white or striped, ie. each one has all the three .phenotypic expressions.

The above experiments clearly show, that the iojap character, once inherited through the female parent maintains itself in the cytoplasm, irrespective of the genotype of the plant. Hence the striped phenotype (iojap) may have any one of the genotypes - *IjIj, Ijij, ijij.*

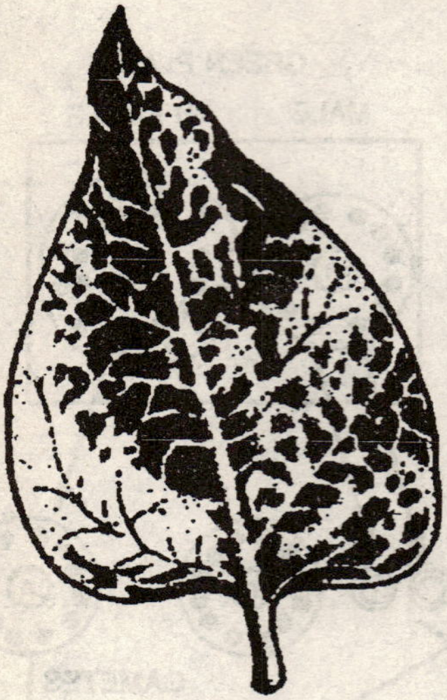

Fig. 17.3 Cytoplasmic Inheritance
Variegated leaf of mirablis jalapa

Male sterility in plants : Sterility in male may be influenced by nuclear genes, cytoplasmic genes or by both cytoplasmic and nuclear genes acting in co-ordination. We shall briefly discuss all these three.

Male sterility by nuclear genes : A single dominant gene on the chromosome controls the fertility, while its recessive allele brings about sterility. In a cross between the two, the F_1 individuals are heterozygous fertile. Selfing of the F_1 individuals to obtain F_2 shows a typical 3:1 seggregation of fertile and sterile plants.

Cytoplasmic male sterility : In many of the crop plants notably maize, pollen grains degenerate even though the ovules are normal and fertile. Marcus Rhodes made a detailed study of the male sterility in maize. He conducted breeding experiments extensively and was successful in replacing all the ten chromosomes of a male sterile strain with those of a male fertile strain. Inspite of this replacement of all the chromsomes, the progeny of this plant continued to be male sterile. This indicated that the nuclear genes did not play any role in determining the male sterility. Since male sterility was more when male sterile plant was used as the female parent in any cross, it is obvious, that the male sterility factor must be present in cytoplasm. A reciprocal cross in which the male sterile plant was used as the male parent and the male fertile pant as the female parent proved this tact (Although it may seem a paradox to use a male sterile plant as the male parnet, some pollen grains are fertile even in a male sterile plant).

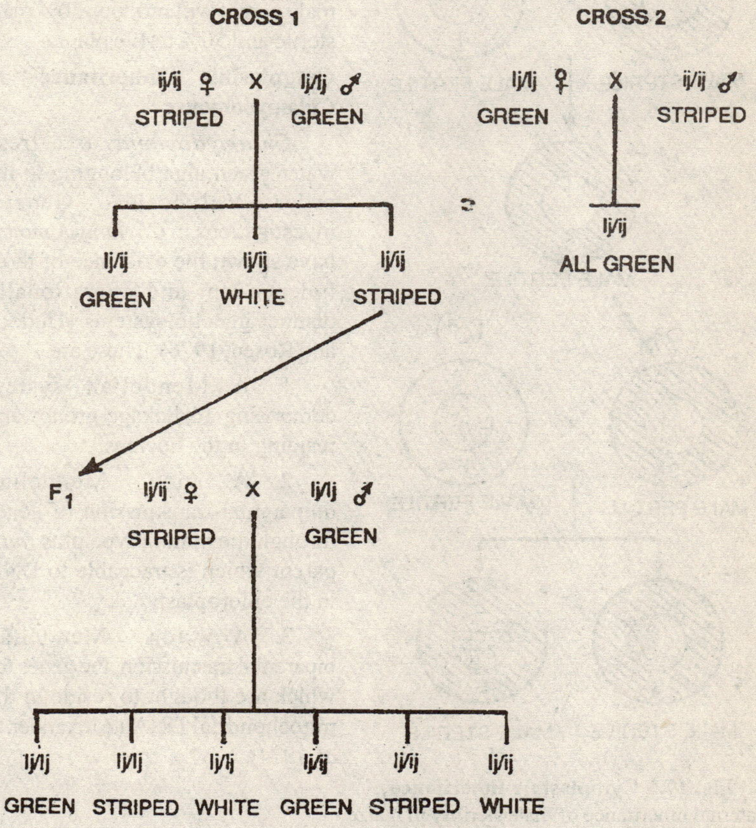

Fig. 17.4 Cytoplasmic Inheritance
Results of reciprocal cross between iojap and normal in maize

Cytoplasmic and nuclear male sterility : In certain instances cytoplasmic induced male sterility may be reversed by a fertility restorer gene in the nucleus. For example, if the female parent in a cross is male sterile, then the genotype (nuclear) of the male parent will decide the phenotype of the F_1 progeny. The male sterile female parent will have the recessive genes (rr) while the restorer gene is dominant (R). If the male parent is homozygous dominant, the F_1 progeny will be heterozygous (Rr) and fertile. On the other hand if the male parent is rr all the F_1 progeny will be also male sterile. A test cross between F_1 hybrid (Rr) and double recessive male parent will produce 50% male sterile and 50% fertile plants.

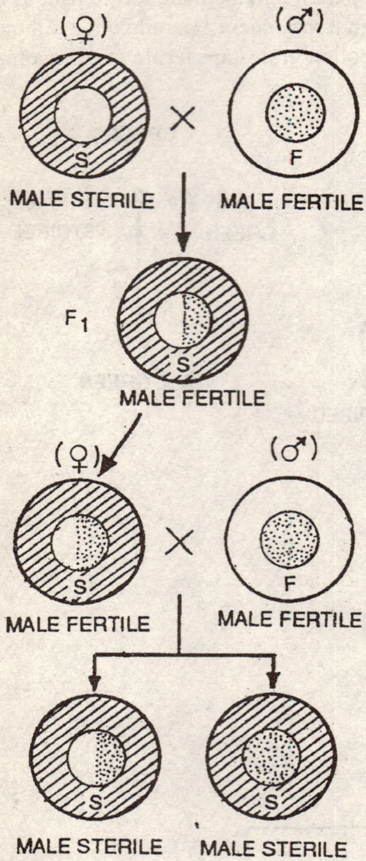

Fig. 17.5 Cytoplasmic Inheritance
Maternal inheritance of male sterility in maize

Cytoplasinic inheritance in Chlamydomonas

Chlamydomonas is a fresh water green alga belonging to the order Volvocales. Genetic investigations in *Chylamydomonas* have shown the existence of three independent and operationally distinct genetic systems (Hudock and Rosen, 1976). These are

1. A Mendelian system comprising 16 linkage groups and residing in the nucleus.

2. A non Mendelian uniparental transmission of genes through the mating type plus *(mt^+)* parent which is traccable to DNA in the chloroplast.

3. A non Mendelian biparental trasmission, the genes for which are thought to reside in the mitochondrial DNA (Alexander *et al*, 1974).

We will study the second category of inheritance which is cytoplasmic in nature. The pioneer in the field of plasma gene studies in *Chylamydomonas* is Ruth Sager (1954, 1964,1970) who has studied the inheritance of streptomycin resistance in *C. reinhardtii.* Seven gene pairs have been identified on the chloroplast gcnome. Ruth Sager (1972) has proposed a circular model for the chloroplast. DNA. Cytoplasmic inheritance in *Chlamyomonas reinhardtii* is studied using mutations for various chemicals; such as *ac* (acetate requiring mutant), *Sniz* (streptomycin resistant), *ery* (erythromycin resistant), *tim* (temperature sensitive) etc. In *C. rcinhardtii,* sexual reproduction is isogamous, hence both the gametes are supposed to contribute equal amount of cytoplasm and as such it is difficult to assess the maternal origin for any cytoplasmic factor. In higher organisms, with oogamous reproduction, the female gamete always contributes more cytoplasm, and the male gamete very little or none. Ruth Sager has identified two races of C. *reinhardtii,* which she designated as mt^+ and mt^-. Of these, it was found out by radiolabelling that only the mt^+ race can donate its chloroplast genome to the zygote and not the mt^- race. On the basis of this even though sexual reproduction is isogamous, the mt^+ race was called maternal and *mt'* race paternal. Hence chloroplast genes of onlv the mt^+ race are inherited.

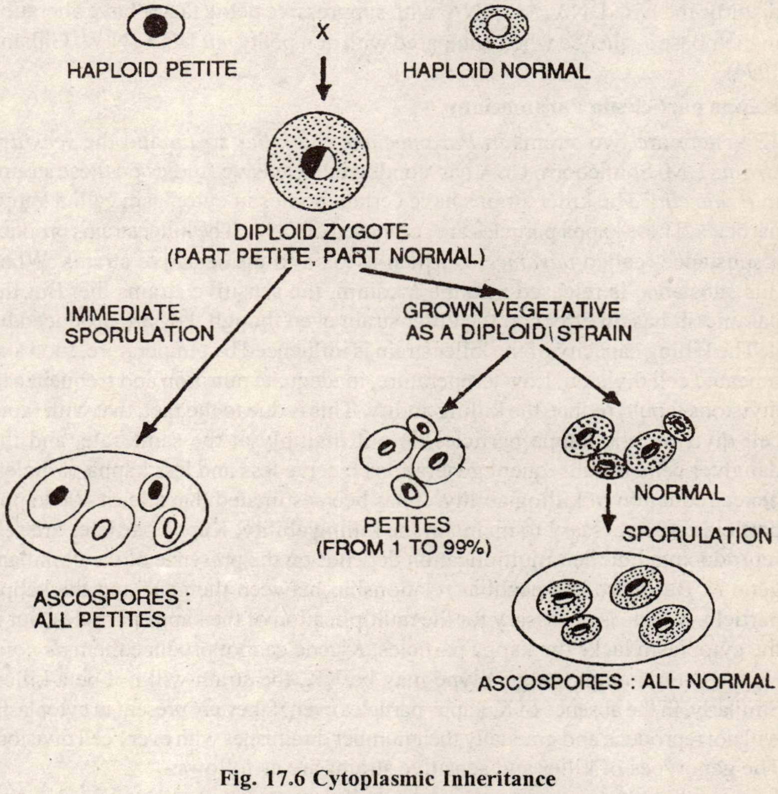

Fig. 17.6 Cytoplasmic Inheritance
Inheritance of petite character in yeasts

Petite character inheritance in Yeasts

Petite character in Yeasts refers to slow growth of mutants in. aerobic medium. The petite yeasts develop into small colonies when compared with the normal one, if the medium is oxygenated. The petite yeasts have a defective aerobic respiratory mechanism. Some of the characters of petite yeasts are as follows a) they are insensitive to cyanide poisining (affecting the aerobic path way) b) Absence of cytochrome a and cytochrome a-?) Incompletely formed mitochondria d) non stainability of petite mitochondria with Janus green etc. The genetic basis of petite character is a cytoplasmic factor , which is either defective or absent in petite yeasts. Thus in petite yeasts p is p or p' (defective or suppressive). The p' cytoplasmic factor is known to be transmitted through the mitochondrial DNA. Evidence for petite factor to be linked with mitochondrial DNA comes from the fact that ethidium bromide, inducing petite mutations disturbs the *mit* - DNA. *Mit* DNA with suppressive petite factor have alteration in their base sequence when compared with non petite *mit* DNA (N.W. Gilham, 1974).

Kappa particles in Paramecium

There are two strains in *Paramecium,* the *killer strain* and the *sensitive strain.* T.M. Sonneborn, USA has conducted extensive studies on these strains in *P. aurelia.* The killer strains have certain bodies in cytoplasm called kappa particles. These kappa particles are composed of DNA. The killer strains produce a substance called *paramecin,* which is toxic to the sensitive strains. When this substance is released into the medium, the sensitive strains die. But the paramecin has no effect on the killer strain even though they are produced by it. The killing capacity of the killer strain is influenced by temperature, food and repeated cell division. Low temperature, inadequate nutrition and frequent cell divisions would reduce the killing ability. This is due to the fact, that with rapid cell division, the kappa particles do not multiply at the same rate, and the daughter cells in subsequent generations receive less and less kappa particles, hence reduction of killing ability. It has been estimated that atleast 400 kappa particles are necessary to maintain the killing ability. Kappa particles are self reproducing, but their multiplication depends on the presence of the dominant gene *K.* But there is a peculiar relationship between the gene and the kappa particle. *K* gene is necessary for the multiplication of the kappa particles, but if the cytoplasm lacks the kappa particles, *K* gene cannot produce them *de now.* Hence even though the genotype may be KK, the strain will not be a killer. Similarly, in the absence of *K,* kappa particles even if they are present in cytoplasm will not reproduce and gradually their number diminishes with every cell division. The genotypes of killer and sensitive strains are as follows.

Killer strain *KK* or *Kk*
Sensitive strain *kk*

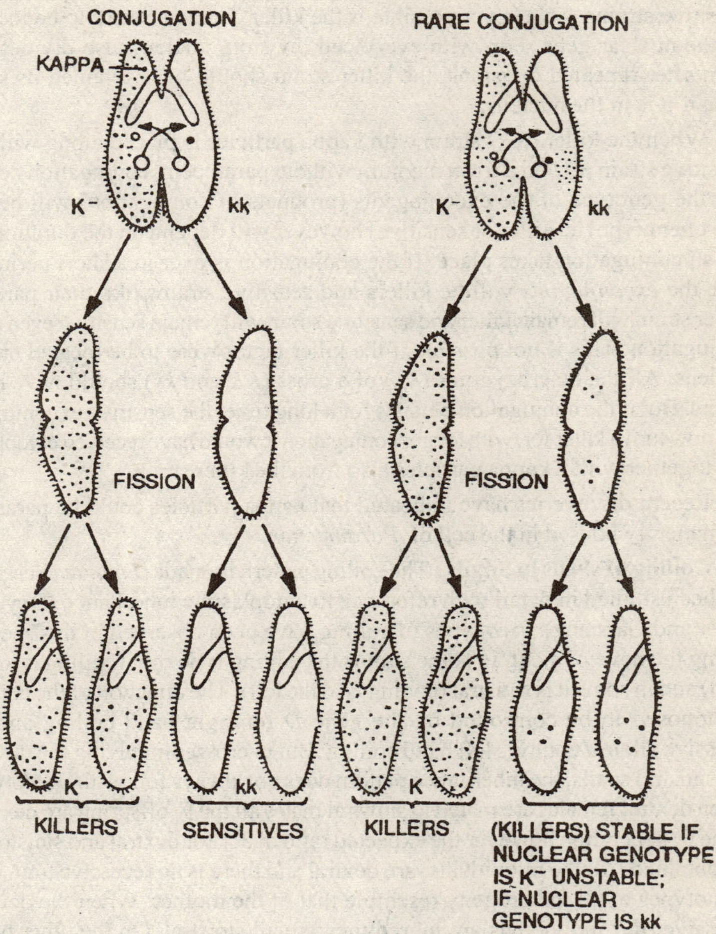

Fig. 17.7 Cytoplasmic Inheritance
Inheritance of kappa particles in Paramecium

By repeated culturing, it is possible to induce a rapid cell division in the killer strains with either *KK* or *Kk* genotypes. The kappa particles can not keep pace with this division and consequently after several generations, the progeny would be without kappa particles, even though they are genotypically KK or Kk and their parents were killers. These progenies (*KK* or *Kk*) would now be sensitive strains. This is not possible if the killer character were to be located on the nuclear gene. For, with every cell division, nucleus also divides and even after repeated divisions, the killer strain should have retained its killer gene if it is in the nucleus.

When the killer *(KK)* strain with kappa particles is placed along with the sensitive strain *(kk)* on a fresh medium without paramecin, conjugation occurs and the genotype of the exconjugants (products of conjugation) will be *Kk*. The phenotype (ie. killer or sensitive) however will depend on the duration for which conjugation takes place. If the conjugation is over in a short period of time the *exconjugants* will be killers and sensitive strains like their parents. Killer strain will remain killer and sensitive strain will remain sensitive even after conjugation. This is not possible if the killer factor were to be located on the nucleus. All the heterozygotes (*Kk*) of a cross (*KK* and *kk*) should have been killers. But if the conjugation persists for a long time, the sensitive exconjugant will now turn a killer for, with longer conjugation it would have received cytoplasm and together with it kappa particles also from the killer strain.

Recent discoveries have indicated that kappa particles could be parasites permanently housed in the cell of *Paramecium*.

Coiling of shells in Snails : The coiling pattern in snails *(Limnaea peregra)* has been studied in detail with reference to cytoplasmic inheritance (Boycott, Diver and Garstang). *Two* types of coiling have been observed in this species during the development. In some strains the coiling is dextral (coiling is to the right) and in some it is sinistral (coiling is to the left). The direction of the coiling is supposed to be controlled by the gene *D* for right hand coiling and its recessive allele *d* controls left hand coiling. But in crosses involving the dextral and sinistral snails, the inheritance pattern does not always follow the genotype. When dextral females are mated to sinistral males all the F_1 offspring are dextral. In the F_2 generation however the expected ratio of 3:1 for dextral and sinistral is not obtained. All the individuals -are dextral and there is no recessive trait. The phenotypes of all the progeny resemble that of the mother. When the double recessive *(dd)* individuals are inbred they are all sinistral. On the other hand when *DD* (dextral) was crossed with Dd (dextral), there appears to be no seggregation and all the offspring are dextral. When a sinistral (recessive) female is crossed to a dextral (dominant) male, the offspring are all like the mother - sinistral.

Investigations have shown that, the coiling is influenced by the orientation of the spindles formed during the cleavage of first metaphase. The spindle is shifted to the right in dextral and to the left in sinistral. This is controlled by the maternal genes (not nuclear) and the paternal genes do not seem to have any influence.

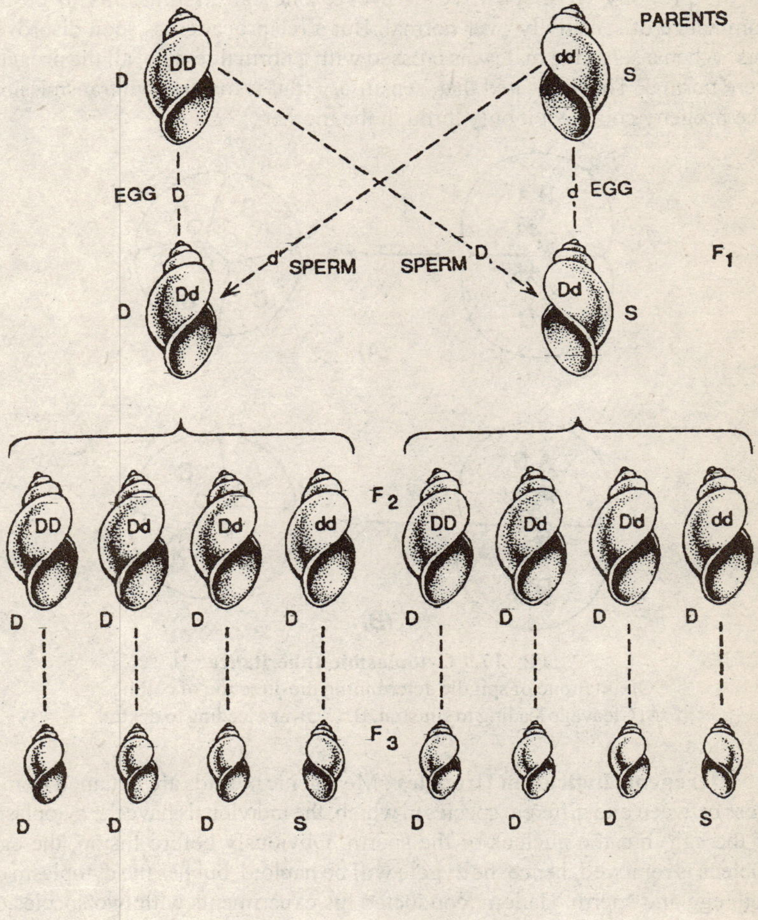

Fig. 17.8 Cytoplasmic Inheritance
Coiling of shells in snails (Limnea peregra)

Carbon dioxide sensitivity in Drosophila : Heritier and Teissier have described a strain of *Drosophila,* which is very sensitive to carbon dioxide than others. Such strains get immobilized on exposure to a high concentration of carbon dioxide. By breeding experiments, Heriteir and Teissier obtained a true breeding strain for carbon sensitivity and established the trait to be heritable. They further proved that this heritable trait does not follow the chromosomal inheritance. When sensitive female strains were crossed to normal male strains, all the progeny were sensitive. However one can assume this to be the dominance of sensitivity over normal. But a reciprocal cross soon disproved this. When a sensitive male was crossed with a normal female, all the progeny were normal. This indicated that, sensitivity trait is maternal in transmission. The progeny could get it only through the mother.

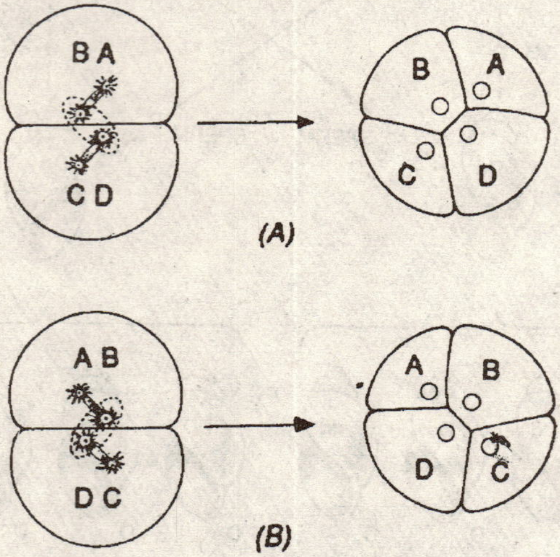

Fig. 17.9 Cytoplasmic Inheritance
Oreintationo of spindle determining the direction of coiling,
A. Cleavage leading to sinistral, **B.** Cleavage leading to dextral

Merogenic hybrids in Urodeles : Merogenic hybrids are obtained from a cross between two different species in which, the individuals have the cytoplasm of the egg, but the nucleus of the sperm. Obviously before fusion, the egg nucleus is removed, hence the zygote will be haploid, but has the cytoplasm of both egg and sperm. Hadom, conducted his experiments with two species of urodeles *Triton palmatus* and *T.cristatus* which differed in the nature of the epidermal cells. The egg of *T.palmatus* was fertilised by the sperm of *T.cristatus.* The zygote was haploid as it had only the sperm nucleus and developed up to the blastula stage. When a portion of the tissue (which would develop into epidermis) from this embryo was grafted on to the larva of another species, the tissue developed into epidermis characteristic of *T.palmatus,* which contributed cytoplasm, through the egg. There was no resemblance to the epidermis of *T.cristatus,* which contributed the nucleus.

Cytoplasmic inheritance in Ephestia : Ephestia is the common flour moth, that occurs in old and stale flour. In one of the species, *E.kuhniella* a clear instance of maternal inheritance has been observed. The dark and the light skin colour is known to be transmitted through the cytoplasm of the mother. The dark skin pigmentation is known to be governed by the gene *A,* while its recessive trait *a* brings about light skin character. Homozygous *AA* individuals are dark, while homozygous *aa* individuals are light. In a cross between, *aa* females with males, half of the progeny are dark and the other half are light skined. In a reciprocal cross (with *Aa* female and *aa* males) however all the progeny irrespective of the genotype are dark, because they receive the precursors of the pigment Kynurenine from the egg cytoplasm. However, when the larvae moult, the progeny without the gene *A* would gradually become pigmentless, as the gene *(A)* is necessary for pigmentation. Transplantation experiments of ovary have comfirmed that a diffusible substance from ovary influences pigmentation. The following chart gives the results of reciprocal crosses.

1 *aa* female **(No larval pigment red eyed in adult)** X *Aa* male **(Larval pigment present dark eyed in adult)**

Progeny

aa (50%) **Unpigmented** — *Aa* (50%) **Pigmented**

2 *Aa* female X *aa* male

Progeny
(All with larval pigment)

aa (50%) **Red eyes in adult)** — *Aa* (50%) **(Dark eyes in adult)**

Other instances of cytoplasmic transmission : Besides the above mentioned examples, which are studied in detail there are also a number of less known instances of cytoplasmic transmission of characters.

Epilobium is a member of the family Onagraceae and has been studied in some detail by Lehmann, Renner, Michelis and others. There are two species of

Epilobium, E.hirsutum and *E.roseum,* which differ in some morphological characters. Reciprocal crosses between these two species produces some interesting results. In a cross where *E.hirsutum* is the female parent and *E.roseum,* the male parent, the progeny are nearly sterile with reduced anther size. In a reciprocal cross, where the *E.hirsutum* is the male parent and *E.roseum,* the female parent, the offspring are normal with little or no sterility. Michelis produced a progeny [by repated back crossing of the F_1 female plant *E.roseum* (female) x *E.hirsutum* (male)] with *E.hirsutum* males, where the cytoplasm was derived from *E. roseum,* while all the chromosomes belonged to *E. hirsutum.*

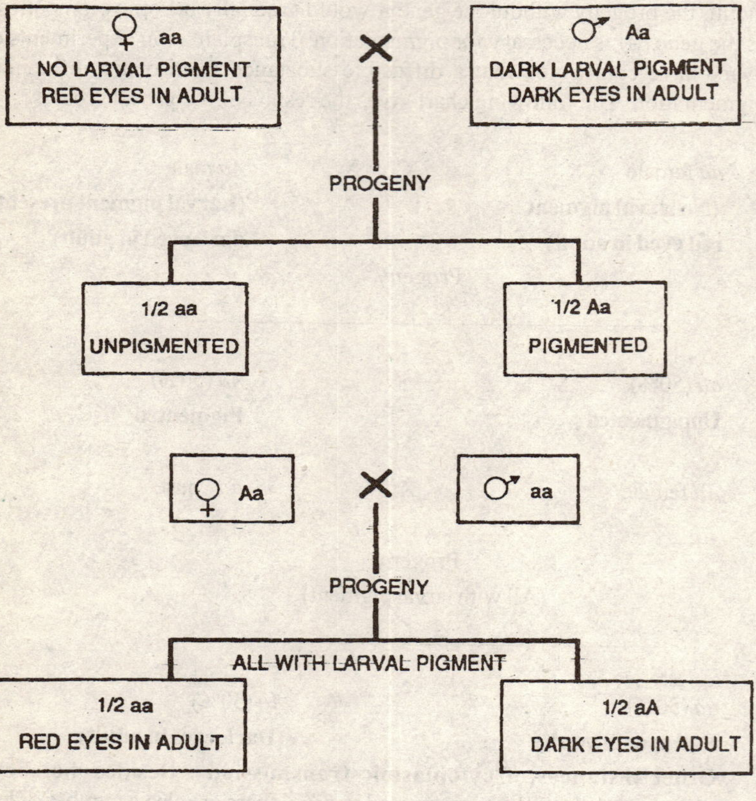

Fig. 17.10 Cytoplasmic Inheritance
Maternal inheritance in flour moth (Ephistia Kuhniella)

When this type was crossed with a typical *E. hirsutum,* the results were same as those obtained between a pure *roseum* and *hirsutum* clearly indicating that the differences (sterility etc) are clearly cytoplasmic in origin. Lehmann explained this due to the changed behaviour of the nucleus in a changed environment.

A similar case of maternal cytoplasmic inheritance has been reported by Wettstein in *Funaria* (a genus of mosses). Reciprocal crosses between *F.hygrometrica* and *F. mediterranea* proved that many of the traits followed the maternal line *ie*. repeated the characters of the female parent.

The above instances of cytoplasmic inheritance will clearly indicate, that while in a large majority of the cases, the nuclear genes no doubt play a predominant role in inheritance, a cytoplasmic environment is very essential for its proper functioning. Sometimes cytoplasmic factors may even mask or alter the effect of the nuclear genes.

18

PLANT AND ANIMAL BREEDING

Ever since its origin, life has maintained itself on this planet because of its capacity of self perpetuation or reproduction. Of the two types of reproduction known in organisms namely asexual and sexual, generally the latter has a higher selective value as it brings about genetic variety. Reproduction takes place randomly or selectively in nature depending on various circumstances. This act of nature of bringing together two individuals so as to produce offspring has been imitated by man, by selectively mating two individuals of desirable quality. This phenomenon wherein human beings interfere in the process of reproduction to allow only selective mating with the idea of producing an individual with required characters is called breeding (as against natural reproduction).

Breeding in domesticated animals and cultivated crops has a history which perhaps began with the changed habit of human beings from the hunter gatherer stage to agricultural settlements. A continuous attempt is made since then and continuing even now to obtain better quality animals (egg production, milk production, meat quality and quantity etc) and better quality plants (increased yield, disease resistance, early maturity etc). With the discovery of laws of inheritance by Mendel and the development of Genetics as an important science, refined tools and techniques have been made available to the plant and animal breeder. Earlier techniques of plant and animal breeding were a touch and go affair. The understanding provided by Genetics however has vastly changed the scenario. Plant and animal breeders are sure of what they want to produce and how to produce the desired type of progeny.

PLANT BREEDING

Cultivation of useful plants, which meant selection also started in prehistoric times, when man gave up the hunter gatherer life and started settlements near the river banks. Wheat, rice and barley are the oldest among the cereals cultivated on this planet. Asian settlements of early man cultivated, pear, oats rye, sugarcane etc, while his new world counterparts were growing maize, cotton, tomato, potato etc.

Ever since man began cultivating the plants, attempts have also been made to improve their yield, quality and other desirable traits. Early man mainly used selection as the principal and only method of crop improvement. Since plants generally have variations in terms of growth, yield, size etc-.he picked the ones that were good in these respects and cultivated them. It is by using this method, that Luther Burbank (1849-1926) succeded in cultivating the stoneless plums.

Selection however is not the best method of crop improvement, because variations noticed in a particular individual may or may not be heritable. At best it is only a hit or miss chance. But in order to bring about improvement, the characters chosen must have genetic basis. Plant breeding gained impetus after the rediscovery of Mendelian laws in 1900, because it provided an understanding as to how the characters are passed on from one generation to another. Breeding of plants is now an important aspect of World agriculture in its fight against hunger in mankind.

Aims and objectives of plant breeding : The principal objective of the plant breeder is to combine as many desirable traits as possible in a single individual which are originally distributed among many individuals. The following are some of the main objectives.

1. Increased production : Plants are the main source of food for man either directly or indirectly. Even the animal foods like egg, butter, milk, meat etc.,are ultimately traceable to plants, hence the popular adage 'All flesh is grass'. The World agricultural output however is scarcely sufficient to feed the ever increasing human population. Even with improved methods of Agriculture, scientific cropping pattern, use of fertilizers, pesticides etc, there is always a food shortage in several countries of the third world. Besides the geopolitical reasons for such uneven distribution of food, there is also a genuine shortage. It is therefore no wonder, that scientists are always looking for varieties and stocks of plants, with increased yield or production. Breeding programmes are undertaken to increase the per hectare yield in maize, rice, wheat and other cereals. If one can recall what, the King of Brabdingnong told Gulliver (in Gulliver's Travels by Jonathan Swift) during his imaginary trip to that country (The King is supposed to have said that he would prefer a man, who can make two blades of grass grow, where one grew before than to any body else); the same may be repeated as the aim and objective of the plant breeder. Just as in many other centres all over the world, in India also scientists at Indian Agricultural Research Institute, New Delhi, Central Potato Research Institute, Simla, Regional Rice Research Institute, Cuttack, Sugarcane Research Institute, Coimbatore, and Agricultural Universities in all the Indian states have been engaged in the production of high yielding varieties.

2. Improved quality : The quality of plants in terms of height, size or shape is another character sought after by the plant breeder. Many of the garden plants are highly prized for their shape, density, size, bright colour of the flowers, early blooming or late blooming etc. Similarly fruit size, nutritional quality, taste etc, are also qualities that are known to be improved by breeding. To mention one or two examples - Long staple cotton has been produced by crossing two varieties of Egyptian cotton. Similarly breeding has improved the sugar content in sugar beet from 7% to about 16%. *Sharbati sonora* wheat is produced as a result of induced mutation in wheat (Sonora 64). This variety is known to have a higher protein content than sonora 64.

3. Resistance to disease and pests : One of the greatest impediments for higher Agricultural output is the plant disease. A variety of causes bring about plant diseases. Fungi, bacteria, nematodes, insects and many other agencies cause untold havoc to agricultural output. There have been instances where plant diseases have brought about a complete change in crop pattern or migration of people from one country to another.. In the years 1845-1847 there was virtual destruction of the potato crop in Ireland due to the late blight disease caused by *Phytophthora ifestans.* As a result many thousands of Irish people migrated to USA. Similarly the impact of coffee rust influenced plantations to switch over to Tea cultivation from coffee in Sri Lanka.

Plant breeders are constantly trying to evolve varieties which can impart genetic resistance to the diseases. In our country particularly, more than the high yielding varieties, disease resistance in crop plants is a primary necessity. In evolving disease resistant varieties, plant breeders usually choose a high yielding variety and cross it with a wild relative which is hardy and resistant. The resultant progeny in many instances will not only have a higher yield, but will also be resistant to the disease.

Disease resistant wheat, sugar cane and many other crops have been evolved through breeding programmes. C250, C253 and C228 are wheat varieties resistant to yellow rust. In grams (pulses) also - varieties G24, and G17 are resistant to gram wilt.

4. Varieties suited to particular soils and climates : All crops cannot be cultivated in all types of soil and environmental conditions. It is essential therefore, that varieties, which are at home in a given environmental set up have to be evolved through breeding in order to achieve a higher yiled. For instance a particular variety may grow well in a hilly area, but may not grow well in plains. But by cross breeding; the same crop may be cultivated even in plains. The cultivation of groundnut was virtually unknown in Punjab during the early decades of this century. But a variety of groundnut PG_1 has been evovied and it is now cultivated extensively in Punjab in sandy soils. Some other new varieties of ground nut, with increased oil content are C117, C145, C158 etc.

5. Varieties resistant to lodging : Lodging means collapsing on the ground. Many of the crop plants at the time of their maturity can not withstand the weight either of the ears or fruits due to weak stem and collapse on the ground. This will greatly reduce the yield as the fruits or grains coming into contact with soil start decaying. The harvest also becomes difficult. Breeders try to evolve varieties, with strong stems or decreased height in order to prevent lodging. A notable mention among wheat varieties which do not lodge in the Mexican drawf.

6. Novel or exotic varieties : Another trait, that the plant breeder is constantly looking for in any plant are unusual features. This is particularly so in horticultural or ornamental crops. Production of novel or exotic characters in plants will not only create a new variety, but also will be in great demand bringing economic benefits to the grower. Seedless grapes, seedless oranges and seedless pomegranates are some examples of novel varieties among the orchard crops. Among the ornamental plants, new varieties of roses, *Petunias, Hydrangia, Philodendrons, Authuriums,* orchids etc command a high price because of their attractive foliage or flower or both.

METHODS OF PLANT BREEDING

Plant breeding is a slow and long process involving several steps and. processes. In a way plant breeding may be defined as both an art and science practised for pleasure and profit. The following are the three main steps of plant breeding - Introduction of variations, selection and hybridization.

Introduction of variations : Presence of a variety of characters is a prerequisite for selecting the plants for a breeding programme. The variations may be present in natural populations or they may have to be introduced or induced artificially. The following are the chief sources of variations among natural populations.

Mendelian variations : Spontaneous mutations bringing about variations in traits get stabilized due to recombinations. Natural hybridizations occuring frequently bring in some more variations. Most of these variations are heritable.

Hybridization : Another source of variation is the introgressive hybridization, that occurs normally between varieties, or even species. This type of hybridization many a time will not breed true, but can be propogated by vegetative means.

Polyploidy : This refers to increase in chromosome numbers from the normal diploid. Increased ploidy in most instances brings in change in the phenotypic traits, like increased growth, size, yield etc. This is one of the principle sources of variations. Polyploidy can even be induced artificially. Polyploids are quite common among flowering plants.

Selection : Selecting plants with favourable or suitable variations is the second step in hybridization. In fact, in earlier days, selection was the only method of breeding. During the pre Mendelian era, selection was primarily based on phenotypic variations. But as we know to day, phenotypic selections may not breed true, for they could be heterozygotes.

Selection practised now a days is exact and based on the genetic mechanism for a particular trait. Among the various individuals of a species growing in a Field, few are picked based on their phenotype. Subsequently they are interbred and several generations of progenies are raised in order to find out whether the plant breeds true for the chosen character. There are two types of selection - Single plant selection and mass selection.

In single plant or pure line selection, several individual plants with superior phenotype are selected. Usually a large number of plants are selected and are sown in separate lines. From these progeny, again individual plants are selected with the desired character. This is called *Progeny testing.* Seeds from these are sown separately again and selection continued in this way for several generations. Finally a progeny is selected possesing the desired qualities. The entire process may take about 5-8 years. Wheat varieties pv-18 and *Kalyan sona* are developed by selection process described above.

In mass selection, many similar plants are selected for each desired trait. The seeds from these are sown together (not separately as in single plant selection) and harvested. The seeds are mixed again forming a composite bulk and used for raising the next generation. The main difference between mass selection and single line selection lies in mixing the seeds and allowing interbreeding, so as to obtain a different genotype in the mass selection, which is not there in single line selection. Plants selected by mass selection possess fewer genotypes than the original because of recombination but more variety in the genotype could be produced than in single line selection.

The two types of selection mentioned above are called artificial selection as against natural selection. The interference of human beings selectively allows perpetuation of some desirable traits, and at the same time eliminates the undersirable ones. This artificial selection may follow the natural selection or as it happens in most of the times it may work exactly opposite. In other words, traits which would have got selected under natural selection maybe eliminated or *vice versa.*

HYBRIDIZATION

Plants that are selected on the basis of possession of favourable traits may be large, as a result the desired traits are distributed in many individuals. The idea of the plant breeder is to put together as many good traits as possible in a single individual. Hence the plants have to be hybridized to put together the traits in a single individual. In addition to this, hybridization provides further variety and improvement. For instance a pure line plant with a good trait may have another undesirable trait in the recessive condition. But by hybridization, this recessive trait can be masked. Hybridization in plants is usually of two basic types *Inbreeding* and *Outbreeding*.

Inbreeding : Mating between closely related individuals is called inbreeding. There may be different degrees of inbreeding, the extreme case being represented by self pollination in a bisexual flower. Johanssen (1903) recognised that inbred plants possess identical characters, when grown under similar environmental conditions. He called such populations as pure lines. In his experiments concerning garden beans, he selected weight as the main criterion and obtained 19 progenies. He found that the seeds have the some mean weight with some minor variations. As a result of his experiments, Johanssen concluded that selection becomes non operative in a pure line as there is no change in the genotype.

Inbreeding experiments in maize, which is normally cross pollinated has revealed, that, there will be decline in quality, vigour and yield as a result of continued inbreeding. East and Jones have conducted intensive investigations in maize plants and have demonstrated Inbreeding depression'. After about five generations of inbreeding, they found that, there was decrease in height and yield. Such degenerative changes increased with the increase of inbreeding ultimately leading to the formation of non viable seeds. To summarise, the following will be the genetic effects due to inbreeding -

1. Pure lines are produced, Homozygosity for many characters increases.
2. Recessive traits get a chance to appear phenotypically.
3. Rate of physiological activities generally comes down.
4. Vigour, yield, growth etc get reduced.
5. Lethality will increase.

Outbreeding : Outbreeding refers to crosses between plants which are not closely related. This increases the vigour, growth, yield etc., in the progeny. But while cross breeding one has to work within a set parametre. If a cross is made between two diverse individuals, there will be genome non homogenity resulting in sterility, even though such individuals may be vigourus. In such an instance the only method of propagation is vegetative. Such individuals however can be made to reproduce sexually by doubling the chromosomes and reintroducing homogenity (see polyploidy for details). Hence it can be said that outbreeding may produce hybrid sterility or hybrid vigour or Heterosis depending on to what extent the parents involved in crossing are related. The phenomenon of outbreeding and hybrid vigour have been noticed since a long time. Hybridization in outbreeding is of three types.

1. Intraspecific : Individuals belonging to the same species, but with different variations are selected as parents. This may be called *Intervarietal* crossing.

2. Interspecific : Individuals belonging to two different species, but belonging to the same genus are chosen for crossing. This may be called *Intrageneric* crossing.

3. Intergeneric : This is the widest parametre within which a cross is possible. Beyond this, the crosses will not succeed. The individuals belong to two different genera, but belong to the same family *(Raphanobrassica* - see chapter on Chromosomal aberrations).

HETEROSIS

Also known as hybrid vigour, this refers to the improved morphological trait of an individual in terms of growth, vigour etc, produced as a result of cross between two individuals not closely related. It is outbreeding that generally produces heterosis, because, the cross involves two different strains or stocks. Heterosis has been noticed both in plants and animals bringing about alround improvement in terms of production, germination, resistance and quality (of meat, egg, milk, taste etc). Heterosis or hybrid vigour has been observed since a long time. Kolereuter, a German plant breeder of the pre Mendelian period,- had observed, that hybrids in tobacco plants were more vigourous, than their parents. Beal (1880) demonstrated a similar behaviour in corn. Shull (1908), East (1908), Jones, Hayes and others, who have made detailed studies in maize, have also come to the conclusion of hybrid vitality, after comparing progenies obtained by self and cross pollination. Outbreeding of various crop plants like, wheat, sugar cane, potato etc., have been practised to yield a better progeny.

Extensive experiments on hybrid vigour in maize have been conducted in USA resulting in the yield per hectare of about 75 Ibs. Besides yield there was improvement of other traits also like size of ears, resistance to drought, disease etc. Hybridization experiments involving two varieties of *Nicotiana* - One measuring 31" and the other 54", have yielded progenies with a height of 64".

Instances of cross breeding, resulting in hybrid vigour are not as numerous in animals as in plants possibly because of the sex chromosomes. The cross between horse and ass resulting in the production of mule is a classical example of outbreeding. But the animal is sterile even though it is stronger and swifter than both the parents. Vicari of USA working on white rats has reported, that the offspring of a cross between two different races, had a better mental ability, and learned more quickly as to how to run through a maze than their parents. This type of heterosis is often described as *Psychological heterosis.*

According to Buchholz, physiological heterosis has been noticed in Pines *(Finns* spp) due to outbreeding. Similarly it has been reported in guinea pigs, that crossing the domestic variety *(Cavia cobaya)* with the wild variety produces offspring of a bigger size.

In sheep also, hybrid vigour is clearly demonstrable. The *Rambovillet* variety has fine short wool, while the *Lincoln* variety has good meat. The product of these two known as *Columbia breed* has intermediate wool and high quality of meat. Likewise, a cross between black faced Hampshire and Rambovillet sheep produces a hybrid with many desirable traits.

There is also a repot on heterosis noticed in *Drosophila melanogaster* (Clarke and Smith, 1955), wherein cross breeding produces a hybrid female with the capacity of higher production of eggs.

Causes of Heterosis : Two types of heterosis have been noticed in plants and animals. These are called *positive* and *negative* heterosis. In positive heterosis, there is alround improvement, while the reverse is true in the case of negative heterosis. Heterosis of the positive type is of considerable economic importance both in plant breeding and animal husbandry. Hence several techniques are adopted to obtain positive heterosis.

Several theories have been put forward to explain the reasons for hybrid vigour. These are mainly based on two interpretations viz. Cytoplasmic interactions and nuclear interactions. According to the cytoplasmic interaction, the cytoplasm by itself or interacting with the chromosomes brings in the hybrid vigour. But many of the geneticists do not attribute any significant role to cytoplasm as causing heterosis. They opine that, it is primarily the genes, which are responsible for heterosis; of course in a suitable environment. Many a time, chromosomal aberrations, both structural and numerical also contribute to heterosis. Two types of heterosis have been recoginsed, based on gene interactions. These are - *Monogenic heterosis* and *multigenic heterosis*. In the former, heterosis is due to the effect of a single gene, while in the latter, it is due to the interaction of many genes. Most of the instances of heterosis are due to multigenic effects.

There are several instances of monogenic heterosis as has been reported in barley (Gustafsson), *Antirrhinum majus* (Stubbe 1953), in *Drosophila* (Stern 1958, Crew 1960) etc.

Superdominance theory : This theory has been proposed by Shull and East (1908). According to them, the grouping together of two different alleles in the hybrid increases the metabolic rate by physiological stimulation. It is quite probable that dominant and recessive genes produce separately different metabolic products. Heterozygotes produce these different substances together in an individual resulting in improvement. This phenomenon is called over dominance or super dominance, where in heterozygote has better qualities than even the homozygote dominant. This phenomenon has been repoted in

Antirrhinum, wherein the normal variety (++) grows to a height of 33.9 cms, while the mutant homozygous called *luteus* (II) grows to a height of only 11.7 cms. The hybrid (I +) grows to a height of about 41.7 cms.

Dominance hypothesis : According to this, heterosis is brought about due to the combined action of many genes. For instance, among the two strains taken for hybridization, the dominant genes responsible for superior quality are distributed in both. Hybridization brings together all these genes in the F_1 hence the fiybrid vigour. However, when these F_1 individuals are self bred the genes get seggregated once again, and the hybrid vigour is lost. But this explanation does not seem to be completely correct, for even in a cross between F_1 individuals, one line of F_2 at least must one again possess all the dominant genes retaining the hybrid vigour. In such a case selfing of these individuals (with dominant genes) must maintain hybrid vigour. But as has been noticed, hybrid vigour is not permanent and there is a gradual decline in generations subsequent to F_2 and it is not possible to maintain hybird vigour.

Jones, who is a supporter of the multiple gene hypothesis to account for hybrid vigour gives an explanation to accout for the absence of any heterosis in the F_2 generation. According to him, the F_1 hybrid between diverse parents brings together many dominant and recessive genes, many of which are linked in their original parents. The hybrid shows heterosis due to the presence of dominant genes. In the F_2 progeny produced as a result of selfing of the F_1, most of the individuals will be homozygous for one to several unfavourable genes; as a result the progeny will be less vigourous than the F_1.

Physiology of heterosis : Kiesselbach (1922) studied hybrid vigour in maize from the point of view of physiology. Increased weight of the kernel, embryo, endosperm, seed coat etc were attributed to rapid assimilation and respiration. According to Ashby (1937), the hybrid would have an embryo greater in size than the parents and it is this "initial capital" that is responsible for the alround superiority of the hybrid. According to Whaley (1950), the hybrids in maize have a more efficient protoplasm than the inbred lines. Bernstein (1943) found that starch digestion and accumulation of sugars would proceed rapidly in the hybrids. He also opined that the endosperm was more in extent in the outbred stock than in inbred lines. Extracts of the hybrid grains of maize have been found to promote the growth of the fungus *Ashbya gossypii,* than those from the inbred grains.

Experiments of Robins on tomato roots in tissue culture have shown that excised roots of hybrids grow faster than the inbred roots.

Techniques of hybridization : Plant hybridization is both an art and science and a breeder must possess not only the deft touch of an artist but also the precision of a scientist. The following are the main steps involved in hybridization.

(a) Selection of parents : The plants suitable for crossing must possess most of the desired traits that the breeder wants to combine in a hybrid. Of the two parents one must be selected as the male and the other as the female. In the case of self pollinated crops, the next step is to prevent self pollination. The anthers in the case of the female parent (in a hermaphrodite individual) should be removed before the ovary is mature. This is called *emasculation*. Physical removal of anthers is possible in the case of large flowers, but in the case of small flowers aggregated into inflorescences, other methods are employed. These include subjecting the flowers to cold or hot treatment and chemicals which selectively destroy the pollen. In *Sorghum,* dipping the inflorescence in hot water (5°C) for 10 minutes is known to destroy all the pollen. In *Ragi,* a test tube lined with moist filter paper is inverted over the inflorescence for some time. The anther sacs stick to the filter paper and can be easily removed. Chemicals such as 2-4 D (50 ppm), maleic hydrazide, Gibberellins etc., are known to cause male sterility. In squash and wheat Sikka and Swaminathan (1956) have successfully employed maleic hydrazide to induce male sterilty.

After emasculation, the female flowers are to be protected by paper or polythene bags untill the stigma is mature and receptive for the pollen. Similarly, the male flowers are also to be protected by bags in order to prevent their contamination from foreign pollen.

The next step to be followed is artificial pollination. Pollen from the designated male plant is collected and dusted on to the stigmatic surface of the female parent. After pollination, the female flower is bagged again until the time of seed setting. In plants like *Sorghum,* the male and female inflorescences are brought together and bagged until seed setting. Large number of identical plants are to be used in artificial pollination, in order to account for chance failure of fertilization, non viability of seeds etc.

BREEDING IN SELF POLLINATED CROPS

The following breeding methods are employed in the case of self pollinated crops guch as cereals, pulses, garden plants, vegetables etc.

(a) Pure line selection : From among the population with variable characters, many single plants are to be selected in large numbers of individual traits. The seeds from these are sown separately and again single plants are selected.

(b) Mass selection : Previous pages in the same chapter

(c) Pedigree method : Plants with desired traits are tested for homozygosity and two such plants are crossed and seeds obtained to raise the F_1 population. Large number of F_1 individuals are raised and self pollination is allowed among plants with dominant traits. Selection again is carried out among the F_2 population. Good ones are again selected and sown. In this way progenies up to F_4 or F_5 are raised, when individuals become almost homozygous for the desired trait. The seeds are now ready for use. Pedigree method is suitable for plants, where traits can be easily observed as in case of tobacco, cotton, soya beans etc.

(d) **Bulk method :** Several plants are selected as the parents and cross pollination is carried out among them. The F_1 progeny is allowed to self pollinate and large number of F_2 individuals are raised. (In pedigree method cross pollination is carried between two selected individuals). The F_2 seeds are sown in bulk (not separately). Natural selection is allowed to c perate in all these crosses and the desired ones are selected at the end of the F_6 or F_8 generations. Bulk method is suitable for small grained crops.

3. **Back cross method :** This is also called recurrent crossing. Characters which are desirable are selectively transfered from one individual to the other in this method. For example, traits such as disease resistance frost resistance etc. present in a variety where the yield is not good are sought to be transfered on to a variety with a high yield but is easily susceptible for the disease. Back cross is done as follows.

Let us assume plant *A* is a high yielding variety but susceptible to the disease and plantB is hardy but with less yiled. In order to bring together high yield as well as hardiness, the two plants are crossed and an F_1 progeny is obtained. F_1 individuals with both the desired traits (high yield and resistance) are selected and crossed with the original parent A. The F_1 products of this back cross are again crossed back to A. This will be done a number of times until the characters of B are selected. Finally these selected plants are selfed to make the traits of B homozygous. In this way, the desired traits of B are introdced into A plant.

The main objects of back cross are -

(a) Reduction of unnecessary variations in further generations.
(b) Increasing the proportion of the desired, gene in the progenies.
(c) Increasing the fertility by back crossing.

Multiple crosses : Multiple crossing also known as compound crossing involves crossing several varieties simultaneously to combine the desired traits. If we assume that crosses are to be carried out in eight stocks viz *a, b, c, d, e, f, g* and *h* a series of individual crosses are conducted first as follows.

(a x b), (c x d), (e x f), (g x h)

In the next step a series of bridging crosses are made -

[(a x b) x (c x d)]; [(e x f) x (g x h)]

The third series of crosses are as follows

[(a x b) x (c x d)] x [(e x f) x (g x h)]

The resultant progeny from the above cross is used as the starting point for selection. Selection from this stock is made either by pedigree method or bulk method. Plants with desirable combination of traits only are selected.

Multilineal crosses : This technique has been developed by Dr. Norman Borlaug, who is often called the Father of green revolution. In this technique developed for wheat, a high yielding variety is crossed with a number of varieties. Progenies (each one) are back crossed with the original variety and selections are made to obtain the combination of both the traits. These are crossed among themselves and the progeny selected showing greatest resistance to the rust disease. By using multilineal crosses, Borlaug obtained day neutral varieties of wheat which could be cultivated in all areas of the world. He was also successful in transfering the dwarf genes of the mexican wheat (which prevents lodging) to Japanese strains to evolve a very successful variety.

BREEDING OF CROSS POLLINATED CROPS

Most of our cultivated crops are generally cross pollinated in nature. Many of the cereals (Particularly maize), forage crops, vegetables and fruit crops belong to this category. These plants are heterozygous and posses a highly complex genotype and carry harmful recessive genes in the genome pool. In such plants, inbreeding is deleterious, as it brings together recessive genes in the homozygous condition. The methods employed in breedng of cross polinated plants are diverse and many a time cannot be clearly defined as in self pollinated crops. There are three important steps in the breeding of these plants. These are *Selection, hybridization* and *production of composite varieties.*

Selection : Mass selection is usually followed. In addition to this, progeny selection and recurrent selection is also done. In progeny selection, selected offspring are grown in separate plots to ascertain the breeding behaviour of these plants. Seeds from many of these plants are grouped together and progenies are selected from these. In recurrent selection, plants with desired traits are selected and selfed. The seeds from these are sown in rows and are intercrossed in all combinations. Hybrid seeds obtained from these are put in a bulk to produce a mixed population. Seeds from suitable plants from these are again sown in rows (seeds from a single plant are sown in a row). Cross pollination is allowed and seeds obtained. In this way, interbreeding and cross breeding are alternatively followed to finally select a progeny for further breeding.

Hybridization : This is done in cross pollinated crops as follows -

1. **Single cross method :** Two inbred lines A and B are crossed and the hybrid is used for raising the crop.

2. Three way cross method : Three inbred lines are involved in this (A, B and C). At the first stage, the stocks A x B are crossed and the progeny of this is crossed with C. (A x B) x C. In the second cross the F_1 of the first cross is usually used as the female parent.

3. Double cross method : Four inbred lines A, B, C, and D are used in this. At the first stage crosses are made between A x B and C x D. The F_1 of each of these crosses are crossed to obtain the progeny used for further selection. The crosses may be symbolically represented as follows.

(A x B) X (C x D)

Double cross method has been widely exploited in the case of maize which has resulted in a very high yield. This method has been widely employed in USA with phenomenal success. In our country also work on these lines have been going on at IARI, Delhi and Punjab Agricultural University, Ludhiana. Some of the well known double cross varieties are -

Ganga 101, Ganga 2, Ganga 3 etc., in maize
HBI variety and NB 21 of Bajra
CHS1 and CHS2 of Sorghum.

Top cross method : In this method widely used in maize, many inbred lines are chosen and back crossed with the original variety. There are two types of top crosses viz, *single top cross* and *double top cross.*

In single top cross method, two different inbred lines are crossed with each other and the F_1 crossed with the original variety. Individuals with desired traits are selected. In double top cross method F_1 hybrids of two different lines are crossed and the product crosed with one of the parents. This is as follows.

(A X B) (C X D)

F_1 X F_1

F_2

F_2 x F_1

Synthetic or composite varieties : A number of selected genotypes are crossed and a synthetic variety is produced after a series of crosses. Only the desirable traits from a large number of plants are put together in the synthetic variety. A synthetic variety may be defined as a strain developed as a result of crossing and combining together many clones, in which seeds are harvested in bulk and replanted in successive generations.

A synthetic type is different from mass selection in that, in the latter there is no controlled crossing and no progeny selection. In mass selection the plants are selected based on a superior phenotype. In synthetic variety however, there is controlled pollination and genotype is carefully selected. Several synthetic varieties of maize have been produced in our country. Some of these are - Jawahar, Amber, Vijay, Vikram, Kissan, Sona etc. Synthetic varieties grown away from local varieties, could be used again and again to produce seeds for the next season. In the case of hybrid varieties, seeds have to be produced afresh (after crossing) for every crop.

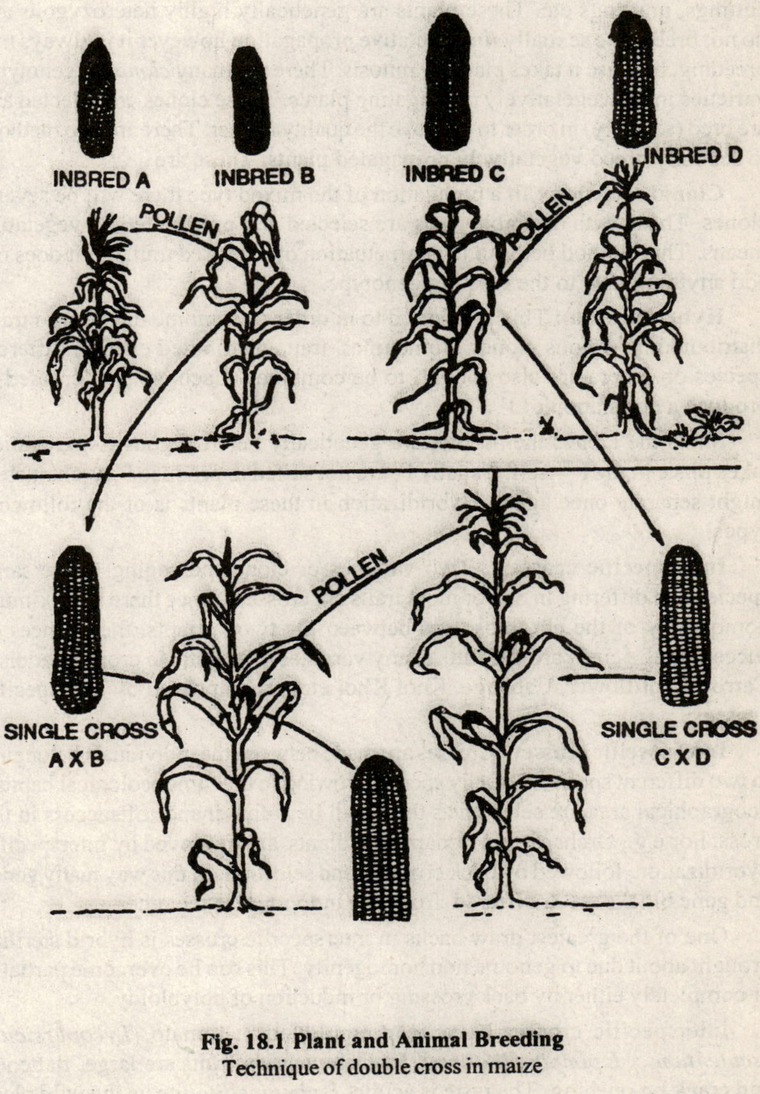

Fig. 18.1 Plant and Animal Breeding
Technique of double cross in maize

BREEDING OF VEGETATIVELY PROPAGATED CROPS

Some of the economically important crop plants normally reproduce asexually and propagate through, runners, stolons, bulb, corm, rhizome, tuber etc. Many others like roses, apple, pear, plum, mango etc are cultivated through cuttings, graftings etc. These plants are genetically highly heterozygous and do not breed true sexually. In vegetative propagation however it is always true breeding, because it takes place by mitosis. There are many *clones* or genotypic varieties in the vegetatively propagating plants. These clones are selected and are bred (sexually) in order to improve the quality further. There are two methods to sexually breed vegetatively propagated plants. These are

Clonal selection : In a population of the mixed type there will be several clones. Those with desirable traits are selected and propagated by vegetative means. This method helps in the perpetuation of a desired trait, but it does not add anything new to the existing genotype.

Hybridization : This is resorted to in order to combine the desired traits distributed in various clones. Sometimes, traits distributed even in different species or genera are also sought to be combined. Each clone is crossed to produce a population of F_1.

Since the clones themselves are genetically heterozygous, seggregation takes place in the F_1 itself. Usually F_1 are not suited to produce F_2 as characters might separate once again. Hybridization in these plants is of the following types.

Intraspecific crosses : Two varieties or clones belonging to the same species and differing in one or more traits are crossed. Since there is maximum homogenity of the chromosomes between the two variants, the chances of success in the cross are definite. Many varieties of vegetable crops (Raddish, Carrot, Cauliflower, Cabbage, Knol Khol etc) are improved by intraspecific crosses.

Interspecific crosses : Crosses are made between the individuals belonging to two different species. Usually species growing in the same ecological habitat, geographical area are selected as there will be a fair chance of success in the cross. For e.g., Orchard, and Ornamental plants are improved by interspecific hybridization, followed by back crossing and selection. In this way many genes and gene blocks are transfered from one individual to the other.

One of the greatest draw backs in interspecific crosses is hybrid sterility brought about due to genome non homogenity. This can be overcome partially or completely either by back crossing or induction of polyploidy.

Interspecific crosses have been employed in tomato ***(Lycopersicum esculentum*** x ***L.pimpinellifolium)***. In ***L.esculentum*** fruits are large, flattened and crack on opening. The taste is acidic. ***L.pimpinellifolium*** is the wild plant possessing small reddish fruits. The plant is also disease resistant. The hybrids between these two plants are known to possess a combination of many desirable traits.

In *Sorghum,* a cross between *(S.helpense* X *S.durra)* x *S.durra* had yielded a hybrid with increased height and girth of the stem, panicle, leaf size etc. Similarly in cotton also a cross between *Gossypium arboreum* X *G.herbaceum* has yielded a variety of cotton (H 190) useful in many respects.

When a plant can be propagated vegetatively, hybrid sterility is no hinderance as the plant need not reproduce sexually. F_1 iindividuals are propagated by means of cuttings, graftings etc. Roses, Plums, Cherries etc are propagated by this method. In sugar cane also *(Saccharum officinarum* x *S.spontaneum)* crosses between species have yielded useful hybrids.

Intergeneric crosses : When a cross is made between two different genera it is known as *intergeneric (Raphanussativus* X *Brassica oleracea).* Hybrid non viability and sterility are much more pronounced in intergeneric crosses than in interspecific ones as the genomes are entirely different. Usually intergeneric crosses are not employed as the chances of success are very meagre. Polyploid individuals however have a fair degree of success. Due to the sheer size of the genome, in a cross with a related genus, there is likliehood of some amount of chromosomal homology, resulting in a successful hybrid. In maize, wheat etc., crosses have been made with related genera to obtain successful hybrids. The genus *Euchlaena* has two species *E.mexicana* and *E.perennis* which have partial homology with the chromosomes of maize. An intergeneric cross between maize and *Euchlaena* has helped in transfering the disease resistant gene to the maize. Crosses of similar type have been attempted in wheat which have helped in tracing the origin of the common bread wheat (For details see chapter on Chromosomal aberrations).

Breeding of Cotton

Cotton is one of the most important fibre yielding plants in our country used extensvely in textile industry. Cotton belongs to the family Malvaceae of dicotyledonous flowering plants. The genus *Gossypium* has several species of which about four are grown in our country. These are long staple American cotton *(G.hirsutum),* Egyptian cotton *(G.barbadense)* and short staple *desi* varieties *(G.herbaceum* and *G.arboreum).* Approximately more than two hundred lakh hectares are under cotton cultivation in our country. The Indian Counci of Agricultural Research has been conducting research for improvement both in terms of yield and quality of the fibre in the cotton plant (particularly in long staple varieties).

Breeding in long staple cotton : The main objectives of breeding in long staple cotton are increase of the mean length of the fibre (28.4mm), better spinning quality and higher ginning percentage. Other desired traits in this plant are resistance to Jassid and early maturity. The mean fibre length of some varieties are given below -H 14- 23.7 mm. H 183 - 27.3 mm, H 162 - 29.1 mm. Of these three - H 183 and H 162 also give a higher yield than H 14 (grown in Haryana). Another variety H 183 - 13 (H14 x AC138) has a mean fibre length of 28-2 mm. sympodial in its habit and matures earlier than H14.

Variety 320F cultivated in the Abohar region of Punjab has a mean fibre length of 24.4mm. There are some local varieties A231 and 218, which have a mean fibre length of 28.4 mm and they also have a higher yield than 320F. A231 has a much branched shoot system and it also matures early and thus escapes frost.

Resistance to Jassid is another quality that plant breeders look for in cotton. A new variety J34 evolved as a result of a cross between 45F x L55 is under cultivation in Punjab and Haryana. F34 also has a higher yield than 320F. Several other strains of J series are J 124, J 135, J 136, J 140, J 148 etc are under experimental cultivation and they seem to be quite promising.

Breeding in short staple cotton : There are two principal objectives in the breeding program for the desi varieties of cotton. These are - a) To obtain harsh staples with increased yield and ginning capacity b) to obtain high yield as well as good lint. The normal variety of desi cotton cultivated is 231R. New varieties Gl and G27 have proved to be better yielding than 231R. These two varieties are short statured, much branching and have a rough fibre. Among Gl and G27 the latter seems to be more promising due to its higher yield than the other two varieties. The plants of G27 mature early, resistant to water logging and pink boll worm. The lint is also of a very high quality. G57 is another high 'yielding variety of cotton.

Breeding in maize

Maize *(Zea mays)* belongs to the family of grasses (Gramineae) and is an important food crop of our country. It has unisexual flowers, but the plant itself is monoecious. Both self and cross pollination generally occur in nature in maize plant. The crop is cultivated extensively in northern Indian plains. In addition to the local varieties, many hybrid varieties have been introduced in the last 20 years. Hybrid varieties were introduced for the first time in 1960. These (Ganga 101 for plains and V154 for hilly tracts) varieties proved to be highly beneficial to the farmers as Ganga 101 had an astonishing 86% more yield per hectare than the local varieties. Some more varieties were evolved in 1964 - Ganga 2, Ganga 3 and Himalaya 123. Ganga 2 was white grained while Ganga 3 was yellow grained. Ganga 3 with the highest possible yield per hectare at that time became very popular with the north Indian farmers.

Further hybridization to get more yield resulted in Ganga 5, EH 238 and EH 2461. Of these, Ganga 5 yielded, 20% more than Ganga 3. Crop breeding work at

IARI, New Delhi has produced several useful varieties which are better than the Ganga varieties. Some of these are 485 and 486. The hybrid varieties yield up to 3,700 kg per hectare as against 1500 kg for the local varieties.

Composite varieties in maize : In producing a composte variety suitable to Indian conditions, races from different maize growing countries like USA, Mexico, Peru, Cuba, Columbia, Venezula have been selected and several crosses conducted between them to combine as many desirable traits as possible. Careful hybridization followed by selection conducted by ICAR in their research stations have resulted in the production of many synthetic or composite varieties.

In the year 1967 ICAR released the following varieties as suitable for cultivation in areas mentioned against their names.

(a) Sona, Vijaya and Jawahar - Punjab, Haryana and West UP.

(b) Kissan and Jawahar - Bihar, Bengal and East UP.

(c) Kissan and Vikram - Gujarat, Rajasthan,

(d) Ambar and Jawahar - Andhra Pradesh, Karnataka, Madhya Pradesh.

(e) Ambar - Hilly regions of UP, Himalayan belt.

The varieties mentioned above not only have a higher yield potential than the Ganga varieties but also resistant to pests, diseases and drought. Vijaya vareity has an yield of 4090 kg per hectare.

Another synthetic variety evolved in 1968 at the Punjab Agricultural University, Ludhiana is perhaps the best breed evolved in India. It has a potential yield of 4225 kg per hectare. Gradually, the hybrid varieties are being replaced by the composite varieities as the latter combine a highly complex genotype and are endowed with many desirable traits. Composite varieties combine, traits like disease resistance, higher yield, drought resistance, early maturity etc.

Besides, composite varieties breed true, so the farmer can use the seeds for next sowing. In hybrid varieties however, the seeds are to be produced afresh from carefully maintained inbred lines. No wonder then composite varieties are being prefered to hybrid varieties.

Breeding in Sugar cane : Botanically known as *Saccharum officinarum,* sugar cane a member of the family Gramineae, is the principal source of raw material for sugar as well as gur manufacture in our country. The other source of sugar - sugar beet is not popular in our country.

There are several research stations in India engaged in sugar cane breeding, but the most important one is the sugar cane breeding Institute of Coimbatore in Tamilnadu. This institute has been engaged in sugar cane improvement. The objectives of sugar can breeding are

(a) Increased yield per hectare.

(b) Early maturity or late maturity depending on the area of cultivation.

(c) Resistance to plant pathogens and pests.

(d) Increased sugar (sucrose) content in the juice.

There are three varieties in sugar cane based on the maturing time.

These are - early season, mid season and late season variety OCo 1266. An early maturing variety has a higher yield than the norami Col 29. P 12091 and Co 1318, two new varieties produced at Coiambatore and released for cultivation in Punjab area have a better yield than Col 29.

Among the mid season maturing canes, the standard variety CoL9 has bepn replaced by Co J76 and Co 975. These not only have a higher sucrose content but also resistant to frost. Experimental cultivations conducted a Jullundur, Kheri etc have proved Co 975 to be superior to the other varieties.

In the late season group a new variety Co 1148 (P 4383 x Co 301) has been shown to be better than the regularly cultivated CoJ 46. Co 1148 has many desirable traits like, high yield, late ripening, resistant to frost with moderate resistance to red rot disease. This variety however is not suitable for gur production.

Several other varieites released for cultivation in Punjab viz. Co 62401, Co 740, P 11996 etc seem to have a higher sucrose content and increased cane output. The late maturing variety Co 1148 cultivated in the Gurudaspur region has 15.6% sucrose content whereas Co 62401 has 15.9% sucrose content. P 11996 is the highest yielder among the late maturing varieties.

The sugar cane breeding Institute has also developed many varieties (among the late maturing ones) which have a sugar content as high as 22 percent.

In addition to the varieties mentioned above which are suitable for cultivation in the plains, many varieties suitable for the sub montane region have also been developed.

Among the sub montane varieties Co 1266 and P 12235 have a better yield and a high content of sucrose. Co 1318, P 12235, Co 1266 are early maturing varieties.

Varieties Co 1307, and Co 975 are midseason canes among the sub montane plants. The other varieties are Co-S 245, and Co 1158 have a high sucrose content.

The Institute at Coimbatore has also developed many frost reistant and red rot resistant varieties. The red rot disease takes a heavy toll of the crop in south India. The varieties resistant to frost are Co 1328, Co 975, Co 1148. Co 1244 is red rot resistant. Varieties resistant to smut disease have also been evolved at Coimbatore. These are - Co 290, Co 449 and Co 617.

The sugar cane breeding Institute at Coimbatore has been rendering yeomen service to the cultivation of improved sugar cane varieties with the result, varieties developed at the Institute have been under cultivation in several parts of the world.

ANIMAL BREEDING

This may be said to be as old as human civilization. Even before written records are available, animal breeders were experimenting and most of the domesticated animals today are a product of selection and breeding. Horse, goat, sheep, pig, fowls, cattle, dogs etc., are the best examples of domesticated animals wich have been bred for desired characters.

Aims and Objectives of Animal Breeding : Animals are mainly used for the following purposes.

1. Most of the domesticated animals are used either for milk or for meat. Goat, sheep, pigs, fowl etc., are used as meat producing animals. The milk of cow and bufallo is very nutritious and also used in making of butter, cheese etc. Eggs of poultry is another good source of nutrition for human beings. The purpose of breeding is to obtain better quality meat, high yield of milk, better quality egg etc. Another purpose of breeding is to establish disease resistant stock particularly in poultry.
2. Animals like donkeys, oxen, mules etc., are reared and bred for improved strength for load bearing in agriculture.
3. Other domesticated animals like sheep, rabbit, and cattle are bred for improved quality of fur, skin etc. which find extensive use as clothing, foot wear etc.
4. Horses are also bred for improved speed particularly for racing purposes.

Methods of animal breeding

The following are the various methods employed in animal breeding.

1. Selection of Characters : Desired characters are chosen in an animal used as a parent stock. In breeding usually a parent in chosen based on not one but many desired characters. This is called artificial selection.

2. Progeny test : Generally in some animals only one sex is commercially useful, for e.g. in cattle cow for milk production and in poultry hen for egg laying etc. But the male also equally contributes to the quality of egg, yield of milk etc. If a proper female is chosen and bred with any type of male desired results are not obtained.

Hence the selection of a proper male is also necessary. But the selection of a proper male for a maternal character is difficult. This is usually done by progeny test. A female with a desired character is a chosen first and is bred with a number of males. The resultant progeny is tested for the desired trait. In whichever cross, the progeny has the desired character, that male parent is selected.

Inbreeding : Production of offspring from closely related parents is called inbreeding. Various degrees of inbreeding occur among animals of different phyla, while in some, self fertilization seems to be more prevalent. Generally however nature also does not prefer inbreeding. Inbreeding seems to be the best method of perpetuation when an ideal gene combination is present in an organisms.

Robert Bakewell, a poineer breeder has inbred horses, cattle, sheep etc. to the best advantage. The experiments of Ritzema Bos (1884) and Weismann on breeding of rats, however have clearly revealed the decrease in vigour as a result of continued inbreeding. Bos inbred rats for over twenty generations, and observed a decreased capacity of reproduction among the young ones. The rate of litter production, which was about 7.5 fell down to 3.5 in the last ten generations. Brother sister matings in Poland China swine however did not show any decreased vigour even after eight generations.

The experiments of Castle on inbreeding in *Drosophila melanogaster* for nearly 60 generations did not reveal any harmful effects. Similarly, the experiments of Sewall wright on guinea pigs for over 15 years have revealed no side effect, expect a slight decline in vigour.

In human beings, most human societies, prohibit incest. In some ancient races, incest was a regular practise among royal families. The ptolemies of Egypt, in order to maintain their 'pure blood' practised brother sister marriages. The famour Cleopatra was also a product of inbreeding. The ancient Egypt provides one more example of inbreeding. The Pharaohs and Hebrews practised marriages among brothers and sisters, obviously with no side effects. Even during the present time, many societies and many countries envourage cousin or nephew neice marriages. An understanding of the mechanism of inheritance, however clearly shows that, inbreeding does result in recessive genes coming' together and enhances the possibility of increased manifestation of genetic disorders if any. On the other hand, distant marriages will enhance the chance of a recessive gene getting the protection of a dominant gene and thus reduces the manifestations of disorders. Some of the genetic disorders like idiocy, insanity etc., (atleast in some cases) may be traced to close inbreeding.

Outbreeding : The term outbreeding refers to crossing individuals which are not closely related. The process is also generally known as hybridization. Due to hybridization, the gene combination becomes varied and the drawbacks one sees in inbreeding like the homozygosity of the recessive genes will not be there. But hybridization between individuals which are very distant may often lead to hybrid sterility as there is absolutely no homogenity in their genomes. Hybrid sterility is of common occurrence in interspecific or intergeneric crosses. But outbreeding between individuals of the same species but differing in many characters in many instances produces a strong and vigorous progeny. This phenomenon is called Hybrid vigour or Heterosis.

It may seem to be a paradox, that outbreeding may produce both hybrid sterility as well as hybrid vigour. But one has to bear in mind, that outbreeding is advantageous and brings in vigour due to recombination of genes within the parametere set by the genome of a species. Any outstepping of the limit will result in non identical genomes and hence production of non viable eggs or sperms leading to sterility Outbreeding in plants is practised to a greater extent than in animals. Many interspecific crosses are also successful in the case of plants. A properly organised and controlled outbreeding even in animals can certainly lead to individuals of better quality like high quality of milk meat, egg, etc. A classical example of interspecific cross is mule, obtained by a cross between an ass and horse. The mule combines the qualities of both horse and ass like speed, strength and lack of excitability. But the mule is sterile.

Outbreeding in sheep has helped in obtaining better quality meat and wool. Two lines of sheep viz. Rambouillet and Lincon varieties have been crossed to obtain a new variety of sheep combining the qualities like gregarious habit and short fine wool of the Rambouillet stock and long coarse wool but good quality of meat of the Lincon stock. The new breed is called the Columbia breed.

Outbreeding in rabbits in known to increase the weight of the progeny, when compared with the inbred lines. Outbreeding of Hereford cattle increases the weight of the progeny as much as 30 kilograms. Similarly a cross between the white short horn and a black Angus cattle produces a blue roan hybrid which exhibits vigour, growth and good quality of meat.

In a cross between the Indian Brahman bull and cattle of European origin, a hybrid with greater adaptability to tropical climate has been produced. The following is a comparison of salient features between inbreeding and outbreeding.

	INBREEDING	OUTBREEDING
1.	Generally, vigour, yield and other vital characters decrease	Vigour, growth and other vital characters improve
2.	Pure lines are created due to continuous inbreeding.	Pure lines are eliminated. Hybrids are produced.
3.	Homozygous individuals increase in number	Heterozygous individuals increase in number.
4.	Recessive genes get a chance for morphological expression as they lack the wild gene.	Recessive genes are generally suppressed due to the presence of the wild gene.

INBREEDING	OUTBREEDING
5. The number of recessive genes in a population generally decrease due to their exposure. Individuals possesing lethal genes die.	Recessive genes are suppressed and protected due to non exposure, individuals heterozygous to the lethal genes survive.
6. Morphological expression of recessive genes does not always expose harmful effects; it may bring out even good qualities	Irrespective of the trait, recessive genes do not have a chance of morphological manifestation as they are generally masked by the effect of dominant genes.
7. Recessive genes are exposed to the effect of natural selection.	Recessive genes are shieleded from the perview of natural selection.
8. No alteration is possible in the existing genotype. Genotype becomes highly exclusive.	Genotype will not be stabilized; alteration is possible.
9. Genotype becomes rigid without any variety and plasticity.	Genetic variety is brought about due to hybridization.
10. Individuals will not have an evolutionary future, but may be highly successful in a static environment. (But the environment is not always static).	Genetic plasticity assures the adaptive potentiality to individuals and are assured of evolutionary future.
11. Continuous inbreeding may result in reduced reproductive potentiality.	Outbreeding between two widely unrelated individuals may bring sterility.

In conclusion it may be said that from the point of view of individual species survival and long range evolutionary future, both inbreeding and outbreeding have their own role to play. In a situation, when an individual has achieved ideal gene combination and is most successful to a given environment, any outbreeding will certainly disturb the gene combination. In such a situation inbreeding is ideal. On the other hand, total abandonment of outbreeding will rob the individual of its potential of genetic variety and plasticity, which is necessary as it provides adaptive radiation. From the evolutionary stand point, a limited inbreeding with regular outbreeding will produce variety among organisms.

19

GENETIC CODE

Proteins are the fundamental biological constituents of the protoplasm. They form 15% of the body in living organisms and are important building material of the cells. They play a significiant role in the physical and chemical activities of the cells. They are involved in the structural and functional organisation of the cell. The structural proteins form the various cellular organelles. The functional proteins like enzymes and hormonės control the metabolic, biosynthetic, biogenetic, bio-energetic, growth regulating, sensory and reproductive functions of the cell. The 'gene actions' take place by means of enzymes. The enzymes are the important catalysing agents in most biochemical reactions. Thus proteins through their particular structure, composition and enzyme activity form the most important biochemical compounds through which 'hereditary traits' are expressed in the organism.

Proteins are giant molecules formed of polypeptide chains of several hundred amino acids. About 20 and odd number of amino acids are known to occur in the cells. Amino acids are formed of a basic amino (NH_2) and an acidic carboxyl (COOH) groups. The variety of cells in an organism and multiple variety of organisms represent myriads of proteins. Different types of proteins are synthesised by different cells of the body. Different combinations of amino acids produce different proteins.

Synthesis of Protein

The process of protein synthesis is the most complicated biological activity. Basically it is governed by the *genetic information* carried in the genes (DNA) of the chromosomes. Specific amino acids are linked in particular sequence or order to form a polypetide chain of protein. The various cell organelles and chemical compounds involved in the synthetic proces are

1. Deoxyribonucleic acid .... DNA
2. Three type of ribonucleic acids .... RNA
3. Amino acids
4. Enzymes and
5. Ribosomes

The discussion above will clearly reveal that proteins are the representative of the master molecule of the cell DNA to carry out and regulate all the metabolic activities. Proteins are important in another way also. They are important for the existence of DNA itself. A number enzymes (proteins) are necessary for the replication of DNA itself. When proteins are of such fundamental biological importance, no wonder then the cell machinery to synthesize them (proteins) is not only complicated but precisely regulated.

Which molecule(s) present in the cell can regulate the synthesis of proteins? Obviously there cannot be another compound than DNA. The structure and properties of the DNA molecule are eminently suited to exercise such a regulation over the synthesis of proteins.

Having conceded that DNA directly is involved in the regulation of protein synthesis we may now try to answer the two following questions - which aspect of protein structure is controlled by DNA? And how and by what mechanism DNA regulates the assembly of amino acids to synthesize the proteins?

Proteins are extremely complicated biological macromolecules. There are different dimensions for its structural complexity and integrity. These are theprimary, secondary, teritary and quaternary structures (for details - see later in protein synthesis). DNA molecule specifies only the primary structure, while othe ther dimensions of protein structure like folding etc is controlled by proeins themselves.

The primary structure of proteins involves the following aspects - quality, quantity and sequence of amino acids and it is this that is regulated by DNA.

What is the mechanism adopted by DNA to regulate the synthesis of proteins? Obviously proteins cannot be synthesized *in situ ie* within the nucleus, because all the components needed for proteins-amino acids - ribosomes etc are not present in the nucleus. It is not possible also for the DNA itself to migrate to cytoplasm to synthesize the proteins. The only alternative is for DNA to send a messenger or representative which carries the message to specify the quality, quantity and the sequence of amino acids to be asembled to produce the protein. This message is called the genetic code, because it specifies in genetic language the amino acids to be assembled.

The language of genetic code

A code is said to be a cryptic or hidden language carrying a message and upon deciphering or translation, the message is understood. In the genetic code, the message is translated as the type of aminoacid to be assembled. What is the composition of the genetic code that comes out of DNA? To answer this we must first understand the manner in which genetic information exists in the DNA molecule.

It is well known that eventhough the DNA molecule has three components namely sugar, phosphate and nitrogen bases, it is the last one that is unique to each DNA molecule in the sequence of their arrangement. The nitrogen bases vary from one DNA segment to another in arrangement so the information is based upon the sequence of their arrangement. The sequence of nucleotides is then the code in which the DNA sends the message. How is the message sent? The DNA molecule replicates in a particular segment and the replicated segment in the form of RNA now called mRNA carries the genetic message in the form of nucleotide sequence (for details see protein synthesis). The sequence of nitrogen bases have been found to be identical to the linear sequence of amino acids in a peptide chain. In otherwords there is colinearity between mRNA and polypeptide chain (see later in the chapter for details of colinearity).

It is thus clear that the genetic code is in the language of nitrogen bases and the reading of the code is in their sequence of arrangement.

Amino acids involved in protein synthesis

A large number of amino acids - almost upto 150 are found in nature. Of these however quite a number of them remain as free amino acids in the sense they do not join together to form a molecule of protein. It has been found out that only about a little more than 20 amino acids are protein amino acids in that all the known proteins are made up of only these amino acids. Some amino acids however are found in a almost all protein chains while a few others are found only in very few proteins. For example cystine is present only in proteins which have a disulphide linkage. Hydroxylproline is another amino acid found only in few proteins.

The code is triplet (basis of crypto analysis)

A DNA molecule from every source contains only 4 types of nucleotides-adenine, guanine, cytosine and thymine. On the other hand the basic building blocks of proteins namely amino acids are more than 20 types. A basic problem that one has to analyse before finding about a genetic code is how many bases specify a unit of amino acis. Sevral opinions have been put forward in this regard.

Singlet code. According to one of the opinions each nucleotide will code for one amino acid. But this would be insufficient to code for all the 20 amino acids as there are only 4 nucleotides. With 4 nucleotides only 4 amino acids can be coded. What about the rest?

Doublet code. This asumes that each code is formed of two letters i.e., 2 nucleotides. In other words, 2 nucleotides will specify one amino acid. In this type of a code all the 20 amino acids cannot be coded but 16 codes (4 x 4) are possible. But there will be a number of ambiguous determination of amino acids.

Possible singlet, doublet and triplet codes of mRNA

Single Code (4 words)	Double (16 words)				Code Triple Code (64 words)			
					AAA	AAG	AAC	AAU
					AGA	AGG	AGC	AGU
					ACA	ACG	ACC	ACU
					AUA	AUG	AUC	AUU
					GAA	GAG	GAC	GAU
					GGA	GGG	GGC	GGU
					GCA	GCG	GCC	GCU
A	AA	AG	AC	AU	GUA	GUG	GUC	GUU
G	GA	GG	GC	GU	CAA	CAG	CAC	CAU
C	CA	CG	CC	CU	CGA	CGG	CGC	CGU
U	UA	UG	UC	UU	CCA	CCG	CCC	CCU
					CUA	CUG	CUC	CUU
					UAA	UAG	UAC	UAU
					UGA	UGG	UGC	UGU
					UCA	UCG	UCC	UCC
					UUA	UUG	UUC	UUC

Triplet code. This was first suggested by the physicist George Gamow (1954). According to this 3 bases (nucleotides) will code for one amino acid. In other words each code will have 3 nucleotides which will specify the particular amino acid. These triplets of codes are given the name codons. With triplet codes the possibilities would be 64 (4x4x4) codons. This would be more than the number of amino acids (which are only 20). Obviously then each amino acid will have more than one code. Experimental evidence shows that the code is a triplet and about 61 of the 64 codes are used to specify amino acids during protein synthesis.

The maximum possible number of codons in the singlet, doublet and triplet codes

Type of code	Number of bases in codon	Number of codons	Ambiguous/ degenerate
Single code	1	4	Amgiguous
Double code	2	4 x 4 = 16	Amgiguous
Triplet code	3	4 x 4 x 4 = 65	Degenerate (more than required number)

Properties of code

1. The code is non overlapping

The DNA molecule is a very long chain and has series of nucleotides. There is gap between the nucleotides. Naturally a question arises if three nucleotides constitute a codon will there be any gap between two successive codes or do the codes overlap. In otherwords is the code overlapping or non overlapping? If the code is over lapping from where the reading will begin. Because the beginning of the code reading will alter the nucleotide combination and hence will alter which amino acid is specified by the code. When Gamow proposed the code he assumed it to be overlapping. Many people attempted to rationalise the excess number of codes i.e., 64 for 20 amino acids by assuming that the codes are overlapping and the codons can be reduced to about 20. But this involves a lot of problems. If we take for instance the codes for lysine (AGG and AAA) and codes for phenyl alanine (UUU and UUC). The code letters of these two amino acids are mutual exclusive i.e., lysine can not follow phenyl alanine and *vice versa* in any protein. This constitutes a forbidden combination of amino acids and proteins. But on the other hand these amino acids are found in proteins proving that the genetic code is non overlapping. Further the overlapping code assumes that a nucleotide is read twice in different combinations to code for amino acids. If this is true the entire precision of code would be disturbed. Further, any mutational change in an overlapping code would affect more than one code thus disturbing a number of amino acids.

Mutational studies have shown that the code is non overlapping. In TMV (Tobacco Mosaic Virus) the change of one base in the DNA due to mutation would alter the composition of protein by a single amino acid proving that the code is non overlapping. If the code is overlapping change of one base should have disturbed more than one amino acid. Studies on normal and sickle cell haemoglobins have shown that single base mutations result in the replacement of only one amino acid.

2. The code is degenerate

(Synonym codons). As it has been mentioned above there are 64 possible codons considering the code to be a triplet one. Of these 64 codes about 61 code for amino acids. As they are only 20 amino acids which form the constituents of proteins, it is obvious that the number of codons far exceed the number of amino acids. This leads to the conclusion that each amino acid must have more than one code. Of the 20 amino acids only tryptophan and methionine have a single codon each while all the others have more than one codons. *Phenylalanine, tryosine, histidine, glutamine, asparagine, lysine, aspartic acid* and *glutamic acid* have two codons each (see the codon table). *Leucine, argenine* and *serine* have 6 codons each. Thus there is no specificity as to the number of codons that decide an amino acid. The number of codons (whether one or many) specifying the amino acid possibley have been evolved over a long period of time during the process of evolution. The variability in the number of codons perhaps may explain the differential distribution of amino acids in proteins (those with multiple codons occur more frequently).

When there are multiple codons for an amino acid, it must be noted that these codons are not totally different. Synonym codons specifying an amino acid have the first two bases of the triplet being constant. Whereas only the third will vary. For instance proline is coded by the following codons - CCU, CCC, CCA and CCG. It is obvious here in these synonm codons the first two bases are common.

The multiplicity or degeneracy of the code may pose a question as to why nature has provided alternate codons for an amino acid where a single codon would have been more precise and specific. One possible reason for the degenrecy of the codes is that multiple codons protect the organism from mutations which might eliminate an amino acid altogether if there were to be only one code.

Number of codons coding for different amino acids

	Amino acids	Number of codons
1.	Tryptophan, methoionine	1
2.	Phenylalanine, tyrosine, histidine, glutamine, asparagine	2
	Lysine, aspartic acid, glutamic acid, cysteine	2
3.	Isoleucine	3
4.	Valine, proline, threonine, alanine, glycine	4
5.	Leucine, agrinine, serine	6

3. Polarity of the code

It is very essential that a particular gene shoule specify an amino acid always and in all situations unless it undergoes mutational changes. It is necessary therefore that the code must be read between a fixed beginning point and a fixed end point. These points are referred to as the initiation and termination codons respectively. Another necessity is the reading of the direction of the code because any change in the direction would alter the amino acid. All these features clearly point out that the code must have a polarity i.e., a fixed start, a fixed end point and a predetermined direction. For instance if the codon direction as given below varies the composition of the amino acids would completely vary.

Leucine	Isoleucine	Valine	Serine →
UUG	AUG	GUG	UCG
← Valine	Leucine	Iso Leucine	Alanine

It is obvious from the above that the direction of reading the code would alter the sequence of the amino acids and obviously changes the composition of the proteins. Available molecular biological evidences indicate that the message in mRNA is readin 5' →3' direction. Based on this message the polypeptide chain is synthesised from the direction of amino group to carboxyl group.

4. The code is comaless

One of the most interesting questions with reference to the non overlapping code is, are there any gaps between the codes in the form of punctuation marks so that one code is separate from the other. In genetic terms this means that there could be bases between codes indicating where one code ends and the other begins. For instance codes with intervening punctuation marks can be represented as follows -

UUG	X	AUG	X	GUG	X	UCG
Valine		Leucine		Leucine		Alanine

In the above X can be regarded as a base separating the two codons. If a mutation occurs in any one of the codes, it will not affect other codes and consequently the disturbance in the protein synthesised would be to the extent of only one amino acid. On the other hand if the code is commaless (no punctuation mark-base between codes) mutation in one base would result in a drastic change of the genetic message. Researches of Dr.Khorana and others had clearly indicated that the code is commaless i.e., there is no delimiting point between one codon and other. Khorana and his associates used artifically synthesised long polynucleotide chains which had repeating sequences to produce polypeptide chains. For example the repeating sequence CUCUCU contains the codons for leucine (CUC) and serine (UCU). When this sequence was used for producing the proteins neither amino acid was incorporated with the protein unless the other one is also present. This clearly explains that the triplet code has to be commaless and only then there would be alternate translation of the codes into leucine and serine.

5. Universality of the code

The code was first deciphered and worked out in microorganisms but subsequent researches have clearly shown that these codes are same in their amino acid specification from bacteria to man. Thus, the code is said to be universal. Marshall Caskey and Nirenbrg (1967) have shown by their experiments that diverse organisms such as *E.coli* (bacterium) *Xenopus laevis* (amphibian) and Guinea pig which is a mammal use the same code for their amino acyl tRNAs.

Gene mutations provide additional evidence for the universality of codes. These mutations result in the substitutionof one amino acid for other. Studies have indicated, gene mutations bringing about amino acid substitutions affect the same amino acid in TMB, *E.coli* and also in man. For instance a single point mutation, changes the amino acid in the coat protein of TMV, alpha chain of tryptophan synthetase in *E.coli* and also in the haemoglobin of man.

Another remarkable feature of the code is not only that it universally occurs in all organisms but it has also remained probably without any change ever since it evolved in some bacteria a few billion years ago. Any mutation that occurs would change the composition of mRNA and consequently the amino acid composition in the protein. Changes such as these apparently have proved to be harmful to the organisms and as such there will be a strong selection pressure against the occurrence of such mutations. Hence natural selection has persisted with the codes perhaps ever since they originated.

Ambiguity in the genetic code

There is no evidence to indicate that the genetic code is ambiguous *in vivo*. Ambiguity means that a single codon may code for more than one amino acid. The only exception to the non ambiguity is the AUG codon in prokaryotes -it codes for formyl methionine at the initiation site while at other positions it specifies methionine. It is not clear as to how this distinction is always met precisely but it is believed that the secondary structure of the mRNA at the initiation site may have got something to do with the coding for formyl methionine. In *in vitro* conditions however genetic codes sometimes appear to be ambiguous. For example poly-U codon is known to incorporate some amounts of leucine in addition to phenylalanine. Treatment of ribosomes with streptomycin is known to introduce ambiguity to codons. For example in addition to coding for phenylalanine UUU is also known to code isoleucine, serine and leucine.

Codons and anticodons

During the process of translation the message carried in the mRNA would be converted into the sequence of amino acids which are picked up by tRNA. This is achieved by the process of binding. For this binding to take place, obviously then there should be a specific relationship between the nucleotide of mRNA and those of tRNA. In otherwords the nucleotides of mRNA should be complementary to the nucleotides of tRNA. The nucleotide sequence of mRNA is called the codon and that of tRNA is called anticodon. The reading of mRNA is in the 5'→ 3' direction and the codons are also written in the same direction. For example codon AUG is written as 5' AUG 3'. The corresponding anticodon and tRNA should therefore represented as 5' CAU 3'. In such a configuration the first nucleotide of both codon and anticodon would be the ones at the 5' end and third nucleotides would be at the 3' end.

Very often the anticodon is written in the 3' → 5' direction so that it will be easy to correlate between the bases of codon and anticodon.

Initiation codons

In most of the polypeptide chains the first amino acid which begins the chain is methionine in eukaryotes and N-formlymethionine in prokaryotes. Methionine or N-formylmethionine tRNA complex specifically binds to the initiation sites in mRNA containing the codon AUG which codes for methionine. The AUG code therefore is referred to as the initiation codon. Less frequently however GUG (code for valine) may also serve as the initiation codon in bacterial protein synthesis. In the bacteriophage MS2, GUG is the initiation codon for the protein referred to as A protein. Researches have indicated that the GUG may replace AUG as initiation codon when the latter is lost due to chromosomal abbreation. It has also been found out that chain initiation by GUG is not as efficient as AUG possibly because the former has less affinity for formyl methionyl tRNA.

Termination codons (nonsense codons)

It has been mentioned above that AUG (occasionally GUG) initiates the synthesise of a protein chain. The natural question would be which codon specifies or signals the end of termination of the synthesisof the protein chain. It has been found out that three of the 64 codons do not specify any tRNA and as such they cannot assemble any amino acid. As such these codons whenever they are found in mRNA would signal the end of the chain. They are called termination codons as they terminate the synthesis of the polypeptide chain. They are also called ***nonsense codons*** as they donot specify any amino acid. The nonsense codons are UAG (*amber*) UAA (*ochre*) and UGA (*opal*). Of the three termination codons UAG was the first termination codon to be discovered. It was named amber after a graduate student in Germany named Bernstein (means amber in German). This graduate student helped in the discovery of the class of mutations. The other two termination codons were obviously given the name of the colours only to maintain uniformity.

Termination codons found in mRNA will not specify any amino acid and as such stop the process of translation and bring about the release of the peptide chain from ribosomes. No tRNA molecules have anticodons complementary to the termination codons found in mRNA. Termination codons seem to have some affinity to proteins called release factors which bring about the release of the protein chain. In prokaryotes there are three release factors RF-1, RF-2 and RF-3. RF-1 recognises the amber and ochre codons while RF-2 recognises ochre and opal codons, RF-3 stimulates RF-1 and RF-2 ultimately releasing the newly synthesised peptide chain. In eukaryotes there is a single factor (RF protein) which is capable of recognising all the three termination codons.

Evidence for genetic code (deciphiring the code)

Earlier to the pathbreaking experiments of Nirenberg, Matthai and H.G. Khorama, work on the genetic code was largely speculative and restricted to development to theoritical concepts. The great physict George Gamow who proposed the triplet code gave the comprehensive theoritical concept for various aspects of genetic code. The main features of his proposals are -

1. The code is a triplet
2. Translation is a direct procedure between codon and amino acid
3. Translation of codes is of overlapping type
4. Code is degenerate
5. Nuclei acid and the peptide chain are colinear
6. Code is universal

The works of Brenner (1957) showed that the triplet code is of non overlapping type. Gamow's idea of the direct translation process became unacceptable when Crick proposed adoptor hypothesis. As per this hypothesis during the translation process some mediator molecules intervene between amino acids and nucleic acids. It is now known that the intervening molecules are tRNA.

Experimental evidence for the existence of genetic code may be obtained by two basic approaches - *in vitro* approach and *in vivo* approach. In *in vitro* method nucleotide sequence are compared with the amino acid residues of the proteins in a culture medium. In *in vivo* method proteins and nucleic acids are obtained from intact cells and then compared.

The *in vitro* approach has the following four methods

1. Genetic analysis of deletion mutatants of a cistron
2. Incorporation of amino acids by synthetic polyribonucleotides
3. Binding of known triplets of aminoacyl tRNA.
4. Amino aicd sequence generated by mRNA transcribed from synthetic tRNA of known nucleotides sequences

1. Genetic analysis

Genetic analysis of deletion and insertion mutants (spontaneous as well as induced) in phage T4 was reported by Crick *et al* in 1961. This deletion or insertion of a nucleotide in a DNA chain leads to a frame shift mutation after the point of deletion or insertion. As a result of this, the reading of the codon subsequent to the mutation gets altered. Obviously then the amino acid composition of the resultant protein would be different. As a result, the protein may be functionally inactive. All the mutations tested by Crick *et al* produced a phenotype called mutant II. It was further observed by Crick *et al* that a series of three mutations was necessary to supress the effects of a previous mutation. In other words three supressor mutations would nullify the effect of three frame shift mutations and bring back the original phenotype. This is a clear evidence to show that the altered codon reading would return to the normal state after three point mutations thus indicating that the codon must have three nucleotides.

The study also indicates that the code is commaless. If there were to be a punctuation mark between the two codes a deletion or insertion of a base would change the number of bases between two commas adjacent to the point of insertion or deletion.

2. Incorporation of amino acids by synthetic polyribonucleotides

Synthetic polyribo nucleotides were used as mRNA by Nirenberg and Matthai to determine the meaning of codons. They produced a synthetic RNA by using the enzyme polynucleotide phosphorylase discovered in 1955 by Grunberg. Manago and Ochoa. This enzyme does not use DNA as a template and can incorporate ribonucleotides in a random order. The first synthetic RNA used for protein in a cell-free system (the *in vitro* system consists of ribosomes, tRNA's and other necessary factors for protein synthesis) was poly U i.e., the mRNA consists of only one nucleotide namely U in a series. This can be called a homopolymer as it is a polymer of only one nucleotide. The poly U mRNA was able to synthesis a homopolymer of a polypeptide chain containing only phenylalanine residues. This proved that the triplet code UUU specifies phenylaline. Subsequently many such homopolymer species of mRNA were synthesized and were directed to produce polypeptide chains. For example AAA was shown to code for lysine and CCC specified proline.

Nirenberg and Ochoa subsequently used heteropolymeres of mRNA to produce polypeptide chains. A heteropolymer includes a mixture of two, three or all the four nucleotides in mRNA. This yielded further information on the possible codons for certain amino acids. For example poly CG directs the incorporation of arginine and alanine in addition to the proline coded by poly C. Some additional information on the assignment of codons to individual amino acids was obtained by varying the ratios of different nucleotides in the synthetic mRNA. In this experiment the code assignment was at best ambiguous since all the four bases were not required for the incorporation of any of the amino acids.

3. Binding of known triplets to aminoacyl tRNA

A triribonucleotide cannot direct the synthesis of a polypeptide but it leads to binding of specific aminoacyl tRNA to the ribosomes. Nirenberg *et al* used this property for assigning specific codons of specific amino acids. Their technique is known Nirenberg - Leder technique. Conventionally a trinucleotide with 5' terminal phosphate are more active and those lacking this phosphates in inducing the binding of aminoacyl tRNA to ribosomes. On the otherhand those with 3' terminal phosphate are inactive. This shows that the codons must be triplet. In the Nirenberg - Leder technique trinucleotides with 5' terminal phosphate are added to a cell free system containing a mixture of 20 amino acids bound to their respective tRNA. One of the 20 amino acids had radioactive carbon. For different experiments different labelled amino acids were used but with the same trinucleotide after the synthesis of protein the cell free mixture containing ribosomes were analysed to detect radioactivity confirming the binding of aminoacyl tRNA to the ribosomes. These studies showed that UUU, CCC and AAA induced the binding of phenylalnine, proline and lycine respectively to ribosomes. Using this technique Nirenberg *et al* assigned most of the codons to their respective amino acids.

FIRST LETTER	SECOND LETTER: U	C	A	G	SECOND LETTER
U	UUU-Phen	UCU-Ser	UAU-Tyr.	UGU-Cys	U
	UUC-Phen	UCC-Ser	UAC-Tyr.	UGC-Cys	C
	UUA-Leu	UCA-Ser	UAA-Ochre	UGA-Nonsense	A
	UUG-Leu	UCG-Pro	UAG-Amber	UGG-Trip	G
C	CUU -Leu	CCU-Pro	CAU-this	CGU-Arg	U
	CUC-Leu	CCC-Pro	CAC-This	CGC-Arg	C
	CUA-Leu	CCA-Pro	CAA-Glu	CGA-Arg	A
	CUG-Leu	CCG-Pro	CAG-Glu	CGG- Arg	G
A	AUU- Ile	ACU-Thr	AAU-Aspn	CGU-Ser	U
	AUC-Ile	ACC-Thr	AAC-Aspn	AGC-Ser	C
	AUA- Ile	ACA-Thr	AAA-Lys.	AGA-Arg	A
	AUG Met	ACG-Thr	AAG-Lys	AGG-Arg	G
G	GUU-Val	GCU-Ala	GAU-Asp	GGU-Gly	U
	GUA-Val	GCC-Ala	GAC-Asp	GGC-Gly	C
	GUA-Val	GCA-Ala	GAA -Glu	GGA Gly	A
	GUG-Val	GCG-Ala	GAG-Glu	GGG-Gly	G

Fig. 19.1 Genetic code

The codon dictionary

4. Amino acid sequence generated by mRNA transcribed from synthetic tRNA of known nucleotides sequences

H.G. Khorana and his associates used the above technique for codon assignment in *in vitro* conditions. Known as Khorana technique in this method long specific DNA sequences are first synthesized. These are then transcribed to mRNA molecules using the DNA directed RNA polymerase enzyme. These mRNA molecules which have known sequences of nucleotide are directed to synthesize polypeptides. The polypeptides were then subjected to sequential degradation to know the amino acid sequences. The nucleotides sequence is then compared with the amino acid sequences. The nucleotide sequence is to deduce specific codons for different amino acids. Using this technique almost all the codons for amino acids were designated. In this technique Khorana and associates also confirmed many other characters of the code such as degenerecy, commaless nature, non overlappingand triplet nature also.

In Vivo codon assignment

In the cell free systems, genetic codes have been deciphered with reference to their amino acid affinity but a doubt may arise whether these codes are the same in living systems also. In otherwords whether the living systems use the same codes for protein synthesis. In order to prove the similarity of codes in both in *vitro* and *in vivo* three different techniques were used by three different molecular biologists.

(i) *Amino acid replacement studies*

(ii) *Frame shift mutation studies*

(iii) *Comparison of a nucleotide sequence of a cistron and the amino acid sequence of the polypeptide produced by it*

Amino acids replacement studies on the synthesis of tryptophan synthetase in *E.coli* (Yanofsky, 1963) have clearly indicated that the codons for the replaced amino acids and for the amino acid replacing it prove the specificity of a codon for a particular amino acid. Frame shift mutations on lysozol enzyme of T4 bacteriophages have also shown the affinity between a specific codon and a particular amino acid.

The direct in vivo evidence for the genetic code comes from a comparison of the base sequence of a cistron and the amino acid sequence in a polypeptide chain produced by it. Such a study has been done with RNA bacteriophage MS2 which has only three cistrons. One of these cistrons produces the coat protein having 129 amino acids. The cistron responsible for it has 387 nucleotides. There is a total agreement between amino acid sequence expected from the base sequence of the cistron and the actual amino acid sequence of the head protein. In othewords each codon of the cistron precisely designates the same amino acids as expected from the coding dictionary.

Wobble hypothesis - for details see protein synthesis

Colinearity of the gene structure and its product

The gene is an unbranched chain of nucleotide pairs in a particular sequence. The polypeptide chain is also unbranched and is made up of amino acid residues attached in a linear series. Thus a linear relationship between the gene and the polypeptide chain produced by it can be indicated. Yanofsky *et al* (1964) established this colinearity in their study of tryptophan synthetase enzyme of *E coli.*

The enzyme tryptophan synthetase is made up of two chains α and β. A genetic map of the α chain gene was established by determining the recombination percentage of mutations for the amino acid tryptophan. The complete amino acid residues of the α chain of the enzyme tryptophan synthetase was thus established. Subsequently the location of amino acid substitutions in the chain for 10 mutations was determined. It was then found out that the order of mutations corresponded with the order of amino acid substitutions in the α chain of the polypeptide.

Sarabhai et al (1964) came to the same conclusion in their study of nonsense mutations in bacteriophage T4.

Pattern of the genetic code

A distinct pattern emerges when one analyses the amino acid structure and the type of codons that specify them. Amino acids with similar structural properties tend to have related codons. For example codons for aspartic acid (GAU and GAC) are similar to the codons for glutanic acid (GAA and GAG). Same relationship is found between the codons of phenylalanine, tyrosine and tryptophan - all these begin with uracil. It is believed that this feature of the code is evolved to minimise the consequences of mistakes that may arise during translation and base substitutions due to mutation. In other words if an amino acidin a protein is replaced by another with almost similar properties the protein may still remain functional.

Another pattern that is seen in the code isthat for synonym codons (multiple codes for the same amino acid) the first two bases are always constant whereas only the third one varies. The flexibility of the third nucleotide of the codon is another method to help minimise the harm posed by mutations. Crick (1966) has called this wobbling and proposed a hypothesis called Wobble hypothesis (see protein synthesis for details).

New genetic codes in mitochondria and ciliate protozoa

It has been mentioned above that the code is universal and ever since it originated it has remained static. However during 1980s it was observed that the genetic codes of mitochondrial DNA in yeasts may be different from the others. In yeast mitochondria UGA codes for tryptophan while in nuclear genes in the same organism UGA is the termination codon. This however is not to say thatin all mitochondria of all organisms the UGA codes for tryptophan. For example in maize cytochrome oxidase tryptophan is coded by CGG. This code in nuclear genes codes for arginine. There are also indications that AUA which codes for isoleucine in nuclear genes codes for methionine in *mit* DNA of mammals, yeast, *Drosophila* etc.

A different genetic code in DNA is perhaps necessiated because of the small *mit* genome size. T.H. Jukes (1966) presented a concept called *archetypal code* which will allow one anticodon (of tRNA) to pair with 4 different codons due to wobbling at the first base of anticodon and the third base of codon.

In 1986 a different genetic code was shown to be working in a ciliate member of Mycoplasma (*Mycoplasma capricolum*). In the genetic code of this organism UAA and UAG are not nonsense codons but code for glutamine.

Evolution of genetic code

Many of the features of the genetic code like degeneracy, non overlapping, commaless nature etc have led to a suggestion that the present version of the genetic code has evolved from a more primitive version which are perhaps a doublet than a triplet. It is believed that this shifting from doublet to triplet occurred very earily in the origin of cellular life. It is not certain however whether all the codes for all the amino acids were evolved simultaneously or the codon dictionary gradually arrived at the present stage of 64 is not certain. One thing however is certain eversince it came into existence in the present form the biological necessity of it imposed such a selection pressure on it that it has remained unchanged upto to the present day.

20

PROTEIN SYNTHESIS

Protein Structure And Classification

Of the two important macromolecules that mastermind all the activities of the living systems, proteins are one, the nucleic acids being the other. Proteins are present all over the cell and are important both structurally and functionally.

The name protein was first suggested by Berzelius (1838). *Protein* in Greek means 'First rank'. Proteins are highly complex organic molecules with molecular weight ranging upto many millions. Chemically proteins are madeup of C, H, O and N. In addition to these major elements, some proteins may also haave sulphur, phosphorous, iron zinc, iodine etc as components. The ratio of major elements in proteins are C= 50-55%, O=20.23%, N=15-18% and S=0-4%.

Proteins are made up of building blocks called amino acids (i.e. on hydrolysis, proteins yield these units). The idea that proteins are built up of amino acids was first proposed by Emil Fischer.

Amino acids are carboxylic acids which have atleast one COOH group and one NH_2 group. Other functional groups may also be present. There are atleast 22 different types of amino acids encountered in plants.

The amino acids are bound to one another in a protein chain by means of linkages or bonds called peptide linkages. Peptide linkages are formed between the COOH group of one amino acid and the NH_2 group of the other, with the elimination of a molecule of water. Several amino acids combine together with the peptide bond and form a peptide chain. Several of these peptides constitute a polypeptide chain. The polypeptide chain folds and refolds in a characteristic fashion to form a protein molecule.

Peptides

These are made up of amino acids linked with CONH (peptide) bonds. Peptides are intermediate compounds produced during the synthesis or degradation of proteins.

Amino acids ——— peptides ——— proteins

Proteins

These are thefinal productsin the N_2 metabolism, and are made up of folded peptide chains which have many additional linkages (depends upon the point of folding) in addition to the CONH bond. Proteins have a three dimensional configuration and have very high molecular weight reaching upto 10^4 - 10^-.

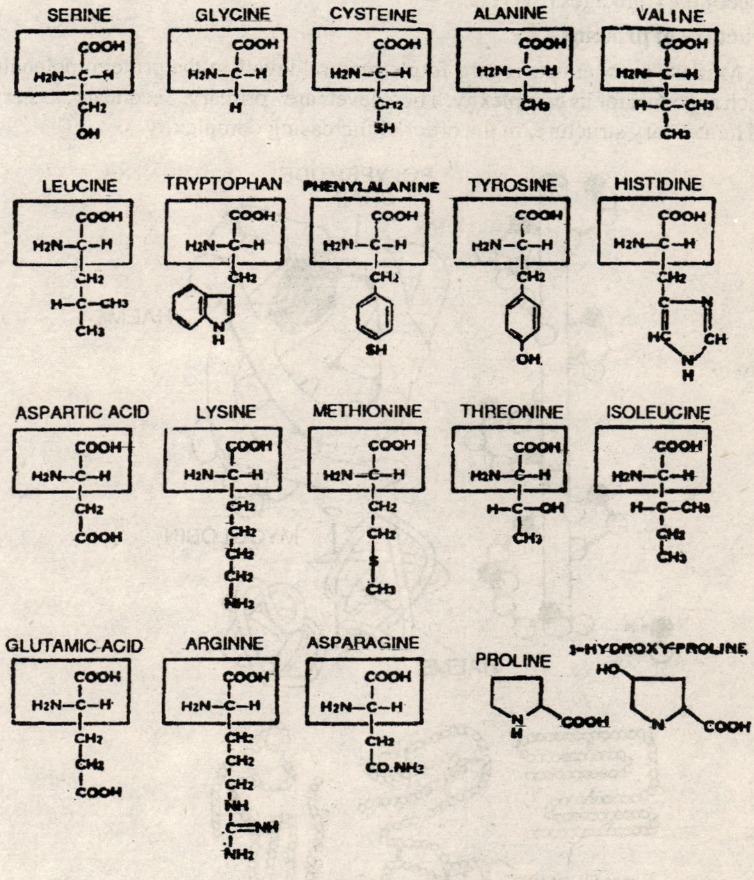

Fig. 20.1 Protein synthesis
Structure of the amino acids

Although proteins contain not more than 20 amino acids, they are of immense variety and complexity due to variations in combination of amino acids. In general the three following aspects pertaining to the amino acids decide the type of protein. These are - the quality, quantity and sequence of amino acids in the peptide chains.

In other words, the type of amino acid, its quantity and the sequence in which these acids are arranged forms the basis for the categorization of proteins. Besides, proteins may differ in the number of peptide chains per molecule, type of secondary linkages (SH) etc.

Structure of proteins

Modern biochemists regard four structural levels in the protein molecule which accounts for its complexity. These levels are - primary. Secondary, tertiary and quaternary structure, in the order of increasing complexity.

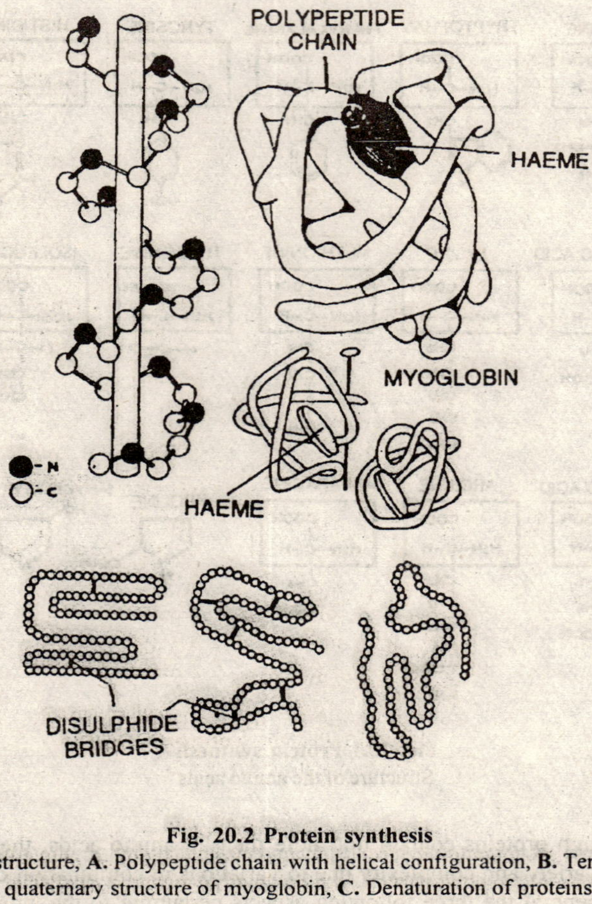

Fig. 20.2 Protein synthesis

Protein structure, A. Polypeptide chain with helical configuration, B. Tertiary and quaternary structure of myoglobin, C. Denaturation of proteins

Primary structure

This is the simplest and the most basic structure and refers to the linear peptide chain. Besides the CONH bond, disulphide bonds (-S-S-) are found or among the peptide chain linkage in the sulphur containing amino acids.

Secondary structure

The primary polypeptide chain spirally coils forming the L helical chain. The characteristic bonds of the secondary structures are hydrogen bonds between the carbonyl and amino groups of peptide links, salt linkages and Vander Wall's forces which help maintain the helical structure.

Tertiary structure

Folding and superfolding of the helical chain in a three dimensional orientation constitutes the tertiary structure. Interaction between the amino acid residues situated far apart in the chain brings about the folding.

Quaternary structure

This consists of more than one identical sub units (poly peptide chain) which associate with one another to form a functional unit. Individually each subunit is non functional. Such complicated structures are usually seen in enzymes. For example the enzyme phosphorylase has two sub units, which are inactive individually, but as dimers, they are active. A protein with identical sub units in the quaternary structure is known to be homogenous or if the subunits are dissimilar it is known as heterogenous. A protein with more than one sub unit (monomer) is referred to as an oligomeric protein.

Classification of Proteins

As the proteins possess, a very complex strucuture, their classification also poses a problem as many categorizations are possible based on structure, function etc. The following is a generalized classification. The major groups are recognized in proteins based on their solubility and chemical properties.

I. Simple proteins
II. Conjugated proteins and
III. Derived proteins.

I. SIMPLE PROTEINS

Chemically these have only amino acids. No additional compounds are present in the molecule. Simple proteins are of the folowing kinds -

1. Albumins

These are soluble in water, dilute salts, acids and alkalies. Heat denatures the protein structure by coagulation. Some of the commonly occuring albumins are Legumelin (from legume seeds), Amylase (from barely), Leucosin (from cereals) etc.

2. Globulins

Less soluble in water than albumins but soluble in less concentrated salt solutions. Heat coagulation is seen in globulins also. Eg. Legumin (pears), Tuberin (potato) etc.

3. Glutelins

Insoluble in water and salt solutions, but soluble in weak acids and alkalies. Glutelins are generally found in plants and are heat immune. Seed proteins found in cereals like Wheat (*glutenin*) and rice, *oryzenin*) are best examples of glutelins.

4. Prolamines

These proteins are water insoluble, but dissolve in 70-80% alcohol. Prolamines have a high concentration of the amino acid proline and other amides. E.g. Gliadin (Wheat), Hordein (barley) and Zein (maize)

5. Scleroproteins

These are fibrous proteins found as an integral part of the structural framework of plants. These proteins are insoluble in most of the solvents.

6. Histones

Most of the nucleoproteins, hemoglobin and globins are histones. They are insoluble in water but insoluble in dilute ammonia. Histones have a high concentration of lysine and arginine.

7. Protamines

These are soluble in water, dilute acids and ammonia and do not undergo heat coagulation. Basic amino acids are rich in protamines, while tryptophan and tyrosine are completely absent. Eg. Nucleoproteins of sperms in fish.

II. CONJUGATED PROTEINS

In these proteins, non amino acid components are associated with the protein molecule. The non amino components are called prosthetic groups. There are seven major categories of conjugated proteins.

1. Nucleoproteins

Proteins are found in combination with nucleic acids. Hydrolysis can separate nucleic acids and simple proteins. Nucleoproteins are water soluble.

2. Glycoproteins

Also called mucoids, these are conjugated with carbohydrates like macromolecular polysaccharides, sugars, sugar phosphate etc. Glycoproteins are found in cell membranes.

3. Chromoproteins

These constitute the pigments and are coloured, the coloured appearance is due to the presence of metals such as Cu, Fe, Mg etc. Chlorophylls, flavoproteins, carotenoids, cytochromes etc are typical examples of chromoproteins.

4. Lipoproteins

Proteins in conjugation with lipids are called lipoproteins. Lecithin, Cephalin etc are the lipids found in combination with proteins. Lipoproteins are an integral part of all cell membranes.

5. Metalloproteins

Certain types of enzymes which require metals as activators belong to this group. Many of the respiratory enzymes belong to this group.

6. Phosphoproteins

These are proteins with phosphoric acid as the prosthetic group. Phosphoproteins are insoluble in water, but soluble in alkalies. E.g. milk and egg protein (casein and viteline).

7. Lecithoprotein

Proteins with lecithin as the prosthetic group (E.g. white of egg) belong to this group.

III. DERIVED PROTEINS

These are degradation products of proteins. Primary proteins on hydrolysis with acids or alkalies yield derived proteins.

(A) Primary derived proteins and
(B) Secondary derived proteins

A. Primary derived Proteins

There are two categories of primary derived proteins. These are metaproteins and Coagulated proteins.

(i) Metaproteins : These are insoluble in water but dissolve in dilute salt solutions, acids and alkalies. Hydrolysis of natural proteins on long treatment with alkalies or acids yield metaproteins.

(ii) Coagulated proteins: Treatment with heat or alcohol of natural proteins yields these proteins.

B. Secondary derived proteins

Three types of secondary derived proteins have been identified. These are protoeses, peptones and peptides.

(i) Proteoses : Prolonged hydrolysis of metaproteins yield proteoses (eg. Albuminoses from albumin). These are water soluble but immune to heat treatment.

(ii) Peptones : Peptones are obtained by continued hydrolysis of proteoses. Like proteoses, these are also water soluble and heat insensitive.

(iii) Peptides : Prolonged hydrolysis of natural proteins yields peptides. These are also water soluble and not coagulated by heat.

Functions of proteins

Most of the vital activities of the cell are controlled by the two master molecules namely proteins and nucleic acids. Proteins are important both from the point of view of structure and function of the cell. Structurally proteins constitute in integral part of membranes, pigments etc. Functionally in the form of enzymes, proteins play such a vital role in cell physiology, that without proteins (enzymes) no metabolic reaction is possible. Even the synthesis of DNA is regulated by proteins. In the form of Chromoproteins (Chlorophyll, Cytochromes etc), proteins mediate all energy transformation reaction. It is because proteins are so important that the nucleic acid directly regulates the protein synthesis.

Protein structure is highly complex (as has been pointed out earlier) as well as specific. The primary structure is determined by the quality, quantity and the sequence of amino acids. Even an alteration of the position of one amino acid would alter the structure of the protein, and if it happens to be an enzyme regulating an important reaction, the entire reaction is disturbed leading to several abnormalities. Hence it is but natural that there is direct control of DNA in the synthesis of proteins. DNA, RNA and ribosomes of the cell are involved in the synthesis of proteins.

The central dogma : The basic mechanism of protein synthesis is that the nuclear DNA regulates the assembly of amino acids in the ribosomes to produce a polypeptide chain. Since DNA cannot move out of the nucleus it sends a messager - mRNA which carries the message in the form of sequence of nucleotides. This mRNA forms a template on the ribosomes. Another type of RNA, tRNA found in cytoplasm (whose nucleotide sequence is complementary to that of mRNA), picks up the amino acids and assembles them on the ribosomes to produce a peptide chain.

This may be briefly expressed as follows :

DNA Replication → DNA Transcription → RNA Translation → Proteins translation. Transcription is the copying of a complementary messenger RNA strand on a DNA strand. In translation, the genetic information present in mRNA (in the form of sequence of nucleotides) directs the sequence of amino acids to be assembled. We shall study these events in detail.

Transcription

Copying of a complementary strand of mRNA requires the following - a template, activated precursors, a divalent metal ion and RNA polymerase.

DNA molecules serves as a template for the production of mRNA. Of the two strands of DNA only one strand called the 'sense' or the 'coding' strand transcribes mRNA. Single stranded DNA also can serve as a template.

The activated precursors required for mRNA synthesis are - Adenine triphosphate, Guanine triphosphate, Uracil triphosphate and Cytosine triphosphate (ATP, GTP, UTP and CTP)

Mg^{++} or Mn^{++} are the divalent metal ions required for mRNA synthesis.

The enzyme RNA polymerase is necessary for transcription. The nucleotides of mRNA are assembled together with the help of RNA polymerase. The enzyme consists of two parts - a core enzyme and a sigma factor. The sigma factor initiates transcription of mRNA on the DNA template and the core enzyme continues transcription. The DNA base sequence are thus transcribed into mRNA base sequence.

Genetic Code

This is the message in mRNA in the form of nucleotide sequence. Three nucleotides code for one amino acid. It is called a triplet code or codon. There are 64 codons for the 20 odd amino acids. i.e., there is more than one code for each amino acid. These alternative codes are helpful in the cae of random mutations which may alter a code (nucleotide).

The nucleotides of mRNA are complementary to the nucleotides of tRNA (present in cytoplasm). The triplet nucleotides of tRNA are called anticodons. Each tRNA has three nucleotides. The pairing between the codon and anticodon (mRNA and tRNA) follows the A-U, G-C combination. For example if mRNA consists of the first code UUU, it pairs with a tRNA having an anticodon. AAA. Thus the series of codons of mRNA determine the series of anticodons of different molecules of tRNA and hence the amino acids (Each tRNA molecule is specific to a particular amino acid). Since the triplets of mRNA are determined by the base sequence of DNA, it follows that the DNA molecule decides the sequence of the amino acids and hence the structure of the protein molecule.

Some triplets do not code for any amino acid (UAA and UAG). These are called nonsense codes. The so called nonsense codes are actually terminator codons and are now called ochre and amber (UAA and AUG). Code AUG is called initiator codon since it initiates the synthesis of a polypeptide chain. (See earlier in the same chapter for details)

The triplet codes for all amino acids collected together is called a codon dictionary. The dictionary was first proposed by Nirenberg (1965) and subsequently worked out in further detail by Khorana H.G.

The mRNA is released out of the nucleus into the cytoplasm where it gets. attached to the smaller sub unit of the ribosomes. Many ribosomes are connected by a single mRNA molecule, constituting a polysome or polyribosome. The mRNA attaches itself to the ribosomes in such a way, that its bases remain free (to be able to undergo paring with the bases of tRNA). The whole structure (polyribosomes + mRNA) is called mRNA complex.

tRNA (transfer RNA) : This is present freely in cytoplasm. Also called sRNA (soluble RNA) is the smallest among the various types of RNA molecules found in the cell. Although the tRNA is single stranded like other types of RNA, it appears double stranded because of coiling. Complementary base pairs of the same strand form pseudo bondings of hydrogen due to folding. There are two regions which are free without bonding - one at the acceptor and which always has CCA base pair sequence and the other in the middle region of the molecule called the anticodon region, where there bases turn out of the folded portion and remain free. The types of tRNA is based on the types of these free bases. tRNA has the following functions.

(i) Attach to a particular amino acid at the acceptor and (CCA) with adenine nucleotide. The choice of amino acid however depends on the type of free bases present at the anticodon end.

(ii) to attach itself at a specific site on the mRNA and

(iii) to free the amino acid after it gets attached to another amino acid by means of peptide linkage.

The Wobble hypothesis

The triplet code or codon is degenerate i.e., there are many more codons than there are amino acids. Only 20 amino acids are involved in protein synthesis, while there are 64 possibilities or types of codons (43). Hence more than one codon can code for an amino acid. It is interesting to find out as to why the codes are degenerate? There could have been only so many codons as there are amino acids. But there is problem here. If there were to be only one code for an amino acid, what happens if there is a mutation at that site in DNA? Obviously the code changes and the amino acid cannot be incorporated in the protein leading to abnormalities. On the other hand, if there are alternate codes, they act as a protection against mutation in a specific base. Hence degeneracy of codes is a must.

Regarding tRNA present in cytoplasm, since they have to bind themselves to a specific codon, there should have been as many tRNA's as there are codons. But the number of tRNA is only as many as there are amino acids. This means, the anticodons of the tRNA's must be able to 'read' more than one codon of mRNA. How is this reading possible when bonding between base pairs is highly specific?

Crick (1966) proposed **'the Wobble hypthesis'** in order to solve this apparent dilemma. According to this hypothesis, only the first two bases of the codon have a precise pairing with the bases of the anticodon while the third one may Wobble (non specific). The pairing in the third base is ambigous. Thus a single tRNA can pair (bind) with more than one mRNA codon differing in only the third base. For example the anticodon UCG of tRNA can read codons AGC and

AGU of mRNA. The pairing between UGC and AGU is a perfect pairing as per the Crick and Watson pattern. But in the second case i.e., between UGC and AGU, the pairing between the first two bases is normal, while between G and U is against the normal pairing pattern. This unsual bonding G and U is called Wobble pairing.

The degeneracy of the code is not totally randon. Multiple codons for an amino acid always carry the same bases in the first two positions in a triplet with only the third 'Wobbling'. For example all the four codons for Valine have the first two bases - GU and for alanine it is GC.

Valine - GUU, GUC, GUA and GUG.

Alanine - GCU, GCC, GCA and GCG.

Translation

The process of translation consists of activation of amino acids, transfer of activated amino acid to tRNA, initiation of synthesis of polypeptide chain, chain elongation and chain termination.

Activation of amino acids

Before amino acids (20 of them) get themselves attached to the specific type of tRNA they have to be activated (energized). The activation is carried out by the ATP molecule in the presence of the specific enzyme called aminoacyl synthetase with Mg as the cofactor. The reaction produces aminoacyl adenylate (AAA) or aminoacyl AMP. Pyrophosphates arereleased in the process.

Amino acid + ATP + Enzyme ———— Enzyme AA> AMP complex + Ppi

Transfer of activated amino acids to tRNA

The activated amino acid (aminoacyl AMP) is transfered on to a specific tRNA, during which AMP and the enzyme (aminoacyl synthetase) are released. The amino acid gets attached to the CCA and tRNA.

Enzyme AA. AMP + tRNA ———— AA. tRNA + AMP + Enzyme

Initiation of Polypeptide chain synthesis

This involves two steps viz., preparation of the site of protein synthesis and initiation of the polypeptide chain.

(i) Preparation of the site of synthesis

Ribosomes in cytoplasm are the actual sites of protein synthesis. These are usually separated into their subunits (50s and 30s), when they are not participating in protein synthesis. The mRNA usually attaches to the 30s subunit through its 5' end carrying the AUG codon. In the process of attachment certain substances called initiation factors (IF) help. These factors are of three types in prokaryotes (IF1, IF2, IF3) and are of six types in eukaryotes (eIF2, eIF2al, eIF2a2, eIF2a3, eIFa4 and eIF3).

The attachment of the mRNA to the 30s submit requires the help of IF3 and Mg^{++}. The IF3 probably unwinds the rRNA (ribosomal RNA), so that it can bind to mRNA. After the attachment of mRNA, an mRNA - 30s complex is formed.

The starting amino acid in a polypeptide is methionine *(met)* in the case of eukaryotes and N-formly methionine *(f-met)* in the case of prokaryotes. The amino acid (met or f-met) tRNA complex attaches to the initiation codon (AUG) on the mRNA 30-s complex through its anticodon (UAC). This forms the 30s initiation complex and requires the participation of IF2, IF3 and GTP (energy donor).

(i) 30s + mRNA $\xrightarrow{\text{IF3}}$ mRNA - 30s complex

(ii) mRNA - 30s complex + met tRNA ——— 70s - mRNA - met - tRNA

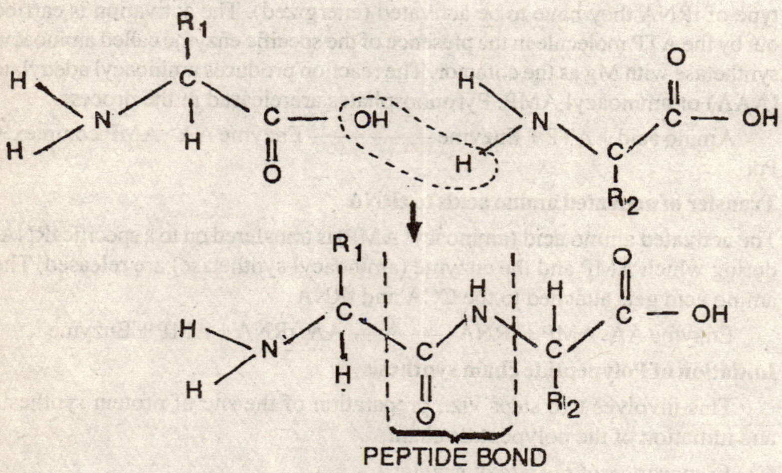

Fig. 20.3 Protein synthesis
Formation of peptide linkages

During the formation of the initiation complex the 50s subunit combines with the 30s subunit to form the 70s unit. This union is facilitated by the participation of IF1. With the formation of the 70s ribosome) the initiation of the polypeptide chain gegins.

(ii) Initiation of the polypeptide chain

Each ribosome has two cavities - P site (polypeptide site) and Asite (aminoacyl sites). AA tRNA complex occupies the A site, while the met - tRNA (tRNA with the initiator aminoacid - methionine) will be at the P site. This occupation requires a molecule of GTP and the participation of IF_1. The energy of GTP is utilized for the formation of the peptide linkage.

Peptide linkage occurs when the carboxyl (COOH) group of peptidyl tRNA (met. tRNA) present at the P site reacts with the amino group (NH_2) of AA tRNA at the A site. The enzyme peptidyl transfers catalyses the formation of peptide bond. Later the AA+tRNA moves from A site to the P site in the presence of GTP and IF_2

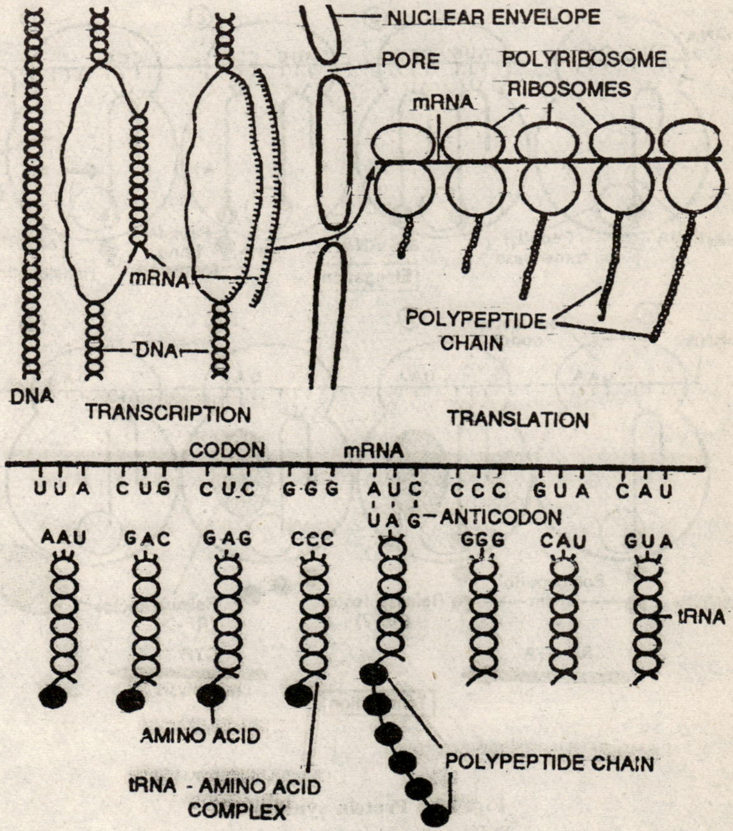

Fig. 20.4 Protein synthesis
General scheme of protein synthesis

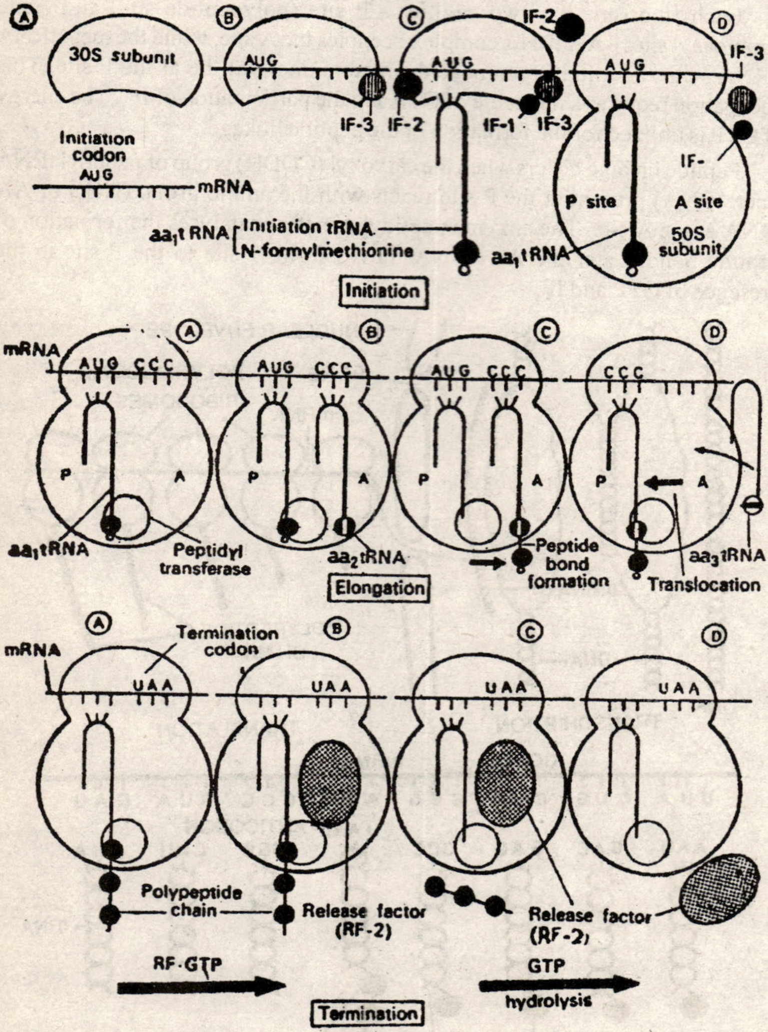

Fig. 20.5 Protein synthesis
Different stages of translation

Formation of the polypeptide chain

A specific type of tRNA (which has bases complementary to the codon of mRNA) linked to a particular amino acid gets attached to a specific site on mRNA when its anticodons can form a pairing with the first codon of the mRNA. Soon after a second tRNA with its amino acid joins the second site (triplet) on mRNA. The first and the second amino acids attached to different tRNA form a peptide linkage as both are linked to mRNA *via* the anticodons of tRNA. A molecule of water is released during the formation of the peptide linkae

$$COOH + NH_2 \xrightarrow{\hspace{4em}} CONH + H_2O$$

Peptide bond

As soon as the peptide linkage is formed the tRNA is made free and comes back to cytoplasm. This whole process in which a specific tRNA carries its amino acid to a specific site is called translation i.e. the code (triplet) is translated into an amino acid. Here the sequence of bases in tRNA will be identical with the base sequence of that part of DNA coding for mRNA.

Chain elongation

Elongation of the chain requires the participation of certain factors called elongation factors (EF). These are EF-Tu, EF-TS and EF-G in prokaryotes and EF-1 and EF-2 in eukaryotes. After the first amino acid tRNA complex has moved from the A site of the ribosome to the P site, a second AA. tRNA complex now occupies the A site. The codons are recognized enzymatically. This requires the participation of Ef-Tu, GTP and Mg^{++}.

Peptide linkage takes place between the two amino acids and the AA. tRNA complex migrates to the P site rendering the A site vacant. Now a third amino acid tRNA complex occupies the A site and theprocess continues. The shifting of th AA. tRNA complex from A site (releasing site) is called translocation. At the P site the tRNA is released from the ribosome while A site has a peptide chain liked to a tRNA which has brought in the last amino acid of the peptide chain. During translocation, the ribosome moves relative to the mRNA in the 5'-3' direction.

Chain termination

The elongation of the chain continues by the alternate occupation and vacancy at the A site by the AA. tRNA complexes until a termination codon (UAA, UAG or UGA) reaches the ribosomes. The termination codon sends signals to the ribosomes to attach release factors (RF-1, RF-2 and RF-3 in prokaryotes and RF in eukaryotes).

The release factors interact with the enzyme peptidyl transferase (which catalyses the formation of peptide bond) resulting in the hydrolysis of the bond between the polypeptide chain and the tRNA (linked to the last amino acid of the peptide chain at the site) and the former is released from the ribosome. Other events that occur at the termination of the polypeptide chain are -

(i) Release factors get disassociated from the ribosomes due to the hydrolysis of GTP.

(ii) tRNA is also released.

(iii) Ribosomal sub units (30s and 50s) get disunited.

(iv) The polypeptide chain is processed by the removal of the methionine residue from the chain. Depending upon the circumstances the chain may get cleaved into two or more pieces.

In eukaryotes, the polypeptide chain passes through a tunnel between the two subunits of the ribosome into the cavity of the cisterna of the endoplasmic reticulum.

Rate of Protein synthesis

The rate of transcription in *Escherichia coli* DNA for the enzyme controlling trypotophan synthesis is 28 nucleotides per second at 39°C. The speed of translation is 7 aminò acids per second. For the haemoglobin molecule, the rate of translation is 4 aminoacids per second.

DIFFERENCE IN PROTEINS SYNTHESIS BETWEEN PROKARYOTES AND EUKARYOTES.

No..	Character	Prokaryotes	Eukaryotes
1.	Ribosomes involved in protein synthesis	70s, with 30s and 50s sub units.	80s with 40s and 60s sub units.
2.	Occurrence of transcription and translation	Translation begins even while transcription is still going on in mRNA	Translation begins after complete transcription and mRNA comes out of the nucleus.
3.	Migration of mRNA	Ribosomes pull out mRNA from the DNA	mRNA moves out of the nucleus through the pores in the nuclear membrane.
4.	Sites of initiation of protein synthesis in mRNA	many	one
5.	Initiator amino acid for protein synthesis.	N-formyl-methionine	Methionine
6.	Initiator factors	IF1, IF21 and IF3	eIF2, eIFwa1, eIF2a2 eIF2a3 and eIF3
7.	Elongation factors	EF-Tu, Ef-Ts and Ef-G	Ef-1, Ef-2
8.	Release factors	Rf-1, Rf-2 and RF-3	Rf (single factor)

21

GENETIC REGULATION

All the activities of an organism, be it unicellular or multicellular, are ultimately controlled by the genes. In multicellular organisms, where cells differ widely in structure and function all of them carry the same genes, since all of them are traceable to a single cell viz., zygote. This poses an interesting question as to the function of genes. How do similar genes function differently? The answer to the question lies in *differential gene action*. In other words net all genes are active at all times. The genes are *switched* and *switched off* at different times. This differential gene action is also responsible for the synthesis of different types of proteins (enzymes) at different times. Not all enzymes are required at all times. Enzymes required during early stages of development may not be required at later stages in the life cycle and *vice versa*. The metabolic products produced may induce or repress the enzyme synthesis.

Genetic control on protein synthesis is exercised at three stages - transcription stage, translation stage and at the release of polypeptide chain (post translation stage).

The control mechanism ensures that the cell is not unnecessarily flooded by the enzymes which are required only at particular times and only in particular quantity. Depending on the requirement the enzyme synthesis can either be induced or suppressed. Genetic regulation is seen both in prokaryotes and in eukaryotes. While the purpose of genetic regulation is same in both prokaryotes and eukaryotes, the mechanisms differ. In prokaryotes, the mechanism of genetic regulation is simple when compared with the eukaryotic organisms. The reasons for this are not far to understand. As the eukaryotic organisms are far more complex they do require a very sophisticated mechanism of genetic regulation. In this chapter we will discuss genetic regulation in both prokaryotes and eukaryotes.

GENETIC REGULATION IN PROKARYOTES

Induction and Repression

In *E.coli* the synthesis of the enzyme β *galactosidase* has been studied in considerable detail. This enzyme breaks up lactose into glucose and galactose. If lactose is not supplied to *E.coli* cells, the presence of the enzyme β galactosidase in hardly detectable, but as soon as the substrate (lactose) is added the production of the enzyme β *galactosidase* increases by as much as 10,000 times. The production of enzyme again gets reduced if lactose is removed from the system. Such enzymes whose sythesis can be increased many times by the presence of the substrate are called **inducible enzymes.** The genetic system responsible for synthesis of such enzymes is called the *inducible system.* The inducible enzyme is an example of adaptive enzyme in the sense its (enzyme) synthesis gets increased due to the presence of the substrate.

In some other systems the reverse of the inducible system occurs for instance in a culture of *E.coli* if no amino acids are supplied from outside the cells can produced all the enzymes required for the production of amino acids. On the otherhand if a particular amino acid like histidine is added to the system the production of histidine synthesising enzymes will fall down. In these systems the addition of a product of a synthetic pathway will check the production of enzymes responsible for the synthetic pathway. In otherwords increased presence of a substrate would reduce the synthesis of an enzyme which has the enhancing effect of the production of that substate. Systems such as these are called *repressible systems* and the enzyme whose synthesis gets checked is known the as the **repressible enzyme.**

Inducer and Co-repressor

It has been mentioned above that an enzyme gets induced or repressed by the presence of a particular substrate. The substance which induces the synthesis of an enzyme is called the inducer and the substance which supresses the synthesis of the enzyme is called the repressor. In the synthesis of β *galactosidase,* lactose acts as the inducer and in the supression of histidine synthesising enzyme histidine acts as the repressor.

Enzyme induction or repression is generally brought about by the substrate on which an enzyme can act. But in some instances there will be molecules which resemble the substrate which also can act as the inducers. A typical example of this kind of induction is IPTG (isopropyl thiogalactoside). IPTG resembles lactose and can induce the production of the enzyme β *galactosidase.* Such inducers which are not substrates themselves but can bring about induction because of similarities with the substrate are known as **gratuitious inducers.**

In the above paragraphs we have discussed as to how in the absence of lactose there is no synthesis of β *galacotosidase.* This means then in the absence of the inducer the genes responsible for the production of the enzyme protein do not function. It will be interesting to find out as to why the enzymes do not function in the absence of lactose and how in the presence of lactose the genes regulating the enzyme synthesis get activated. It has been found out that a group of molecules called *repressors* are present in the cell and they check the activity of the enzymes. In the presence of the inducers the repressors get inactivated. In some instances ordinarily the repressors are inactive but they become active in the presence of another group of molecules called co-repressors. The induction and repression is supposed to work in the following manner.

1. Inducible system : active repressor + inducer = inactive repressor
2. Repressible system : inactive repressor + corepressor = active repressor

The operon concept

F.Jacob and J.Monod (1961) the Nobel Laureates have studied in detail the inducible system in the synthesis of the enzyme β *galactosidase* in *E.coli.* In order to explain the induction and repression of enzyme synthesis they have proposed the involvement of a group of genes along with the presence of cytoplasmic inducers and repressors. Their model of gene action is popularly called the operon model. This scheme of gene action proposed by Jacob and Monod as originally conceived by them consisted of an operator gene and a number of structural genes. As per the current understanding however the operon system consists of a structural gene, operator gene, promoter gene, regulator gene and repressor, inducer and co-repressor. The following is an account of the components of the operon model.

Structural genes

There are many structural genes associated in an operon system. These direct the synthesis of the mRNA and govern the sequence of amino acids in a protein molecule. Each structural gene might produce a particular kind of protein or all structural genes might regulate the production of a single protein. The activities of the structural gene(s) are controlled by the promoter and operator site of the operon system. The most well studied structural genes (*z*,*y* and *ac*) are those of the lactose operon system in *E.coli.*

Operator gene

The operator gene is situated adjacent to the first structural gene. It switches on or switches off the functioning of the structural gene (protein synthesis). In case a structural gene has to be suppressed, a repressor attaches itself to the operator to form an Operator-repressor complex. In the case of protein synthesis, the operator-repressor complex prevents the transcription by blocking the movement of RNA polymerase.

Promoter gene

The promoter gene is continuous with the operator gene and is believed to lie left to it. It is suggested that RNA polymerase binds to the promoter site during transcription. Three regions have been recognised in the promoter site. These are (a) recognition site, initial binding site and the mRNA initiation site (operator site).

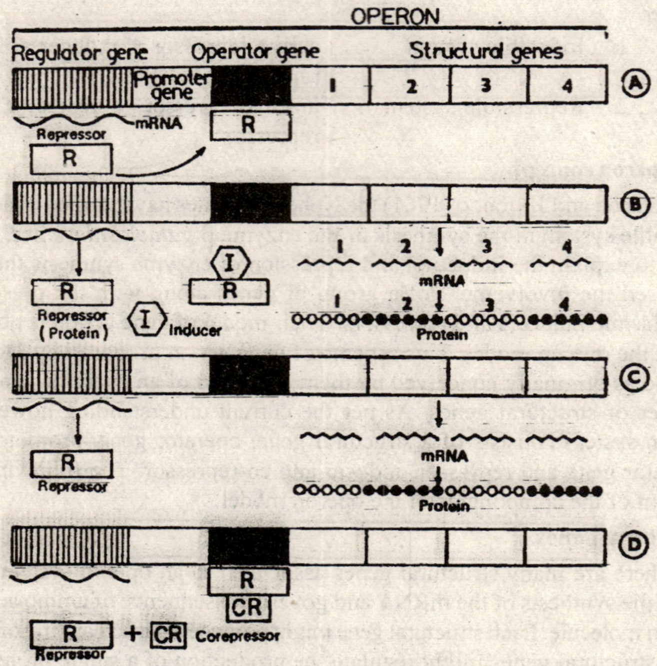

Fig. 21.1 Genetic regulation
Genetic regulation of protein synthesis in prokaryotes
(the Operon system of Jacob and Monod, 1961)

(i) Recognition site

Also called the *cga* site (catabolic gene activator site), it consists of certain palindromic sequence of DNA. These symmetrical sections of DNA are recognised by proteins having symmetrically placed sub units. This site, also called the CRP site (cyclic AMP receptor protein site) binds a Carotenoid protein to the promoter gene and thus facilities the binding of the enzyme RNA polymerase. It has been found that in *E.coli*, CRP combines with cAMP (cyclic adenosine monophosphate) forming a CRP + cAMP complex which binds to the promoter enhancing the binding of RNA polymerase and activates transcription. This regulation is called positive control.

(ii) Initial binding site

This consists of seven bases (DNA) to which the RNA polymerase binds.

(iii)RNA initiation site

The site where transcription begins is called initiation site. This is the region overlapping with the operator region.

Regulator gene

The regulator gene directs the activity of the operator gene by producing inhibitor proteins called repressors. This repressor protein binds to the operator gene and blocks the path of RNA polymerase, thus preventing transcription. If an inducer is present in the system, it binds to the repressor which undergoes conformational change and becomes inactive. As the inactive repressor cannot bind to the operator, the structural genes get activated and protein synthesis continues.

In a repressible system, if only a repressor is present, it is inactive by itself and cannot attach to the operator gene and hence transcription continues. However when another protein called corepressor is present it attaches to the repressor forming a *repressor-corepressor* complex, which blocks the operator gene thus preventing transcription.

Types of regulatory mechanism

Earlier in the chapter it has been mentioned as to how the presence or absence of a substrate can induce or supress the synthesis of the enzyme protein. Here we shall study in some more detail the various regulatory mechanisms that are involved in the synthesis of enzymes.

Induction. It has already been mentioned that in inducible systems the inducible enzymes are normally present in small quantities and their synthesis can be increased manifold by the presence of the inducer. Such an example of inducer in *E.coli* is lactose and the inducible enzyme is β *galactosidase.* In the absence of lactose only one ore two molecules of the enzymes β *galactosidase* may be present in the system. When the inducer is added, within three minutes about 3,000 molecules of the enzyme are synthesised by the gene.

When the inducer is absent the repressor protein will block the production of the enzyme by not allowing transcription of mRNA by the structural genes. The repressor protein actually blocks the operator gene. When the inducer is present the active repressor binds to the inducer to form a repressor inducer complex. As a result the repressor gets inactivated. An inactivated repressor cannot bind to the operator and hence the operator will allow the structural genes to transcribe mRNA and the enzyme is synthesised.

Repression. The presence of a metabolite inhibiting the synthesis of an enzyme in the system is called repression. It has been mentioned already that histidine acts as a repressor and blocks the production of the enzyme responsible for histidine synthesis. This is called enzyme repression. Another example of repression is the blocking of the production of the enzyme tryptophan synthetase by the substrate tryptophan. The enzyme tryptophan synthetase is produced only when the bacterium (*E.coli*) is cultured in a tryptophan free medium.

In the repressible system, the protein produced by the regulator gene is an inactive repressor (*aporepressor*). On combining with a corepressor (effector) the aporepressor molecules get activated due to a conformational change. As a result of this the aporepressor becomes active and binds to the operator gene. As a result of the operator genes getting blocked the structural genes cannot transcribe mRNA. However when the corepressor is absent, the aporepressor is inactive and by itself cannot bind to the operator gene. The operator gene being free will allow the structural genes to transcribe mRNA. The following is a summary of the regulation of enzyme synthesis is inducible and repressive systems.

I. Inducible system

1. ***Inducer present :*** Regulator gene → Active repressor + inducer → repressor inactive → operator gene free → structural genes transcribe mRNA → synthesis of enzyme protein.
2. ***Inducer absent :*** Regulator gene → active repressor → binds to the operator gene which becomes inactive → no mRNA transcription → inhibition of enzyme synthesis.

II. Repressible system

1. ***Corepressor present :*** Regulator gene → inactive repressor + corepressor → active repressor → binds and inactivates operator gene → structural genes do not transcribe mRNA → inhibition of enzyme synthesis.
2. ***Corepressor absent :*** Regulator gene → inactive repressor → operator gene not blocked → structural genes transcribe mRNA → enzyme protein synthesised.

Negative control

In the inducible and repressive systems, protein synthesis is allowed to take place when the operator gene is free and it (protein synthesis) stops if the operator gene is blocked. In otherwords, gene expression is possible only when the operator is free. Such a controlled mechanism of protein synthesis is said to be of a negative type. A typical example of negative control is the production of the enzyme protein in the presence of lactose and in the absence of glucose. The presence of glucose actually inhibits the production of the enzyme β *galactosidase* while the presence of lactose promotes the production of the eyzyme.

In negative control the regulator protein acting as the repressor prevents the transcription of mRNA by structural genes. The main controlling factor is the operator gene.

Positive control

In this control, the regulator protein functions as an activator and increases the enzyme synthesis. The activator binds itself to DNA in a location called the initiator site. Here the initiator site need not necessarily be the operator gene. As the regulator protein enhances the transcription of mRNA by structural genes this kind of regulation is called a positive control. A typical example of a positive control is the arabinose operon seen in *E. coli* (see later for details).

Replication of DNA is also an example of positive control. The bacterial genome is made up of replicating units called replicons which are capable of independent duplication. One of the structural genes of a replicon is known to produce an activator protein which in turn is induced by some cytoplasmic factors. The activator binds to a specific site on the replicon called the replicator and initiates replication from this point.

Catabolic repression

The works of Magasaine and others have shown that the presence of glucose inhibits the synthesis of enzymes involved in the breakdown of sugars such as lactose, arabinose or glactose. This phenomenon of repression is known as catabolic repression. This has been seen in many microorganisms including *E.coli,* yeasts etc. For instance when a culture of *E.coli* maintained on lactose is supplemented with glucose it has been seen that the synthesis of β *galactosidase* enzyme becomes suppressed as long as glucose is present in the medium. The inhibitory effect of glucose is due to a marked drop in the intercellular levels of a nucleotide–cyclic AMP. The studies of Zubay and Beckwith (1970), have shown that glucose suppresses the level of cyclic AMP which in turn inhibits the transcription of mRNA.

In vitro studies of Eron, et al (1971) have indicated that lactose operon transcription requires not only cyclic AMP but also a protein called CAP (catabolic activator protein). CAP binds to the cyclic AMP. Thus catabolic repression has two steps at the first stage CAP binds to cyclic AMP and at the second stage this complex (CAP cyclic AMP) exerts its effect on the transcription process.

Feed back inhibition

In some instances the final product of a particular biosynthetic pathway gets accumulated if it is not utilised for metabolic activities. Such a kind of accumulation many a time will cause the stoppage of further synthesis of the substance. For instance if the normally growing *E.coli* cells are supplied with isoleucine (an amino acid), it has the effect of blocking the isoleucine synthesising enzyme. This inhibition is due to the binding of isoleucine to enzyme *threonine deaminase.* This kind of inhibition is called feed back inhibition. Feed back inhibition may be defined as the inhibitory effect of the final product on the enzyme involved in the first step of production when a synthetic pathway is made up of several steps and is controlled by the activity of specific enzymes. Feed back inhibition has an advantage in the sense if the enzyme of the first step is blocked there is no necessity to block the intermediary enzymes as in any case they would not get the substrate.

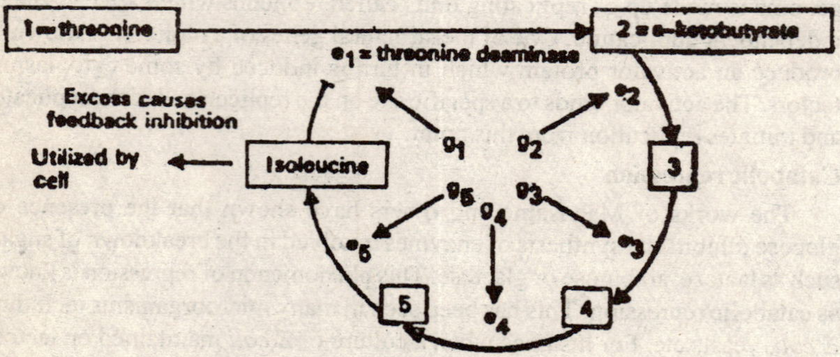

Fig. 21.2 Genetic regulation
Feedback inhibition in *E.coli* (after Stansfield, 1969)

Feed back inhibition is mostly through the allosteric transformation of the enzyme so that its active site gets inactivated. Feed back inhibition is different from repression in that in the later there is no mRNA synthesis and hence no enzyme synthesis. Feed back inhibition is actually a case of control of gene expression after translation.

Role of Leader sequences in genetic regulation

Gene expression in prokaryotes is controlled both at the level of transcription as well as after the transcription. In the mechanisms which operate after transcription a prominent role is played by leader sequences and attenuators. For example in the tryptophan operon of *E.coli* the mRNA of gene *trp E* (gene for anthranilate synthetase) has a sequence of 162 bases between initiator codon and the promoter operator region of this gene. This sequence of 162 bases is called leader sequence and is thought to exercise post transcriptional control. This leader sequence of the gene *trp E* has a mechanism which allows transcription when synthesis is needed and stop the transcription whenever synthesis is not needed.

Regulation by antisense RNA

Some of the recent researches have shown that regulation of protein synthesis can be controlled at the translational level by using RNA which has complementary bases to mRNA. When such a RNA is introduced it binds to mRNA forming RNA mRNA hybrid and prevents the translation, it (RNA) is this RNA is in complementary to mRNA and interferes in the translation which and it (RNA) is called antisense RNA. Antisense RNA can be used in experimental conditions to stop the translation of mRNA. In *in vivo* conditions also antisense RNAs are known to regulate the translation of mRNA. In transposon Tn 10, the production of the enzyme *transposase* is prohibited by antisense RNA. The production of antisense RNA is controlled by a promoter which directs transcription in a direction opposite to the transposase gene thus producing antisense RNA.

Role of antisense RNA in regulating gene expression has also been demonstrated in the case of the two genes involved for the synthesis of outer membrane protein.

Examples of a few operon systems

The lac operon of E.coli. The lac operator consists of three structural genes.

1. Gene *z*. This is made up of 3,063 base pairs and codes for enzyme β *galactosidase* which is active as a tetramer and breaks lactose into glucose and galactose.
2. Gene *y*. This is made up of 800 base pairs and codes for the enzyme β *galactoside permease* which is a membrane bound protein and helps in the transportation of metabolites.
3. Gene *ac*. This consists of 800 base pairs and codes for β *galactoside transacetylase* an enzyme that transfers an acetyl group from acetyl coA to β *galactosides.*

In addition to the structural genes the lac operon consists of a regulator gene *i*, an operator gene *o* and a promoter gene *p*. These six adjacent cistrons (genes) constitute the lac operon system. An operon can be defined as an integrated genetic unit.

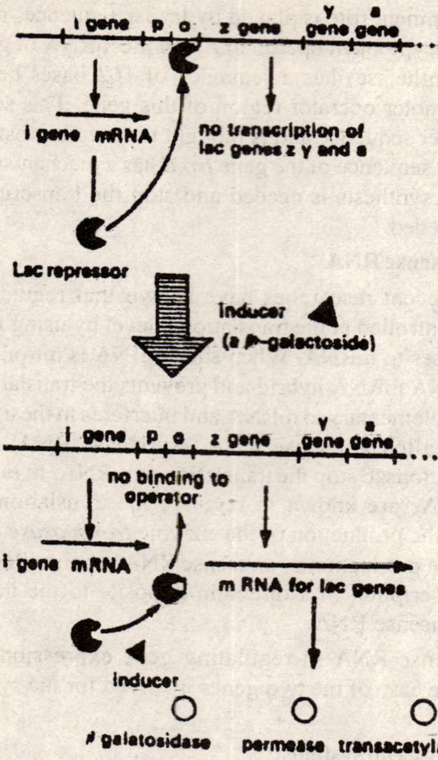

Fig. 21.3 Genetic regulation
Lac-operon model

In lac operon, the gene *i* produces a repressor (protein) which inactivates the operator by binding with it. Subsequently an inducer such a lactose binds with the repressor molecule there by inactiviting it. As a result the operon gene *o* is free from the repressor and becomes active. When the operator gene is active mRNA is produced from the structural genes *z, y* and *ac.* The production of mRNA starts from the promoter gene. It has been found at that all the three structural genes produce a single mRNA molecule which codes for the sequence amino acids for all the three enzymes - β *galactosidase, permease* and *transacetylase.* Thus equal amounts of all the three enzymes are produced and the first message translated is for β *galactosidase;* this is followed by the synthesis of *permease* and then followed by *transacetylase*. Thus the operons show polarity. This has been proved by mutational studies. Mutations in the *z* region will reduce the quantities of all the three enzymes. While mutations in *y* locus will have no effect on β *galactosidase* but will reduce the quantities of other two enzymes. Such mutations are said to be **polar mutations.**

The gal operon system

In the gal operon systen in *E.coli* the sequence of three structural genes are *gal E*, *gal T* and *gal K*. These genes are directly responsible for the sequence of the enzymes produced namely *galactokinase*, *galactose-1-phosphate uridyl transferase*, and *uridinediphospho-galactose-4- epimerase*. These enzymes are responsible for the degradation of galactose into glucose-1-phosphate and UDP glucose.

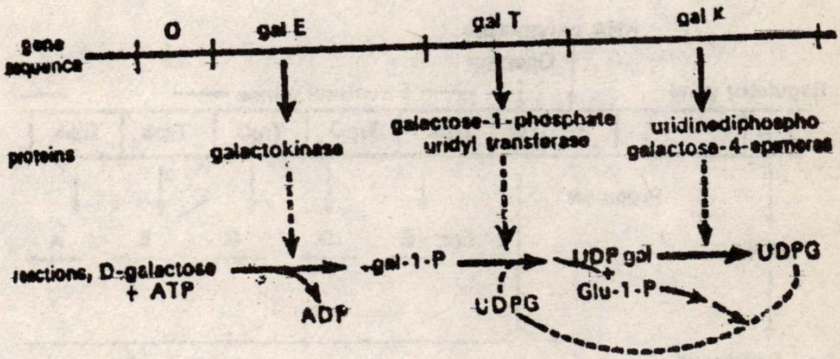

Fig. 21.4 Genetic regulation

The galactose (gal) operon of E.coli. Abbreviations : O-perator, Gal-1-galactose-1-phosphate, UDPG-uridine diphosphoglucose; UDP GAl - uridine diphosphogalactose; Glu-1 P=glucose-1-phosphage (after Goodenough and Levine, 1974)

Tryptophan operon system (trp operon)

The *trp* operon is also seen *E.coli* and consists of five structural genes ABCD and E. These genes code for the following enzymes :

1. Genes A and B code for *tryptophan synthetase*.
2. Gene C codes for *PRA isomerase* and *IGP synthetase*.
3. Gene D codes for *phosphoribosyl pyrophosphate anthranilate transferase*
4. Gene E codes for *anthranilate synthetase*.

The levels of these enzymes is low when the amount of tryptophan is more and the level high when the amount of tryptophan is less. All these enzymes are regulated in a coordinated fashion. The operator and promoter are overlapping and are located next to *trp* E gene. The regulator gene (R) is located away from the operon and the repressor produced by it is inactive until it combines with tryptophan. All the enzymes are produced constitutively if the repressor is either absent or fails to combine with tryptophan. All the structural genes are translated together and form a polycistronic mRNA. This polycistronic mRNA besides the transcription of the bases of structural genes has a 160 nucleotide long leader sequence. This contains the attenuator site to which the substrate tryptophan can get attached and thus reduce the rate of transcription. Thus in *trp* operon there are two sites of regulation - the regulator gene and the attenuator site in the mRNA itself.

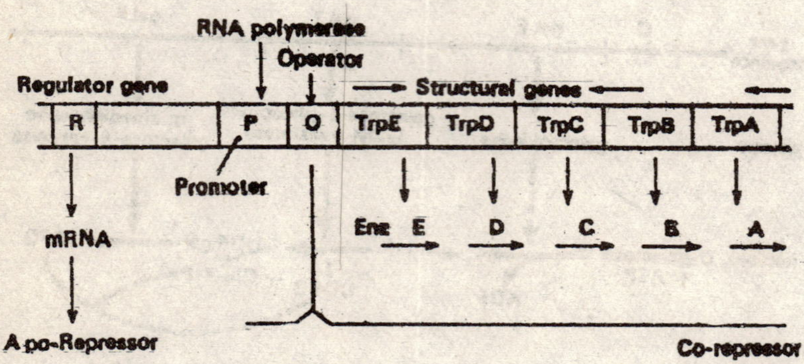

Fig. 21.5 Genetic regulation
Tryptophan operon

The *trp* operon thus seems to have a dual control-a control by regulator and also by attenuator. In addition to this feed back regulation is also seen in *trp* operon.

Arabinose operon

This is also seen in *E.coli* and is an example of positive control. Like the lac operon the arabinose operon also consists of three strcutural genes. These are

(i) *ara* A gene codes for *arabinose isomerase*

(ii) *ara* B gene codes for *L-ribulokinase*

(iii) *ara* B gene codes for *L-ribulose-5-phosphate epimerase*

These structural genes are located together on the *E.coli* chromosome. Their expression is under the regulation of a regulator gene C. This gene C called activator must be present for transcription of the arabinose operon. The product of C gene binds to the operator in the presence of arabinose and forms the activator protein. As a result of this, transcription takes place in the arabinose genes. If the activator is not bound to the arabinose or if the arabinose is absent, the operon is not expressed because the regulator protein binds to the operator gene (*ara* o) and functions as a repressor. In arabinose operon the gene C acts both as an activator and repressor. In this way arabinose operon is different from lac operon.

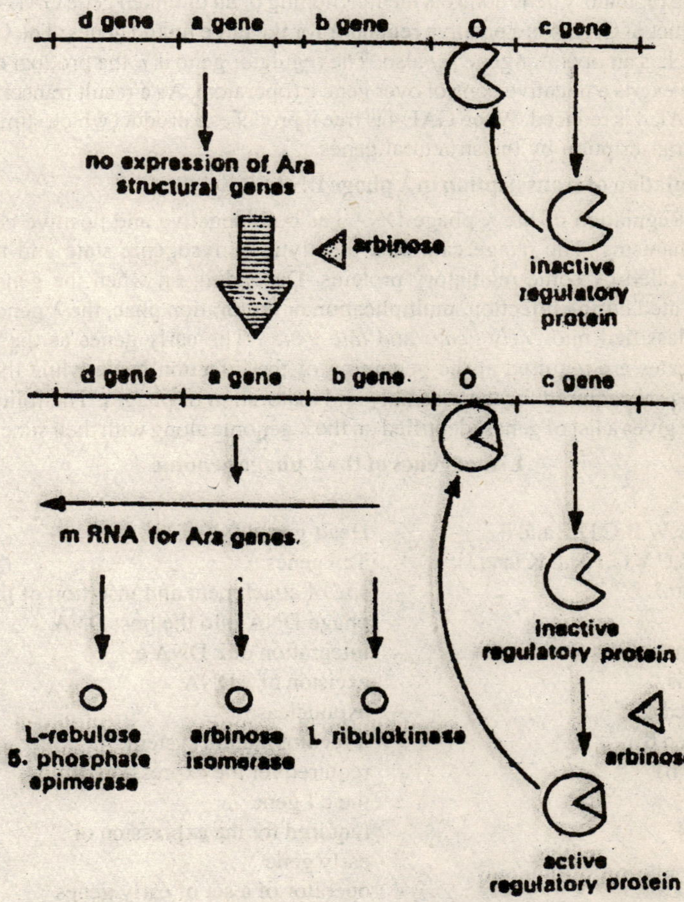

Fig. 21.6 Genetic regulation
The L-arabinose operon of E.coli

Gal genes in yeasts

In yeasts galactose if fermented by the activity of three enzymes-kinase, transferase and epimerase. These are coded by the three structural genes GAL 1, GAL 7 and GAL 10. The regulator gene is located away from the structural genes. If a mutation occurs in a regulator gene all the three enzymes are synthesised without control indicating thereby that the product of the regulator gene is a repressor. The regulator or gene of gal in yeasts is very much similar to the gals in *E.coli*. A detailed genetic analysis has revealed that the product of the regulatory gene controls the functioning of an unlinked gene GAL 4. The product of GAL 4 is a positive regulator for the three linked genes. The GAL 4 gene has an operator gene *(c)* also. The regulator gene is *i,* the product of this gene exerts a negative control over gene c (operator). As a result transcription of GAL 4 is reduced. When GAL 4 is free it produces a product which stimulates the transcription by the structural genes.

Regulation of transcription in λ phage DNA

Regulation of the λ phage DNA has both negative and positive control mechanisms. The phage can exist in a lytic or lysogenic state and this is controlled by some regulatory proteins. Depending on when the genes get activated during infection, multiplication or muturation phae, the λ genes can be classified into *early genes* and *late genes.* The early genes as the name indicates are required at the beginning of the infection cycle while the late genes are required for the assembly and maturation of phages. The following table gives a list of genes identified on the λ genome along with their functions.

List of genes of the λ phage genome

A,W,B,C,D,E and F	-	Head genes
Z,U,V,G,T,H,L,K,Iand J	-	Tail genes
att λ	-	site of attachment and insertion of the phage DNA into the host DNA
int	-	integration of λ DNA e
xis	-	excision of λ DNA
red α	-	exonuclease
red β	-	λ recombination system
c III	-	required for the expression of the c I gene
N	-	required for the expression of early gene
OL	-	operator of a set of early genes
rex	-	restriction of trowth of T4 R II
c I	-	λ repressor

OR	-	operator of another set of early genes
tof	-	negative regulator of c I transcription
c II	-	required for the expressions of the c I gene
ori	-	point of origin of replication
O	-	required for λ replication
P	-	required for λ replication
Q	-	stimulates transcription of late genes
pl	-	promoter of late genes
S	-	required for host lysis
R	-	required for host lysis

The cI gene codes for the repressor which binds to the operator genes thereby blocking the transcription of both the early operons. The repressor can bind to the operons blocking its integration and replication resulting in immunity due to a negative control exerted by a repressor. The product of gene N however acts as a positive regulator and allows transcription. The product of the N gene is known as antiterminator because instead of stopping it allows transcription. Another example of positive regulation is the influenceof Q gene product on late genes. This product combines with the coat transcriptase enzyme of *E.coli* and acts favourably on the promoter of the late genes. Thus in the λ phage there are both negative and positive regulatory mechanisms to control the initiation and completion of lytic or lysogenic cycle. This is very necessary for an organism which has to survive in a continuously changing environment such as the bacterial cell.

GENETIC REGULATION IN EUKARYOTES

The mechanism of gene regulation of protein synthesis explained above illustrates the phenomenon in prokaryotes, whereby a repressor protein transcribed by regulator genes may activate or prevent the protein synthesis depending on the presence of inducer or corepressor.

In Eukaryotes, genetic regulation takes place by a slightly different mechanism. Two types of proteins associated with the DNA of the chromosomes possibly play a role in gene regulation. These are histones and non histone chromosomal proteins (NHC proteins). Since histones of different organisms have similar amino acid composition it is unlikely that in they can selectively repress gene action. At best, histones may probably bring about a general (non specific) repression. It is believed that histones under certain situations bring about supercoiling of DNA preventing the movement of RNA-polymerase and thus blocking transcription. This is known by the fact RNA precursors are incorporated only in those regions where chromatin is diffuse (no super coiling).

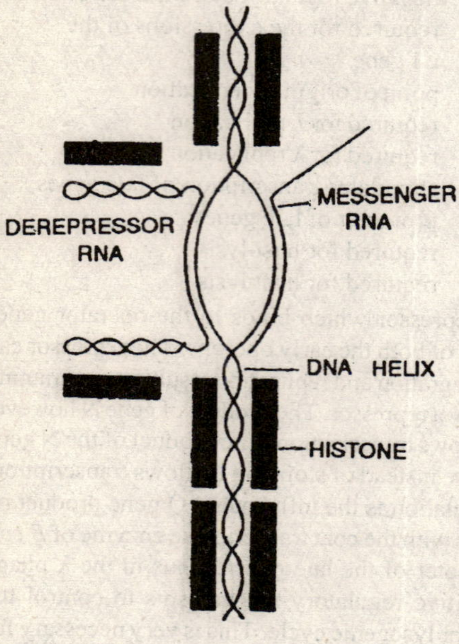

Fig. 21.7 Genetic regulation

Genetic regulation of protein synthesis in Eukaryotes0Frenster's model of gene regulation

Three models have been proposed by various scientists to account for gene regulation in eukaryotes. These are - 1. Frenster's model, 2. Non histone derepressor model and Britten and Davidson's model.

Frenster's model

This is also called gene specific derepressor RNA model. As has been pointed out earlier, histones bring about non specific repression of transcription. Derepression (initiation of transcription) is brought about when nuclear polyions separate histones from DNA at certain specific parts (of DNA) and form complexes with histones.

Non histones derepressors

The model proposed by Paul et al (1971), is similar to Frenster's model except the derepression is brought about by NHC acid proteins instead gene specific RNA. The fact that NHC proteins are of immense variety in different organisms, and also at different stages of growth even in the same individual goes to show that they can undertake selective derepression at specific gene loci. Derepression is brought about when NHC proteins bind themselves at specific loci to histones forming complexes. This complex separates itself from the DNA and allows it to transcribe, only at those specific loci.

Britten Davidson Model

Also known as operon operator model, this is somewhat different from the other two models. As per this model, four types of genes are involved in the regulation process. These are sensor genes, producer genes, integrator genes and receptor genes.

1. ***Sensor genes***

Comparable to the promoter genes these are sensitive to the metabolic status of the cell. The sensor gene is stimulated by various metabolic substances.

2. Producer genes

These regulate the output of metabolism and control the formation of enzymes, cell organelle, membranes etc.

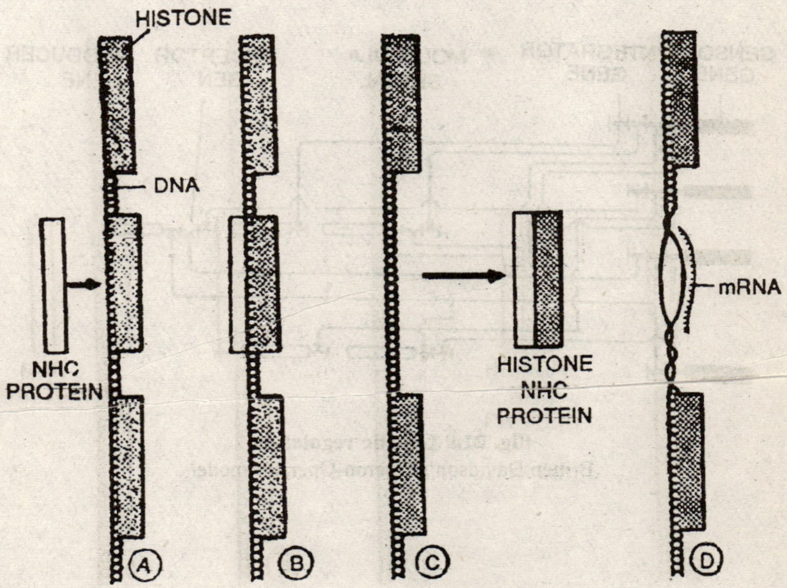

Fig. 21.8 Genetic regulation

Gene regulation by NHC proteins, **A.** Non specific repression by histones, **B.** Specific binding of NHC Proteins to histones, **C.** Removal of histone by NHC proteins, **D.** De repression of DNA, leading to transcription.

3. Integrator gene

As the name suggests, the gene integrates the activities of other genes. The integrator gene sends specific molecular signals to other genes as to whether the sensor gene is activated or not. Each sensor gene may be associated with a single or a group of integrator genes. In the latter case, a sensor gene may send a variety of molecular signals to other genes through its various integrator genes.

4. Receptor gene

This acts as an intermediate between the integrators and the producers. When the molecular signal reaches the receptor gene, it inturn activates the producer gene. A producer may have one or a group of receptor genes associated with it in the same way as sensors have seveal integrators. This helps, not only in the variety of origin of molecular signals, (from sensors) but also variety in reception of these signals (by receptors). Perhaps multintegrator gene complex and multireceptor gene complex may have a specific multichannel relationship.

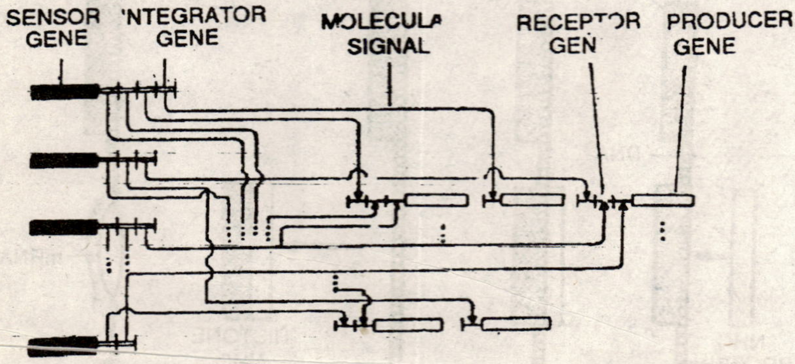

Fig. 21.9 Genetic regulation
Britten Davidson's Operon-Operator model

22

MICROBIAL GENETICS

Genetical studies in microorganisms is extremely difficult as they are very minute in size and do not posses any variability in their phenotype which can be subjected to genetic analysis. Another difficulty of microbial genetical studies is that microorganisms reproduce a sexually to multiply their number and microbiologists thought that microbes like bacteria do not reproduce sexually. Extensive and repeated reseaches were made to explore the possibility of Sexual reproduction in bacteria. Most of the earlier attempts were unsuccessful, because they were based purely on morphological observation of cell fusion. When Luria and Delburck established the assay procedure for obtaining the meaningful results, bacteriologists knew that their approach towards bacterial sexuality should change and a new technique is necessary for the analysis of sexuality in bacteria. The first successful experiment in bacterial genetics was performed by Joshua Lederberg and E.L. Tatum. These two collaborated in 1946 and using K_{12} strains of *E.coli* conducted what can now be called a classical experiment in bacterial crossing. They were able to demonstrate, that in *E.coli,* exchange of biochemical traits is possible. For their work on bacterial genetics, lederberg and Tatum shared with G.W. Beadle, the Nobel prize in medicine, for the year 1958.

With the establishment of the fact, that bacteria do exhibit sexuality, a vast area of microbial genetics opened up for geneticists. Prokaryotic organisms like bacteria were favoured for genetic experiments because -

1. Large amount of material could be handled as they are small
2. Several generations could be obtained within a short period
3. Pure cultures could be easily obtained for analysis.

With the advantages mentioned above, microbial genetics has made rapid strides in the last few decades.

Types of genetic material transfer

As in any other organism in bacteria also, sexuality involves transfer and recombination of genetic material from one bacterial cell to the other. Three methods of genetic recombination have been demonstrated in bacteria. These are conjugation, transformation and transduction.

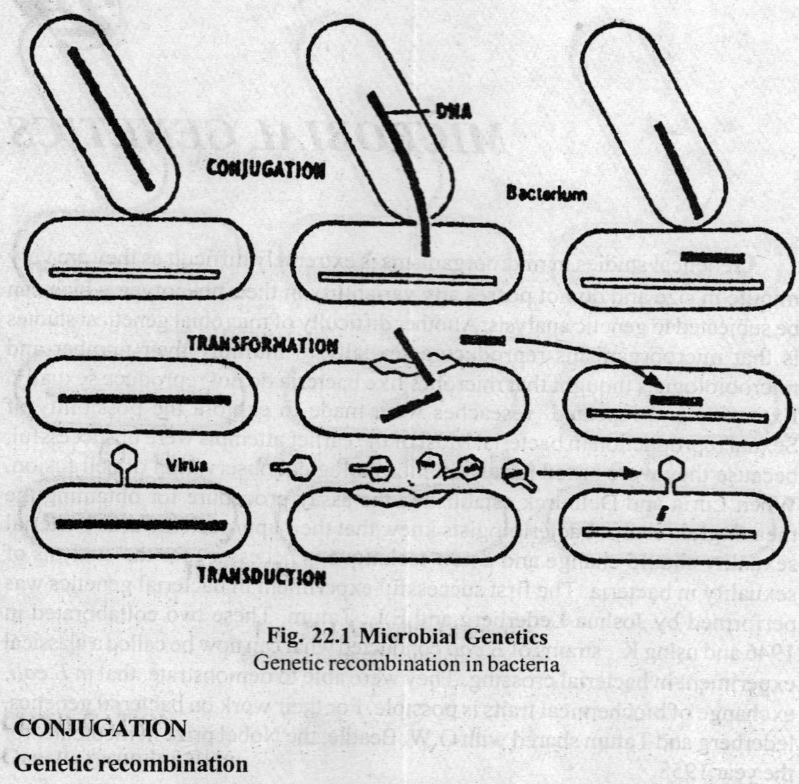

Fig. 22.1 Microbial Genetics
Genetic recombination in bacteria

CONJUGATION

Genetic recombination

Lederberg and Tatum (1944) demonstrated this in experimenting with the biochemical mutants of *Escherichia coli.* These bacteria require the following four nutrients 1. Biotin 2. Methionine 3. Leucine 4. Thereonine. But they can be grown on a minimal medium (a medium containing only agar and carbohydrates) because, by using carbohydrates they can synthesize all the above four nutrients. They are called 'Paratrophs' and can be genotypically designated as follows :

$$B^+ M^+ L^+ T^+$$

In this, letter stands for the nutrient (B = biotin etc) and the sign + stands for the capacity to synthesize that particular nutrient.

By subculturing in the laboratory, the paratrophs undergo mutation and lose the capacity to synthesize one or more nutrients. The mutants are called

Auxotrophs. By careful isolation, Lederberg and Tatum obtained two complementary polyauxotrophic varieties of *E.coli*. They can be designated as follows

1. $B^+ M^+ L^+ T^+$
2. $B^- M^- L^- T^-$

(The sign-stands for the loss of the synthesizing capacity. For ex : L means leucine cannot be synthesized and hence it has to be added to the culture).

It is obvious that both strains 1 and 2 cannot be cultured on a minimal medium. Strain 1 cannot be cultured because it cannot synthesize leucine and theronine. Strain 2 cannot be cultured because it cannot synthesize biotin and methionine.

But when both of them are kept on a minimal medium curiously they survive (normal expectation is, they should not live). On nutritional analysis, it was revealed that they were Paratrophs. The formation of paratrophs from two polyauxotrophic varieties can be explained only onthe possibility of sexual recombination between strain 1 and 2.

$B^+M^+L^+T^+$ $B^-M^-L^-T^-$
1 2

Because of recombination of 1 and 2 the following combinations may be obtained.

$B^-M^-L^-T^-$ and $B^+M^+L^+T^+$
(a) (b)

Of the above (a) will not survive because it has lost the capacity to synthesize all the nutrients but (b) will survive because it has become a paratroph.

Mechanism of conjugation

The exact mechanism of genetic exchange was worked out by three groups of scientists led by Lederberg in Wisconsin USA, Hayes in London and Woolman in Paris. Genetic transformation was not involved in the process was confirmed when cell free extracts of one bacterium failed to transformer other cells. It was demonstrated that the two bacterial cells physically come together and DNA from one passes into the other through the conjugation tube.

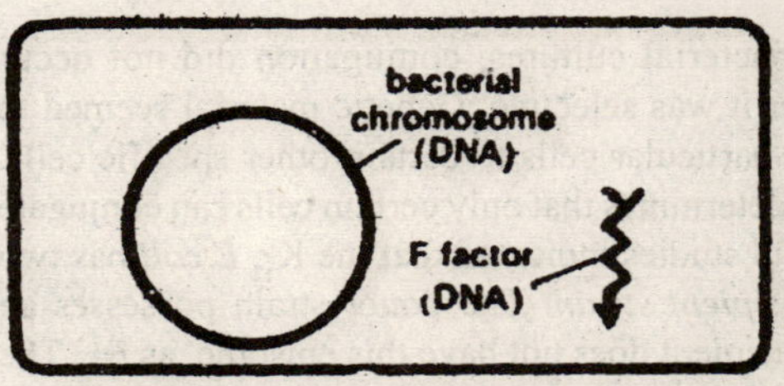

Fig. 22.2 Microbial Genetics
A bacterial cell showing circular DNA and F factor

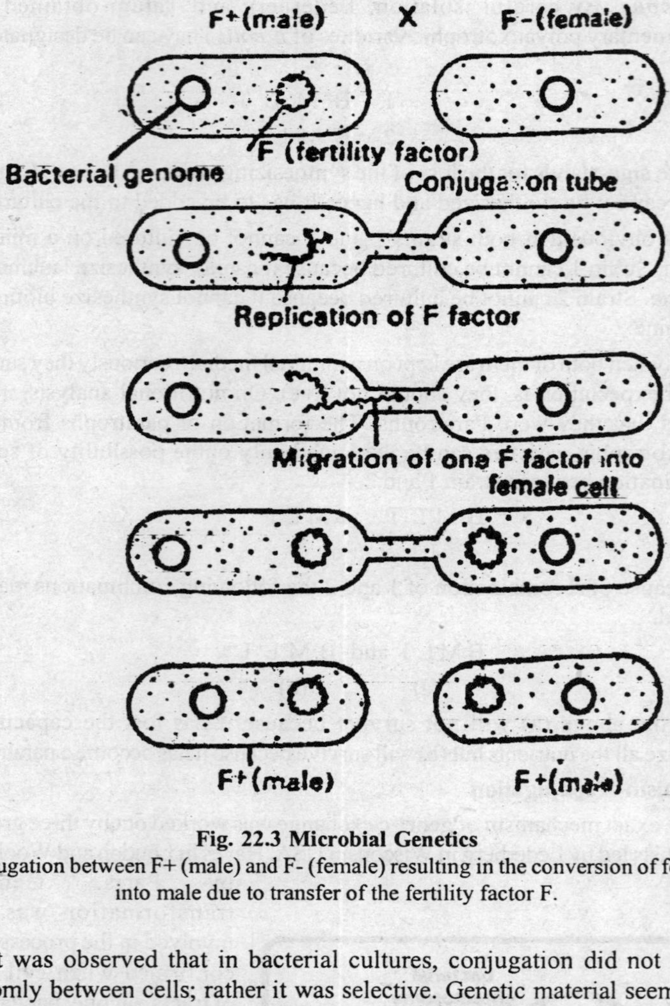

Fig. 22.3 Microbial Genetics

Conjugation between F+ (male) and F- (female) resulting in the conversion of female into male due to transfer of the fertility factor F.

It was observed that in bacterial cultures, conjugation did not occur randomly between cells; rather it was selective. Genetic material seemed to migrate selectively only from particular cells to certain other specific cells. What is this specificity? What determines that only certain cells can conjugate while the others cannot. Careful studies indicated that the K_{12} *E.coli* has two strains - *Donor strain* and *recipient strain.* The donor strain possesses an episome (plasmid) while the recipient does not have this episome, as F+. The recipient strain does not have F factor and can be designated as F-. The donor strain may also be called male and the recipient female.

The fertility factor is free of the main genome of the bacterium and lies freely in cytoplasm. It is made up of a small DNA molecule having a molecular weight of 2,50,000. Normally only one F factor is present in a cell andit replicates along with the main genome during cell division.

When conjugation occurs between F and F cells, the main genome is not involved. Consequently chromosomal genes are not transfered from donor to recipient cell. In normal conjugation, the F factor of donor replicates and one copy of the F factor migrates along the conjugation tube tothe recipient cell. As a result both the cells now have a F factor. Consequent to this transfer, even the original recipient cell now becomes a donor as it has got an F factor. In other words both the cells are now F^+. This means that the female cell has become male. The newly converted donor cell can now transfer its F factor to other recipient cells by *infecting* them with F factor.

If the entire conjugation process were to be limited to only transfer of the F factor with chromosome genes not being involved, it would have been perhaps of little genetic interest. But the discovery of another K_{12} *E.coli* strain by Cavalli-the *Hrf* (High fertility) strain changed the entire approach to the phenomenon of bacterial conjugation.

What is a *Hfr* strain? The F factor in the donor cell exists freely in cytoplasm - a point that has already been stressed. Occassionally however, the F factor gets integrated with the chromosome (main genome). The F^+ cell that has an integrated F factor (with the chromosome) is now called a *Hfr* strain as it can increase the rate of recombination many fold. So a F^+ male that brings about recombination has now been converted into a supermale (High fertility male). Integration of F factor into the chromosome involves a break (in the circular chromosome) and attachment of F factor. As a result of this integration, the chromosome along with its F factor becomes linear with two free ends. It is this chromoome. As the F factor becomes a part of the chromosome and as the chromosome has free ends one end enters the other bacterium through the conjugation tube.

When a *Hfr* cell conjugates with a F cell, the latter receives the chromosomal genes. Which end of the chromosome of Hfr cell enters the F-cell? It has been found out that when F+ joins the chromosome with a single nick it will be at one end. This end can be called posterior and the other and anterior. Usually chromosome movement from *Hfr* to F begins at the anterior end and the F factor enters the F strain only when conjugation is complete. This however rarely happens as conjugation and the F factor remains in the Hfr due to partial conjugation. Two possibilities exist here.

1. Complete conjugation

Total transfer of genome along with F factor from *Hfr* to F. As a result not only the F acquires the genetic traits of *Hfr*, it becomes a Hfr. This is total recombination.

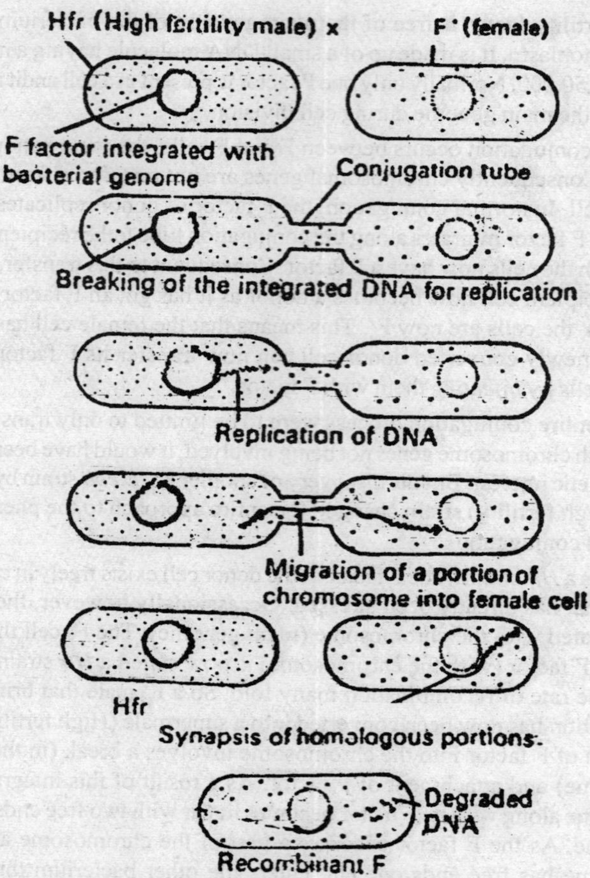

Fig. 22.4 Microbial Genetics

Conjugation between high fertility male (Hfr) and female (F-) cells, resulting in production of recombinant female

2. Interrupted or partial recombination

Here chromosome entry from *Hfr* to F stops in the middle. As a result F remains female (F) only, but acquires new chromosomal genes as a result of partial recombination. Whichever genes have entered from *Hfr* to F, they express themselves i.e., the F acquires new phenotype.

The F factor attachment to the chromosome is not at any fixed locus. There are several loci at which the chromosome can have a single break and the F factor can integrate to change the cell into a Hfr from F+. In otherwords, the integration of F factor into the chromosome may take place at any one of the possible loci. This interesting observation has led to the conclusion of the existence of several Hfr strains categorized on the basis of locus of attachment of F factor to the chromosome. This can be further clarified as follows-let us suppose that the bacterial genome has genes A to Z on it. Theoretically, the F factor can attach between A and B or Z and A, Ç and A and soon. The point of attachment of F factor can be proved by the fact, that if gene A appears first in the recombinant followed by B, then the attachment is between A and B. The F factor always forms the rear end of the genome. For different Hfr strains, the recombination values of various genes in a population vaires. But when once, the recombination frequency for a gene is known, the frequency of other genes is always fixed. In otherwords, in a chromosome from Hfr which evergene may enter first, its distance from other genes will not vary. This aspect has been exploited for mapping the genes on bacterial chromosome.

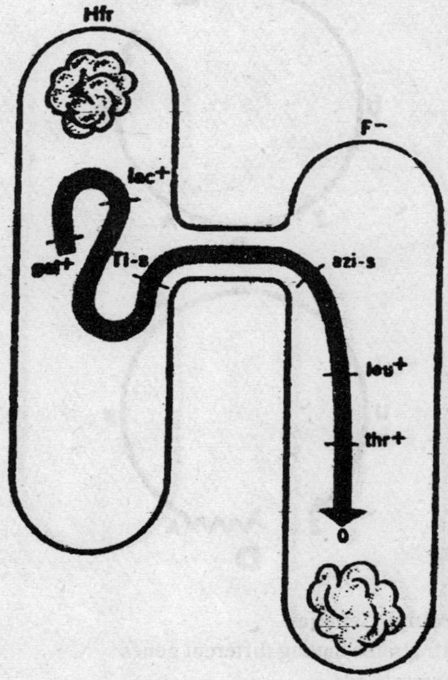

Fig. 22.5 Microbial Genetics
Transfer of genes from Hfr to F in a definite linear order

Interrupted conjugation and chromosome mapping

It has been pointed above, that in a mating between *Hfr* and F, the process of conjugation is rarely completed. More often it is interrupted by several environmental factors and as result only few genes of the *Hfr* chromosome get transfered (after duplication) to F. This can be tested as the recombinant acquires a new phenotype (as it has genes obtained from *Hfr*). This interruption of mating can be artifically induced in a culture medium and the recombinant tested for acquiring the new trait. By carefully controlling the duration of mating one can observe, the series of new phenotype acquired by recombinant. Let us suppose, after 5 minutes of conjugation *gal* - gene enters the recombinant, and after 10 minutes *lac* - gene enters followed by leu-gene after 15 minutes, it is obvious that the genes are located in the following sequence.

gal- ____________ lac- ____________ leu-

By following the method of controlling conjugation time, one can map all the genes on a bacterial chromosome.

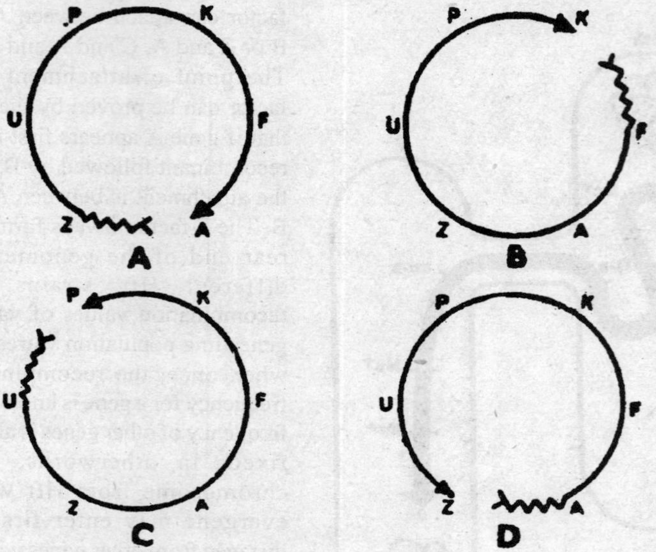

Fig. 22.6 Microbial Genetics
(A,B,C,D). Four hypothetical Hfr strains having different genes at their proximal ends

Jacob and Woman (1957) used the technique of "interrupted mating" between a *Hfr* strain and a F strain. At different time intervals, the mating mixture was diluted and agitated on a waring blender to separate the mating cells forcibly, thus interrupting conjugation and then plated on selective agar media. They demonstrated a lag period of 8 minutes before the first recombinant appeared. The recombinants then appear for other genes in a linear order in relation to the time allowed for conjugation. From this Jacob and Wolman concluded that the latent period of 8 minjutes is required for the conjugating cells to make contact, whereafter the genetic material from *Hfr* is transfered to F in a linear order. They showed that 89 minutes are required for the complete transfer of the chromosome form *Hfr* to F. The bacterial chromosome is therefore 89 time units long. Wolman and Jacob in 1956 produced the first genetic map of a bacterial chromosome in a *Hfr* strain.

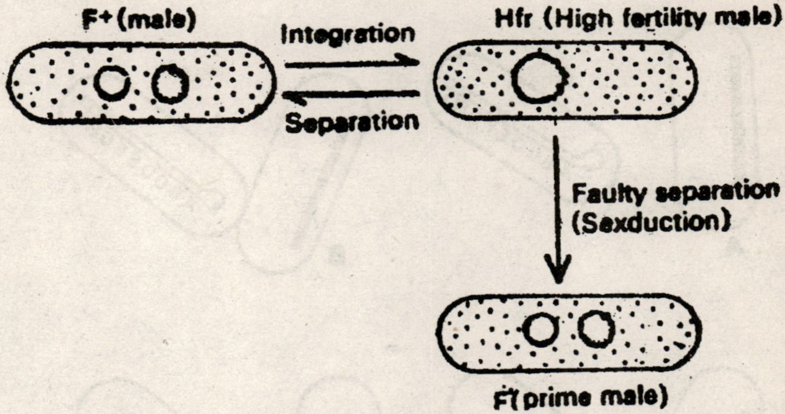

Fig. 22.7 Microbial Genetics
The showing interconversion between male and high fertility male. Faulty release of the fertility factor results in Sexduction and production of F' (Fprime) male.

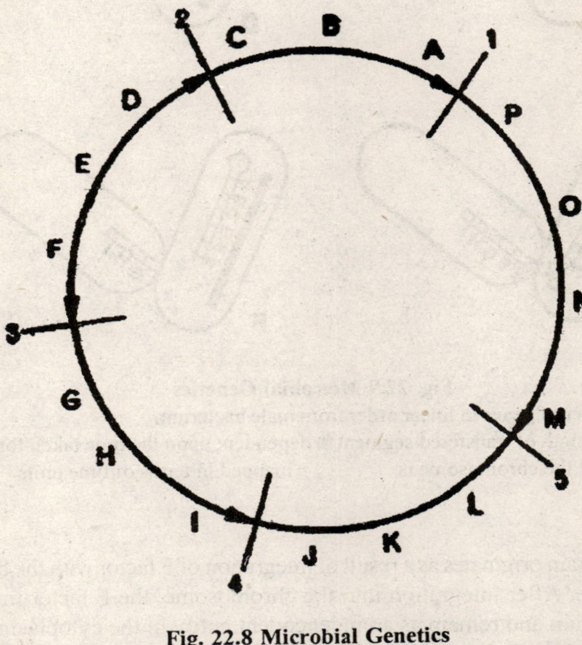

Fig. 22.8 Microbial Genetics
The linear order of genes in five hypothetical Hfr strains, resulting due to breaking of bacterial strain at different sites and subsequent orientation acquired by the resulting linear chromosome

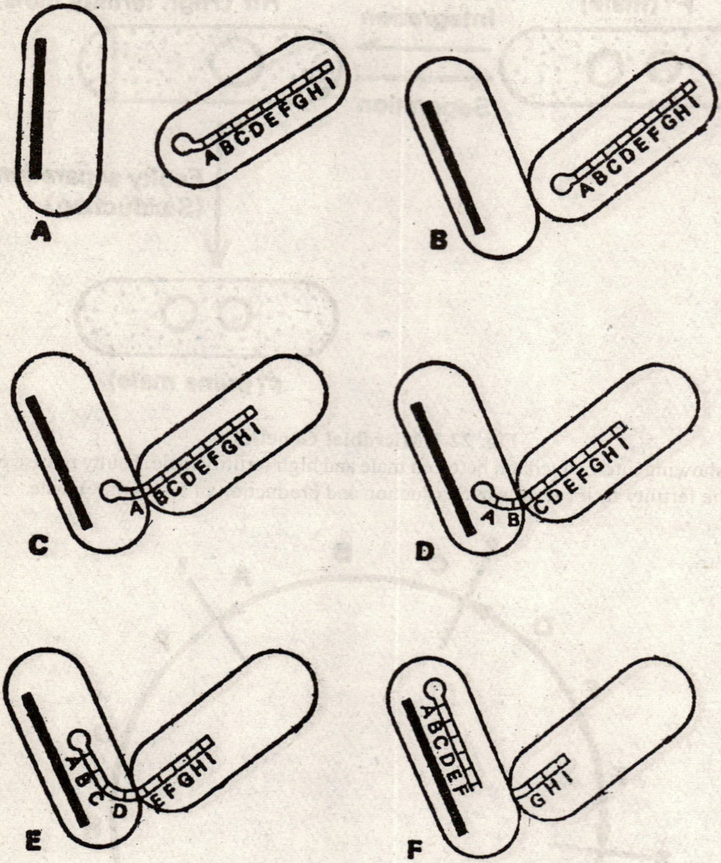

Fig. 22.9 Microbial Genetics

The transfer of genes in linear order from male bacterium female; the length of transfered segment is dependent upon the time taken for transfer and the chromosome is, mapped in terms of time units

Sex duction

A *Hfr* strain originates as a result of integration of F factor with the bacterial chromosome. After integration into the chromosome, the F factor might get separated again and remain as an independent entity in the cytoplasm. If this happens, the *Hfr* strain would change into a F^+ strain. In otherwords *Hfr* and F^+ strains are interconvertible.

In some unusual cases, when an integrated F factor gets detached from the chromosome, it may carry along with it some of the chromosomal genes (some porition of the chromosome gets torn and remains attached to the F factor). Such an independent F^+ factor is given the name F^1 (F prime). An F^1 cell is male and like the F^+ except that the F factor has some genes of the chromosome.

When a F^1 (male) cell conjugates with a F cell, the recipient cell on getting the F^1 becomes a donor. In addition it becomes diploid for certain genes of the chromosome which are present in the F^1. Because these genes are present on the chromosome as well as an F^1. This phenomenon is known as *sexduction* (Jacob and Alderberg, 1959). The recipient cells become *paritial diploids* for the genes introduced by the F^1.

GENETIC TRANSFORMATION

Every individual born out of Sexual reproduction will have the mixture of traits of both the parents. In genetic terms, this means that there is genetic recombination in the offsping. Genetic recombination or transformation which is an index of genetic change has also been reported in bacteria.

Genetic transformation i.e., change of one genetic type to other was first reported by British bactyeriologist F.Griffith (1928) while working with pneumococci (*Diplococcus pneumoniae*).

There are two strains in *Diplococcus pneumoniae.* One is capsulated and the other one is Non capsulated ones form glistening smooth (S) colonies on the culture medium while the non capsuleated ones form dull, rought (R) colonies. Further, the capsulated (S) strains are virulent while the non capsulated (R) strains are non virulent i.e., do not produce toxins. The ability of producing or not producing a capsule is a genetic character.

Griffith injected experimental mice with R strains of pneumococci and found that they survived but when S strains are injected the, mice died. When heat killed (killing the bacteria by applying heat when DNA gets denatured and will not produce toxin) 'S' strains were injected the mice survived. Griffith next injected both R strain and heat killed 'S' strain to the same experimental mice and they (mice) died. Blood analysis of the dead mice (which were infected with R strain and heat killed S strain) showed the presence of 'live' S strains. There are three possibilities how the heat killed 'S' strains can become live again.

1. Heat killed S strain might have become alive in the body of mice-this is an impossibility.
2. A mutation might have occured in the R strain converting them to S strain. This is also not possible because mutations will not occur frequently, but everytime the experiment showed the presence of capsulated S strains in the blood of the dead mice.

3. Some factor in the head killed strain has transferred the genetic information for capsule synthesis to R strain making them produce the capsule. In other words they become S strain. This is the only way a live S strain could be found in the blood of mice. Griffith (1928) thought that the transforming principle was a bacterial polysaccharide. But Avery *et al* (1944) demonstrated that the transforming principle was DNA.

This experiment clearly demonstrates that a piece of DNA responsible for capsule synthesis recombined with the DNA of the R strain inducing it to produce a capsule. This can be called a natural method of genetic engineering.

Mechanism of transformation

This involves the following steps - competence, binding, penetration, synapsis and integration.

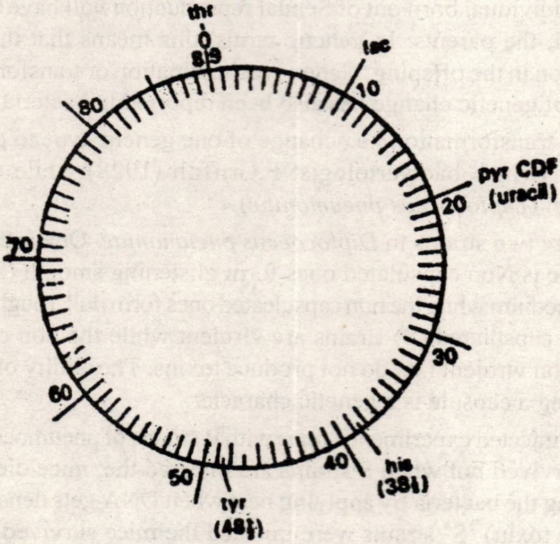

Fig. 22.10 Microbial Genetics

Circular linkage map of *Escherichia coli* chromosome, the units of recombination shown as minute required for transfer

Competence

The recipient bacteria must be competent if they are to accept the foreign DNA and undergo transformation. Competence of recipient bacteria depends on several factors such as age, physiological condition etc. The duration and time of occurrence of competence varies with species also. During growth, competence is observed during the end of logarthmic phase and just at the

beginning of stationary phase. Experiments of Euphrissi-Taylor and Freed (1964) have shown that in *Pneumococcus,* competence developed in 90-100 minutes old culture and lasted for just 7-15 minutes. In *Bacillus subtilis* competence lasts for several hours, but only a few cells in the culture become competent. Several external factors are known to induce competence in an otherwise non competent cells.

Binding

DNA of the transforming bacterium comes into contact with the cell surface of recipient cells as a result of random collision. Subsequently the DNA binds to the surface at places called *receptor sites* which appear to be associated with mesosomes.

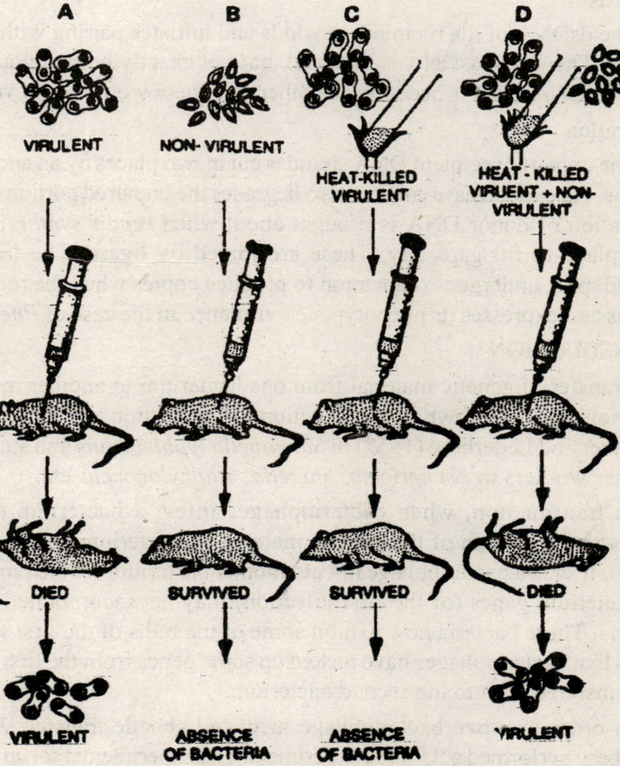

Fig. 22.11 Microbial Genetics

Schematic representation of Griffith's experiment to demonstrate transformation in *Diplococcus pneumoniae*

Penetration

After binding itself to the cell surface, the DNA penetrates the bacterial cell. It is believed that the double strand DNA (dsDNA) becomes single strand DNA (ssDNA) on entering into the recipient cell in *pneumococcus*. According to one of the theories when one end of dsDNA enters the cell, an endonuclease enzyme of the recipient digests one of the strands, while the other strand is pulled into the cell. Labelling experiments have shown, half the labelling is present in one strand of DNA, while the other half is in the degraded strand. The ssDNA of the donor migrates from the periphery to the chromosome of recipient. In *Bacillus subtilis,* this takes 15-60 minutes. Mesosomes seen to play a role in carrying the ssDNA on to the chromosome.

Synapsis

The dsDNA of the recipient unwinds and initiates pairing with the donor ssDNA. The donor ssDNA is identical, but not exactly homologous with the recipient DNA. This is necessary as otherwise there would be no variation.

Integration

The unpaired recipient DNA strand is cut in two places by an endonuclease enzyme. An exonuclease enzyme also degrades the unpaired portion of ssDNA. Integration of donor DNA is brought about when *repair synthesis* of DNA takes place to fill gaps any. These are joined by ligase. The transformed heteroduplex undergoes replication to produce copies when the recipient cell divides and expresses its phenotype ie., virulence in the case of *Pneumococci.*

TRANSDUCTION

Transfer of genetic material from one bacterium to another mediated by bacteriophages is known as transduction. Transduction was first discovered by Zinder and Lederberg (1952) in *Salmonella typhimurium* and subsequently by other workers in *Escherichia, Shigella, Staphylococcus* etc.

In transduction, when bacteriophages infect a bacterium they often incorporate a portion of the genetic material of bacterium into their genetic system. If such a bacteriophage infects another bacterium (of the same species) the bacterium genes (of the first infection) may get incorporated into these bacteria. These bacteria now exhibit some of the traits of the first strain. This shows that bacteriophages have picked up some genes from the first bacterium and transfered it on to the second bacterium.

In order to prove bacteriophage mediated genetic transfer. Zinder and Lederberg performed a 'U' tube experiment. The experimental set up consists of a 'U' tube where the two arms are separated at the base by means of a sintered glass filter (Bacterial filter). Zinder and Lederberg (1952) grew two different strains of bacteria *Salmonella typhimurium* in the two arms. One strain was infected with bacteriophages. A little later when the bacteria in both the arms of the 'U' tube were analysed it was noticed that the strains in both the arms had become recombinants. Since the bacterial filter does not allow the migration of bacteria, the only way for transfer of genetic material was through bacteriophages since they can move across bacterial filters.

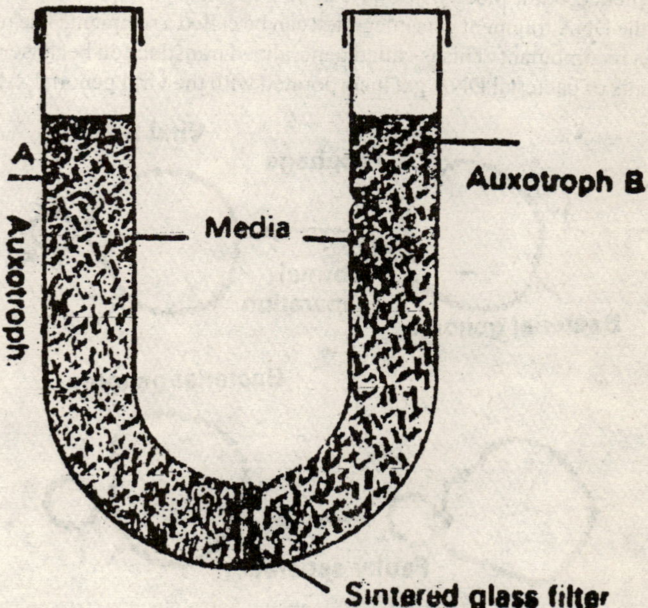

Fig. 22.12 Microbial Genetics
The Transduction (U tube) experiment of Zinder and Lederberg

Types of transduction

There are two types of transduction - Generalized transduction and special or restricted transduction.

Generalized transduction

Phage mediated transfer of small segment of DNA from any part of bacterial chromosome is called generalized transduction. Bacteriophages of P1 of *E.coli*, P22 of *Salmonella* and SP10 and PBSI of *Bacillus subtilis* sometimes make mistakes during their lytic infection cycles. At the end of the lytic cycle when phage particles are packaged into protein coats and the host chromosome is getting degraded, a small piece of host DNA, usually the same length as the phage chromosome, gets incorporated into the phage and becomes a part of phage DNA. The virus particle now infects a second bacterium. In this bacterial cell, the fragment of DNA (which has been picked up by the virus) can be inserted into the bacterial chromosome. The first bacterium from which the phage picked out a piece of DNA can be called a donor, and the second in which the DNA fragment gets integrated can be called a recipient. The recipient will bea recombinant. This is called generalized transduction because random fragments of bacterial DNA get incorporated with the viral genome.

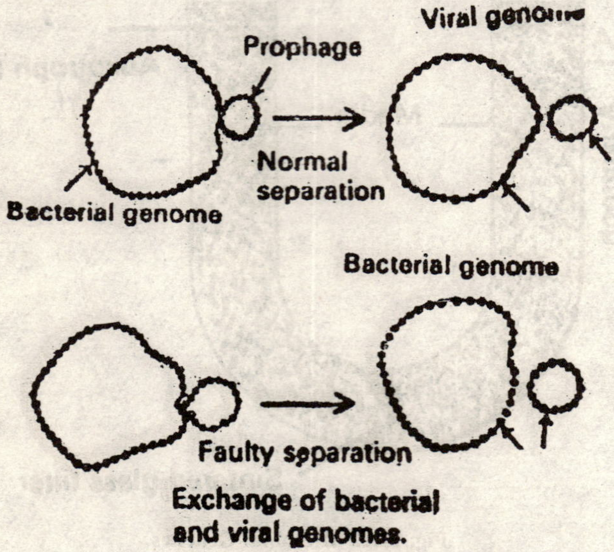

Fig. 22.13 Microbial Genetics

Showing normal and faulty separation of phage DNA from bacterial genome. A piece of bacterial DNA is incorporated into the phage DNA and vice-versa.

Specialized transduction

Also called restricted transduction, in this the phage is able to transduce or transfer only certain segment of the bacterial genome. Specialized transduction takes place as follows.

When prophages are induced to leave the bacterial chromosome, the viral genome caries with it only some bacterial genes covalently linked to the viral genes. This hybrid DNA packed in the phage coat is called *special transducing particle* because it can transfer from one bacterium to another only certain genes - genes that are adjacent to the prophage attachment site. Specialized transduction is induced by λ prophage, ϕ 80 prophage which usually occupy a fixed site on the bacterial chromosome. The site is called prophage site. In *E.coli,* the prophage site is flanked on one side by bacterial genes gal K, T and ε genes of the galactose gene cluster and on the other side by block of genes involved with the synthesis of biotin - bio A,B,F,C and D. Thus λ prophage can transduce only *gal* or *bio* genes.

The total length of hybrid DNA in a transducing prophage is exactly equivalent in length to the normal viral genome (as otherwise it cannot be packedinto the coat) which means to accomodate the bacterial genes, a corresponding length of viral genome should be missing. As such these phages are called defective paste (they lack some viral genes).

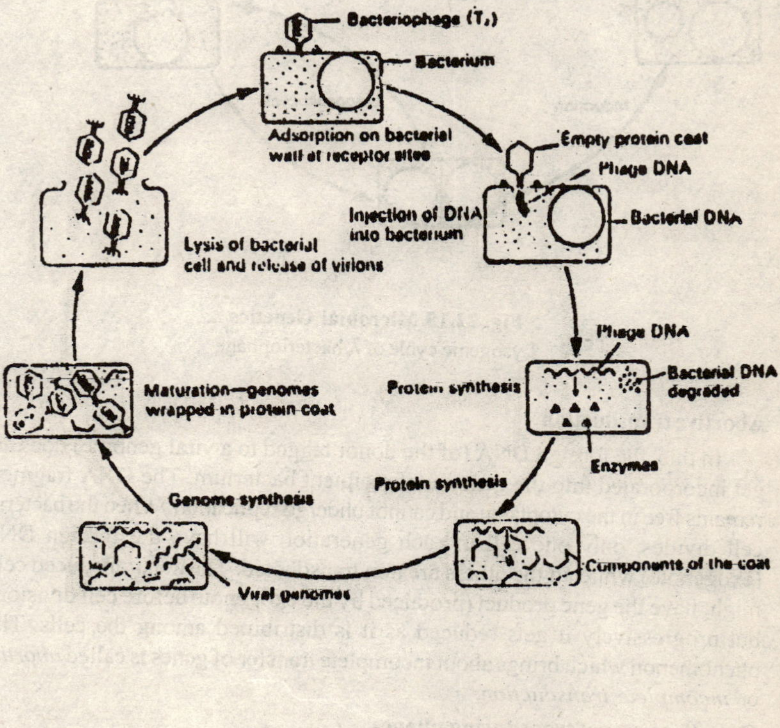

Fig. 22.14 Microbial Genetics
Lytic cycle of a bacteriophage (T_2)

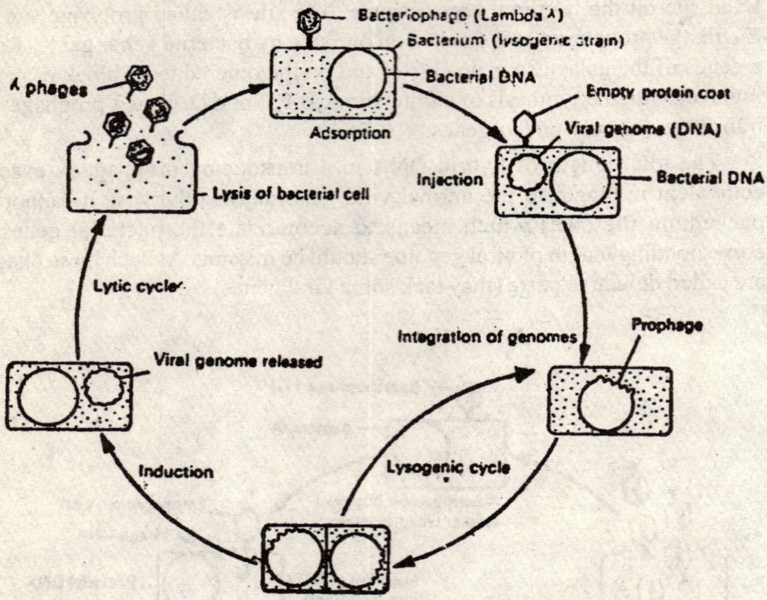

Fig. 22.15 Microbial Genetics
Lysogenic cycle of λ bacteriophage

Abortive transduction

In this, the foreign DNA (of the donor tagged to a viral genome) does not get incorporated into the genome of recipient bacterium. The DNA fragment remains free in the cytoplasm and cannot uhdergo replication. When the bacterial cell divides, only one cell in each generation will have the foreign DNA (exogenote) while all the others are non transducted. The non transduced cells might have the gene product (produced by the exogenote before cell division), but progressively it gets reduced as it is distributed among the cells. This phenomenon which brings about incomplete transfer of genes is called *abortive* or *incomplete transduction.*

Growth phases of transducing phages

Bacteriophages whicha bring about transduction can be divided into two groups based on their growth cycles. These are **lytic cycle** and **lysogenic cycle.**

Lytic cycle

This is seen is phages called virulent phages typified by T series phages. Here soon after infection the host cell lyses releasing the newly formed viral particles. The lytic cycle seen in Tphages infecting *E.coli* bacterium has the following stages.

Adsorption

The phage attaches to specific receptor sites on the bacterial surface.

Injection

The tail fibres hold the phage in position and a pore is formed in the bacterial wall, through which the viral DNA is injected inside the host cell.

Protein synthesis

Phage DNAm 'takes over' the synthetic machinery of the bacterial cell and forms viral mRNA and through this the viral proteins.

Genome synthesis

Viral DNA replicates and produces several copies of the viral genome.

Maturation and release

Viral genome gets packed into the newly formed coats, thus assembling new phage particles. At a particular time, the host cell lyses (breaks up) releasing the phage particles.

Lysogenic cycle

This is seen in λ phage. The phages are also called temperate phages (as they show lysogenic cycle). Lysogenic cycle was first discovered by Andre Lwoff. The characteristic feature of this cycle is that the host cell do not lyse as a result of infection by the phages. But the phages will remain in the host cell in a sort of an association. The lysogenic cycle is as follows.

The DNA of the phage, after adsorption and injection, enters the bacterial cell. But instead of starting its degrading activity, the phage genome gets integrated with the host genome. This integrated condition of the viral genome is said to be **prophage.** When the bacterial cell divides, the integrated genome replicates in the normal way. The viral genome may be said to be in a hibernating state as it is not trying to express itself. Occasionally, the viral genome gets separated from the bacterial genome and is released into the cytoplasm where it separated from the bacterial genome and is released into the cytoplasm where it starts multiplying and causes the lysis of cells. The dissociation of viral genome from bacterial genome (with causes lysogeny to become lytic) is called *induction*.

23

GENETIC DISEASES

Disease caused by genetic disorders are called genetic diseases. Malfunctioning of a gene is called a genetic disorder. For instance a gene is supposed to produce a particular enzyme and that has to participate in a reaction producing a specific product. If for some reason the gene gets altered i.e., undergoes mutation, then the gene product-enzyme can not be producedand this may block a particular metabolic pathway resulting in the non formation of a product. If this product is an important one it leads to diseases known as genetic diseases.

The discovery of Beadle and Tatum (1940) in *Neurospora* that mutational changes in genes can be linked to losses of specific enzymes paved the way for further studies of many unexplained diseasesin human beings.

A.E. Garrod (1908) was the first to study genetic diseases connected to distrubed metabolic pathways. He used the term *'inborn errors of metabolism'* to denote the genetic disease *Alkaptaneuria* or dark urine disease. The phenomenon of inborn errors of metabolism may be understood clearly by understanding *metabolic blocks*.

Metabolic block

A biosynthetic pathway normally consists of several steps with each step and the formation of anintermediary product under the influence of an enzyme which in turn is controlled by a gene. If a mutation occurs in any gene, either the production of normal enzyme is stopped or a defective enzyme (phenotype) produces a defective characer. Such an alteration of normal phenotype due to alterarion of metabolic pathway is called *metabolic block*.

Metabolic blocks or metabolic errors produce a number of defective characters in human beings and provide an opportunity to understand the relationship between genes, enzyme and phenotypes. This helps us to unravel the genetic regulation of biochemical pathways. Such a field of study is known as biochemical genetics. Biochemical genetics may be defined as analysis of genetic control of biosynthetic pathways.

Defects in bio synthetic pathways are of various types. These are -

1. Defects in the metabolism of aminoacids
2. Defects in the metabolism of lipids
3. Defects in sugar metabolism
4. Defects in the production of Haemogiobin etc,

In this book defects in aminoacid metabolism and haemoglobin are discussed.

Defects in the metabolism of aminoacids

Metabolic pathways involving (a) phenylalanine - Tyrosine, (b) Tryptophan (c) Arginine serve as good examples to study the genetic defects and associated phenotypic alterations. Here we shall study the metabolic pathway involving the amino acids Tyrosine and phenyl alanine.

Metabolism of phenylalanine

Phenylalanine is an important constituent of proteins in our diet. During digestion of proteins, the amino acid (phenyl alanine) is released into the digestive tract and then gets absorbed by the body cells. Within the cell there are three pathways for the metabolism of phenyl alanine as follows -

(i) It may combine with other amino acids to form proteins
(ii) Can convert itself into phenyl pyruvic acid.
(iii) Can convert itself into Tyrosine.

We shall now consider the possible abnormalities in the (ii) and (iii)

Phenyl Ketonuria

The conversion of phenyl alanine to tyrosine is under the control of the enzyme phenyl alanine hydroxylase (present in liver) which is in turn regulated by the gene *P*. In homozygous recessive condition genes *pp* will not produce the enzyme and hence there is accumulation of phenyl alanine as it cannot convert itself into tyrosine. As a result there is abnormal increase in the level of phenyl alanine and also its product (in another pathway) phenyl pyruvic acid. Both these - phenyl alanine and phenyl pyruvic acid accumulate in the cells in large amounts and most of these is excreted through the urine or may get accumulated in the blood. This condition is known as phenylketonuria (Pku).

Normal persons will have a plalsma phenylalanine level of 1-2 mg/100ml while Pku persones will have 15-64mg/100ml.

Similarly the urine level phenyl alanine in normal humans is 30mg/100ml while Pku persones will have 300-1000mg/100ml.

Complications of Pku include brain damage leading to mental retardation (with an IQ level below 20). High quantities of phenyl alanine seem to interfer with the development of brain cells. Persons suffering from Pku are called *Phenylopyruvic idiots* as they have very low IQ.

Effects of Pku will be noticed a few months after birth. Affected babies may show eczema of skin, defective enamel of teeth and bone deformations.

Treatment of Pku includes phenyl alanine free diet which can prevent brain damages. The diet however should include fixed amount of phenyl alanine also as it is an essential amino acid.

Tyrosine metabolism

Tyrosine is another key amino acid involved in various metabolic pathways. It may be obtained by conversion of phenyl alanine or by the direct break down of proteins. In the normal human beings the metabolism of Tyrosine proceeds as follows -

(a) It may combine with other amino acids and become part of cellular proteins.

(b) It may combine with Iodine in the thyroid gland to produce thyroid hormones - Failure of this results in insufficient thyroid hormones producing a defect called *genetic goitrus cretenism.* This is characterised by physical and mental retardation.

(c) Tyrosine gets converted intodihydroxy phenyl alaline (DOPA) which inturn leads to melanin formation. Failure of this leads to *Albinism.*

(d) In the fourth pathway tyrosine gets degraded in a stepwise fashion to CO_2 and water as follows :

(1) Tyrosine (2) Parahydroxy phenyl pyruvic acid (3) Dihyrdoxyphenyl pyruvic acid (4) Homogentistic acid (5) $CO_2 + H_2O$.

Failure of conversion of 2 to 3 (as shown above) leads to a disease called *tyrosinosis.* Failure of degradation of Homogentisic acid leads to its excretion along with urine and the disease is known as *Alkaptoneuria.* Urine of Alkapataneurics turns black on exposure to air. Hence it is called black urine disease.

Albinism

As has already been pointed out Albinism is a result of failure of metabolism of Tyrosine. In normal human beings metabolism of Tyrosine leads to the formation of melanin pigmentation which gives the normal colouration to the skin. The normal metabolic pathway is as follows-

$$\text{Tyrosine} \rightarrow \text{DOPA} \rightarrow \text{DOPAquinone} \rightarrow \text{melanin.}$$

Albinism results due to the absence of the enzyme *Tyrosinase* (which normally acts on tyrosine and produces DOPA). There are two types of albinism.

(i) Ocular albinism - only eye pigments are absent.

(ii) Genral albinism - no pigments in both eyes and skin.

In normal human beings the enzyme tyrosinase is present in the structures called melanosomes present in melanocytes. In albinos the enzyme is not produced due to a defective gene.

Metabolic effect in theproduction of haemoglobin

Haemoglobin in the blood is necessary for gaseous exchange particularly to absorb oxygen. A normal haemoglobin consists of four polypeptide chains each associated with a single haeme group. Out of the four chains two are called *alpha* chains and are common in children and adults. The remaining two chains are different at different ages in human beings. Each polypeptide chain is coded by a different gene.

Defects in the haemoglobin chain may be divided intothe following groups-

(i) Thallassaemia caused by reduction in globin chain synthesis

(ii) Sickle anaemia

(iii) Hereditary persistance of foetal haemoglobin

We will study sickle cell anaemia in some detail.

Sickle cell anaemia

The name is derived from the anaemic condition (destruction of haemoglobin) owing to abnormal condition of the haemoglobin. In patients suffering from sickle cell disease, most of the erythrocytes (RBC's) of the blood lose their normal disc shape and become sickle shaped. These sickled cells increase the viscosity of the blood. Their presence in small vessels leads to blockage of capillaires. The sickle erythrocytes are fragile and easily get destroyed in the spleen. This leads to anaemic condition and a blood test will reveal the presence of sickle RBC's.

Sickle celled anaemia is caused due to abnormal haemoglobin called sickle haemoglobin. In sickle haemoglobin *alpha* and *beta* chains undergo structural variations due to replacement of amino acids. This in turn is due to mutations in the structural genes. Linus Pauling 91949) discovered the difference between normal haemoglobin and sickle haemoglobin. Tugram (1957) showed clearly that a single amino acid substitution is the difference between the normal and sickle haemoglobin.

Normal haemoglobin is controlled by the gene *ha* and the mutated form is *hs*. Disease manifests in the following combinations.

h*a* h*a* - Normal individuals

h*a* h*s* - Mild form of sickle cell anaemia (heterozygous)

h*s* h*s* - Severe form of sickle cell anaemia (homozygous)

Hameophilia

This is another irregularity of the blood and is a genetic disorder. Commonly called bleeder's disease, in this, blood fails to clot on exposure to air. In haemophilicss the gene to produce vitamin K necessary for clotting will be defective, hence even in a minor wound there is continuous bleeding which may be fatal. This is a sex linked charater. (For details see chapter 16)

GENETIC ENGINEERING

Recombinant DNA technology or Genetic engineering as it is popularly known, is the newest tool that is available in the human arsenal of knowledge in man's quest for a better human life. What is genetic engineering or recombinant DNA technology?

Imagine a situation of chronic diabetic patients being able to get back the capacity of synthesis of insulin; patients suffering from incurable diseases getting an injection of gene therapy-lo and behold they are cured of their diseases; consider a situation which is at present in the realms of fantasy of making man producing his own food just like the green plants do from natural sources; or visualize a situation wherein revolution in agricultural technology would make the use of chemical fertilizers completely redundant or going to the extreme, culturing a human being of the desired trait on a medium of nutrients i.e., man made to order. The scope is fantastic; possibilities are immense; it is as if the role of creator has been for once given to human beings. Well this is genetic engineering or recombinant DNA technology, the most powerful biological technique which the human beings can use either to make or mar the society. It can be used either for progress or for destruction. Using the techniques of genetic engineering you can create deadly pathogenic bacteria and unleash them on human beings; you can produce varieties of agricultural crops which are disease free or you can introduce pathogens into the crops and totally destroy them. Genetic engineering used judiciously can be a harbinger of new revolution but used injudiciously may produce many prototype of criminals, antisocial elements, boot leggers etc. In this chapter we shall briefly discuss some of the fundamental aspects of genetic engineering and how to use them for betterment of human life.

Genetic engineering may be defined as the method of artificial synthesis of new genes and their subsequent transplantation in the new genome of an organism, by molecular biological techniques. Recombinant DNA is achieved by constructing molecules outside the living cells by joining natural or synthetic

DNA molecules that can replicate inside a living cell. Recombinant DNA technology involves several stages or steps.

The main aspects of genetic engineering (gene cloning) are the following -

1. Identification and isolation of the gene to be cloned.
2. Insertion on the gene into another piece of DNA called vector which will allow it to be taken up by microorganisms like bacteria and replicate within them as the cells divide.
3. Transfer of the recombinant vectors into bacterial cells.
4. Selection of those cells which have the desired recombinant vectors.
5. Growth of the microorganisms to get increased quantity of cloned DNA.
6. Expression of the desired gene to obtain the desired product.

Outline procedure of Genetic engineering

Genetic engineering of a desired gene and gene product involves the following procedure. First of all the desired gene has to be obtained from a source which then has to be identified and isolated.

(i) The living cells from which the genetic material is to be obtained has to be broken open. One popular method is to shear the cells in a blender and treat them with a suitable detergent.

(ii) The genetic material from the cell is to be removed. Several techniques are available to remove the DNA. The DNA molecules can even be spooled on to a glass rod. The glass rod bearing the DNA molecules is then lifted up from the debris of the cells.

(iii) The next step is to cut away the specific genes of interest from the DNA molecule. Restriction enzymes popularly called molecular scissors are used to cut and separate the desired gene from the DNA helix.

(iv) In the next step the specific sections of DNA are incorporated into cloning vectors or vehicles such as plasmids, phages etc. These cloning vehicles are then introduced into a rapidly multiplying living system such as bacteria where multiple copies of the cloned DNA can be obtained. The cloned DNA also called chimeric DNA contains the desired foreign gene. The coloned DNA is also called recombinant DNA.

(v) In the final step which is a very delicate process the cloned gene is allowed to express itself in the bacterial cell. Gene expression here means production of a desired gene product. For instance if a human insulin gene is coloned in a plasmid and is inserted into a bacterial cell, the bacterial cell along with its metabolic products also will produce insulin. This insulin may than be separated by the normal methods of chemical purification and isolation.

RESTRICTION ENZYMES (restriction endonucleases)

The first account of restriction enzymes was given by Werner Arber while studying the bacteriophages. He found that in some instances as soon as the viral DNA entered into a bacterial cell it (viral DNA) was cut into bits and destroyed. Based on this observation Arber opined that the bacterial cell must possess certain specific DNA destroying enzymes that could infect only the viral DNA but not the host DNA. In otherwords the enzyme should be such that it should be able to distinguish between foreign DNA and its own DNA. He gave the name restriction enzymes and hypothesized that these restriction enzymes can recognise and act at specific sites on the viral DNA.

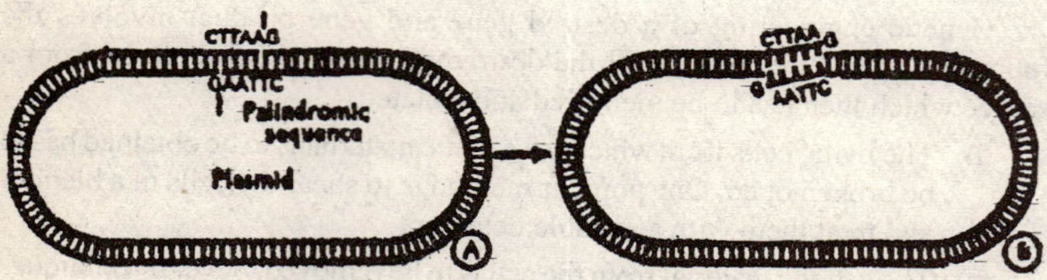

Fig. 24.1 Genetic Engineering
Action of restriction enzymes

The next step in the discovery of restriction enzymes was taken by Smith *et al* (1970) when they isolated a restriction enzyme from the bacterium *Haemophilus influezae.* Smith showed that the restriction enzyme can cut the viral DNA at specific sites. All the DNA termini were pGpTpPy-3' and 5' pPupApCp, showing that these were cut from the double stranded DNA having the following sequence

5'pGpTpy | pPupApCp-3'
3'pGpApPu | pPypTpGp-5'

The above example shows that the restriction enzyme from *Haemophilus influenzae* can cut the DNA molecule which exhibit a two fold symmetry i.e., with a palindromic sequence (same sequence running in opposite directions). Some restriction endonucleases, there source, recognition sequence and sites of cleavage (indicated by arrow) are given below.

Enzyme	Source	Recognition sequence and clearing site
Eco R1	*Escherichia coli* Ry13	↓ G.AA TTC GTT AAG
Hind II	*Haemophilus influenzae*	GTPy ↓ PuAC CAPu ↓ PyTG
Hind III	*Haemophilus influenzae* Rd	↓ A AG CTT TTC ↓ GA A ↑
Hpa I	*Haemophilus parainfluenzae*	GTT ↑ AAC CAA ↓ TTG
Hpa II	*Haemophilus parainfluenzae*	CC GG GG CC ↑ ↑
Bam HI	*Bacillus amyloliquefaciens*	GGA TCC CCT AGG ↓ ↑
Bgl III	*Bacillus globigi*	A GA TCT TCT AG A ↓ ↑
Hae II	*Haemophilus aegyptius*	PuGG GCPy PyCG ↑ CGPu
Hae III	*Haemophilus aegyptius*	GG ↓ CC CC ↑ GG ↓
Hha I	*Haemophilus haemolyticus*	GC GC CG CG ↑
Pst I	*Providencia stuartii*	CTG CA G ↓ GAC GTC ↑ ↓
Sma I	*Serratia marcescens*	CCC GGG GGG CCC ↓ ↑
Taq I	*Thermus aquaticus*	T C GA AG CT ↑

Bal I	*Brevibacterium albidum*	TCG	↓	CCA
		ACC	↑	GGT
		↓		
Sal I	*Streptomyces albus* G	GTC		GAC
		CAG		CTG
				↓↑
Xor II	*Xanthomonas oryzae*	CGA		TCG
		GCT		AGC
		↑		
Alu I	*Arthrobacter luteus*	AG		CT
		TC		GA
			↓	
Msp I	*Moraxella* sp.	CC		GG
		GG	↑	CC
		↓		
Mbo I	*Moraxella bovis*	GA		TC
Sau 3 Al	*Staphylococcus aureus* 3A	GA	↓	TC
		CT	↑	AG

Subsequent work by Daniel Nathans (1971) showed that the restriction enzyme discovered by Smith can cut the monkey virus DNA into eleven well defined pieces. By using specific restriction enzymes it is also possible to map the DNA which they cut as their specificity is known. Arber, Nathans and Smith were awarded the 1978 Noble prize in physiology and medicine for their work on restriction enzymes.

In many microorganisms restriction enzymes are a means of protection against intrudent viral DNA. In the working of the restriction enzyme the nucleotide sequence of the host DNA is identified and methylated to avoid degradation. As a result of this the DNA gets the protection while the foreign DNA with the same sequence will not be methylated and consequently subjects itself for degradation. The whole mechanism is called the RM system (restriction modification) and is wide spread in bacteria.

Classification of restriction enzymes

Restriction enzymes are able to recognise specific nucleotide sequence in the double stranded DNA and cleave both the strands. To date more than 150 restriction enzymes have been discovered which are known to recognise 40 different nucleotide sequence. Some restriction enzymes however may not cut DNA at specific sites. Based on this restriction enzymes are classified into two categories type 1 and type 2. Type 1 restriction enzymes recognise a specific sequence of DNA molecule but the cut is made elsewhere whereas type 2 enzymes make a cut only within the restriction site and produce two single strand breaks, one break in each strand. Type 2 enzymes are most important because they produce broken chain of nucleotides with a palindromic sequence. The following table gives a summary of the difference between type 1 and type 2 enzymes.

	Type 1	Type 2
1.	Non-specific in cleavage	Cleavage is site-specific
2.	M.W 300,000	Lower MW (20,000 - 1,00,000)
3.	Has non-identical subunits	Has two identical subunits
4.	Require ATP, Mg ++ and generally S-adenosyl	Require only Mg ++ as co-factor
5.	Examples : EcoB, EcoK, EcoPi	Example : EcoRI

Nomenclature of restriction enzymes

The names are designated according to the following principles.

(1) Name of the organism is identified by the first letter of the gene's name and the first two letters of the species name to form a three letter abbreviation in italics. For example *E.coli* = *Eco* and *H.influenzae* = *Hin* etc.

(2) A strain or type identified is written as a subscript. For example *E.coli* strain k is written as Eco_k.

(3) In cases where the restriction modification systems are genetically specified by a virus or plasmids the extra chromosomal element is identified by a subscript as *Eco RI, Eco PI* etc.

When a particular strain has several restrictions and modification systems these are identified by Roman numerals. For example Hin dI, Hin dII, Hin dIII etc.

Cleavage brought about by restriction enzymes

Restriction enzymes have an ability to recognise a particular sequence and cleave DNA molecule at that site. Most of the sequences recognised by these enzymes are tetranucleotide or hexanucleotide pairs which show a characteristic two fold symmetry i.e., palindromic sequence. The Eco RII site is very unique as it contains 5 base pairs with the axis of symmetry passing through the middle AT pair as shown below.

CCTGG
CCACC

Some times restriction enzymes from unrelated species can recognise the same nucleotide sequence. For instance GGCC sequence specific enzymes have been discovered in *Bacillus subtilis, Haemophilus aegypticus* etc. Such enzymes are called isoschizomers.

Cleavage sites may be even or staggered. In even cleavage the breaks on the two strands are exactly opposite to each other. Whereas in staggered breaks the breaks on the two strands are a little away from each other. Even breaks donot produce unpaired terminal nucleotides whereas staggered breaks may produce sticky ends.

Use of restriction enzymes

The use of restriction enzymes has proved to be a highly useful tool for the sequence analysis of DNA. It also plays a significant role for gene cloning and amplification in genetic engineering.

The DNA molecule from bacteriophages and many other viruses consists of 5,000 to 50,000 base pairs. It is of fundamental importance to know the sequence of these bases to understand the gene structure and regulation and also for decoding the information stored in these genes. By the use of several restriction enzymes it is possible to cut fragments of DNA as small as 300 bp. These fragments can be used for sequence analysis and mapping.

The DNA segments produced by restriction enzymes can be covalently linked to the plasmid DNA and such recombined DNA can be inserted into bacteria such as *E.coli* for transformation. The transformed cells can now be cultured as separate colones.

The ability of restriction enzymes to locate and cut at a particular sequence is of great help in identifying and isolating a particular gene.

Identification of a required DNA piece (gene)

Theoritically, identification of a gene involves, the reading of the message back in protein synthesis. During protein synthesis DNA produces mRNA and this in turn identifies and allows the alignment of amino acids to synthesize a protein. In the identification of a gene responsible for the production of a particular protein, the process has to be followed backwards. Let us take an instance of the human insulin which is a protein.

The steps involved in the identification of the gene or segment of DNA responsible for insulin are as follows.

(a) Isolation and purification of the protein

(b) Sequential degradation of the protein : In sequential degradation, not only the qualitative composition of the amino acids are known, but even their sequence of arrangement in the polypeptide chain will be known. After ascertaining the sequence of amino acids the next step would be :

(c) Identification of codes for each amino acid : This can be done easily as we know the triplet codes for each amino acid. This would give us a length of the mRNA segment equivalent to the length of the polypeptide chain. (For example if the protein consists of 25 amino acids, the length of the mRNA should be 75 nucleotides).

The nucleotide sequence in mRNA can be easily substituted for the complementary DNA segment. We now have a gene or a segment of DNA which governs the production of insulin.

ISOLATION OF SPECIFIC DNA SEGMENT (GENE)

The DNA of an organism whose specific gene is required for the purpose of expression in another organism contains thousands of genes. The first problem therefore is to separate the required gene from the DNA of the organism. There are several techniques to isolate the required gene from the DNA molecule.

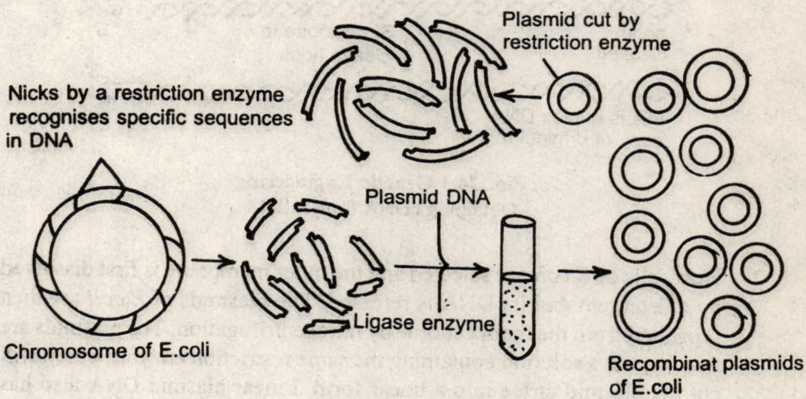

Fig. 24.2 Genetic Engineering
Isolation and recombination of genes using shot gun method

Shotgun method

In this, the entire DNA of the organism is subjected to the action of restriction enzymes and is broken down into a number of fragments. Each of these fragments is then combined with the DNA from a suitable vector to produce recombinant DNA molecule. Subsequently these recombined DNA molecules are inserted randomly into the host cells such as *E.coli*. These host cells are cultured separately and grown into colonies. The following are the steps of the shotgun method.

1. Using specific restriction enzymes the isolated DNA from a particular organism is cleaved into many bits. As the restriction enzymes may bring about even or staggered cuts many sticky ends are left. The resultant DNA fragments are of different length.

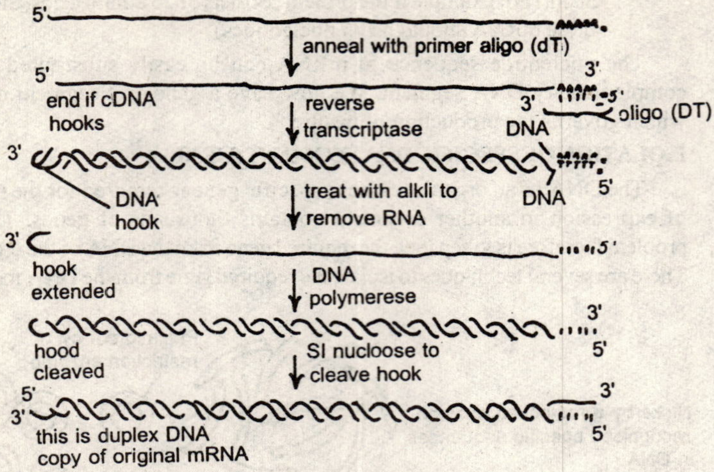

Fig. 24.3 Genetic Engineering
Obtaining cDNA from mRNA

2. Host cells of *E.coli* are selected and the outer membrane is first dissolved by a detergent and its DNA is released. The plasmids of *E.coli* are then separated from the main genome by ultracentrifugation. The plasmids are then kept in a solution containing the same restriction enzyme which will cut the plasmid circle into a linear form. Linear plasmid DNA also has overlapping sticky ends.
3. In this step isolated DNA and linear plasmid DNA are mixed. As a result random association occurs between the foreign DNA and the plasmid DNA. Subsequently the foreign DNA gets integrated into plasmid DNA to form a long linear DNA molecule which then becomes a circle due to covalent joining. The resultant DNA is a recombinant or chimeric DNA.
4. The chimeric DNA molecules are now placed in a solution of calcium chloride which also has *E.coli* cells. On heating suddenly upto 42°C the membranes of bacteria become permeable to chimeric DNA molecules. Thus the *E.coli* cells incorporate the chimeric DNA plasmids.
5. The bacterial cells containing the chimeric plasmids are then cultured on a medium. The cells express not only their genes but the genes of the chimeric plasmids also thus producing a desired product. All these cells are produced by the division of the original bacterial cell having a single chimeric plasmid. Hence they are called clones. Insertng a chimeric plasmid into a bacterial

cell is of very rare occurrence; it has been estimated that only one in 10^5 of 10^6 cells are capable of undergoing transformation.

In shotgun method several genes can be cloned at a time and it is an omnibus method because the genes to be cloned are not picked and identified before.

Obtaining DNA from mRNA

In shotgun method gene cloning is a general one and not specific. As the genes to be cloned are not identified and isolated before, the chances of inserting a particular gene by this method are very rare. Another specific method of isolating gene is to first obtain the messenger RNA transcribed by that particular gene and then obtain DNA from mRNA. DNA from mRNA can be obtained by the following two methods.

Hybridization method

When DNA transcribes and forms mRNA a complex is formed. The hybridization method depends on this mechanism. At the first step the total DNA from an organism is isolated and treated with heat or alkali to convert it into a single stranded form. These single strands are then mixed with the specific mRNA obtained from the gene. Obviously the mRNA chains pair with that section of DNA which has complimentary nucleotides to it thus forming aDNA-RNA hybrid. This complex can be isolated and the DNA can be separated from the RNA. The single stran DNA can be converted into a double strand DNA by enzymes such as polymerase I. This method is highly useful for isolating ribosomal genes.

Reverse transcriptase method

In the normal transcription the flow of information is from DNA → RNA → proteins. Transcription of RNA from DNA is catalysed by the enzyme transcriptase also known as DNA dependent RNA polymerase. Temin and Baltimore independently discovered that occasionally the genetic information may flow in the reverse direction also (from RNA to DNA) in some RNA tumour viruses. They named the enzyme *Reverse transcriptase* (RNA directed DNA polymerase). This enzyme catalyses the synthesis of a single strand DNA using an RNA template. This discovery has proved to be highly useful for isolating particular genes.

In reverse transcriptase method, purified mRNA segments of the required gene are used as a template to produce a fragment of single stranded DNA under the influence of the enzyme reverse transcriptase. As this single strand DNA is complementary to mRNA it is called complimentary DNA or cDNA. Hydrolysis of RNA template will separate a single strand DNA. This single strand DNA is converted into double strand using the enzyme DNA polymerase.

Another enzyme S1 nuclease breaks the covalent linkage between two DNA strands.

VECTORS (Carriers or Vehicles)

Vectors are defined as those DNA molecules that can carry a foreign DNA fragment inserted into them without any disturbance in their expression. Vectors are also called vehicle DNAs. Vectors are obtained from a number of sources. These are grouped into categories such as plasmids, bacteriophages, cosmids and phasmids.

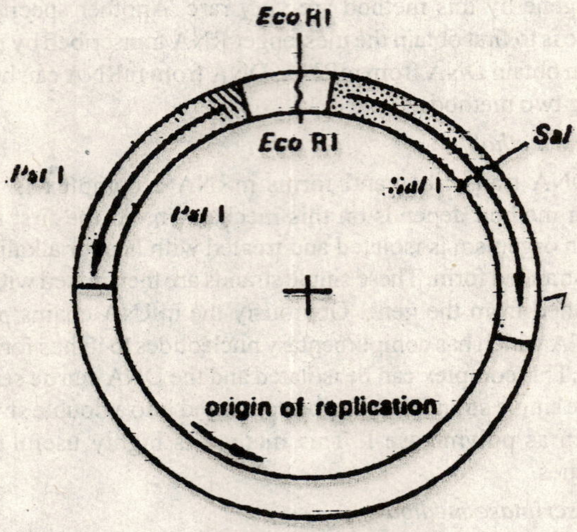

Fig. 24.4 Genetic Engineering
Genetic map of plasmid pBR 322

Plasmids

These are extra chromosomal, self replicating and double stranded covalentaly closed circular DNA molecules present in the bacterial cell. A number of plasmids are present in bacterial cells that have sufficient genetic information for their replication. Eventhough they are not necessary for the survival of the bacteria they carry such necessary information as drug resistance, metal resistance, toxin production, nitrogen fixation etc. Naturally occuring plasmids can also be modified by *in vitro* techniques such as code transformation. Use of plasmids as a vector for DNA cloning was reported for first time by Cohen et al (1973).

Plasmids are used as cloning vehicles when they posses the following features.

1. It can be readily isolated from the cells
2. It possesses a single restriction site for one or more restriction enzyme(s)
3. Insertion of a linear molecule at one of these sites does not alter its replication properties.
4. It can be reintroduced into a bacterial cell and cells carrying the plasmid with or without the insert can be selected or identified (Bernard and Helinski, 1980).
5. They do not occur free in nature but are found in bacterial cells.

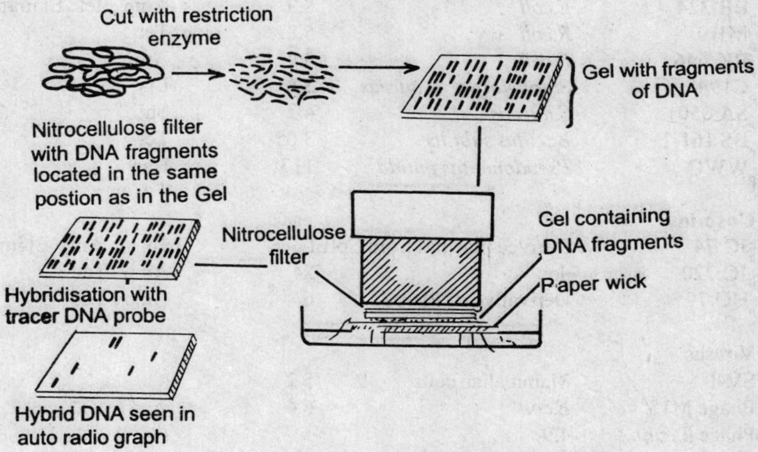

Fig. 24.5 Genetic Engineering
The Southern blotting technique

In many instances the main objective of coloning is the insertion of a particular fragment of DNA into a suitable plasmid vector and its amplification. Amplification is a process of increasing the number of plasmids in a bacterial cell. In this process, a cell containing a relaxed plasmid is treated with a drug to inhibit protein synthesis. Consequently replication stops and the relaxed plasmid (eg pBR 322) continues to replicate despite the drug treatment. Addition of chloramphenicol causes the plasmid BR 322 to increase its number to 3,000 per cell. In order to replicate and clone a piece of foreign DNA, it is necessary to possess a sequence of nucleotides which is recognised by the host bacterium as origin of replication. The origin of replication occurs naturally in plasmids. In naturally occurring plasmids due to exchange of genetic information between plasmids and bacterial chromosome new genes originate in the plasmids.

Therefore plasmids have been artifically developed with specific sequence of genes so that they would integrate foreign DNA without any problem.

Some cloning vectors

Cloning vectors	Natural occurrence	Size (Kb)*	Selective marker**
Plasmids			
pACYC 177	*E.coli*	3.7	Amp^r, Kan^r
pBR 322	*E.coli*	4.0	Amp^r, Tet^r
pBR 324	*E.coli*	8.3	Amp^r,, tet^r. El imm
pMB9	*R.coli*	5.8	Tet^r
pRK 646	*E.coli*	3.4	Amp^r
pC194	*Staphylococcus aureus*	3.6	Ery$_r$
pSA 0501	*S.aureus*	4.2	Str^r
pBS 161-1	*Bacillus subtilis*	3.65	Tet^r
pWWO	*Pseudomonas putida*	117	Kan^r
Cosmids			
pJC 74	Derived plasmid from ColEL		16 Amp^r El imm
pJC 720	do	24	Amp^r, Tet^r
pHC 79	Derivative of PBR 322	6	Amp^r, Tet^r
Virusus			
SV40	Mammalian cells	5.2	-
Phage M13$^+$	*E.coli*	6.4	-
Phage *E.coli*	4.9		-

* 1Kb (Kilobase pairs) = 1,000 base pairs = 0.66 mega dalton;

**. Resistance of ampicillin (Ampr), tetracycline (Tetr), erythromycine (Eryr), streptomycine

(Sttr), Kanamycin (Kanr), rifampicin (Rifr), and colicin production (EL imm).

The plasmid BR 322 is such an artifically constructed plasmid using two plasmids of *E.coli* - PBR 318 and PBR 322. This plasmid contains the origin of replication *(ori)* derived from a plasmid related to naturally occurring plasmid Col E1. As a result the BR 322 plasmid replicates at a rate faster than bacterial genome. It also possesses genes confering resistance to antibiotics such as ampicillin and tetracyclin. It also has a unique recognition site for 20 restriction enzymes. Certain restriction sites, for example Bam HI in the *tet* gene of the plasmid is present within the gene in such a way that the insertion of foreign DNA will inactivate the *tet* gene. As a result, the recombinant plasmid will allow the cells to grow only in the presence of ampicillin but will not protect them against tetracyclin. This antibiotic resistance will allow the selective isolation of cells which can be cultured on a medium supplemented with ampicillin.

In addition to the *E.coli* plasmids a plasmid of gram negative bacteria called RK2 plasmid has been developed which has a very broad host range and has a single restriction site which can be acted upon by several endonucleases.

Isolation of bacterial plasmids

The following steps are ncessary for isolating the bacterial plasmids

1. Treat the prokaryotic cells with detergents which will release plasmid DNA and chromosome from the bacterial cell along with other molecules. This mixture is known as lysate.
2. Treat the lysate with potassium acetate or acetic acid solution. This precipitates chromosomal DNA and some protein molecules.
3. Remove the precipitate from the lysate by high speed centrifugation. The supernatant contains plasmid DNA along with RNA, protein and some DNA debris of the chromosome.
4. Treat the lysate with RNAase, this will digest the RNA.
5. The lysate is treated with phenol and as a result two layers are formed - phenol layer and water layer. The water layer contains plasmid DNA and the other contaminants are found in the phenol layer.

Bacteriophages

A virus which attacks the bacteria is called a bacteriophage. A number of bacteriophages with different genetic materials have been reported so far from a variety of bacteria. Some of these phages are ϕ x 174, phages λ,.M13, Fd11, R209 etc. Phages also can be used as cloning vectors like plasmids. Of all the phages the λ phage perhaps is the one that has been used very frequently as a cloning vector. The λ phage contains a proteinaceous head and a long tail. The head portion has 50 genes in its 49 kb genome of which about half of the genes are essential. On attachment to the host (*E.coli*) the linear DNA molecule is injected into the cell. The linear double stranded molecule of DNA becomes a circle by joining through the single strand of 12 nucleotides commonly known as *cos* site. This *cos* site is a very important feature of λ DNA.

The λ phage has two kinds of life cycles - the lytic phase and the lysogenic phase in the bacterial cell. In the lytic pathway early in the infection the circular DNA replicates by a rolling circle mechanism and produces long molecules of DNA. At the same time the phage DNA directs the synthesis of proteins to produce the head. In order to pack the DNA into the head it undergoes cleavage to yield the fragments of such sizes as to fit in the head. Eventually a tail is attached to the head. In the lysogenic pathway the phage genome integrates with the bacterial genome at an attachment site (*att*) where it replicates along with the bacterial genome.

The following are the advantage of using phage as cloning vectors - 1. DNA can be packed *in vitro* into phage particles and transduced into *E.coli* with high efficiency, 2. Foreign DNA upto 25 kb in length can be inserted into phage vector, and 3. Screening and storage of recombinant DNA is easier (Dahl et al., 1981). Before using the λ phage vector it will be essential to remove the genome from the restriction sites for the enzymes commonly used for cloning. Two types of phage cloning vectors have been constructed - these are the *insertion vector* and the *replacement vector.*

Insertion vector. These have unique cleavage sites into which a relatively small piece of foreign DNA can be inserted. These fragments do not affect the functioning of the phage. The upper and lower limits of DNA that may be packed into the phage particles is between 35-53 kb. The maximum size of a foreign DNA that can be inserted is about 18kb.

Replacement vector. These vectors have cleavage sites present on either side of the length of non essential DNA. As a result of cleavage left and right arms are formed and each arm has a terminal *cos* site and a longer stiffer region (the non essential region) which can be substituted by foreign DNA. The maximum size of foreign DNA that can be inserted into this vector depends on how much the phage DNA is non essential. It has been estimated that about 25-35kb of genome can be replaced with foreign DNA segments. Example of substituted vectors are-gt, WES and λ 1059.

Cosmids

These may be defined as the hybrid vectors derived from the plasmids which contain *cos* site of λ phage. Reported for the first time by Colins and Hohn (1975) cosmids lack genes for encoding viral proteins. Therefore neither viral particles are formed in the host cell nor cell lysis occurs. Special features of cosmids similar to plasmids are origin of replication, a marker gene coding for antibiotic resistance, a special cleavage site for the insertion of foreign DNA and the small cells. Characters of cosmids dissimilar to plasmids are presence of extraphage DNA, and the *cos* site.

Phasmids

When plasmids are inserted into the genome of λ phage they are said to be phasmids. The process of insertion of the plasmid DNA into the phage genome occurs in the same way as a phage genome is inserted into the bacterial chromosome. Insertion of plasmid into λ phage is done with a view to have a specific site responsible for recombinational insertion of the phage into bacterial chromosome.

Phasmids may be used in many ways. They can be used as a phage cloning vector from which a recombinant vector may be released.

CLONING ORGANISMS

The vectors that are chosen as vehicles to carry the foreign DNA must be cloned in an organism that multiplies rapidly thereby producing the gene product in a large quantity. Such organisms into which the vectors are inserted for the purpose of gene expression are known as cloning organisms. A number of microorganisms have been used for the purpose of cloning. The most important among them are the various strains of the colon bacterium *E.coli.* The strains of *E.coli* used as cloning organisms are HB101, h303 and RR1. The cloning organisms should normally be deficient in DNA recombination as it will reduce undesirable hybridization of DNA. Another essential feature of the cloning organism is it should lack restriction enzymes that might degrade foreign DNA. Strains of bacteria that can bud off mini cells are highly useful if the gene expression is the purpose of experiment (mini cells are those which contain all the elements of gene expression except chromosome).

For a long time *E.coli* has been the most favourite cloning organism in recombinant DNA studies. Of late yeasts are also being used as cloning vehicles and they have some advantages over bacteria. They do not live in human beings and are non pathogenic. Fink et al (1974) for the first time introduced a bacterial gene for the production of leucine into baker's yeast. A snail enzyme was used to induce the yeast to take up bacterial DNA.

Techniques used for identification of clones

Several techniques are employed to identify the isolated clones using a specific molecular probe. Some of these techniques are described below :

1. Polyacrylamide gel electrophoresis

When the genomic DNA extracted from a particular source is digested by a specific restriction enzyme it is broken into several fragments. These fragments of different sizes can be separated through a technique called gel electrophoresis. This separation is necessary to identify a specific gene that is required for use. After these are separated a specific molecular probe can be used to detect the segments which have sequences similar to those in the probe. For instance if a gene with a specific nucleotide sequence is required to be separated from a mixture a probe is prepared with nucleotide sequence complementary to the gene. These (molecular probes) are then allowed to hybridize and the particular gene to be identified.

In gel electrophoresis the DNA molecules migrate from one end of the gel to the other. The gel is usually a cylindrical structure or occasionally even may be a slab. The rate of movement of fragments of DNA on the gel is inversely proportional to the size of the molecules. Heavier fragments will remain at the beginning while lighter fragments will move away. Fragments of different sizes appear as discrete bands on the gel and can be isolated for further study.

Separation of DNA molecules using PFGE (pulsed field gel electrophoresis)

Gel electrophoresis is suitable for only small fragments of DNA which can easily get separated. Large size molecules of DNA however cannot be separated using this technique. A new technique called PFGE is used for the separation of large sized DNA fragments, some times representing even whole chromosomes. Using the PFGE technique separation of DNA molecules belonging to each of the sixteen chromosomes of yeast has been made possible. In this technique short pulses of electric current are used in two different directions and the DNA is embedded in Agarose plugs to avoid fragmentation. Using this technique genomes of several fungi have been resolved into chromosomal bands.

Blotting techniques

Gel electrophoresis helps in the separation of fragments of DNA or RNA. The separated bands can be stained and absorbed on the gel. This technique however will only help in the separation of fragments of DNA but will not tell as to which fragment contains the desired gene. For this purpose a molecular probe (which is a DNA fragment) consisting of nucleotides complimentary to the gene are used for hybridization and the required gene is identified. For easy identification and detection, the probe is radioactively labelled. To facilitate hybridization the bands of the genome are usually transferred to a nitrocellulose membrane in a technique called blotting. Blotting technique was first invented by E.M. Southern and is known as the Southern blotting technique. Two other blotting techniques discovered subsequently are named Northern blotting technique and Western blotting technique. These are described briefly below.

Southern blotting technique. The DNA sample is first cleaved with a restriction enzyme and the sample is loaded on to gel electrophoresis for separation. The DNA bands that appear in the gel are denatured into single strands using an alkali solution. Later the gel is laid on top of a buffer saturated filter paper placed on a glass plate with its two edges immerged in the buffer. A sheet of nitrocellulose membrane is placed on top of the gel and a stack of many paper towels along with a weight are placed on this membrane (see figure). The buffer solution is drawn up by the filter paper folds and passes through the gel and to the nitrocellulose membrane. Finally buffer moves up to the paper towels. While passing through the gel the buffer carries with it the fragments of single stranded DNA and binds them on to the nitrocellulose membrane as it passes through it (membrane) to the paper towels above. For the complete migration of the buffer it may take a few hours. Subsequently the paper towels are discarded, the nitrocellulose membrane with the single stranded fragments of DNA attached to it in different positions is baked at 80°C to fix the strands permanently on it. This membrane now has the fragments of single stranded DNA fixed on to it in the same position in which they were on the gel. In otherwords the nitrocellulose membrane is the replica of the gel with its attached DNA fragments. The nitrocellulose membrane is now dipped in a solution containing labelled gene that is present on the membrane. The radio labelled probe hybridizes with the complimentary fragment of DNA on the membrane. The filter subsequently is removed from the solution and washed thoroughly to remove any unbound fragments of DNA. Later the filter is placed against a photographic film. Wherever the probe has hybridized with the DNA fragments there will be markings like black dots. This can now be compared with the original gel and the corresponding DNA band can be identified as the required gene.

Northern blotting technique. This is used to identify the required RNA bands. The technique of southern blotting used for DNA transfer from the gel to the nitrocellulose membrane could not be used for transfer of RNA because RNA would not bind with the nitrocellulose membrane. Alwin *et al* (1979) devised a technique in which the mRNA bands from the gel were blot transfered to a chemically reactive paper prepared by diazotization of aminobenzyloxymethyl paper. RNA fragments can bind themselves on to this paper and the paper can be used for hybridization with radiolabelled DNA probes. Subsequently by autoradiography the hybridized bands can be identified. Some of the researches of Thomas (1980) however have shown that mRNA bands can also be blotted directly on to nitrocellulose membrane using special techniques.

Western blotting technique. This technique is used to detect proteins of a particular speciality. Discovered by Towbin *et al* (1979) in this technique newly coded proteins by a transformed cell can be identified. In this method however nucleic acid probes are not used. This technique involves the following steps:

(a) Electrophoretic separation of the required protein on a polyacrylamide gel

(b) Transfering of the separated peptide chains on to a nitrocellulose membrane

(c) Using radiolabelled antibodies as probes the required peptide chain may be hybridized. (The probe consists of antibodies which bind to the antigenic protein)

(d) Autoradiographic identification of the required hybridized protein

CONSTRUCTION OF CHEMERIC DNA (insertion of DNA into vector)

Chimeric DNA molecules are produced by the insertion of a foreign DNA segment into a DNA molecule of the vector. These chimeric DNA molecules are the means of the cloning genes or other small DNA sequences. Basically production of chimeric DNA molecules involves breaking open the vector DNA and insertion of foreign DNA followed by joining of the ends. There are three techniques available for the construction of chimeric DNA. These are - pallindromic sequences (cohesive ends) and staggered cleavage. dAdT tailing and blunt end ligation.

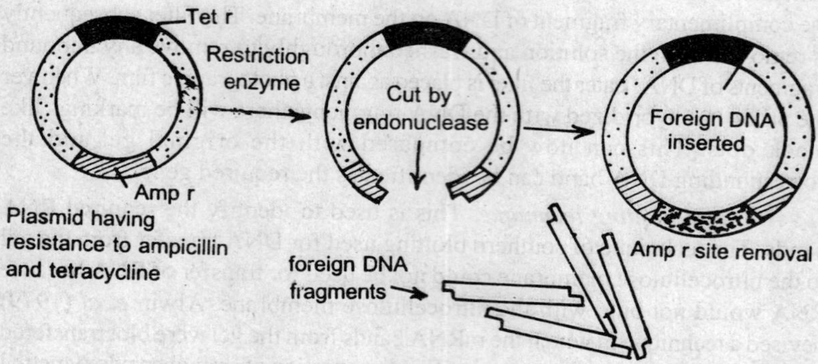

Fig. 24.6 Genetic Engineering
The concept of cloning of foreign DNA in a vector

1. Pallindromes and staggered cleavage (cohesive ends). It has already been explained that a pallindromic sequence has complimentary sequences at the two ends of a single strand. Restriction enzymes cutting the pallindromic sequences may have an even cut or a staggered cut. Result of the staggered cut is DNA fragments with sticky ends are formed. When another DNA molecule (a foreign DNA molecule) is cut similarly and when the two DNAs are mixed both DNAs will combine forming a chimeric DNA

Discovered for the first time by Boyer and Cohen, this mechanism has an advantage of easily combining two different DNA molecules. Further it also produces two restriction sites in the chimeric DNA. There are some disadvantages in this method. For instance, the two sticky ends of a vector DNA or of a foreign DNA may themselves join without allowing for the insertion of one into the other.

dA - dT tailing (the terminal transferase method)

In this method DNA can be cut at the desired position both in the vector and in the clone without staggered cleavage. Using the precursor dATP polydA is added at both the 3' cut ends of the vector with the help of the enzyme terminal transferase. Similarly using the precursor dTTP poly dT is added at both the 3' cut ends of the DNA sequence to be cloned. The vector and clone can then be joined by anniealing the polydA with polydT tails and then lygating them using the DNA lygase enzyme. In this technique there is no possibility of the two cut ends of the same DNA molecule joining together because they have same nucleotides. There is one disadvantage in this technique because it will not be easy to retrive the cloned DNA as the recognition site of the enzyme is lost due to the addition of poly dA and poly dT. It has been found out that use of poly dG and poly dC will help in the restoration of the recognition site.

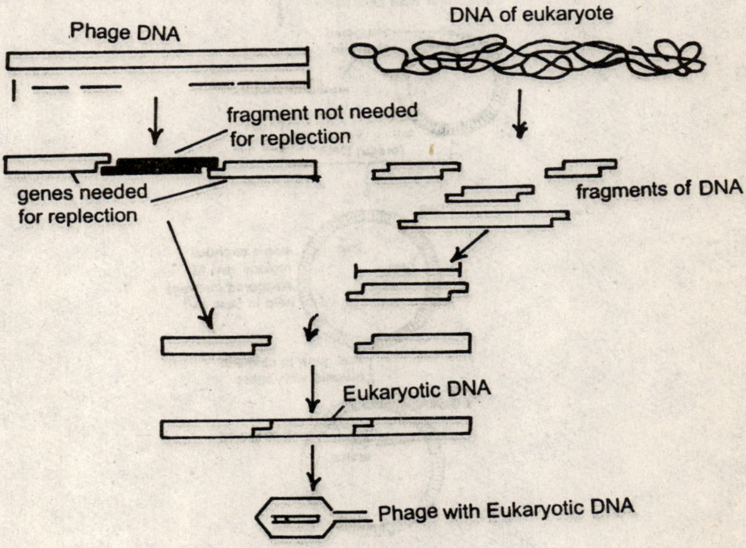

Fig. 24.7 Genetic Engineering
Use of λ phage for cloning

Blunt end ligation

In this technique a restriction enzymes is used to cut a duplex DNA at the same site in both the strands. The broken ends are then used for joining with the two ends of foreign DNA molecule irrespective of the sequences present at the broken ends of the two molecules. The blunt end ligaton is made possible by the use of the T4 DNA lygase. This technique also has a disadvantage in that the broken ends of the same DNA molecule may join together.

Construction of genomic and cDNA libraries

In order to isolate required gene or genes from a genome a mixture of clones each carrying DNA fragments derived either from the natural genome or from cDNA is prepared. This mixture contains thousands of clones and is collectively called genomic library. Similarly when cDNA clones are collected it is known as cDNA library.

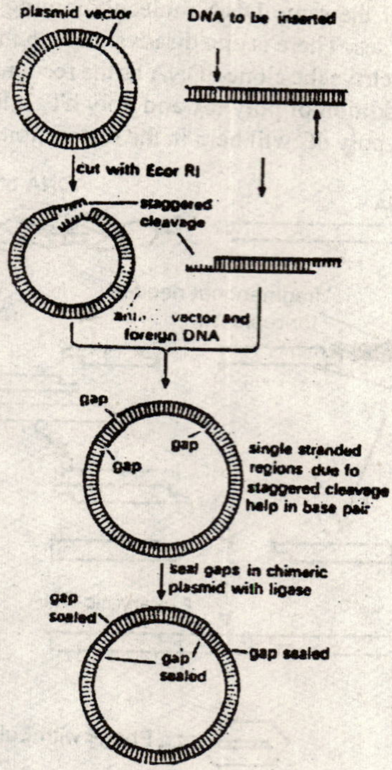

Fig. 24.8 Genetic Engineering
Cloning of a segment of DNA by staggered cleavage

Construction of genomic library

Cloning an entire genome in the form of fragments mixed randomly is known as genomic library. This may be done by a method known as shotgun method (see earlier in the same chapter for details). With a genome library clones can be perpetuated indefinetely in a plasmid vector and retrived when ever necessary.

Genomic libraries can also be prepared by using a number of restriction endonucleases one at a time so that one will have fragments of different sizes with cuts at different places. This has a disadvantage in that many a time the inciscion site many be within a gene so that complete genes may be difficult to obtain. This may be overcome by using restriction enzymes which have very short recognition sequences so that the fragments that are obtained will be long and the chances of splicing within a gene are avoided.

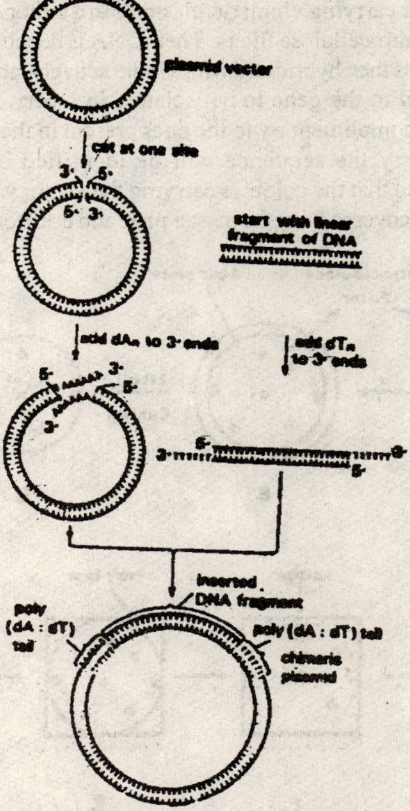

Fig. 24.9 Genetic Engineering
Cloning of DNA segment by dA-dT tailing

cDNA library

It has already been explained above as to how to obtain a cDNA using its complimentary mRNA under the influence of the enzyme reverse transcriptase. When once a cDNA molecule is obtained it can be made double stranded by the use of DNA polymerase. A collection of such cDNA molecules will constitute cDNA library.

Screening of the library

When a genomic or cDNA library is available it can be used for the isolation of a specific gene sequence. For this the DNA library has to be screened. This is done with the hlep of a technique known as Colony hybridization. In this technique bacteria carrying chimeric plasmids are cultured into colonies and are then lysed on nitrocellulose filters. Their DNA is denatured *in situ* and fixed on the filter which is then hybridized with a radio actively labelled probe carrying a sequence related to the gene to be isolated. In otherwords, the probe will have nucleotides complimentary to the ones present in the gene to be isolated. Colonies that carry the sequence will be identified by dark spots after radioautography so that the colonies carrying the vector with the desired gene sequence can be recovered from the master plate and used for further experiment.

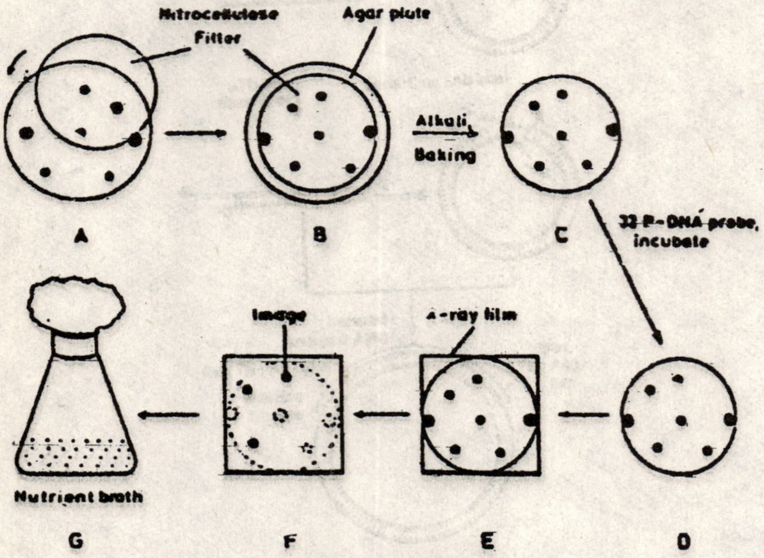

Fig. 24.10 Genetic Engineering
Colony hybridization technique

Transfer of the recombinant DNA into a cloning organism

When once a mixture of recombinant DNA is obtained it has to be transfered to a suitable cloning organism for the purpose of expression. Several techniques are used to transfer the recombinant DNA into suitable cloning cells. Transforming the cloning cells with recombinant DNA is a difficult process as the cells of bacteria *(E.coli)* have restriction enzymes which will immediately degrade the foreign DNA. To escape from degradation exponentially growing culture of *E.coli* is pretreated with $CaCl_2$ at low temperature and thereafter the DNA is mixed up. This treatment is known to sufficiently prevent the action of restriction enzymes. When the recombinant plasmids get established in the cells of *E.coli* the cells are said to be transformed.

Instead of plasmids even λ phages could be used as transforming elements. The entry of the phage into *E.coli* is usually termed transfection (a combination of transfermation and infermation).

Not all the cells will accept recombinant DNA and get transformed. It has been estimated that about 10^5 transformats per microgram of cloned circular plasmid can be generated. The cells which have been transformed will grow into colonies along with other non transformed ones. Colonies with transformed cells can be identified with suitable techniques.

Expression of cloned DNA

The purpose of genetic engineering is not just to separate and clone the genes in a suitable organism. Isolation and multiplication of genes is only a means ultimately to obtain the gene product namely the required protein. Hence the recombinant DNA molecules should be allowed to express in the new environment (*E.coli* cells) and produce what ever protein they were producing. For instance if an insulin gene from human beings is transfered into *E.coli* the gene should be able to produce insulin molecules using the protein synthesizing machinery of the bacterium. Expression of a cloned gene is a verydifficult process. This is more so when a eukaryotic gene is inserted into a prokaryotic organism. As the protein synthesizing genetic machinery of prokaryote is different from eukaryotes, the eukaryotic gene should be provided with the necessary ingredients of a prokaryote to produce the protein. The factors that are necessary for eukaryotic gene to express in the prokaryotic environment are as follows :

(i) Supply of prokaryotic promoter necessary for expression of eukaryotic gene

(ii) Supply of ribosomal binding sites for the cloning vector

(iii) Removal of introns from mRNA obtained from the eukaryotic genes

(iv) Inhibition of bacterial gene responsible for degradation of the protein produced by the eukaryotic gene.

Recovery of the gene product

This is the final step in genetic engineering techniques. After all the hurdles are passed and the eukaryotic gene has successfully expressed itself in the prokaryotic cell, the required product namely the eukaryotic protein is produced. This can be identified by antigen antibody reaction (for details see genetically engineered insulin later in the same chapter). The protein produced can be purified by standard chemical processes.

APPLICATIONS OF GENETIC ENGINEERING

Scope of genetic engineering (Biotechnology)

The possibilities are immense and sky seems to be the limit for future biotechnologists. The following are some of the applications of genetic engineering.

I. Gene therapy

A new branch of curative medicine is opened up due to genetic engineering. Many genetic disorders like hemophilia, alkaptoneuria, galactosemia etc., which are due to defective genes can be cured by replacing them (defective genes) with correct genes. Plasmid or virus mediated genes may be incorporated into human systems.

II. Cheap production of drugss

Many of the drugs like vitamins, antibiotics, hormones are now being produced chemically or produced from higher organisms which is a slow and costly process. If the genes for the production of these are introduced into rapidly multiplying bacterial cells, we have virtually myriads of tiny living factories turning out the medicines at a fraction of their original production cost.

III. Gene for new diet

Some of the plants or plant products are presently non edible for want of enzymes in the human system to digest them. For ex wood, grass, etc. If the genes that code for the digestive enzymes (for materials like wood etc) could be introduced into the human system, wherein there would virtually be no famine on earth. Another possibility, (which sounds unbelivable at present) could be to introduce genes that can produce the chlorophyll pigment in the animal or human system, wherein we would be solving the food problem once for all !.

IV. Role of genetic engineering in Agriculture

The following are some of the advantages of gene recombination in crop improvement.

(a) Production of new varieties

New varieties of plants that are not present in nature can be produced by the introduction of new genes.

(b) Somatic hybridization

Two crop plants with important characters, which could not be hybridized sexually due to genome incompatibility can be hybridized through protoplast fusion. Production of *Pomato* (Tomato x Potato) is one such example.

(c) Increasing photosynthetic efficiency

Ribulose diphosphate carboxylase (Rubisco) is a key enzyme in the dark fixation of CO_2. Modification of *Rubisco* to reduce photorespiration (Osmond 1981) by elimination of oxygenase activity would increase-the CO_2 fixation rate. The enzyme has two sub units and is known to be coded by seven genes. If these genes could be altered, resulting in the changed *Rubisco,* it will increase the photosynthetic efficiency.

(d) Nitrogen fixation

The roots of leguminous plants normally possess nitrogen fixing nodules, induced by various strains of *Rhizobium*.m As a result, leguminous plants require little or no nitrogen fertilizer. Arable crops require about 100 kg of nitrogen per hectare. If this can be replaced by N_2 fixing genes, it would lead to a lot of saving in terms of fertilizer cost. Nitrogen fixation is catalyzed by the ATP dependent electron reduction of dinitrogen to ammonia by nitrogenase. If it is possible to introduce the gene to higher plants, it would bring about a revolution in agriculture. This may be achieeved by one of the following ways.

1. Transfer of nitrogen fixing gene (*nif*) from the living bacteria like *Klebsiella, Azatobacter* etc., to higher plants. This would enable the plants to fix the N_2 directly. This is still in the experimental stage, as the *nitrogenase,* produced by the *nif* gene is highly oxygen liabile and gets degraded in higher organisms.
2. Expansion of host range of symbiosis to crops other than legumes. At present non leguminous plants do not have symbiosis with *Rhizobium.* If it is possible to expand the host range for the bacteria, a lot more plants will have the capacity of N_2 fixation.
3. Increasing the efficiency of symbiotic bacteria to N_2 fixation. By gene manipulation, it may be possible to increase the N_2 fixing capacity of the symbiotic bacteria, which will benefit the plants.

(e) Herbicide resistance, disease resistance etc

By gene manipulation, it will be possible to introduce this character into plants.

In conclusion it may be said, that genetic engineering is a highly potential tool by which man can alter the macromolecule of inheritance and thereby change the biological environment to his choice. But the new technique has to be used judiciously, otherwise it can also create untold harm to human society, if unscrupulous scientists use it to create destructive genes.

A few of the specific applications of genetic engineering are discussed below in some detail.

Nitrogen fixing genes (*nif* genes)

Nodule formation and nitrogen fixation are two of the important biological processes which are genetically controlled in diazotrophic bacteria. From the genome of *Rhizobium,* several genes coding for nodulation (*nod* genes) and nitrogen fixation (*nif* genes) have been identified and isolated. In free living and symbiotic nitrogen fixers, nodule forming and non-nodule forming *nif* genes are present either on the genome or on the plasmids in their cells.

Nod genes

Nodule formign species of *Rhizobium* contain in their cells an extremely large plasmid called *mega plasmid* which consists of a number of *nod* genes and *nif* genes (Rosenberg et al 1981). Bot the genes are closely located.

Kondorosi *et al* (1982) were able to transfer the megaplasmids from one species of *Rhizobium* to other simultaneously transfering the ability of nodule formation.

The nod gene region is of 8.5 kb in nucleotide sequence length and proteins encoded by the 8.5 kb fragment when transfered to *E.coli* has been determined. The *nod* gene is a cluster made up of 4 genes designated as *nod a, b, c* and *d.* A comparison of *nod* genes between different species of *Rhibozium* shows that about 70% of the nucleotides are homologous.

Nif genes

The *nif* genes are present in several species of *Rhibozium* and are located on a megaplasmid adjacent to the *nod* genes. *Nif* genes have also been identified in many cyanobacteria such as *Anabena,* where the *nif* genes are located on the main genome.

Early studies on *nif* genes were carried out in *Klebsiella pneumoniae* and the function of these genes was confirmed by transfering into *E.coli* cells. Researches have also been conducted to identify the product of *nif* gene cluster. The *nif* gene cluster consists of 7 operons.

In cyanobacteria *nif* genes have been located both in vegetative cells as well as in heterocysts. But there is some difference in the nature of the *nif* gene between the vegetative cells and the heterocysts.

Cloning of *nif* genes

Researches are being conducted in many countries to transfer the *nif* genes to higher plants especially to monocots. If this is successful it will be indeed a great boon to agriculture as there will be plenty of saving in nitrogen fertilizers for the plants themselves will be able to fix atmospheric nitrogen. Gene expression of *nif* genes in eukaryotic cells is very difficult because the nitrogenase enzyme required for fixing the nitrogen and controlled by the *nif* gene would get denatured in the preence of oxygen. If this can be overcome *nif* genes can be easily transfered to eukaryotes. *Nif* genes however have been cloned in *E.coli*. One of the methods of transfering *nif* genes is to transfer them into the chloroplast of eukaryotic cells as the translational and transcriptional processes of chloroplasts resemble prokaryotic features. These attempts might succeed because the chloroplasts are able to produce the ATP and reducing power both of which are required for nitrogen fixation (Merrick and Dixon, 1984). But there are major problems for such a transfer of *nif* gene to chloroplasts. These are

1. Lack of chloroplast transfering technique
2. Protection of nitrogenase from oxygen evolved during photosynthesis.

Genetically engineered Insulin

Insulin is an important hormone that plays a vital role in the metabolism of carbohydrates. In patients suffering from diabetes, insulin has to be injected subcutaneously to regulate the blood sugar level. Insulin producing genes can be transfered to bacteria by techniques of genetic engineering and large quantities of insulin may be extracted. This process is cheapter and convenient than the conventional one. We will briefly discuss below the method of procuring insulin by genetic engineering techniques.

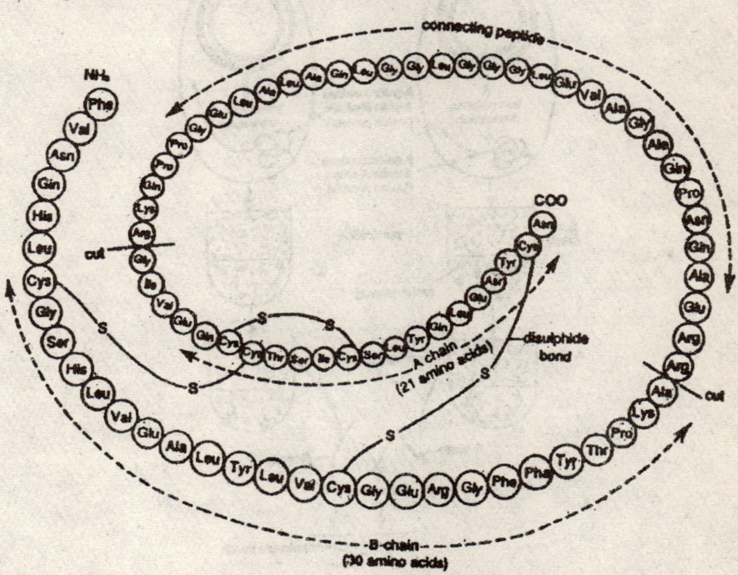

Fig. 24.11 Genetic Engineering
Structure of Insulin molecule

Structure of human insulin

Insulin molecule is composed of two chains - α and β chains of aminoacids. Initially it is produced as a single long chain called *Pre-proinsulin* which is later cut into a shorter chain called *proinsulin* (composed of 84 aminoacid units). Proinsulin then breaks into α and β chains when a piece from the middle is cut off. Chain α is composed of 21 aminoacids and chain β has 30 amino acids - The remaining 33 aminoacids act as a connecting peptide chain.

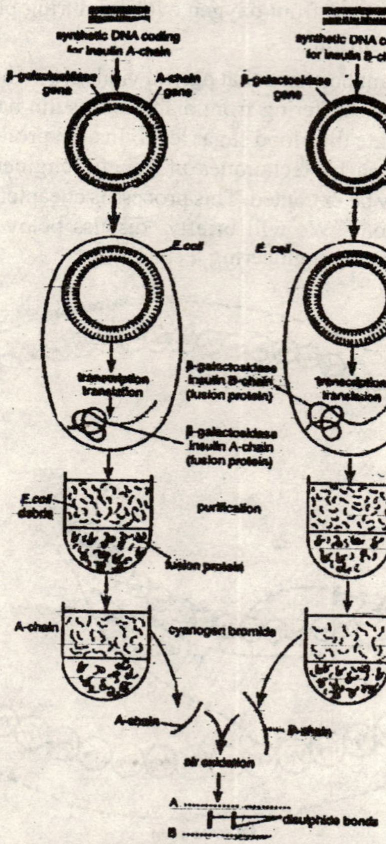

Fig. 24.12 Genetic Engineering
Technique of producing genetically engineered insulin in E.coli

Production of Insulin in *E.coli*

The genes for insulin chain α and β are identified and located. This may be done first by identifying the codons and then the corresponding mRNAs can be reconstructed. Using these mRNA molecules and with the help of the enzyme *reverse transcriptase* the corresponding segmentas of double stranded DNA molecules are produced. Then with the help of the enzyme *terminal transferase,* the ends of the insulin genes (DNA strands) are extended with short sequence of identical bases.

Plasmids obtained from *E.coli* are opened up at specific portions by the use of restriction enzyme. The insulin genes (DNA strands) of α and β chains are added to the plasmids separately forming recombinant DNA plasmids. Gaps if any in the circular plasmids of α and β chains are filled by lac operon gene for switching on the synthetic process. The plasmids with recombinant DNA for α and β chains are inserted into *E.coli* finally.

The recombinant DNA plasmids multiply in *E.coli* and trigger the synthesis of α and β chains of insulin as a genetic expression. Following large scale production cultures, the insulin chains are obtained following specific purification processes. Finally the α and β chains are chemically bonded by disulphide bonds to produce the complete molecule of insulin.

Gilbert and Villakomaroff (1980) isolated mRNA for insulin from β cells of the pancrease of rat and inserted it into PBR 322 plasmid in the middle of a gene normally coding for the enzyme penicillinase and incorporated it into the cloning organism (*E.coli*) *E.coli* cells produced the hybrid protein consisting of penicillinase + proinsulin. Proinsulin was then separated from penicillinase.

Immunological tests to identify insulin producing colonies

On a culture medium there will be colonies which are transformed as well as non transformed. In otherwords colonies with a recombinant DNA and those without recombinant DNA will be there. Colonies with recombinant DNA and successfully expressing the gene will produce the insulin protein. These colonies have to be identified so that they can be picked up for further multiplication. This is done by two immunological techniques - radioactive antibody test and immunoprecipitation test.

Radio active antibody test

In this test a plastic disk to which antibodies of the gene product (insulin) are bound is pressed on to the colonies. If the protein (insulin) is present in any colony it will bind to the antibody and to the disk. The disk is then placed in a solution containing radio active antibody (to insulin). If any required proteins (insulin) are present on the disk the radioactive antibody sticks to the proteins on to the disk. The disk is then washed and the autoradiograph will identify colonies if any producing insulin.

Immunoprecipitation test

This test is also used to identify a protein (insulin) producing colony. In this technique insulin antibodies are added to the agar medium. When the bacterial colonies grow if any of the colonies contain insulin it gets percipitated surrounding the colonies due to the action of the antibodies.

Human insulin humulin produced by the genetic engineering technique was made available to Diabetic patients in September 1982. It was the first therapeutic product to be produced by genetic engineering.

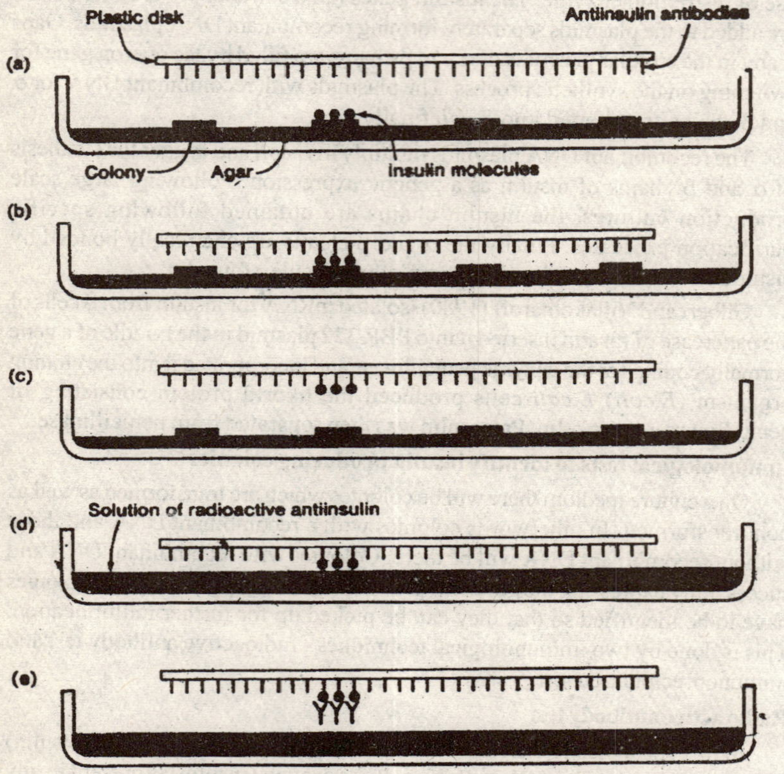

Fig. 24.13 Genetic Engineering
Radioactive antibody test

Human growth hormone (HGH)

Also known as Somatotrophin, this hormone is secreted by the anterior part of the pituitary and is made up of 190 aminoacid residues. The deficiency of this hormones results in dwarffism. For the conventional treatment of dwarfism

HGH is injected into the patients. But the extraction of hormone from the pituitary glands cannot meet the ever increasing demand for this hormone. Genetic engineering procedures have successfully produced somatotrophin.

Double stranded cDNAs were obtained from the mRNA precursors of HGH and then incorporated into bacterial cells where they expressed in non precursor form. The bacteria were unable to convert the peptides of HGH into biological active forms. A recombinant plasmid containing a full length of HGH cDNA is cleaved with restriction enzymes that release fragments containing the complete HGH coding sequence after codon 24. Several overlapping complimentary oligo nucleotides were joined to form a synthetic strand of a small DNA fragment which contains the coding sequence for the first 24 aminoacids of mature HGH. The synthetic DNA and cDNA molecules are joined together to produce a new fragment which has the complete coding sequence of HGH. This is then ligated to a restriction site a little below the *lac* promoter operator gene cloned on a plasmid. These plasmids are cloned in *E.coli*. Synthesis of HGH is induced by an inducer (IPTG) of *lac* operon. The HGH thus obtained is later purified by chemical methods.

About 1 lakh molecules of the hormone per cell of *E.coli* have been produced by genetic engineering techniques. One of the problems in this is the attachment of an extra methionine to the molecule. This has to be removed to make the molecule biologicaly active.

Vaccine for Rabies virus (RV)

Hydrophobia caused by made dog bite used to take a heavy toll of the human life. The credit of discovering a method to cure hydrophobia or rabies goes to Louis Pasteur. Even now however ignorance and not taking the vaccine in time, is causing a number of death of humans and animals in many Asian and African countries. The conventional antivirus vaccine is difficult to obtain and also a tedious process. Researches are being conducted to produce genetically engineered rabies vaccine using *E.coli*. Attempts are made to isolate the mRNA coding for the viral protein from the RV infected cells. The genes coding for the production of a virus glycoprotein coat has been successfully transfered to the cell of *E.coli*. This seems to the first step in the production of antirabies vaccine because this glycoprotein stimulates the production of antibodies in affected individuals. The Eister Institute in Philadelphia USA has developed a new genetically engineered vaccinia virus by inserting a small fragment of foreign DNA. This genetically engineered virus could synthesise antirabies vaccine. The virus however does not cause rabies in those animals receiving the rabies genome but instead activates the immune system against infection. The vaccine has been certified that it can be administered orally to animals.

BIOHAZARDS OF GENETIC ENGINEERING

Recombinant DNA technology popularly called genetic engineering is one of the most potent tools in the arsenal of human knowledge that can be used either for good or for bad. Ever since human civilisation evolved, two developments in the field of science have had the effect of changing the human destiny. One development that took place in the field of physical sciences is that of atomic fission which gave the man a vast amount of energy which when produced can be used for improvement or for destruction. A development similar to this or much more potent than this has taken place in the biological sciences in the form of recombinant DNA technology. With the power and ability to synthesise the gene, to order the alignment of gene and to regulate its expression man indeed has been handed over the very basis of origin and differentiation of life. With this enormously potential tool he can create different types of organisms, vastly modify the existing organisms for his betterment or he can create organisms which are more harmful than the existing ones and can even spell the deathknell of the very nature which has created him.

The brief discussion above will clearly point out to the fact that research in genetic engineering has to be carefully controlled, manipulated and should be encouraged only when it is absolutely necessary and that too with plenty of safeguards. In the paragraphs below we will briefly outline the biohazards of uncontrolled genetic engineering research and what safeguards have to be followed while following the techniques of recombinant DNA.

Harmful aspects

Genetic engineering involves introducing a foreign DNA into another organism so that it gets transformed. Many a time when a gene segment is transfered one may be aware of its expression in the original organism. But one is not too sure as to what kind of expression it may have in the new environment i.e., in the new organism. This kind of recombination many a time creates a dangerous new form either deliberately or accidentally. A harmless microorganism might turn out to be a very harmful one after it acquires new genes from another organism. Eventhough it is true that the genes introduced by themselves may not be harmful in their original combination, but when they are introduced into a new set up they might bring about the potentially dangerous expression. If by chance a transformed organism comes to carry a deadly disease due to genetic manipulation and if that organism escapes out of laboratory one can imagine the uncontrolled horror that the organism might bring about. The genetically manipulated organism might be so potent in its pathogenicity that any of the existing drugs may not be able to combat it. For instance *Streptococcus* a pathogenic organism was never resistant to penicilin originally in nature. For the purpose of genetic engineering research a plasmid with a desired gene is introduced into *Streptococcus* and at the same time to identify the transformed organisms a marker gene such as penicillin resistant gene is itnroduced, when the organism becomes penicillin resistant, the antibiotic now would be useless. If such an organism even though created in the laboratory were to escape one can imagine the dangers caused by it.

Escape of transformed microbes into environment

Inspite of precautions being taken their always exists a possibility that a recombnant orgnanism might escape from laboratory and get permanently entrenched in the ecological system. If the organism in question were to be a parasite it would cause immense havoc to allthose organisms it parasitizes. Microorganisms that live in special ecological niche like hot spring or salt water might not pose such a great problem as they cannot spread widely.

The escape of microorganisms from the laboratory may be by design or by accident. If it is by design then one has to understand that microbes are allowed to escape deliberately to cause harm to the environment outside. Accidental escape of chimeric microbes from the experimental laboratories may take any one of the following routes.

(1) Laboratory personnel such as scientists, attendants, visitors, sweepers etc might inadvertentaly carry the microbes and spread them outside.

(2) Microbes might also find their way out through laboratory facilities such as glassware, drainage of chemicals, spillage of media and such other inanimate objects.

In addition ot the above, non scientific personnel in the laboratory many a time may not be aware of the stringent precautions that have to be mandatorily taken while dealing with pathogenic microbes. Many a time even if they are aware they might just not follow the precautions as they are quite tedious and cumbersome. Laboratory personnel while constantly dealing with pathogenic microbes many a time might acquire immunity and may not suffer from the consequences of contact with pathogens but they act as carriers and others who come in contact with them will have to suffer the consequences.

Unintended escape of microbes and possible creation of new microbes posses perhaps the greatest danger to the environment. In this context it is worthwhile mentioning the opinion of three international experts on AIDS - Dr.John Seale from London. Dr.Robert Strecker from California and Dr.Jacob Segal from Berlin. These scientists claimed in 1987 that the AIDS virus was artificially created by American scientists during laboratory experiments when they were trying to discover a cure for cancer by combining parts of Maedy - visna virus found in the sheep and human T-cell Leukaemia virus type 1. They argued that the scientists or other personnel in the laboratory could have been infected with the new virus through a minute cut or even by inhaling (Ignacimuthu, 1995).

Plus and Minus points of genetic engineering research

A great controversy is going on currently in the International Community involving biologists, social scientists, politicians and religious people regarding the desirability or otherwise of conducting genetic engineering research. While many people argue that genetic engineering research would be a harbinger of prosperity others are equally vehement in opposing that research in genetic engineering would cause untold harm to human life as it is trying to tinker with the very basis of life and evolutionary process. The arguments for and against recombinant DNA technology are summarised below.

Arguments favouring genetic engineering research

1. The transfer of genetic material from eukaryotes to prokaryotes and *vice versa* have been going on even in nature perhaps on a very small scale. If nature were to intend to prevent the transfer of a genetic material, evolution would have surely brought in a perfect genetic barrier preventing such a transfer. In fact ever since the origin of life evolution could proceed only because nature took to genetic engineering.
2. The dangers of genetic engineering research perhaps will receed with time as people and scientists become experienced and accumulate knowledge.
3. Enough safe guards are already available in research laboratories dealing with pathogenic organisms. They can be made much more stringent. In any case the beneficial aspects of combating the disease perhaps far more outweigh the possible dangers.
4. Genetically transformed microbes have been designed with a special purpose. Hence the argument that they would compete with the other normal microbes and perhaps might be picked by natural selection appears to be imaginary. Further with attenuated characters the transformed organisms will not be able to survive unless special conditions such as the laboratory environment are provided with.
5. The idea that by accuring a new gene the microorganisms become parhogenic is not true because in any genetic transformation the host organism will always reject a virulent gene combination and the unwanted genes are generally lysed by restriction enzymes and even if the genes express themselves the gene product namely the foreign protein gets degraded by proteolytic enzymes.
6. All types of genetic engineering research need not be dubbed as harmful and dangerous. For instance research in the field of agriculture, dairy and others will not pose any problem. Researches in the medical field however can be continued with stringent regulations and control. At the same time however one cannot simply push aside the vast benefits that have accrued

to man kind because of improved health care products from genetic engineering. Hence total stoppage of genetic engineering research would weaken the ability of man to understand and control nature and ultimately it is not in the interest of man himself.

Arguments against genetic engineering research

1. Unintended or accidental escape of microbes from the laboratory is possible through many routes. This escape of the transformed organism into the environment will pose great danger.
2. Genetic engineering research actually tinkers with the very basis of the evolutionary process. Nature indeed has been a very efficient genetic engineer and it has been doing this work very slowly and steadily over a period of millions of years. Transfer of genetic material and production of new traits in nature takes millions of years to be achieved. If this is sought to be achieved in a very short period it amounts to short circuiting the normal process and the consequences could be really hazardous. When an individual is fashioned out of natural process it will be a package of both weakness and strength. If we were to tinker with this process it would naturally disturb the fine tuned balance and relationship that is existing between the organisms since millions of years.
3. The intended benefits of genetic engineering research can be actually achieved through other research methodologies. To achieve these goals one need not resort to such dangerous techniques lke genetic engineering. The benefit of genetic engineering research does not justify the cost (not just in terms of money) involved.
4. With the kind of diverse political set up prevailing in different countries of the world where dictators, fundamentalists etc still have a very powerful say, this technique can definitely be misused and there is every possibility that these people might unleash a biological warfare on countries whom they consider inimical to them. For instance water bodies of a country could be infected with new versions of pathogens or their environment might be sprayed with pathogenic microbes. All these possibilities should make one think whether it is worthwhile indulging in this kind of research.

Safe guards in genetic engineering research

The scientific committee at large and biologists in general have been thinking for a very long time as to how to introduce some sense into genetic engineering research. While it may not be prudent to indulge in genetic engineering for problems which can be solved otherwise it is equally true that genetic engineering cannot be totally given up as it indeed has the potential of solving some of the serious problems confronting the human race which other research methodologies cannot hope to solve. The only answer to this being, research in genetic engineering should be properly regulated, monitored and if necessary with stringent international control.

A committee headed by Paulberg (1973-74) an eminent scientist held discussions with other interested persons and published a small bullettin outlining the risks involved in genetic engineering research. In 1975 an International group of scientists who were very much concerned with genetic engineering research convened a meeting in California USA and considered the ethical and safety implications of genetic engineering research. An outcome of this meeting was the formulation of a series of guidelines that sought to regulate and in some cases even prohibit research in recombinant DNA. In the USA, the National Institute of Health (NIH) issued guidelines in the year 1976 for US scientists involved in genetic engineering research. The guidelines required among other things that any research proposal involving recombinant DNA should be submitted to a special committee of NIH for approval. NIH also graded the laboratories into four levels (P1 to P4) where genetic engineering research of different levels were recommended. For instance experiments involving DNA from primates and animal viruses involving harmful genes could be carried out only in extra secure P4 laboratories. In 1982 an advisory panel of NIH - the recombinant DNA advisory committee (RAC) published revised guidelines. According to these new regulations recombinant DNA experiments were graded into 5 classes and of these it is essential that three levels of research must obtain NIH approval even before initiation. These include researches involving drug resistance of microorganisms, toxin synthesizing genes and operations involving release of genetically engineered organisms into environment (as those used for pest control).

On the 26th January 1982 a meeting was held at the parlimentary assembly of the council of Europe in Strasbury and recommended certain guidelines aimed at protecting the individual from the inheritant dangers of genetic manipulation. Three areas were mentioned in particular - genome map of human cells, gene therapy of somatic cells and gene therapy of germ cells. The report of the council concluded that inspite of the possible advantages of genetic engineering research, man made decisions should not substitute the free play of nature and everyone's right not to be genetically manipulated should be affirmed (Ignacimuthu, 1995).

Outside USA, the regulations on genetic engineering research are not actually as stringent as they ought to be. France and Germany are considering whether to restrict research in genetic engineering because of the ethical questions involved. Recombinant DNA guidelines of France are ambiguous about the deliberate release of genetically altered organisms. In Germany however release into environment of genetically altered organisms are strictly prohibited. Many social activist groups are opposing gene therapy and such other genetic engineering parctices in terms of ethical and moral parameters.

In India, genetic engineering research is still in infacy, yet considering the importance of it, Government of India has constituted four committees for this purpose.

1. Recombinant DNA advisory committee (RDAC). To evolve guidelines.
2. Institutional Biosafety Committee (IBSC). For implementation of guidelines.
3. Review Committee of Genetic manipulation (RCGM). To recommend special suitable conditions for experiments and trial.
4. Genetic Engineering approval committee (GEAC). For large scale manufacturing, environmental release of genetically altered organisms/ products and import/export of genetically altered organisms.

The followng may be considered as some of the safeguards that should involve any research in genetic engineering.

1. Harmful genes such as those coding for toxins and antibiotics should not be cloned without extreme precautions.
2. Animal genes, genes of tumour viruses should not ordinarily be cloned in bacteria or others microbes.
3. Laboratory facilities should be such that there should be virtually no possibility of the escape of genetically altered microbe. In addition to scientists even the other ordinarily personnel of the laboratory should be thoroughly briefed about the dangers of carelessness before they are employed. Workshops on precautionary measures should be conducted periodically so that no one violates them. There should be mandatory check of laboratory equipments of cabinets, hoods and other glassware to see that they are microfree when they are taken out of the laboratory. Laboratory should also possess special equipments like negative pressure rooms, safety cabinets, special traps and drinage etc., to prevent the possible escape of the microbe.
4. Use of microbes which can live only in special environmental conditions should be picked up for genetic engineering research because even if these organisms escape into the environmental after genetic alteration they will not survive in the normal environmental conditions so that the chances of their rapid spread are very less.
5. As far as possible cloning vectors should be non conjugative plasmids because even if they are uncontrolled they will not be able to promote their own transfer by conjugation.
6. The cloned vector should be sufficiently modified or altered in such a way that it will not be able to express itself in any environment but can do so

only under special circumstances like a particular host strain that are normally not available The genetic alteration must be such that in case it is transfered to another microbe it should prove lethal to it.

7. The cloning organisms should be modified in such a way that after cloning they depend upon very special conditions of existence which can be provided only in a laboratory and are not available in the environment.
8. Attempts are being made to produce "crippled microbes" for use in genetic engineering research. The genome of these microbes is altered and disabled in such a way that if they escape from the special laboratory conditions they will not survive. The following are some of the instances of crippled microbes for use in genetic engineering research.

Diaminopimelic acid (DAP) is an important component of the cell membrane in *E.coli*. Genetically altered *E.coli* were produced which were DAP deficient. These cannot survive unless supplemented by DAP. Hence these organisms even if they escape outside cannot survive. Such organisms are ideal tools for genetic manipulation. Precautions are however necessary because many a time microbes are known to undergo mutation very fast. In fact in the above example the DAP deficient *E.coli* very soon mutated back and was able to produce DAP. Scientists however discovered that there was more then one gene involved in the production of DAP and deleted that also. But the bacteria would not yield so easily to the manipulation of the microbiologists. The DAP deficient bacteria again survived by producing a sticky substance called Calanic acid around their protoplast. But then the calanic producing gene was again removed. This will clearly reveal that our knowledge on the genome of microbes would always remain incomplete because we will be able to identify a gene only when it express itself after natural selection; for instance calanic acid producing gene was not selected to express when DAP producing gene is there. In the absence of the later the former was selected. Who knows in the absence of calanic acid producing gene which other bacterial gene which is hybernating may get selected and express itself. Afterall life is a struggle and no individual will give up its existence so easily.

Genetic engineering research and Ethics

Man is a product of Evolution and however much hey may think that he is different from other organisms because of his intelligence, the stark truth is that he is definitely a part of biological spectrum whether he likes it or not. Man is neither the first step nor the last step in the evolution of life. The process of Evolution which has produced so many diverse types of organisms has also produced man and all these organisms that from the biological spectrum were not produced within a day. Even the Evolution of human beings took several millions of years. It is quite true that the millions of organisms in the present day biological spectrum are produced out of nature's genetic engineering. But one must realise that these have been crafted painstakingly and patiently over the course of millions of years. Man's attempt of fast genetic engineering seeks to destabilise the delicate balance that has been inbuilt into the relationship of all organisms. Further, the diversity of life and its glorious uncertanity is the spice that makes life meaningful. Present day world consists of beneficial organisms, harmful organisms, bad individuals, good individuals etc. Variety should be there, only then one can understand the difference. If every thing is sought to be made uniform then the very essence of life is lost. Man should seriously think whether it is in the interest of nature and his own interest to pursue with unbridled genetic engineering research. Because as per the process of natural selection the genes that are not expressing in a given set of environmental conditions might express in a new environment and who knows what do they contain.

25

EUGENICS

Human beings constitute an integral part of the biological world. They share with other organisms genetic, physiological and metabolic characters at the basic level. Most of the physiological functions and genetic patterns are common between man and other organisms. In Genetics, particularly the fundamental nature of the genetic material and inheritance pattern of characters is common between man and other organisms. If this is true, then many of the human traits like mental, physical and physiological trait should be hereditary and subject to the evolutionary process. Keeping this in mind one can ask whether the genetic composition of human beings is static or changing. If so what is the direction of the change and can anything be done to guide the course of change. But genetic studies in human beings are beset with many fundamental difficulties, because it is not possible to obtain mating of any individual with any other individual as it is possible with other organisms. There are many sociological and ethical constraints. In spite of these draw backs, however genetic studies have been conducted in human beings and we have a fairly detailed account of human genetic traits, inheritance pattern and the course of Evolution of the human genetic material. Genetic studies conducted in the human genetic potentiality is called **Eugenics.**

History : The term Eugenics literally meaning 'true birth' or good origin was first coined by sir Francis Gallon (1822 - 1911) who opined that man is also subject to same evolutionary forces like other organisms and the human race could be improved both in terms of physical and mental abilities. He defined Eugenics as *"the study of agencies under social control that may improve or impair the racial qualities of future generations either physically or mentally'.* In other words eugenics is the application of the laws of genetics for the improvement of human race.

The idea of genetic improvement of human race is quite old, though its scientifc study is fairly recent. Many ancient, Chinese and Indian writings contain references (mainly imagined) to produce races of good, quality either

to work as slaves or as soldiers. Ancient philosopher Plato opined that, the liberty to live and eat is the right of only those who distinguish themselves in some field of human endeavour. The ancient Greeks had definite ideas regarding Eugenics. In Sparta importance was given to the physical attributes, while the Athenians cared more for intellectual abilities.

The scientific studies of Galton, Pearson etc., revealed that a large number of human traits both good as well as bad are hereditary. As a result of their study, they argued that persons with serious hereditary diseases should not produce any children. In fact, in many countries, a sterilization law is in force to prevent persons with serious health hazards from begetting any children.

Aims and objectives of Eugenics : Aiming towards perfection and maximum harmony with the environment is the ideal goal for human race. But realising this objective is easier said than done, as there are many impediments in implementing genetic principles to human beings. It is an Utopian objective to achieve a human society free of prejudices, sickness, poverty and congenitial disabilities. The following may be regarded as the main objectives set forth for eugenic improvement of human race.

Health : Individuals with optimum health, both bodily and physically are an ideal asset in any human society. Such individuals can contribute for the maximum well being of the society. From the point of view of Genetics, a healthy society consists of individuals who are free from all types of hereditary disorders involving both body and mind. The average age of individuals must reach the maximum possible limit for the human genome.

Intelligence : Man is an integral part of the biological world. From the point of view of body strength, physical attributes etc., he is not the strongest species in the ecosystem. Yet he is the most dominant species today and is in virtual control of the whole of the environment both biological and abiological. This is made possible because of his superior mental attributes. Hence intelligence is an important human trait that should not only be preserved, but also should be improved. The average intelligence of the human individual has been improving no doubt as can be understood from the course of human history. Improvement of human intelligence for the allround welfare of the society is one of the foremost goals of Eugenics.

Moral attributes : Morality in an individual is reflected both in his deeds and words. These should be such as to promote harmony, good will and affection among all concerned. A sense of belonging to the human society and fellowship towards other less preveliged members is a sign of moral evolution among man.

Variability : It is often said variety is the spice of life. In any human society if there were to be a monotony of homogenity, with no scope for variability, that society is bound to be doomed, as the members are not willing participants in the activity of the society. Extensive variability, with basic unity of purpose is an ideal attribute for any human society. Individuals specialized in various fields not only provide an immense array of human attributes in the biological Kaleidoscope, but also contribute their best for the allround development of society. It is the responsibiltiy of every society to provide all its members oppurtunities in an unhindered fashion so that their abilities find full scope of blooming. *Let hundred flowers bloom, with not even one bud withering in the process* is an ideal Eugenic goal.

Racial differences : The term racial difference as used here does not connote the political attitude of one group of individuals to another based on skin colour difference. In a strict biological sense, racial difference (not discrimination) refers to special characteristics of a group of people residing in a particular geographical area. The attributes of people living in an area represents their ability to adjust to the characteristics of the environment and lead a successful life. Skin colour depends on the intensity of sunlight to which people are generally exposed. People living in tropical and sub tropical countries are generally dark skinned than those living in comparatively cooler countries like those of the European and American continent. Many other differences such as shape and size of the skull, facial features, average height, hair colour have all contributed to various human races like Mongoloid, Oriental, Cacusoid etc. While isolation of these races helps the geneticists to understand the genetic mechanism behind their special characters, intermarriages which are quite frequent now a days due to migration of people from one area to another provides an oppurtunity to analyse the interaction of these various genetic potentialities.

Eugenics, Euthenics and Euphenics : There are several stages or several aspects in the genetic improvement of human race. While Eugenics deals with the prenatal study of human individuals for genetic purposes, Euthenics deals with the improvement of human beings after birth. Euphenics on the other and mainly concerns itself with the symptomatic treatment of genetic diseases (See later for details).

Euthenics hopes to bring in improvement by concentrating on the education and health and hygine of the individual by placing them in the most suitable environment. Eugenics however tries to bring in better progeny into this world by manipulation of the parentage. Eugenics and Euthenics however are not distinct by themselves because they cannot work in isolation. A total and allround improvement is possible only when Eugenics and Euthenics work in coordination.

Types of Eugenics : Broadly speaking, the Eugenic method of human improvement can be classified into positive and negative. Positive Eugenics deals with the identification of virtues or good attributes in the human race and devises methods to preserve, improve and perpetuate them; Negative Eugenics on the other hand identifies harmful or undesirable traits in the human race and devises methods to suppress them so that they do not get perpetuated. Positive Eugenics is also called *Constructive Eugenics,* while negative Eugenics is called *Restrictive Eugenics.*

NEGATIVE EUGENICS : Among the two types, the negative Eugenics is the more difficult one to employ. While any Eugenic method has to be largely voluntary, it is more so with negative Eugenic methods. The production of progeny, marriage etc., in human beings are not regarded purely as biological phenomena, but have got themselves involved in social, emotional and such other personal parametres. The following are some of the methods recommended to eliminate the undesirable genotypes from the human gene pool.

Sexual separation of the defective : There are several incurable hereditary diseases such as hemophilia, epilespy, diabetes, feeble mindedness, idiocy etc. It is generally advisable not to allow two such persons to marry among themselves. By avoiding such marriages, the defective gene gets gradually eliminated from the gene pool. In some instances, two individuals who are seemingly normal maybe heterozygous for either sex linked or autosome linked defective genes. The children of such couple or atleast a good majority of them are likely to inherit the disease as the recessive genes would get a chance to express themselves. If in such a couple, the first child expresses the defective trait they should realise that they are heterozygous and should take a decision whether to have the second child. In such a situation it is better not to opt for a second child. Perhaps the best thing for the would be couple, would be to go to a genetic counsellor with their family history and seek his advice. But then again, this is not always possible; several considerations like, emotional attachment, monetary considerations, commitment of the elders play a large role in the life of the would be bride and groom and genetics takes a backseat.

Several other physical attributes apart from mental illness merit the separation of individuals carrying defective genes. One of the most significant problems is the inheritance of Rh factor. This factor present in the blood of some individuals (Rh positive) and absent in some (Rh negative), poses a problem when a Rh positive male marries a Rh negative female. Usually about 85% of the population are Rh positive and 15% Rh negative. Assuming a random marriage, about 11% would be intermarriages. The children of such couple are likely to suffer a disease known as *Erythroblastosis foetalis* (For details see chapter on Multiple alleles). The first child may be spared, but the subsequent ones may be still born. In order to avoid such a situation, the would be couple (before an alliance) should have a blood test done to ascertain the Rh factor.

In order to achieve the aims of selective separation of defective individuals, the following are some of the measures suggested, it should be noted however that some of them are too harsh and can be implemented only in a regimented society. In a democratic society however, it should be left to the conscience of the individuals concerned.

Eugenic sentiment : Davenport, one of the geneticists has commented "Dry the stream that feed the torrent of defective and degenerate protoplasm". This is possible only by an enlightened public opinion free of prejudices of any kind. There should be a large scale educational program to make people aware of the eugenic problems like the hereditary diseases and the consequences of a marriage between defective individuals. These persuasive (and not coercive) methods will help to change the mood of the society and make their mind receptive for any genetic suggestion. Considerations like dowry etc. will in a large measure probably go to background. People should be made aware, that while marriages are made in heaven, children have to be brought up on Earth. In this way, it will be possible to develop a 'Eugenic sentiment' in society.

Seggregation : This is a mildly coercive method, wherein individuals with known hereditary defects are not allowed to marry; generally by appealing to their conscience or if it fails by other coercive methods. For a healthy society, it is not desirable that idiots, epileptics and habitual criminals marry and enhance the survival chance of harmful genes in the human gene pool. Seggregation of defective individuals does not and should not mean that socially they should be ostracised. Such individuals should be taken care of by the society as a general responsibility.

Sterilization : This is a coercive method to be adopted, when it is not possible to prevent the reproduction of the highly defective individuals. Individuals of this type are to be sterilized, while they can marry and lead a normal life. Sterilization should be done both in the case of male *(Vasectomy)* and female *(Salpingectomy)*. Many countries have passed sterilization laws. These are USA, Canada, New Zealand, Denmark, Norway, Sweden etc. Compulsory sterilization of individuals with incurable diseases is the best method to prevent the multiplication of a defective gene. This will not prevent marriages or any social obligations.

Birth control and MTP (Medical termination of pregnancy)

One of the less coercive, but largely debatable method is free dessimination of birth control knowledge and popularization of birth control measures. This may particularly work in groups in the lower levels of social order, where there is ignorance due to economic conditions. This will prevent the production of large number of uncared for children who in later years will be a burden on society. Deprived of comfortable home and parental affection, it is children of this type who turn into criminals and indulge in antisocial activities at a later stage.

Many societies (including our own) who are tradition bound, and many religious groups oppose free dessimination of knowledge on birth control methods as they fear, that it would usher in a wave of immorality among the youth, as it may encourage promiscuous behaviour free of the fear of pregnancy (at least among women). They argue that sex is a private and personal affair of two individuals and society has no right to interfere in this. It is true that in measures such as the ones suggested above there is a possible backlash in the form of promiscuous behaviour. But one has to strike a balance, together with the dessimination of the birth control knowledge, the other elements of the social fabric should be strengthened. For instance, children who are loved, who feel wanted and have affectionate parents are less likely to misuse their sexual knowledge than those who become vagabounds by the force of circumstances. Social and religious voluntary groups in general and parents in particular can play a pivotal role in shaping the character of their wards.

In situations, where a pregnancy has occurred it should be terminated so as to prevent further complications due to defective genes.

Marriage among close relatives : (Consanguineous marriages)

This enhances the chances of homozygosity and subsequent morphological expression of the defective genes as they have a common ancestry. As far as possible this should be avoided to prevent further problems. Indeed in many human societies, there is a practise (particularly among south Indian Brahmins) of enquiring the geneology of the prospective groom and bride before finalising an alliance. But of late, other considerations have largely reduced this to a farce.

Genetic counselling : This refers to the advice tendered by experts in the field as to the desirability or otherwise of couples to have a child. This would be a voluntary restriction by the couples who have a choice not to carry serious genetic disorders. For instance if an individual is aware of his father suffering from a serious genetic ailment, he himself would not want his children to suffer the same fate; rather he would not produce any children. Such genetic counselling units exist in many western countries like USA. Unfortunately in our country, such counselling units are woefully less and even when they exist, are not popular. Aso like countries of our own, where people are generally poor, genetic counselling should be dispensed free and ought to be funded by the Government. In the long run, in terms of absence of diseases and other problems, it will pay for itself.

POSITIVE EUGENICS : Broadly defining, positve eugenic methods deal with attempts to increase the production of children only by those with most desirable traits. According to Nobel Laureate H.J. Muller. Individuals with desirable traits should be allowed to produce more number of children than others, to improve the society. He even suggests artificial insemination methods to increase the progeny of such people. But here again the problems of morality and human ethics creep in. Is it desirable from all points of view to produce children from artificial insemination? What will be the emotional attachment of parents to such children. These are problems that should find a satisfactory answer. The following are some of the positve eugenic measures.

Immigration : Modern times are characterised by large scale migration of individuals from one country to another in search of green pastures. Professionals, academicians, scientists and others migrate to another country in search of oppurtunities. These are mostly for monetary considerations. Many a time, these may be to escape harsh social conditions or to free themselves from descrimmative practices of a none too developed society. Advanced countries practise immigration procedures in both positive and negative ways. They prevent the immigration of undesirable elements into their society by banning their entry, as they do not want to disturb the ethnic, social or economic balance. They also do not want epiletic, insance and other form of infirmities to creep into their society and get a foot hold in the form of marriage with the locals. On the other hand people with desirable traits are welcomed with open arms, encouraged and given all types of benefits so that their own society will improve from their contribution. In this connection, the instance of 'brain drain' from third world countries to developed countries may be mentioned.

Early marriage of individuals with desirable traits : It is often seen, that ambitious individuals marry quite late in their age, as they would be devoting best part of their youth in realizing their ambitions. Genetic studies of late marriages have indicated that children born out of late marriages are not genetically very strong (barring exceptions). Hence, poeple with desirable traits and qualities should be encouraged to marry early (not very early of course).

Subsidizing the fit : This is one of the best methods of positive eugenics. Individuals, who are going to be an asset to the society in terms of their traits are to be given more preveliges, so that they need not struggle to obtain the requirements of life. They should be encouraged in their chosen avocation and should be encouraged to produce more number of children. Such children can contribute to society quite a lot. Because, there is a limit to the reproductive potentialities of such individuals, Muller has suggested that such individuals should father large number of children through artificial insemination. Artificial insemination is in practise even now, in order to provide children to women, whose husbands are sterile. In this context in order to prevent complications, the names of donor and recipient will be kept secret.

The outcome of artificial insemination practises has lead to the suggestion by scientists of the establishment of egg and sperm banks. The gametes are frozen in these banks and can be kept alive for a long time. It will be possible by this method to have selective fusion of gametes. Artificial insemination, *in vitro* fertilization and subsequent implantation of the zygote in the womb have all raised the hopes of test tube babies. In quite a few instances test tube babies have been successfull and have come as a boon to supposedly barren women. In many countries, the hypothesis of surrogate mothers - (who accomodate, the egg and sperm of other individuals) has become a reality. In many instances, this has however lead to many legal complications, as to who qualifies as the real mother - the one who provides the genotype or the one who provides the environment? The production of a total test tube baby - starting from fertilization up to the development of a new individual, however has not been successful so far. Another aspect that has to be regarded is the desirability of producing a total test tube baby under the prevailing social conditions.

Education : In order to create a proper environment, a thorough education on biological and genetic principles is a paramount necessity. Children should be educated about health, hygine and other methods of keeping their body and mind ina sound condition. Educating the children and grown ups on these lines need not be done in formal schools only. Voluntary organisations, social councils, temple, church committees etc., have a large and influential role to play in the realization of these aims. Mass media like Radio, television, News papers and even theatre groups could be engaged in inculcating a scientific spirit among men and women.

Improving the scope of individual oppurtanities

Many a time, the best of the germplasm may not be allowed to develop or reproduce due to want of oppurtunities. This leads to the avoidable waste of good germplasm. For instance, the cream of the society like soldiers in terms of physical attributes die at an early age due to war, leaving the continuation of society to less able men. The death of the soldiers is preventable. Benjamin Franklin points out *Wars are not paid for in war time; the bill comes later* meaning that a sick and disabled society is the result of removal of fit genotype as a result off war. Hitler who realized the dysgenic effects off war, had urged the German girls to have babies from soldiers before they went of to war, in order to preserve the best germplasm.

But the present complexity of the Weapon systems possessed by super powers largely makes the above mentioned effect of war redundant. For in any future war (involving nuclear weapons) it is the civilian population and industry that is largely going to be destroyed. Men to men combat is becoming a thing of the past. In a nuclear war there will be neither a victor nor vanquished, because all would be crushed. Hence not only from the point of view of peace for the present generation, but from the future eugenic point of view also, war should be avoided. (One can imagine the strife and sorrow for the civilian and military populace of Iran and Iraq which had waged several years long war).

Improvement of environment : An allround improvement of the biological and physical environment is conductive for the proper development of human genotype. Earnest attempts are needed to maintain the ecosystem balance and maintain natural resources. Plundering of the environment for short range economic gains should stop.

Production of genetic research : Extensive research in human genetics in order to get a comprehensive knowledge about the human genome is a basic necessity for any meaningful eugenic programme. But it is very difficult to analyse the human genome and its functions. A welcome sign of late is the multinational project involving several scientists to map the human genotype involving 23 pairs of chromosomes.and about one lakh genes. When this work gets completed (in future), it would provide a solid foundation for human genetic improvement.

EUPHENICS : The term euphenics is employed for the symptomatic treatment of gentic diseases in man. Most of the genetic disorders, which do not cause any visual genetic abnormality in the physical attributes, but alter the functional balance are called *inborn errors in metabolism.* One of the common examples of inborn errors of metabolism is *phenylketonuria,* determined by an autosomal recessive gene. Individuals suffering from this defect cannot metabolize the amino acid phenylalanine resulting in its accumulation. This in turn causes mental retardation. Once a child is diagnosed of *phenylketonuria,* it can be given a diet free of phenylalanine and the child develops normally.

In all instances however metabolic errors can not be cured, even though causes are known. For instance, albinism can not be cured, but albino individuals can be made to suryive by not exposing themselves to excessive radiation. Some of the possible methods of euphenic treatment are as follows.

Enzyme treatment : Many of the defects such as *Alkaptanuria.* (black urine) are caused due to absence of one or more enzymes. It is worthwhile examining whether intake of such enzymes can bring about relelf. Attempts indeed have been made in this direction with limited success, because of immunological difficulties.

A study of the synthesis of chain of Hemoglobin has helped scientists to understand the reasons for Cooles and Lepore anemia, and one day they hope to rectify the mutated gene providing cure for the suffering individuals.

The role of genetics in human medicine is increasingly becoming important and some of the dreaded diseases like cancer, AIDS etc., may one day be eliminated due to advancement in genetic techniques.